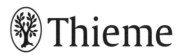

The Grasping Hand

Structural and Functional Anatomy of the Hand and Upper Extremity

Amit Gupta, MD, MSOrth, MChOrth, FRCS
Clinical Professor
Department of Orthopedic Surgery
University of Louisville School of Medicine;
Director
Norton Louisville Arm & Hand
Louisville, Kentucky, USA

Makoto Tamai, MD, PhD
Director and Hand Surgeon
West 18th Street Hand Clinic for Hand Surgery
   and Rehabilitation
Sapporo, Hokkaido, Japan

1184 illustrations

Thieme
New York • Stuttgart • Delhi • Rio de Janeiro

Library of Congress Cataloging-in-Publication Data is available with the publisher.

Important note: Medicine is an ever-changing science undergoing continual development. Research and clinical experience are continually expanding our knowledge, in particular our knowledge of proper treatment and drug therapy. Insofar as this book mentions any dosage or application, readers may rest assured that the authors, editors, and publishers have made every effort to ensure that such references are in accordance with **the state of knowledge at the time of production of the book.**

Nevertheless, this does not involve, imply, or express any guarantee or responsibility on the part of the publishers in respect to any dosage instructions and forms of applications stated in the book. **Every user is requested to examine carefully** the manufacturers' leaflets accompanying each drug and to check, if necessary in consultation with a physician or specialist, whether the dosage schedules mentioned therein or the contraindications stated by the manufacturers differ from the statements made in the present book. Such examination is particularly important with drugs that are either rarely used or have been newly released on the market. Every dosage schedule or every form of application used is entirely at the user's own risk and responsibility. The authors and publishers request every user to report to the publishers any discrepancies or inaccuracies noticed. If errors in this work are found after publication, errata will be posted at www.thieme.com on the product description page.

Some of the product names, patents, and registered designs referred to in this book are in fact registered trademarks or proprietary names even though specific reference to this fact is not always made in the text. Therefore, the appearance of a name without designation as proprietary is not to be construed as a representation by the publisher that it is in the public domain.

Thieme Medical Publishers, Inc.
333 Seventh Avenue, 18th Floor
New York, NY 10001, USA
www.thieme.com
+1 800 782 3488, customerservice@thieme.com

Copyright to all the images used in the book, except for the ones borrowed from third parties, is held by the author, Dr. Amit Gupta.

Cover design: Thieme Publishing Group
Typesetting by DiTech Process Solutions, India

Printed in Germany by Beltz Grafische Betriebe   5 4 3 2

ISBN 978-1-60406-816-0

Also available as an e-book:
eISBN 978-1-60406-817-7

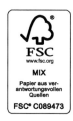

FSC
www.fsc.org
MIX
Papier aus ver-
antwortungsvollen
Quellen
FSC® C089473

Contents

Section IV Regional Anatomy and Function

Contents

Contents

Contents

36   The Interphalangeal Joint 419

Hilton P. Gottschalk and Randy S. Bindra

37   The Nail and Finger Pulp.. 428

Nada N. Berry, Reuben A. Bueno, and Elvin Zook

Section V Epilegomena

38   Imaging and Anatomy.. 441

Herbert P. von Schroeder and Ali Naraghi

Foreword

It is an honor that Dr. Amit Gupta and Dr. Makoto Tamai have invited us, the Zancolli family, to write the foreword for this amazing book *The Grasping Hand: Structural and Functional Anatomy of the Hand and Upper Extremity.*

This is the first time that three generations of hand surgeons, who are so passionate about what they do, have been invited to write a foreword together.

Since the Renaissance, the moment when humans overcame the obscurantism of the Middle Ages, anatomy has been the focus of many brilliant minds.

One could argue that anatomy is already an explored discipline, that all anatomical structures and relations have been described. However, it is a book like *The Grasping Hand* that demonstrates to us that anatomical knowledge continues its evolution and that many of the details that are needed for new surgical techniques can still be highlighted. This book also emphasizes how anatomy can be approached in a totally different way. The book's subtitle "Structural and Functional" suggests that we are dealing with dynamic knowledge.

Surgery of the hand and upper extremity is not only extremely fascinating but also perhaps the most complex of all surgical specialties. Until World War II, four different surgeons were needed to treat war wounds of the hand. An orthopaedic surgeon for the bones, a neurosurgeon for the repair of nerves, a vascular surgeon for blood vessels, and a plastic surgeon for skin coverage. Brilliant minds such as Sterling Bunnell realized that a surgeon with the knowledge of all these four specialties was needed. And that was the birth of what we do and love today.

Knowledge of many different basic sciences like biomechanics, kinematics, and physiology is necessary to become a good hand surgeon. Above all, knowledge of anatomy is of paramount importance. A detailed and three-dimensional anatomical knowledge allows the surgeon to choose the best and most direct approach, not touching structures that are not involved and treating the damaged structures with maximum precision. There is another factor that is enhanced by anatomical knowledge: creativity. It is the basis of imagination and intuition to develop new surgical techniques.

The Grasping Hand shows us in pristine and exquisite detail all the fundamental anatomical structures of the hand. This book has been a labor of love for the authors who worked for over 20 years, dissecting hundreds of cadavers, amassing over 16,000 high-quality photographs of meticulous dissections to bring us this wonderful glimpse into the structural and functional anatomy of the hand and upper extremity.

We hope that you enjoy these dissections and discussions as much as we did.

Eduardo Alfredo Zancolli, MD
Professor
National Academic for Orthopaedics and Traumatology;
Former President
Argentine Society of Orthopaedics and Traumatology
Argentine Society for Surgery of the Hand and Upper Limb
Buenos Aires, Argentina

Eduardo Rafael Zancolli, MD
Ex president of the South American Federation for Surgery
of the Hand;
Private Practice
Buenos Aires, Argentina

Eduardo Pablo Zancolli, MD
Upper Extremity Unit Hospital Universitario Fundación
Favarolo,
Buenos Aires, Argentina

Preface

The quest started about 20 years ago. There was a need for a detailed textbook on the anatomy of the hand and upper extremity describing both the structural and functional anatomy. I had the great fortune of working with Dr. Robert Acland in his Fresh Tissue Laboratory at the University of Louisville. I also had the luxury of being able to observe many hand surgery fellows from around the world.

Both Dr. Acland and I were very impressed with the detailed dissections of Dr. Makoto Tamai who was a hand surgery fellow at the time. I offered him to stay one more year as a research fellow to do the heavy lifting of the dissection work for the book project and I am glad that both he and his father Dr. Susumu Tamai consented to the idea.

Dr. Makoto Tamai spent the next year dissecting many cadaveric specimens with the utmost care and attention to detail to bring out the most intricate anatomy as well as photographing the specimens. After he returned to Japan, I continued with the work and even started a new Fresh Tissue Laboratory with the help of Norton Hospital. We ended up with a collection of over 16,000 photographs of anatomical specimens.

I classified the photographs and sent them to my hand surgery and research friends and colleagues around the world and asked them to write the text of the chapters. I am very thankful to the authors for doing such an outstanding job. I would also like to thank Dr. David Slutsky for putting me in touch with Thieme Publishers. My thanks to Ms. Snehil Sharma at Thieme Publishers for her great effort in the completion of this book.

Our sincere thanks to the Fresh Tissue Laboratory at the University of Louisville. We are deeply indebted to all the people who donated their bodies for science. I would also like to thank the Bioskills Lab at the Orthopedic and Hand Education Center at Norton Brownsboro Hospital.

The fire that started the quest was lit a long time ago by Dr. Eduardo Zancolli and his book, *The Structural and Dynamic Basis of Hand Surgery in* 1978. The fire was sustained by my teachers in hand surgery, such as Professor G.C. Das, Professor Frank Burke, Dr. Ueli Buchler, Professor Harold Kleinert, Professor Robert Acland, Dr. Joseph Kutz, Dr. Thomas Wolff, Dr. Tsu Min Tsai, Dr. Luis Scheker, Dr. James Kleinert, and Dr. Steven McCabe. To them, especially my partners at Kleinert Kutz and Associates and Kleinert Institute at Louisville, Kentucky, I am grateful to them for making it possible for me to undertake this monumental project and for agreeing to the production of this book. I am also thankful to my partners at Louisville Arm and Hand for being supportive of this endeavor and for their contributions. I am especially indebted to Dr. Russell A. Shatford for his constructive criticisms, numerous revisions, and his friendship over the years.

Why is the book named *The Grasping Hand*? In ancient Hindu texts in Sanskrit, *Indriyas* are the medium through which our body perceives and interacts with the whole creation, the medium through which the *Aatma* (Soul) experiences the knowledge of the senses. The *Indriyas* are *Jnana* (Knowledge) *Indriyas* and *Karma* (Action) *Indriyas*. Through the *Jnana Indriyas* (the eyes, ears, nose, tongue, and skin as the sense organ of touch), we gain knowledge of our environment. With the *Karma Indriyas* the body performs tasks. *Pani-tattva* or the **grasping hand** is one of the *Karma Indriyas*. Hence the name of the book: **The Grasping Hand**. Sage Charaka defined the function of the hand as *Grahana* (receive, gather, collect) and *Dharana* (hold). Sage Saankhya defined the function of the hand as *Aharana* (receive) and *Aadaana* (hold). It is amazing how succinctly the function of the hand was defined in ancient times! The whole upper extremity is involved in the function of grasp and manipulation by the hands. We have therefore included the whole upper extremity in **The Grasping Hand**.

We are thankful to Dr. Eduardo Alfredo Zancolli, his son Dr. Eduardo Rafael Zancolli, and his grandson Dr. Eduardo Pablo Zancolli for writing the foreword to this book. This family of hand surgeons has been an inspiration to many surgeons around the world with their dedication to the study of hand anatomy and will continue to inspire many more in years to come.

I would also like to acknowledge my family including my wife Bhavna, my daughter Niki, my son-in-law Marc, and my grandson Roshan without whose love and support this book would not have been possible.

This book has been a labor of love. I have spent 20 years of my life in preparing this book. My sincere hope is that you enjoy it and that the book is helpful in furthering the knowledge of hand and upper extremity structure and function.

Amit Gupta, MD, MSOrth, MChOrth, FRCS

Preface

"It ain't necessarily so!" a pet phrase of Dr. Robert D. Acland that we, the fellows of Christine M. Kleinert Institute for Hand and Microsurgery, would have heard or seen written on the front of the brown apron in his laboratory. Dr. Acland served as the Director of Fresh Tissue Laboratory of the University of Louisville since 1983. I had the privilege of spending some time dissecting fresh cadavers with him for over 2 years from late 2000 to early 2003. Observing him work on the famous *Video Atlas of Human Anatomy* was also a tremendously wonderful experience. That phrase, "it ain't necessarily so," frequently helped me in accepting the existence of unexpected anatomical "differences" on dissected specimens from the drawings or descriptions in past publications.

In 2001, in the latter period of my first year of fellowship, Dr. Amit Gupta proposed that I extend my stay in Louisville for one more year to serve the institute as a senior fellow and to compile the anatomical studies into a book. The main target of this publication are those who are keen to learn the "real" anatomy of hand and upper extremity. The knowledge of anatomy is tremendously important for surgeons and therapists. Anatomical knowledge gives one the confidence to design solutions for any surgical problems.

My anatomical dissections under magnification were carried out at odd hours during the fellowship work. In between, the specimens were dipped into saline and stored in the refrigerator to prevent degeneration. A selection of the photographs I had taken have been presented in the book. In addition, Dr. Gupta performed some important dissections. To show "real" anatomy, we tried to fill the book with as many photographs as possible. These high-quality photographs were taken in "real time" during the dissections, so the specimens still kept their freshness and the photographs could show real colors and textures of the tissue.

There may be some criticism about teaching anatomy using photographs of specimens, especially about the consistency of anatomy. A limited number of specimens cannot represent the standard anatomical features of each structure and their appearance can be altered by the dissecting procedure of each dissector. For example, the capsular ligaments of the wrist joint are buried in the joint capsule covered by the thick reticulum layer outside and the synovial membrane inside, and the collagenous fibers of ligaments also have numerous connections with the surrounding structures like the retinaculum or the tendon sheath. Therefore, it is impossible to show those ligaments without removing the superficial tissues or without severing the connections with those other structures. The appearances of the ligaments will definitely be changed. I would be asking the observers to remember Dr. Acland's words, "It ain't necessarily so!"

Anyway, it is my great pleasure to introduce the book to friends, fellows, and staff of Kleinert Institute, and everyone who expected its publication. On this achievement, I would like to acknowledge Dr. Amit Gupta and all contributors, the Christine M. Kleinert Institute, the University of Louisville Body Bequeathal Program, and especially my father, Dr. Susumu Tamai, for supporting my 2 years' study in the USA and waiting for the publication. I hope this book will help all readers in a deeper understanding of the anatomy of hand and upper extremity.

We dedicate this book to Dr. Robert D. Acland (June 20, 1941 – January 6, 2016) and Dr. Harold E. Kleinert (October 7, 1921 – September 28, 2013).

Makoto Tamai, MD, PhD

"*Qu'ils n'oublient jamais que sans anatomy il n'y a point de physiologie, point de chirurgie, point de médecine; qu'en un mot, toutes les sciences médicales sont greffées sur l'anatomie.*"

"Let them never forget that without anatomy there is no physiology, no surgery, no medicine; that in a word, all the medical sciences are grafted on the anatomy."

(J. Cruveilhier, *Traite d'Anatomie Descriptive*, 1834)

Contributors

Joshua M. Abzug, MD
Associate Professor
Departments of Orthopedics and Pediatrics
University of Maryland School of Medicine;
Director
University of Maryland Brachial Plexus Practice;
Director of Pediatric Orthopedics
University of Maryland Medical Center;
Deputy Surgeon-in-Chief
University of Maryland Children's Hospital;
Director and Founder
Camp Open Arms
Timonium, Maryland, USA

Gregory I. Bain, PhD, MBBS, FRACS, FA (Ortho)
Professor of Upper Limb Surgery and Research
Department of Orthopedic and Trauma Surgery
Flinders University and Flinders Medical Centre
Adelaide, Australia

Nada N. Berry, MD
Assistant Professor
Division of Plastic Surgery
Southern Illinois University School of Medicine
Springfield, Illinois, USA

Randy Bindra, MD, FRACS
Professor of Orthopedic Surgery
Griffith University and Gold Coast University Hospital
Gold Coast, Queensland, Australia

Allen T. Bishop, MD
Professor
Department of Orthopedic Surgery
Mayo Clinic
Rochester, Minnesota, USA

Anders Bjorkman, MD, PhD
Adjunct Professor in Hand Surgery
Department of Translational Medicine
Medical Faculty
Lund University;
Senior Consultant
Department of Specialized Surgery – Hand Surgery
Skåne University Hospital;
Clinical Fellow
Wallenberg Center for Molecular Medicine
Malmö, Sweden

Ethan W. Blackburn, MD
Hand Surgeon
Louisville Arm & Hand
Louisville, Kentucky, USA

Reuben A. Bueno, MD
Professor and Chairman
Division of Plastic Surgery
Southern Illinois University School of Medicine
Springfield, Illinois, USA

John T. Capo, MD
Chief of Hand Surgery
Vice Chairman of Orthopedics;
Residency Program Director
Rutgers-RWJ Barnabas Health
Jersey City, New Jersey, USA

Alain Carlier, MD
Professor
CHU de Liege
Chirurgie de la Main
Liege, Belgium

Indranil Chakrabarti, BMed Sci (Hons), BMBS, FRCSEd (ORTH), MFSTEd
Orthopedic Hand and Wrist Surgeon
South Yorkshire Orthopedic Services
Rotherham, and Thornbury Hospital
Sheffield, UK;
Honorary Clinical Senior Lecturer, University of Sheffield, UK;
Member of Faculty of Surgical Trainers
Royal College of Surgeons of Edinburgh
Scotland, UK

David Elliot, MA(Oxon), FRCSEng, BM, BCh
Former Consultant Hand and Plastic Surgeon
St. Andrew's Centre for Burns and Plastic Surgery
Broomfield Hospital
Chelmsford, Essex, UK

Quentin Fogg, MD
Associate Professor in Clinical Anatomy
Department of Anatomy and Neuroscience;
Faculty of Medicine
Dentistry and Health Sciences
The University of Melbourne
Victoria, Australia

Jan Fridén, MD
Hand Surgeon (Hanchirurgie)
Schweizer Paraplegiker-Zentrum
Nottwil, Switzerland

Marc Garcia-Elias, MD
Hand Surgeon
Hand and Upper Extremity Surgery
Institut Kaplan
Barcelona, Spain

Hilton P. Gottschalk, MD
Hand Surgeon
Central Texas Pediatric Orthopedics
Austin, Texas, USA

Jeffrey A. Greenberg, MD
Clinical Professor
Indiana Hand to Shoulder Center
Indianapolis, Indiana, USA

Jean-Claude Guimberteau, MD (Retired)
L'Institut Aquitain de la Main
Bordeaux, France

Amit Gupta, MD, MSOrth, FRCS, MChOrth
Clinical Professor
Department of Orthopedic Surgery
University of Louisville;
Director
Louisville Arm & Hand
Louisville, Kentucky, USA

Ranjan Gupta, MD
Professor of Orthopedic Surgery
Anatomy and Neurobiology
    And Biomedical Engineering;
Councilor
Zeta Chapter of Alpha Omega Alpha Honor Medical
    Society
University of California, Irvine
Orange, California, USA

Elisabet Hagert, MD, PhD
Associate Professor
Department of Clinical Science and Education
Karolinska Institutet;
Arcademy, H.M. Queen Sophia Hospital;
Musculoskeletal and Sports Injury Epidemiology Center
Department of Health Promotion Science
Sophiahemmet University
Stockholm, Sweden

Peter Hahn, MD
Staff Orthopedic Surgeon
Miller's Children Hospital
Long Beach, California, USA

Hill Hastings II, MD
Clinical Professor Department of Orthopedic Surgery
Indiana University Medical Center
Indiana Hand to Shoulder Center
Indianapolis, Indiana, USA

Antony Hazel, MD
Hand Surgeon
Louisville Arm & Hand
Louisville, Kentucky, USA

Vasudeva G. Iyer, MD
Director
Neurodiagnostic Center of Louisville
Retired Professor of Neurology
University of Louisville School of Medicine
Louisville, Kentucky, USA

Jaehon M. Kim, MD
Hand and Microvascular Surgeon
Mount Sinai Hospital
Icahn School of Medicine
New York, New York, USA

James M. Kleinert, MD
Independent Researcher
New Castle, Kentucky, USA;
Retired Hand Surgeon
Kleinert Kutz and Associates Hand Care Center
Louisville, Kentucky, USA

William B. Kleinman, MD
Clinical Professor
Indiana Hand to Shoulder Center
Indianapolis, Indiana, USA

Scott H. Kozin, MD
Chief of Staff
Shriners Hospital for Children
Philadelphia, Pennsylvania, USA

Krzysztof Kusza, MD, PhD
Professor
Department of Anesthesiology and Intensive Therapy
Poznań University of Medical Sciences
Poznań, Poland

Joanne Labriola, MD
Orthopedic Surgeon
DMG Orthopedics – Bone, Joint and Spine Center
Downers Grove, Illinois, USA

Nirusha Lachman, PhD
Professor and Chair
Department of Anatomy
Mayo Clinic
Rochester, Minnesota, USA

Amy L. Ladd, MD
Hand and Upper Extremity Surgeon
Chase Hand and Upper Limb Center
Stanford University Medical Center
Palo Alto, California, USA

Alexis Laungani
Plastic Surgeon
Department of Plastic Surgery
Mayo Clinic
Rochester, Minnesota, USA

Richard L. Lieber, PhD
Chief Scientific Officer and Senior Vice President
Shirley Ryan Ability Lab;
Professor
Physical Physiology and Biomedical Engineering
Northwestern University Feinberg School of Medicine
Chicago, Illinois, USA

Beng Hai Lim, FRCS
Professor
National University Hospital;
Director and Senior Consultant
Centre for Hand and Reconstructive Microsurgery
   (CHARMS)
Orchard Road, Singapore

Alejandro Maciel-Miranda, MD
Plastic Surgeon
Microsurgery and Breast Reconstruction
Anker Global Oncology
Guadalajara, Jalisco, Mexico

Steven J. McCabe, MD, FRCS(C)
Professor
University of Toronto Hand Program
Toronto Western Hospital
Toronto, Ontario, Canada

Brett McClelland, FRACS
Hand Surgeon
Hunter Hand Surgery
Charlestown, New South Wales, Australia

**Duncan A. McGrouther, MBChB, FRCS, MSc,
   MD, FMedSci**
Senior Hand Consultant
Department of Hand Surgery
Singapore General Hospital
Outram Road, Singapore

Duncan McGuire, MD
Hand Surgeon
Martin Singer Hand Unit
Groote Schuur Hospital
University of Cape Town
Cape Town, South Africa

Steven L. Moran, MD
Professor
Department of Orthopedic Surgery
Mayo Clinic
Rochester, Minnesota, USA

Steven F. Morris, MD
Professor of Surgery
Division of Plastic Surgery
Dalhousie University
Halifax, Nova Scotia, Canada

Mohamed Morsey, MD
Orthopedic Surgeon
Department of Orthopedics
Assiut University
Assiut, Egypt

Chaitanya S. Mudgal, MD, MS, MChOrth
Associate Professor
Department of Orthopedic Surgery
Massachusetts General Hospital
Harvard Medical School
Boston, Massachusetts, USA

Keiichi Murata, PhD
Director
Limb Trauma Center
Nara City Hospital;
Clinical Professor
Department of Orthopedic Surgery
Nara University
Nara, Japan

Ali Naraghi, FRCR
Assistant Professor
Division of Musculoskeletal Imaging
Department of Medical Imaging
University of Toronto
and Toronto Western Hospital University Health
   Network
Toronto, Canada

Nathan Polley, MD
Orthopedic Surgeon
King's Daughters Hospital
Madison, Indiana, USA

Ghazi M. Rayan, MD
Director
Oklahoma Hand Fellowship Program
INTEGRIS Baptist Medical Center
Oklahoma City, Oklahoma, USA

Susanne Rein, MD, PhD, MBA
Senior Consultant
Department of Plastic and Hand Surgery
Burn Unit
Klinikum Sankt Georg
Leipzig, Germany;
Martin-Luther-University of Halle-Wittenberg
Halle (Saale), Germany

Luke P. Robinson, MD
Hand Surgeon
Louisville Arm & Hand
Louisville, Kentucky, USA

Mark Ross, FRACS
Associate Professor of Orthopedic Surgery
University of Queensland
Director
Brisbane Hand and Upper Limb Research Institute
Brisbane, Australia

Michel Saint-Cyr, MD, FRCS (C)
Director
Division of Plastic Surgery
Vice Chairman (Surgical Services)
Wigley Professor in Plastic Surgery
Clinical Professor (Affiliated)
Texas A&M College of Medicine
Temple, Texas, USA

Sandeep Jacob Sebastin, MCh (Plast)
Senior Consultant Hand Surgeon
Department of Hand and Reconstructive Microsurgery
National University Health System
Singapore

Ben Shamian, MD
Attending Physician
Critical Care Medicine
Mount Sinai Hospital South Nassau
New York, New York, USA

Russell A. Shatford, MD MPH, MSEd.
Hand Surgeon
Louisville Arm & Hand
Louisville, Kentucky, USA

Maria Siemionow, MD, PhD, DSc
Professor of Orthopedics
Director of Microsurgery Research
Department of Orthopedics
University of Illinois at Chicago
Chicago, Illinois, USA

David J Slutsky MD, FRCS(C)
Clinical Assistant Professor
Department of Orthopedics
Chief of Reconstructive Surgery
Harbor-UCLA Medical Center
Los Angeles, California, USA;
Private Practice
The Hand and Wrist Institute
Torrance, California, USA

Jacek Szopinski, MD
Department of General, Hepatobiliary, and Transplant
  Surgery
Collegium Medicum in Bydgoszcz
Nicolaus Copernicus University
Torun, Poland

David E. Tate Jr., MD
Clinical Associate Professor
Department of Orthopedic Surgery
University of Louisville;
Hand Surgeon
Louisville Arm & Hand
Louisville, Kentucky, USA

Makoto Tamai, MD, PhD
Director and Hand Surgeon
West 18th Street Hand Clinic for Hand Surgery
  and Rehabilitation
Sapporo, Hokkaido, Japan

Nick A. van Alphen, MD
Plastic Surgeon
Department of Plastic Surgery
Amsterdam, Netherlands

Herbert P. von Schroeder, MD, MSc, FRCSC
Associate Professor
University Hand Program
Toronto Western Hospital
University Health Network
  and Divisions of Orthopedic and Plastic Surgery
University of Toronto
Toronto, Canada

Joost I.P. Willems, MD
Orthopedic Surgeon
Spaarne Gasthuis
Hoofddorp, Netherlands

Jason K.F. Wong, MBChB, FHEA, PhD, FRCS(Plast)
Academic Consultant (Plastic Surgery)
Senior Lecturer in Plastic Surgery
King James IV Professor Royal College of Surgeons of
  Edinburgh
Manchester University Foundation Trust
Edinburgh, Scotland

Dan A. Zlotolow, MD
Professor of Orthopedics
Sydney Kimmel Medical College
Thomas Jefferson University;
Shriners Hospital for Children Philadelphia;
Shriners Hospital for Children Greenville
The Philadelphia Hand to Shoulder Center
The Hospital for Special Surgery
Philadelphia, Pennsylvania, USA

Elvin Zook, MD
Professor Emeritus
Division of Plastic Surgery
Southern Illinois University School of Medicine
Springfield, Illinois, USA

Section I

Prolegomena

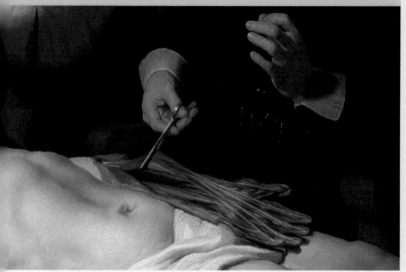

From: The Anatomy Lessons of Dr. Nicolaes Tulp. Painting by Rembrandt 1632. Courtesy of Mauritshuis, The Hague, Netherlands.

1 The Story of Hand Anatomy

David E. Tate, Jr.

Progress in knowledge of anatomy of the human hand has paralleled that of knowledge of human anatomy in general. This chapter will serve as an overview to select areas of a very broad topic.

Scientists and scholars studied anatomy in rather desultory fashion until the 16th century CE, at which time Leonardo da Vinci and Andreas Vesalius ushered in a contemporary era of inquiry based on direct observation. From being scorned or even punished in earlier times, anatomical dissections became honorable, festive civic occasions, best exemplified by Rembrandt's painting *The Anatomy Lesson of Nicolaes Tulp*. Unfortunately, the journey from furtive, forbidden study to grand public occasion has been tortuous, as societal and religious prohibitions eased only grudgingly. However, once the genie of inquiry was released, during the Renaissance, anatomical studies gained momentum, with further refinements in anatomical knowledge arising after the introduction of anesthetics in the 1840s, along with Baron Joseph Lister's antiseptic and later aseptic surgery, in 1867.[1] The ability to patiently operate and dissect, free from fear of infliction of distress or infection, ushered in the era of modern surgical care. Exemplified by Kocher, Billroth, Halsted, Cushing, and Kanavel, modern surgical care became increasingly refined, depending not just on gross anatomy, but also on increasingly fine gradations of functional anatomy. Deliberate pacing of dissection as demonstrated by these pioneers yielded improved results and stimulated still further study. "Smash and grab" surgery on unprepped, unanesthetized patients went by the wayside. Anatomical precision, gross and functional, became paramount to effective operative patient care. While considerable progress has occurred since the 1840s anesthetic advent of William T.G. Morton and Crawford Long, these gains did not occur in a vacuum. Medical inquiry can be traced to Egypt, 4,600 years before Morton and Long presented the world with the possibility of pain-free surgical care.

In keeping with this line of thought, the chapter will discuss not only the gross anatomical study of the hand, but will also delve into various functional aspects of hand anatomy, such as studies of Tinel on behavior of nerve wounds, Destot for carpal mechanics, Kanavel for synovial fluid circulation, Carl Manchot, Michel Salmon, and G. Ian Taylor for circulation of the skin, Harold Kleinert for behavior of flexor tendons, Andrew Koman for dynamics of hand circulation, and Charles Sherrington, Wilder Penfield, and Goran Lundborg for cerebral cortical aspects of the hand, to name a few.

The starting point of any discussion of contemporary medicine is Imhotep. As described in 1913 by Sir William Osler, Imhotep is the "...first figure of a physician to stand out clearly from the mists of antiquity."[2] This Egyptian prodigy was a physician, architect, and vizier to Pharaoh Zoser of the Third Dynasty, circa 2980 BCE. Imhotep was eventually promoted to demigod, and then to the status as a full god of medicine (▶ Fig. 1.1).[3]

The Edwin Smith Papyrus was written around 1500 BCE, but it is attributed to Imhotep, and others, circa 2800 BCE (▶ Fig. 1.2). The papyrus contains the first documented cause-and-effect medical case histories recorded by humans. The papyrus describes nonmagical treatments for these ailments, most of which were head injuries.[4]

In India, Sushruta (circa 600 BCE) ▶ Fig. 1.3 urged doctors to study the human body to become more effective practitioners. Dissection with a knife, though, was prohibited. Sushruta overcame this restriction by wrapping a body in a shroud of grass and then placing it in a river (▶ Fig. 1.4a and b). After 7 days, a grass whisk could sweep away outer tissue layers. Sushruta used his findings to describe "*Marmas*," points on the upper limb, and elsewhere in the body, where penetrating injuries could inflict serious harm[5,6] (▶ Figs. 1.4a, b).

In Greece, Hippocrates and Aristotle studied human illnesses. Hippocrates commented on splinting of upper limb fractures in *The Genuine Works of Hippocrates*: "The forearm is to be placed at right angles to the arm, in a state intermediate between pronation and supination...."[7]

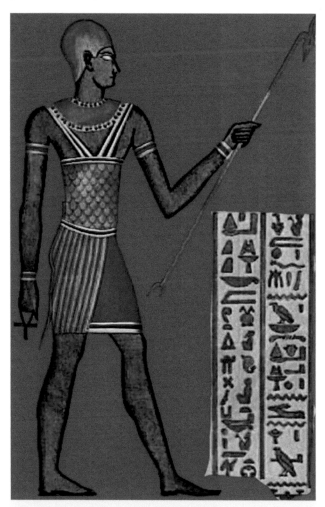

Fig. 1.1 Ancient Egyptian physician Imhotep.

Of all the Greek physicians, Galen of Pergamon is best known. With the dissection prohibitions of his time, he studied human bodies as he could. Galen also made considerable study of animal bodies, thus becoming an early paragon of comparative anatomy. While his diligence was commendable, Galen made many unfortunate and unfounded extrapolations from animal to human anatomy. Galen was considered infallible, so numerous errors persisted to the time of Andreas Vesalius (1514–1564), such as imaginary fibers within veins, sought in vain by Vesalius: "...I had separated the substance of the veins, in search of the fibers, I dissected it raw and boiled, and by Hercules, to tell the truth, the fibers had come from the imagination of our authors (i.e., Galen) ...."[8]

By 476 CE, the Dark Ages descended upon Western Europe. Odoacer, a Germanic chief, defeated Romulus Augustus as the Germanic troops sacked Rome. Leadership in medical studies then passed to Arab physicians. Chief of these Arabic physicians was Avicenna (980–1037 CE). Avicenna was born in Afshona, at the time a town in the Persian Empire, now in present-day Uzbekistan. Aviecenna's *Canon of Medicine* (circa 1020 CE) synthesized medical knowledge of the time, combining Hippocrates and Aristotle with Avicenna's own observations. Translated into Latin, the *Canon* served as a prime medical textbook for several centuries. At present, there is not a full English translation of the work. In the *Canon,* Avicenna made numerous incisive observations pertaining to the hand: "The seven carpal bones in the wrist joint form two rows. Proximal carpal row consists of three bones and the distal carpal row consists of four bones. The three proximal bones taper and form a wedge proximally. They articulate with the lower end of the radius and ulna and provide flexion and extension of the wrist." Avicenna also differentiated between tendons and nerves and cautioned against excessively tight dressings.[9]

As Western Europe's reawakening took hold in the 15th and 16th centuries, a spirit of medical inquiry was part of this scientific and intellectual flowering. Leonardo da Vinci and Andreas Vesalius represent two of the high points of this era. da Vinci (▶ Fig. 1.5) was a spectacular polymath, skilled in art

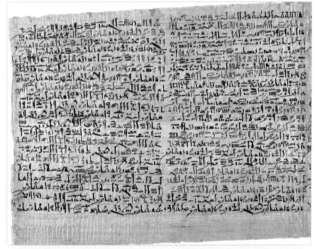

Fig. 1.2 The Edwin Smith Papyrus, written about 1500 BCE, but attributed to Imhotep and others, circa 2800 BCE. (Courtesy of the New York Academy of Medicine Library.)

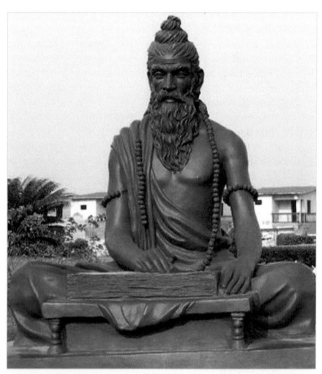

Fig. 1.3 Statue of Susrata in Hardiwar, India. (Alokprasad at en.wikipedia, CC BY-SA 3.0 <https://creativecommons.org/licenses/by-sa/3.0>, via Wikimedia Commons.)

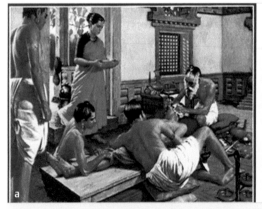
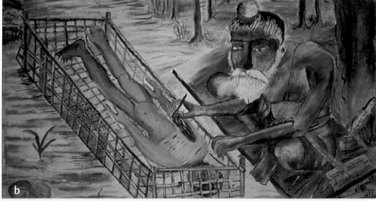

Fig. 1.4 (a) Sushruta performing surgery. (b) Sushruta wraps a body in a shroud of grass and places it in a river. After 7 days, a grass whisk could sweep away outer tissue layers.

and numerous natural sciences, including human and animal anatomy. Based on personal observation and dissection of human specimens, da Vinci started, but did not complete, a survey of the entirety of human anatomy. His plan was outlined, in part, as follows: "This work should begin with the conception of man and describe the nature of the womb and how the child lives in it ... next describe a grown male and female ... composed of vessels, nerves, muscles and bones ...."[10]

At first, da Vinci may have been interested in human anatomy from the standpoint of an artist, but interest in anatomy for its own sake soon developed. In the drawings which he did complete, he drew the same part from four views. He also pioneered the use of cross-sectional images, and injected wax into the ventricles of the brain to better study their shape. da Vinci represents the acme of the artist as an anatomist. Thereafter, the two fields diverged, with anatomists enlisting skilled artists to depict structures of interest. O'Malley and Sanders expertly critique da Vinci's strengths and weaknesses as an anatomist. In their estimation, da Vinci's iconic depictions of bones and muscles were the high point of the work, with depictions of other body areas suffering from flaws and incomplete renderings.[10]

Leonardo da Vinci depicted the hand (▶Figs. 1.6a, b) in a dorsal projection:

"The first bone of the thumb [metacarpal I] and the first bone of the index finger [metacarpal II] are placed upon the basilar bone [multangulum majus] in immediate support ...."[10]

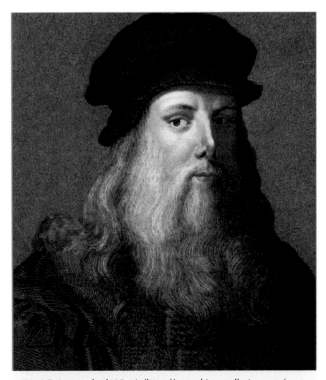

Fig. 1.5 Leonardo da Vinci. (http://www.kingsgalleries.com/wp-content/uploads/2010/07/Leonardo da Vinci.jpg)

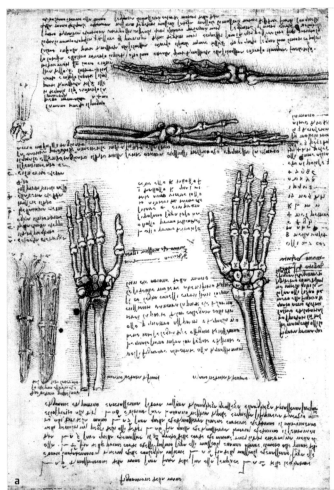
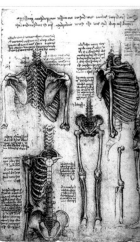
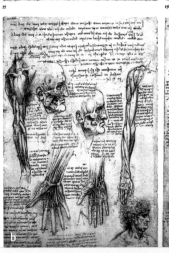
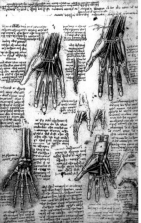

Fig. 1.6 (a, b) Hand drawings by Leonardo da Vinci.

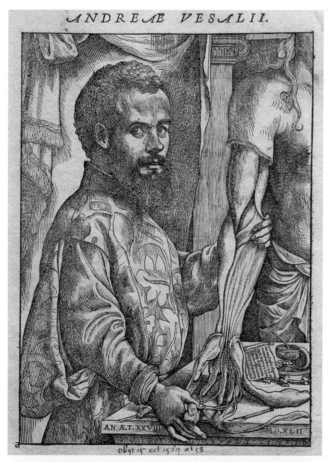

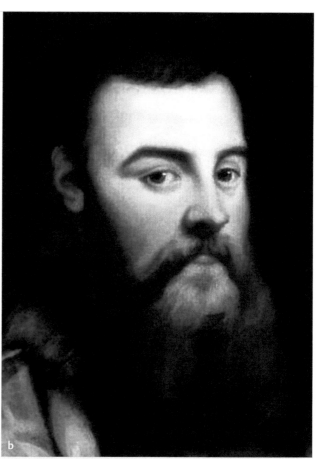

Fig. 1.7 (a, b) Portraits of Andreas Vesalius, creator of the Fabrica. (a: Attributed to Jan van Calcar, Public domain, via Wikimedia Commons.)

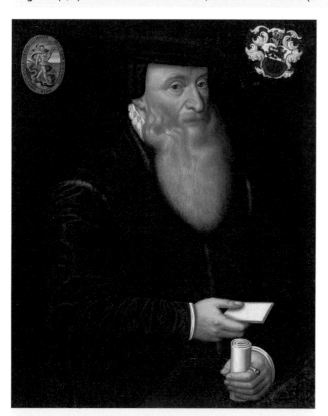

Fig. 1.8 Johannes Oporinus, publisher of the Fabrica. (Hans Bock, CC0, via Wikimedia Commons.)

Similarly, he describes the soft tissues of the hand on the palmar surface, "Show and describe what cord in each finger is the most powerful and the largest ... the cords of the palm of the hand together with their muscles are very much larger than those of its dorsum."[10]

da Vinci's plan to depict the whole of human development remained incomplete, but he was clearly anticipating future directions with the work that he did complete.

Miraculously, the da Vinci drawings survived, drifting around Europe for centuries, making a miraculous reappearance at Windsor castle, not unlike the surfacing of Franz Schubert's unpublished, unplayed musical manuscripts "... shoved in cupboards and drawers all over Europe."

The paradigm for artist-anatomist collaboration was set with anatomist Andreas Vesalius (►Figs. 1.7a, b), and artist Johann van Kalkar in *De Fabrica Corporis Humani* (published in 1543), with their Swiss publisher Johannes Oporinus (►Fig.1.8) setting a similarly exacting standard for superlative printing of an epoch-making book.[11]

A native of Brussels, Vesalius was only 29 when the *Fabrica* was published. From an early age, Vesalius demonstrated an insatiable appetite for primary anatomical knowledge. By age 22, he had robbed a gibbet of the corpse of a deceased criminal in Louvain, Belgium: "... I was ... looking for bones where executed criminals are usually placed along the country roads ... I came upon a dried cadaver .... the birds had cleansed this one ... which had been partially burned and roasted over a fire of straw and then bound to a stake .... I climbed the stake and pulled the femur away from the hipbone. Upon my tugging, the scapulae and arms and hands also came away. After I had surreptitiously brought the arms and legs home in successive trips—leaving the head and trunk behind—I allowed myself to be shut out of the city in the evening so that I might obtain the thorax, which was held securely by a chain. So great was my desire to possess these bones, that in the middle of the night, alone and in the midst of all these corpses, I climbed the stake with considerable effort and did not hesitate to snatch away that which I so desired."[12,13]

With a stroke, the days of a teacher standing on high, droning out of a book, while the lowly barber performed the actual dissection, were over. Instead, Vesalius the teacher was also Vesalius the prosector, front and center, as the famous image from the cover of the *Fabrica* demonstrates (▶Fig. 1.9).

The *Fabrica* is a revolutionary work, covering the whole of human anatomy, based on primary dissections. The work is divided into seven books: Book I: *The Bones and Cartilages* (English translation by William F. Richardson and John B. Carman and published by Norman; ▶Fig. 1.10a), Book II: *The Ligaments and Muscles* (English translation by William F. Richardson and John B. Carman and published by Norman; ▶Fig. 1.10b), Book III: *The Veins and Arteries*, Book IV: *The Nerves*, Book V: *The Organs of Nutrition and Generation*, Book VI: *The Heart and Associated Organs*, and Book VII: *The Brain*.

In discussing the upper limbs in the *Fabrica*, Vesalius uses the terms "radius" and "ulna" for the two forearm bones. The

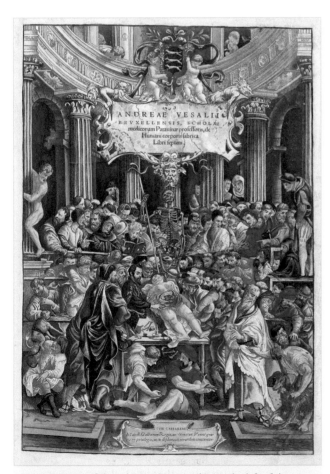

Fig. 1.9 Cover of the Fabrica. Note Vesalius to the left of the dissecting table, demonstrating to the gallery. (Jan van Calcar, Public domain, via Wikimedia Commons.)

teleology of the triangular fibrocartilage is charming: "... Nature did not want the rest of the epiphysis to touch the carpus without the intervention of something else, and she therefore drew out ... a cartilage which ascends the epiphysis of the ulna and separates it from the carpus ... the ulna supports the carpus without touching it ...." Metacarpals are referred to as metacarpals by Vesalius, with various names for phalanges: "The fingers contain three bones each ... sometimes known as internodes, joints, phalanges, cudgels, and knuckles."[14]

For Vesalius, nomenclature of hand-based muscles was numeric, with an explanation for each muscle's function. For example, muscles 26 to 29 are the lumbricals: "... they are thin, rounded muscles that stretch out from the four individual tendons of the second muscle (flexor digitorum profundus) ... they proceed ... and insert into the root of the fingers ... to incline the four fingers sideways toward the thumb ...."[15]

Vesalius depicts the brachial plexus in Book IV: he uses a numeric system to describe the nerves: the median nerve is the third nerve; the ulnar nerve is the fifth. "...the third nerve... sits on the anterior side of the inner tubercle of the humerus ...the fifth nerve...reaches the inner tubercle of the humerus; it bends around the rear of this, having its own special groove through which it may fitly travel into the forearm."[16]

Vesalius and da Vinci are the giants upon whose shoulders all the other anatomy scholars stand, up to and including today. Their insistence on primary investigation and accurate rendering of their results furnished the template for all investigations to follow.

In terms of artistic depiction of anatomic study, Rembrandt's iconic *The Anatomy Lesson of Dr. Nicolaes Tulp* (painted in 1632) documents the prestige associated with quality scientific inquiry (▶Fig. 1.11).

This Dutch painting depicts Nicolaes Tulp, physician, anatomic demonstrator, and Amsterdam civic leader, conducting an anatomical dissection of a recently executed criminal. William Heckscher's book-length study of the painting discusses the history of artistic depictions of anatomic dissections. Heckscher vividly describes the civic atmosphere of the Netherlands at the time, rich with a spirit of logic, learning, and scholarly inquiry.[17] While some, including Heckscher, have reported anatomic errors in the painting, likely based on surveys of anatomy atlases, Dutch surgeons clarified the situation using an actual anatomic dissection to investigate Rembrandt's painted depiction. The famous "misplaced muscle" is likely an accurate rendering of a reflected flexor carpi radialis, although Rembrandt does depict anomalous nerve and tendon structures in the hand (▶Fig. 1.12).[17,18]

A similar artistic-anatomic connection took place in the Netherlands in 1690. The anatomist was Govaert Bidloo, the artist was Gerard de Lairesse, and the engraver was Abraham van Bloetling. While the resulting Atlas *Humani Corpori* was unsuccessful commercially, one of its images has lived on as a memento of a stylish intersection of anatomy and art (▶Fig. 1.13).[19]

Jacob Benignus Winslow (1669–1760) was born in Odense, Denmark but moved to France where he worked for the rest of his life. In France, he changed his name to Jacques Benigne Winslow (Fig. 1.10a). His famous anatomical text "Exposition Anatomique de la Structure du Corps Humain" was published in French in 1732 (Fig. 1.10b) and translated into English by G. Douglas M.D[20]. Apart from the eponymous epiploic foramen

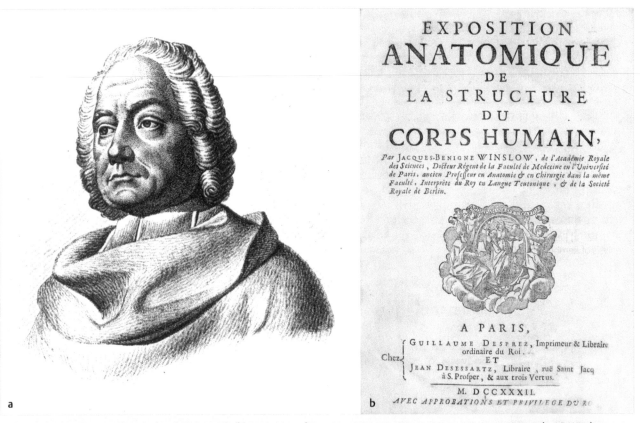

Fig. 1.10 (a) Jaques-Benigne Winslow (1669–1760). (b) Front cover of *Exposition Anatomique De La Structure Du Corps Humain* by J.B.Winslow published in 1732. (a: Ambroise Tardieu, Licence Ouverte, via Wikimedia Commons.)

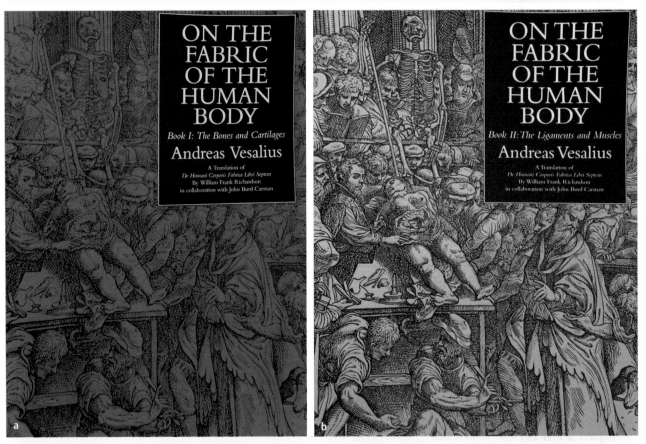

Fig. 1.11 (a) On the Fabric of the Human Body, Book 1: The Bones and Cartilages (Norman Publishing). (b) On the Fabric of the Human Body, (b) Book 2: The Ligaments and Muscles (Norman Publishing.)

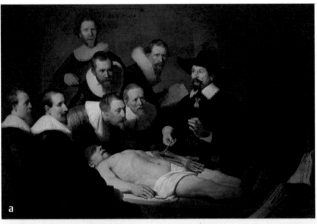
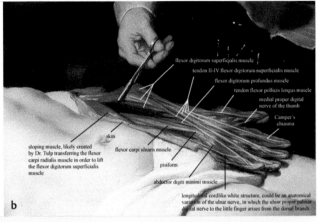

Fig. 1.12 (a) Rembrandt's The Anatomy Lesson of Dr. Nicholaes Tulp. (Rembrandt, Public domain, via Wikimedia Commons) (b) Detailed analysis of Rembrandt's The Anatomy Lesson of Dr. Nicholaes Tulp. (With permission of Elsevier Limited, J Hand Surg 2006, 31A:882–891.)

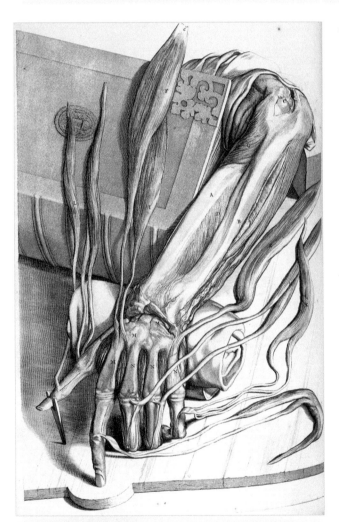

Fig. 1.13 Intersection of art and anatomy by anatomist Govaert Bidloo, artist Gerard de Lairesse, and engraver Abraham van Bloteling. (Gerard de Lairesse, Public domain, via Wikimedia Commons)

in the abdomen, he made important contributions to hand anatomy: he described the extensor tendon rhombus (described in Chapters 2 and 29), the sagittal band (see Chapter 29). Winslow described, for the first time, the trapeziometacarpal

joint as "double ginglymus", that "both curved surfaces in opposite directions".

Another Dutch prodigy in the tradition of Nicolaes Tulp was Petrus Camper. While best known for the eponymous "chiasma" in the flexor digitorum sublimis, Ijpma and coworkers documented the wide range of Camper's interests and intellect in a 2010 article. Camper was a comparative anatomist in the style of John Hunter, lecturing at the illustrious Amsterdam Guild of Surgeons, literally following in the footsteps of Nicolaes Tulp and other luminaries of Dutch medicine. Like Tulp, Camper was also commemorated in a painting during an "anatomy." In the *Anatomy Lesson of Prof. Petrus Camper*, painted by Tibout Regters (painted in 1758), Camper is on the far right (▶ Fig. 1.14).[21]

On the heels of Rembrandt came Josias Weitbrecht, a German anatomist who worked in Russia, sponsored by Peter the Great. His masterwork, *Syndesmology* represents a summation of his life's work, and a partnership with artist Andreas Grecow, along with Grecow's students Gregorius Katschalow and Johannes Sokolow. As Bartoníček and Naňka mentioned in their insightful biographical article of Weitbrecht, the original book was in Latin, featuring "…more than 10 different font styles and sizes. Each paragraph is followed by references to works of individual authors, including a brief commentary. References to figures can be found on the page margins. Each double-page ends in a footnote that contains a word representing the first word of the following page." In addition to the distinctive layout of the book, the anatomic depictions are masterful: "…A number of views presenting individual articular structures have been used in the standard anatomical literature until today…although their names …differed significantly from the current anatomical terminology…." Unfortunately, the book suffered from a series of truncating, subpar translations, shortening the book, and casting aside the illustrations as well. Emmanuel Kaplan redeemed the work with a masterful English translation in 1969 which restored the work to full length, and also reincorporated the illustrations.[22]

Here is Weitbrecht himself, via Kaplan, on the triangular fibrocartilage complex: "A band or very strong retinaculum, which holds the ulna in its lower end, is the intermediate triangular cartilage that covers the sinuosity of the lower end of the radius. It was very well described by Vesalius…the base is so perfectly attached to the radius by a cartilaginous contact that it forms only one sinus. Two of the angles that form the tip of the process of

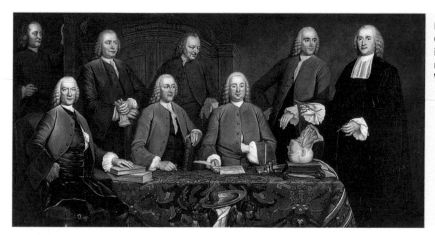

Fig. 1.14 The Anatomy Lesson of Prof. Petrus Camper, painted by Tibout Regters; Camper is to the far right holding dissecting equipment. (Tibout Regters, Public domain, via Wikimedia Commons)

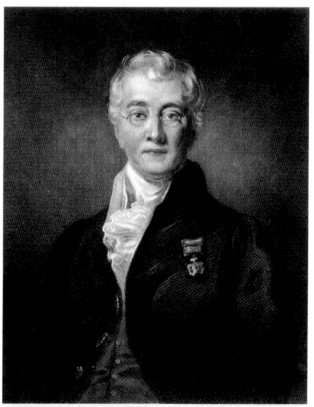

Fig. 1.15 Charles Bell, anatomist, physican and author of *The Hand: Its Mechanism and Vital Endowments as Evincing Design*.

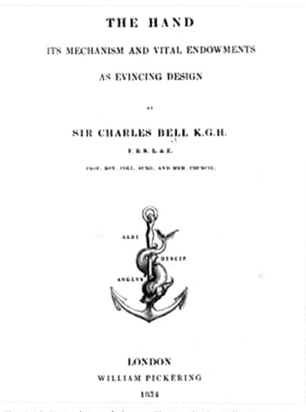

THE HAND

ITS MECHANISM AND VITAL ENDOWMENTS

AS EVINCING DESIGN

SIR CHARLES BELL K.G.H.

LONDON
WILLIAM PICKERING
1834

Fig. 1.16 First edition of *The Hand* by Sir Charles Bell, 1834.

the base of the radius are covered by the short ligaments, which are fused with the capsular ligament that unites the carpus with the radius. That is how it is attached to the ulna. The tip of the cartilage…inserts into the base of the styloid process of the ulna directly opposite to it. This insertion is the center of motion of the radius. A straight line drawn from this insertion to the styloid process of the radial bone represents the radius of this portion of a circle made by the tip of the radial styloid process when it turns around the styloid process of the ulna."[23]

In the spirit of comparative anatomical investigation, Charles Bell (▶ Fig. 1.15) produced a tour de force, in 1833.

The product was *The Hand, Its Mechanism and Vital Endowments as Evincing Design* (▶ Fig. 1.16). It was one of a set of treatises commissioned by the Royal Society for "…a work… On the Power, Wisdom, and Goodness of God, as manifested in the creation.…" Other works in the series included studies of geology, astronomy, and physiology of plants and animals. Bell's book is a masterful survey of the hand, with exhaustive comparative anatomical surveys of humans, horses, bats, anteaters, and various dinosaurs. Take, for example, the upper limb of the bat: " the phalanges of the fingers are elongated…for the purpose of sustaining a membranous web, and to form a wing.…on the fine web of a bat's wing, nerves are distributed, which enable it to avoid objects in its flight, during obscurity of night when both eyes and ears fail.…"

As for the ant-eater: "…the distinctiveness of the spines and processes declares the strength of the muscles…in the development of one grand metacarpal bone, which gives attachment to a strong claw… a very distinct provision for scratching and turning aside the ant-hill.…"

Bell tied in these discussions with the human upper limb: "...When a man strikes with a hammer, the muscle near the shoulder, acts upon the humerus in raising the extended lever of the arm and hammer...." Bell, in explaining his theme of the ingenious design of the hand as reflecting the undoubted input of the creator, offers a quote which encapsulates the essence of the theme: "...Some animals have horns, some have hoofs, some teeth, some talons, some claws, some spurs and beaks: man hath none of these, but is weak and feeble, and sent unarmed into the world—Why, a hand, with reason to use it, supplies the use of all these."[24]

This intellectual tour de force of natural history is also exemplified by brothers and rivals, William and John Hunter. The brothers were predecessors of Bell at London's Great Windmill Street School of Anatomy. Neither of the Hunters studied the hand in particular, but they are luminaries in anatomy's ascent as a vital part of medical science.

Of the Hunters, William was the more polished brother. William was a capable anatomist and teacher, especially in obstetrics. Additionally, William was a sought-after society doctor. In contrast, John was an insatiable and indefatigable master of human and animal anatomy. John was keen to dissect anything on which he could put his hands, and to that end, he was on familiar terms with the underworld of London's pre-Anatomy Act resurrectionists and body-snatchers.

As a sidelight to any discussion of anatomical study, body-snatchers are a fascinating, if repellent, collection of characters, and a necessary digression to this narrative. As there was no provision to legally obtain "material" for human dissections, villainous gangs worked on moonless nights, harvesting the dead. Londoners were terrified of being harvested, and church graveyards were often pockmarked with mazes of empty graves. Children were priced by the inch. Unfortunately, shortage of cadavers for dissection, coupled with a need for expansion of anatomic knowledge, made body-snatching a necessary, if unappealing, feature of London life in the 18th and 19th centuries. Sir Astley Cooper, first a pupil of John Hunter, and later a distinguished surgeon in his own right, characterizes the resurrectionists: "...the lowest dregs of degradation. I do not know that I could describe them better; there is no crime they would not commit...a dissolute and ruffianly gang." While condemning them, Cooper did have to make use of their services as he sought to hone his anatomical knowledge and surgical skill. Cooper testified to Parliament regarding the reach of the body-snatchers: "There is no person, let his situation in life be what it may, whom if I were disposed to dissect, I could not obtain. The law only enhances the price and does not prevent exhumation...."[25]

As surgical care improved, and treatment for more conditions became feasible, refinements of functional anatomy became increasingly important. Across the English Channel from the Hunters, Baron Guillaume Dupuytren (1777–1835) pioneered treatment of a functional anatomical problem, now named for him: Dupuytren contracture. It was first mentioned by Felix Platter, a Swiss physician in 1614, while Henry Cline, an English surgeon, performed dissection on two hands with the condition. Astley Cooper, in 1824, attributed the abnormality to a derangement of the palmar fascia, but the eponym went to Dupuytren. Wylock presents an account by a colleague of Dupuytren at work: "After the hand was fully immobilized, Dupuytren made a transversal incision of 2.5 cm at the MP joint

of the fifth finger in the palm of the hand. After this incision, the aponeurosis was severed with an audible scratching noise. In this manner, a good extension was achieved."[26,27]

Back in England, by the 1830s, a combination of realization of the need for improved anatomic instruction and improved access to anatomical material led to the Anatomy Act of 1832. The Act did not eliminate abuses but did augment the supply of legally obtained corpses. Prior to the act, only bodies of murderers retrieved from the gallows were legally available for dissection. After the Act, bodies from Victorian workhouses that went unclaimed were also made available. This had its own problems with anatomy inspectors pressuring clergy in charge of workhouses to avoid mentioning to residents the option of stating their wishes regarding burial versus dissection; the notion of being dissected rather than being buried was a considerable source of distress in Victorian England.[28]

Regardless of the rather unappetizing manner of obtaining corpses for dissection, the momentum for improved anatomical instruction was unstoppable. This momentum led to the creation of a publishing landmark: *Gray's Anatomy*. This text was released in 1858, and it took anatomic illustration and discussion to a new level of excellence. The book was jointly produced by Henry Gray (writer) (▶Fig. 1.17), and Henry van Dyke Carter (artist) (▶Fig. 1.18).

Using Carter's iconic depictions of dissections by the authors, combined with terse but elegant verbal summation, *Gray's Anatomy* yielded an elegant summation of human anatomical knowledge at that time. The text was revolutionary in its readability, practicality, and visual presentation. The book combined the talents of Gray, Carter, and the publishing house of J.W. Parker and Son, and the printing firm of John Wertheimer, to yield a physical product which became and remains to this day (41st Edition published in 2015), a classic of medical education and medical edification. Indeed, this coalescence of skill to produce *Gray's* is reminiscent of the partnership of Vesalius, Kalkar, and Oporinus in producing the *Fabrica*. In each case, writer, artist, and publisher came together to yield a peerless physical manifestation of knowledge.[28]

Gray's is an overview of all of human anatomy, but the hand receives generous attention from its masterful producers. Carter's drawings had beautifully rendered, hand-lettered labels placed directly upon the subjects, while Gray deftly and logically described the structures in question: "...The articulation between the two rows of the carpus consists of an enarthroidial joint in the middle, formed by reception of the os magnum into a cavity formed by the scaphoid and the semilunar bones, and of an arthroidial joint on either side, the outer one formed by the articulation of the scaphoid with the trapezium and trapezoid, the internal one by the articulation of the cuneiform and the unciform."[29]

Similarly, the interossei are masterfully and clearly represented visually by Carter, while Gray delivers a concise description: "...The interossei muscles are so named from their occupying their intervals between the metacarpal bones. They are divided into two sets, a dorsal and a palmar, the former are four in number, one in each metacarpal space, the latter, three in number lie upon the metacarpal bones...."[29]

Gray's Anatomy is a landmark, as it represents a dramatic elevation in the quality and quantity of anatomical instruction, yielding a product of exceeding high standard, and widely available. It foreshadows such advances as Robert Acland's

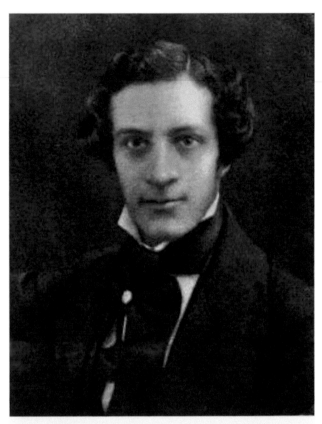

Fig. 1.17 Henry Gray, writer of Gray's Anatomy. (H. Pollock, CC BY 4.0 <https://creativecommons.org/licenses/by/4.0>, via Wikimedia Commons.)

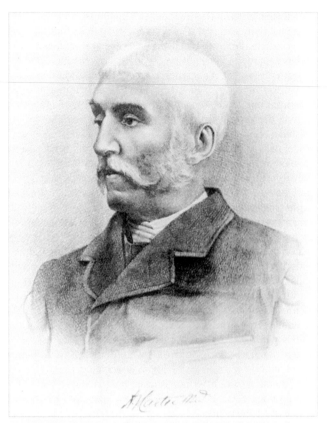

Fig. 1.18 Self-portrait: Henry van Dyke Carter, artist of Gray's Anatomy. (Henry Vandyke Carter, Public domain, via Wikimedia Commons.)

monumental *Practice Manual for Microvascular Surgery*. This course combined written and video instructions, using Acland's microsurgical skill, meticulous presentation standards, and his dry, but droll, verbal narration, to yield a standardized and superlative instructional product which has helped train several generations of microsurgical practitioners, over 100 years after the appearance of *Gray's Anatomy*.[30]

As we note the names of structures in *Gray's Anatomy*, we can shift attention to anatomical nomenclature. Anatomical terminology has slowly become codified; initially each investigator coined a novel name for each bone described, as discussions of da Vinci, Vesalius, and Gray illustrate. In 1895, the introduction of the Basel Nomina Anatomica (BNA) represented an attempt to standardize anatomic terminology. Interrupted by World Wars I and II, a widely accepted BNA revision known as the Nomina Anatomica was ratified in Paris in July 1955. A second edition was released in 2011, representing the latest effort at a worldwide set of terms for human anatomical structures.[31]

For nomenclature of the carpal (Greek, karpos, wrist)[32] bones, McMurrich in 1914 and Johnson in 1990 provide informative and entertaining summaries of the twists and turns of carpal bone nomenclature. Their articles take the journey from the numbers of Vesalius to present-day naming schemes. The origins of today's system of carpal nomenclature originated with Vesalius. He numbered the bones 1 through 8, starting with the scaphoid as 1, lunate 2, triquetrum 3, pisiform 4, trapezium 5, trapezoid 6, capitate 7, hamate 8. Interestingly,

the numbers live on to the time of the ICD-9, with carpal bone fractures classified as 814.01, scaphoid fracture, 814.02, lunate fracture, and onward, up to fracture of the hamate, 814.08.[33,34]

In 1653, Michael Lyser, a German who worked in Denmark, wrote a five-volume anatomy text. The fifth volume contained suggestions for preparing skeletons for display. In this volume, he proposed names for the carpal bones. Starting radially on the first row: cotyloid (Greek: cup shaped), lunatum (Latin: crescent-shaped), cuneiform (Latin: wedge-shaped), ossiculum magnitudine pisi sativi (Latin: a bone small in magnitude like a cultivated pea), then the distal row: trapezoides (Latin: trapezoid), trapezium (Greek: table), os maximum et crassissimum, in postcaparte capitulum obtinenens (a bone large and thick, held against the back portion of the head), and unciform (Latin: possessing a hook). McMurrich documents the popularity of Lyser's book, but also documents ongoing flux and controversy in naming of carpal bones. By 1726, Alexander Monro (primus), a Scotsman, had named the carpals: scaphoiudes/naviculare (scaphion [Greek]: boat; naviculare [Latin]: boat), lunare, cunieforme, pisiforme (cartilaginosum), trapezia, trapezoids, magnum, unciform, with Monro transposing the trapezium and the trapezoid.

Also, in 1726, Bernard Siegfried Albinus named the carpals: naviculare, lunatum, triquetrum, subrotundum (Latin: approximately, beneath the round area), multangulum majus (having many angles, large), multangulus minor (having many angles, small), capitatum (Latin: having or forming a head), and cunieforme. In 1871, Henle, a German anatomist, added hamate to the list (hamulus [Latin]: hook). McMurrich includes a table in his article, while Johnson provides serial drawings of the carpus depicting the evolution of the names[33,34] (►Fig. 1.19).

With the advent of anesthesia (Crawford Long 1842, William TG Morton 1846), applied anatomy took on new importance, as anesthesia eliminated intraoperative pain and allowed for more patient, deliberate, and delicate dissection, as exemplified by Halsted's approach to inguinal hernia.[35-37] The ability to safely render patients insensible of pain was an epochal breakthrough. Coupled with this advance, Baron Lister's antiseptic surgery, later to evolve into aseptic surgery, further freed surgeons to work patiently, and with respect for anatomy, by reducing fear of the scourge of infection.[38] The combination of freedom from intraoperative pain, and reduction of fear of infection, yielded a new importance of not just gross, but functional aspects of anatomy: how do body parts work, and how can their functions be repaired and restored? By 1900, surgical interventions were becoming increasingly sophisticated—improved anesthetic management (Codman and Cushing: "ether chart") with ever-enhanced anatomical knowledge and precision led inevitably from the necessary lightning speed of Victor Horsley (1890s neurosurgery), to Harvey Cushing's meticulous, deliberately paced interventions of 1910. Cushing observed Horsley firsthand: "He found Horsley living in seemingly great confusion, dictating letters to a male secretary during breakfast... patting dogs between letters, operating like a wild man. HC gave him a copy of his paper on the Gasserian ganglion, whereupon Horsley said he would show him how to do a case. They drove off the next morning in Horsley's cab, after sterilizing the instruments in H's house, and packing them in a towel, went to a well-appointed West End mansion. Horsley dashed upstairs, had his patient under ether in 5 minutes, and was operating within 15 minutes after entering the house; made a great hole in the woman's skull, pushed up the temporal lobe, blood everywhere, gauze packed into the middle fossa, the ganglion cut, the wound closed, and he was out of the house less than an hour after he entered it."[39] In contrast, Cushing refined a deliberate approach to operating on the brain: "...chief advances... were of technical nature. The introduction of blood pressure

recording during operations had added to the safety of neurosurgical procedures in general, and he had added a number of ingenious devices for diminishing hemorrhage...."[40]. In addition to neurosurgery, these anesthetic and infection control advances led to broad surgical progress, rendering previously untreatable, virtual death sentences such as breast carcinoma, appendicitis, and cholecystitis into entities which could, in fact, be treated with reasonable hope of success.[32,40,41]

In step with these new surgical vistas, functional systems of the hand became important. The ability to operate in a patient and deliberate manner offered a boon to surgeons and patients but posed new challenges as well. Areas of anatomy, previously inaccessible, and of little interest, suddenly became vitally important.

In association with anesthetic and surgical progress, Wilhelm Roentgen's discovery of X-rays in 1895 "Ueber eine neue Art von Strahlen" (strahlen, German for beam or ray), the discovery of "X-strahlen," became a vital part of the study of functional anatomical systems.[42,43] Etienne Destot of France (►Fig. 1.20) was a prime exponent of the use of this new technology to study the functional behavior of body systems, specifically, the wrist. Within 2 months of the announcement of the discovery of the X-ray of Roentgen, he was "...already making radiographs of patients in l'Hotel Dieu."[44]

Destot masterfully defined carpal behavior, normal and pathologic in his masterwork *Injuries of the Wrist*, translated into English in 1926. In this book, Destot clearly defined various derangements and maladies of the wrist which continue to bedevil surgeons and patients alike to the present day. Among the discussions are those of proximal pole scaphoid fractures, and what would later come to be known as SLAC (scapholunate advanced collapse). "I desire to draw only one conclusion... when we find a fracture of the upper extremity of the scaphoid combined with an alteration of the glenoid cavity of the radius, ...it is not rare to observe stiffness and loss of function passing

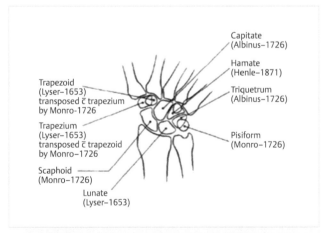

Fig. 1.19 Carpal nomenclature, summarizing origins of current names of the carpal bones. (By permission of Elsevier, J Hand Surg 1990; 15A: 834-838).

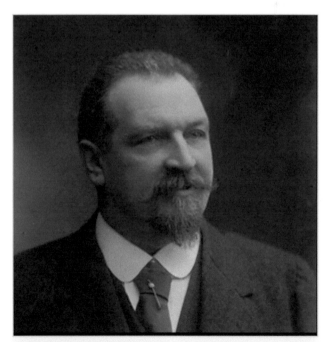

Fig. 1.20 Etienne Destot.

on to anchylosis between the radius and the scaphoid…it is often in these complications in the radius that we must seek for the principal factors in the seriousness of carpal lesions which appear simple."[44]

Across the Atlantic, Kansas-native Allen Buckner Kanavel (▶Fig. 1.21) made his own innovative use of Roentgen's "X-Strahlen." Circa 1900, infection was perhaps the most pressing problem pertaining to the hand. At the time, mechanisms of spread, and methods to treat infections of the hand were sorely lacking. Poorly executed attempts to drain hand infections frequently left patients with a useless hand, no hand, or worse, as surgeons blundered through multiple trips to the operating theater, making multiple ill-advised incisions on the hands of their hapless patients.

Kanavel worked in Chicago, Illinois. Among the many industries in booming Chicago was the meatpacking industry. Centered at the Union Stockyards, the 475-acre complex on Chicago's South Side, it processed as many as 18 million animals a year.[46] Described in rather lurid, but likely not too exaggeratedly, by Upton Sinclair in his muckraking *The Jungle*, the stockyards were a veritable injury factory, featuring speedy transit of large animals, and innumerable blunt and sharp instruments of all varieties. In turn, this recipe for mayhem yielded numerous hand infections, often in advanced stages of distress: "…one constantly meets cases in which the patient has been subjected to incision at some swollen or tender area, under the assumption that if there is not pus there 'the drainage will do good anyway.' A general rule should be laid down not to incise unless the surgeon has an accurate appreciation of the condition and

an absolute diagnosis made." Here, he summarizes a complex case which presented to him: "The immense size to which these infected hands may grow can hardly be believed unless they are seen. I recall particularly a patient who presented himself with such a hand which had been treated for four weeks without the surgeon having diagnosticated and opened a typical middle palmar abscess…the size of the infected hand…could be compared to the appearance of a large turtle. The patient had had ten or fifteen incisions on the fingers and the dorsum of the hand when I saw him. Only one incision—that of the middle palmar space—was necessary for drainage. A cupful of pus was evacuated, and the patient ultimately recovered complete function of his hand…. he had been advised by several surgeons to have his hand amputated."[47]

Using X-rays, Kanavel injected radio-opaque barium paste into flexor sheaths and deep spaces, thereby mapping patterns of synovial fluid drainage. With knowledge of the drainage pattern, a precise and accurate delineation of when to incise, and where, became available to assist the surgeon and patient alike. Instead of dozens, or more incisions, one or two judiciously applied, and carefully planned, incisions would clear tendon sheath and deep space infections. The book graphically demonstrates the contrast between ill-advised, essentially blind attempts at drainage, leaving the patient with a ruined limb, versus the excellent results available in timely, anatomically precise interventions, even in severe infections. Demonstrating his patient, methodical approach, Kanavel documents essential preparation for success: "Operation should always be done under general anesthesia and in a bloodless field."[47] Kanavel is perhaps best known for the "cardinal signs" of flexor tenosynovitis. The first three were described in 1912: "The three cardinal symptoms and signs are: 1. Excessive tenderness over the course of the sheath. This symptom is by all odds the most important. 2. Flexion of the finger. 3. Excruciating pain on extending the finger, most marked at the proximal end." By the fifth edition of the book, in 1925, the fourth cardinal sign had taken its place: 4. "Symmetrical enlargement of the whole finger."[47]

Further refinements of functional properties of the human form came from the landmark studies of cutaneous and muscular circulation, initially by Carl Manchot, of Switzerland, followed by Frenchman Michel Salmon. Both authors performed injection studies. As a medical student, the precocious Manchot performed a survey of the entire human cutaneous circulation, using an unknown dye, and dissecting the injected areas via an open technique in the time before X-rays were known. Manchot demonstrated that cutaneous perfusion is not a random occurrence, but rather that cutaneous perfusion is an ordered set of overlays, each supplied by a named vessel. In France, Michel Salmon took advantage of Roentgen's rays and performed injections with radio-opaque agents, followed by radiographic images, to map perfusion of skin and muscle. Salmon observed: "The cutaneous territory of the radial artery corresponds to the radial side and a smaller portion of the flexor side of the forearm. The remainder of the forearm skin receives its arterial supply from the ulnar artery…Posterior Compartment: in general, these muscles are supplied by the system of interosseous arteries. According to the classic authors, the anterior interosseous artery divides below the pronator quadratus into two terminal branches, anterior and posterior. The anterior… terminates in the pronator quadratus…the posterior branch

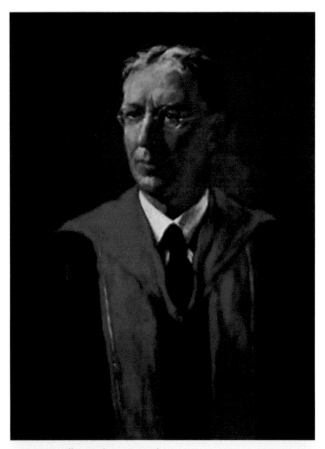

Fig. 1.21 Allen Buckner Kanavel.

pierces the interosseous membrane and enters the posterior compartment of the forearm...."[48,49]

Manchot and Salmon proved to be far ahead of their time, however, and their works languished until more refined clinical techniques could make use of these key observations. As William Morain observed, it is tantalizing to think of what might have been had Sir Harold Gilles, master of the random pattern flap for facial reconstruction in World War I, been able to read French and German, in order to apply the findings of Manchot and Salmon to his clinical cases. Over half a century passed until clinical medicine caught up to these two laboratory paragons, with their work reflected in the world's first free tissue transfer in 1973.[48-50] Taking this work into the 21st century, G. Ian Taylor and coworkers have made spectacular studies of human and animal cutaneous circulation, the angiosome concept: "...each nerve is associated with a longitudinally oriented system of arteries and veins. The 'inductive' effect of the nerves is very obvious, especially in the skin, where the vessels or their branches 'peel off' to accompany the nerve. The nervous system is one of the first to differentiate in the vertebrate embryo, and it is interesting to speculate what role its peripheral fibers may have played in the organization of the germ layers...."[51]

Additional refinements of study have allowed investigation into vessels of increasingly small caliber, along with dynamic behavior of these vessels in health, and in sickness. A leader in these studies is L. Andrew Koman, using modalities including digital plethysmography, laser Doppler flowmetry, and vital capillaroscopy to assess hand perfusion and hand ischemia.[52]

Study of the anatomy of the hand, in the meantime, continued for both gross and functional anatomy. In 1892, Legueu and Juvara of France described a now-eponymous set of vertical fascial septations in the palm at the proximal end of the flexor tendon pulley system. The septae assist with partitioning of flexor tendons and neurovascular bundles in the palm. Bilderback and Rayan presented a further study of these septae in 2004.[53]

In 1861, Jean C.F. Guyon of France described the anatomic passageway of the ulnar nerve at the wrist which now bears his name. "...On the underside of the wrist, just inside the pisiform, at the base of the hypothenar area, there is a small intralaminar section...Another interesting fact when describing this small space is the presence in the cavity of the ulnar artery and the nerve lying on the posterior wall, that is to say, on the anterior ligament of the carpus...."[54] Gross and Gelberman, quoted in Maroukis et al, delivered a landmark follow-up study in 1985, defining three zones of Guyon's canal: "Zone I: Begins from the proximal edge of the palmar carpal ligament and ends distally at the bifurcation of the ulnar nerve. Zone II: Runs from just distal to the bifurcation of the ulnar nerve to the fibrous arch of the hypothenar muscles and contains the deep branch of the ulnar nerve. Zone III: Begins just distal to the bifurcation of the ulnar nerve and contains the superficial branch of the ulnar nerve."[55]

In analogous fashion, Ulrich Lanz of Germany, in 1977 defined vital patterns of variation in median nerve motor branch takeoff. The report documents the seemingly capricious, and potentially hazardous takeoff points of the motor branch: radial, ulnar, proximal, distal, and all points in between.[56] This point is reinforced by Green and Morgan in 2008, a report in which they document that the finding of muscle crossing the midline of a carpal tunnel dissection may portend the presence of an aberrant motor branch of the median nerve.[57] To reinforce the notion of variability of what might be found in the carpal tunnel, Galzio and coworkers documented the presence of the entire ulnar nerve, bilaterally, within the carpal tunnels of a single patient.[58]

A giant in the field of dynamic behavior of peripheral nerves was Jules Tinel of France. Tinel summarized his extensive World War I nerve repair experiences in his 1918 book, *Nerve Wounds*. He described formication (Latin, formica: ant), defined in the Oxford English Dictionary as: "An abnormal sensation, as of ants creeping over the skin." Tinel describes formication as "...provoked by pressure: When compression or percussion is lightly applied to the injured nerve trunk, we often find, in the cutaneous region of the nerve a creeping sensation usually compared by the patient to electricity."[59] Pietrzak and coworkers report that Paul Hoffman of Germany described the sign first, but World War I prevented his work from reaching the global medical community.[60] Much like Newton and Liebniz, Tinel and Hoffman arrived at the same conclusion independently of one another.[61]

J. William Littler (▶ Fig. 1.22), a New York City hand surgeon, devoted much of his lengthy career to the study of the thumb. A gifted surgeon, talented artist,[62] and American Society for Surgery of the Hand founding member, Littler described the refinements of pollicization, and summarized efforts to overcome thumb deficiency in a fascinating 1976 review.[63] Joseph Upton and colleagues recently reported on the unique nature of the thumb and on pollicization. This report summarized Upton's own extensive experience, while offering an elegant synthesis of the early work of Littler and others, works which have led to the theoretical and technical practices for managing thumb deficiency, attempting to replace the irreplaceable.[64]

The 20th century saw a flowering of applied hand anatomy scholarship. Paul Brand (▶ Fig. 1.23) was a brilliant scientist, surgeon, and humanitarian. While working as a missionary surgeon in India, he helped define the pathoanatomy of the hand in leprosy. He also defined numerous surgical correctives for the resultant deformities, to the infinite benefit to these otherwise shunned victims of *M. leprae*. Brand's keen interest in mechanics led to detailed studies of functional properties of muscles. In turn, these studies helped codify a rational basis for tendon transfers. By matching excursion of the fibers, and cross-sectional area of the muscles, Brand optimized techniques for substitution of muscles for one another.[65,66]

Enhanced understanding of peripheral nerve anatomy was spearheaded by Sir Sidney Sunderland. Among his many contributions was a massive study of full-length fascicular architecture of upper limb nerves in 1945.[67] Hand in hand, enhanced understanding of peripheral nerve entrapment also occurred. Learmonth described the now-eponymous submuscular transposition of the ulnar nerve in 1942, McGowan graded degrees of ulnar nerve entrapment in 1950, and Osborne described the ligament that bears his name in 1957.[68-70]

In analogous fashion to these ulnar nerve investigators, G.S. Phalen clarified and advanced treatment for median nerve entrapment in the 1950s and 1960s. Here Phalen describes the test that now bears his name: "In performing the so-called wrist flexion test, the patient is asked to hold the forearms vertically and to allow both hands to drop into complete flexion at the wrist

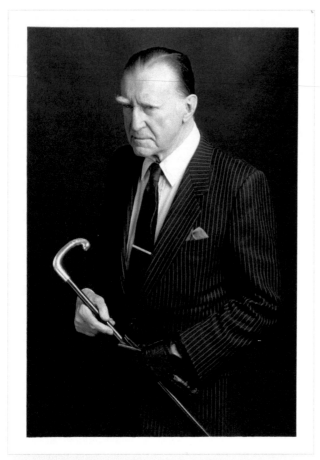

Fig. 1.22 J. William Littler, intelligence, elegance, and elan personified. (Image by kind permission of the New York Academy of Medicine.)

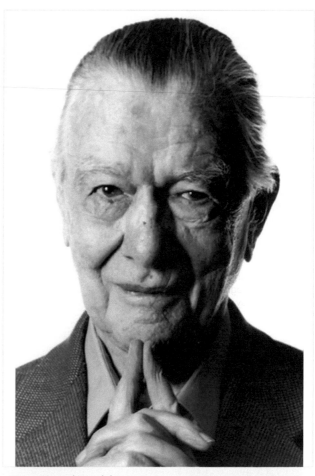

Fig. 1.23 Paul Brand- humanitarian, master surgeon, master mechanic of the hand.

for approximately one minute. In this position the median nerve is squeezed between the proximal edge of the transverse carpal ligament and the adjacent flexor tendons and radius. Maintaining this position for a long time eventually causes numbness and tingling over the distribution of the median nerve in the normal hand. However, when the median nerve is already somewhat compressed within the carpal tunnel, further compression by this maneuver causes almost immediate aggravation of the numbness and paresthesia in the fingers (▶ Fig. 1.24)."[71,72] In an added refinement, Szabo and Gelberman defined pathophysiology of peripheral nerve entrapment in association with distal radius fracture, in 1987, while Green and Rayan studied static and dynamic behavior of the cubital tunnel in 1999.[73,74]

Functional anatomical investigation continued across the full width and breadth of hand anatomy. Flexor tendon injuries have represented, and continue to represent, a severe challenge to patient and surgeon alike. Sterling Bunnell (▶ Fig. 1.25) pioneered and refined techniques for tendon grafting. This focus eventually led to publication in 1944 of his landmark *Surgery of the Hand,* a summary of his life's work not just in tendon repair, but also a virtuoso discussion of comparative anatomy, and a summation of hand care as it existed at the time. This book replaced Kanavel's as the accepted hand surgery resource in English.[75] In addition to his formidable scientific and surgical skills, Bunnell was also a talented organizer and leader.

In World War II, Bunnell oversaw the formation of a set of nine specialized hand surgery hospitals in the United States.[76] In turn, this group of pioneers formed the core of the American Society for Surgery of the Hand, founded in 1946.[77]

Taking Bunnell's work a step further, Harold Kleinert (▶ Fig. 1.26) had a revolutionary vision of direct repair of flexor tendons, with rehabilitation incorporating immediate controlled motion. This concept met with initial skepticism and in fact overt hostility: "...Primary repair in no man's land is not recommended by the authors for the occasional operator in hand surgery. However, the authors concluded that the results were obtainable by the experienced surgeon in selected patients, support their contention that no man's land is some man's land. Dr. J.H. Boyes, in discussing this paper noted that these were the most outstanding results obtained by any one in flexor-tendon repair. One gathered that he questioned the percentage of good results without any failures."[78] In spite of this formidable opposition, the excellence of Kleinert's concepts and clinical skills won the day and created a "one-man revolution in hand surgery."[79] Kleinert, a native of Sunburst, Montana was a charismatic prodigy, urged to attend medical school at Temple ("go as far east as you can, you need the polish"), who was basically self-taught: "...he made his own fellowship, for himself...."[80,81] Kleinert's work in Louisville, KY spanned more than a half-century, spanning a broad spectrum of expertise:

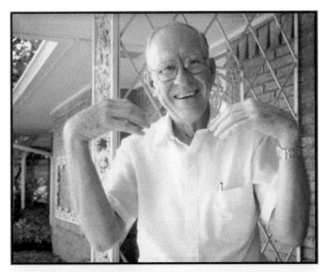

Fig. 1.24 George Phalen demonstarting the Phalen test to Harold Kleinert. Photographed at Dr Phalen's house. Photo courtesy of Sharon Kleinert.

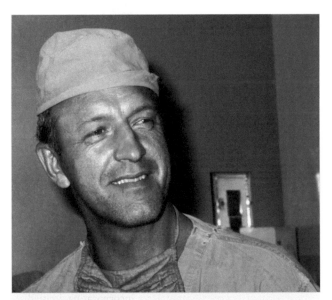

Fig. 1.26 Harold E. Kleinert – pictured in the mid-1960s, giant of hand surgery, mentor and teacher to multiple generations of hand surgeons. (Image courtesy of Sharon Kleinert.)

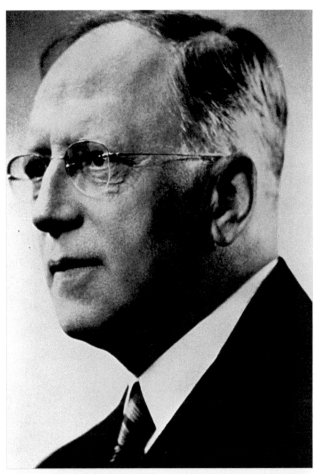

Fig. 1.25 Sterling Bunnell.

high-volume small vessel repair, replantation, free tissue transfers, and a host of other interventions which expanded treatment for the injured human upper limb. Kleinert's startling advances attracted a host of additional skilled teachers and practitioners to Louisville, perhaps none more formidable than Robert Acland (▶ Fig. 1.27).

Acland was a skilled plastic surgeon, microsurgeon, anatomist, and multimedia educational expert. Acland devised instruments to standardize microsurgical care, and an iconic written and video course on microsurgical training, known and loved by generations of microsurgical trainees: "…scenes like this needn't be a part of the human condition; let's see how…." A spectacular postscript to Acland's clinical time

was creation of a video atlas, surveying the entire human frame.[82–88]

Claude Verdan of Switzerland (▶ Fig 1.28), who was also a collaborator of Kleinert, provided standardization of tendon care at the level of organized medicine, and defined the quadrigia effect, a tendon dysfunction seen in certain cases of finger amputation, where a tethered profundus stump of an amputated digit can prevent excursion of flexor digitorum profundus (FDP) tendons of the other three digits in the ipsilateral hand, secondary to their common muscle origin.[89,90]

Other investigators studied dynamic aspect of systems involving combined hard and soft tissue systems. Building on Destot's foundation, Linscheid and Dobyns clarified patterns of wrist injury and consequent deformity, leading to adoption of standardized recognition and terminology for wrist injury, initially dorsal intercalated segment instability (DISI) and volar intercalated segment instability (VISI), later expanded by the Mayo Clinic hand group to include CID (carpal instability, dissociative) and CIND (carpal instability, nondissociative).[90,91] Taleisnik performed a landmark study on wrist ligaments in 1976, while Berger and coworkers from the Mayo Clinic have offered further refinements of such study, with works on magnetic resonance imaging characteristics of anterior radiocarpal ligaments (1994), along with gross and histologic analyses of scapholunate (1996) and lunotriquetral ligaments (1998).[93–96]

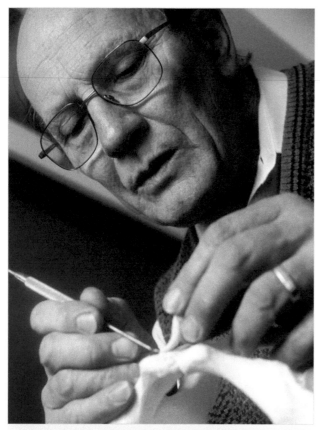

Fig. 1.27 Robert D. Acland: microsurgical teacher and educational icon, here depicted workingh on an anatomical specimen. (Image Courtesy of Bette Levy.)

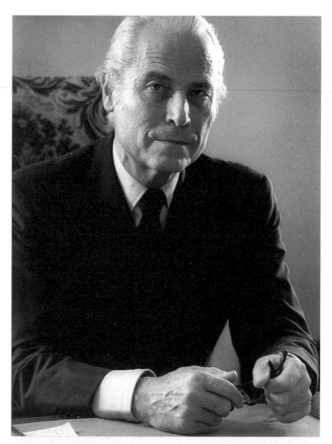

Fig. 1.28 Claude Verdan.

Further expanding microsurgical frontiers, Chase and coworkers documented functional flap transfers, thereby covering damaged structures. Chase summarized his life's work in his 1984 ASSH Presidential Address.[97,98]

Eduardo A. Zancolli of Argentina (▶ Fig. 1.29) defined his own concept of functional hand anatomy, and of hand surgery, in the two editions[99,100] of the iconic *Structural and Dynamic Bases of Hand Surgery*. Cementing his legacy is the spectacular 1991 collaboration with Elbio Cozzi, *Atlas of Surgical Anatomy of the Hand*, a large-format, high-resolution triumph of anatomical exposition.[101] On a smaller scale, but of similar quality, is Lee Milford's 1968 *Retaining Ligaments of the Digits of the Hand*.[102]

While functional anatomical concepts have assumed greater and greater importance, gross anatomy remains a vital focus of interest. To name just a pair, von Schroeder and Botte collaborated on defining studies of juncturae tendinum, and extensor tendons of the digits in the early 1990s—the two articles remain benchmark anatomical references.[103,104]

Another area of functional hand anatomy that is coming into its own is application of cerebral cortical localization. In the late 19th and early 20th centuries, Charles Sherrington performed pioneering cortical mapping via electrical stimulation studies performed on primates. His studies defined reflexes, as well as sensory, motor, and visual parameters of the brain.[105]

In a logical extension of Sherrington's work, Wilder Penfield, a trainee of Harvey Cushing, carried out spectacular human cerebral cortical mapping while performing epilepsy surgery under local anesthesia at McGill University in Montreal, Canada. These findings were summarized in his 896 -page collaboration with Herbert Jasper: *Epilepsy and the Functional Anatomy of the Human Brain* (1954).[106]

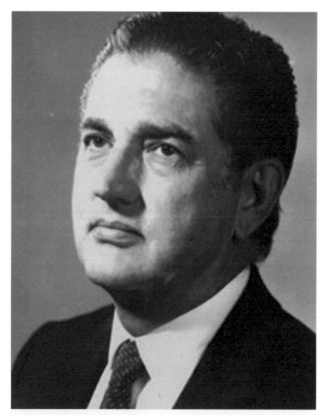

Fig. 1.29 Eduardo A. Zancolli.

Goran Lundborg has studied the hand in relation to its cerebral control center in great detail: "A nerve transection, isolated or in association with an amputation injury, represents an acute deafferentiation with immediate and long-standing influence on the corresponding representational areas in the brain cortex as well as in adjacent cortical territories."[107]

A true new frontier in application of the work of Sherrington and Penfield is the development of "brain-powered" prostheses which can allow bypass of damaged spinal cord or brachial plexus segments. Researchers are now documenting the effectiveness of the "brain-machine interface" (BMI), with a sensor picking and disseminating the signals from the motor strip of the cerebral cortex to motor a prosthesis.[108,109] While motor functions have been an initial focus, Yadav and coworkers describe a proposed interface to transfer artificial sensory information via dorsal column stimulation, in yet another tantalizing advance.[110]

Over time, anatomical knowledge of the hand has advanced in step with anatomy as a whole, from Imhotep and Sushruta to the present, with Vesalius representing a massive leap forward. Since the time of Vesalius, studies have become increasingly refined, directed toward ever-sharpening gradations of topography and function, as the chapter has discussed. While research is always advancing, some truths remain as constants. To paraphrase Harvey Cushing, accidents and injuries will never go away, and we must always be ready to care for them. To do so requires a proper knowledge of anatomy, but medical science is constantly evolving, so there must be a commitment to master and renew what is known, all the while staying abreast of new discoveries. Undoubtedly, much has been left out of this chapter, but I am hopeful that it will serve as a useful overview of the massive efforts over the centuries to understand hand and upper limb anatomy to properly care for conditions of the human hand in disease and health.

References

1. Lancet. vol I, pp. 326, 357, 387, 507; vol II, p. 95, reprinted in The Collected Papers of Joseph, Baron Lister, Volume 2. Birmingham, AL: Classics of Surgery Library; 1867;1979:1–100
2. Osler SW. The evolution of modern medicine. Reprinted by Classics of Medicine Library, Birmingham, AL; 1979:10
3. Hurry JB. Imhotep. Oxford; 1928:3
4. Art of Ancient Egypt. Yale/MMA; 2005:70–115
5. Shin EK, Meals RA. The historical importance of the hand in advancing the study of human anatomy. J Hand Surg Am 2005;30(2):209–221
6. Bhishagratna KL. An English translation of the Sushruta Samhita. Calcutta: Wilkins Press; 1907
7. Genuine Works of Hippocrates. "The Surgery." Classics of Medicine; 1985:472
8. O'Malley CD. Andreas Vesalius of Brussels. University of California Press; 1967:95
9. Afshar A. A brief report about the concepts of hand disorders in the Canon of Medicine of Avicenna. J Hand Surg Am 2011;36(9):1509–1514
10. O'Malley CC, Saunders JB. Leonardo da Vinci: on the human body. Dover; 1983
11. Vesalius A. De Fabrica Corporis Humani. Basel, Switzerland: Johannes Oporinus; 1543
12. Cushing H. A bio-bibliography of Andreas Vesalius. Archon Books;1962:xxiv
13. O'Malley C. Andreas Vesalius of Brussels 1514–1564. University of California Press; 1967:64
14. Vesalius A. On the fabric of the human body: a translation of De Humani Corporis Fabrica Libri Septem. Volume I: The Bones and Cartilages. Translated by William Frank Richardson in collaboration with John Burd Carman. San Francisco: Jeremy Norman; 1998–2009:259–296
15. Vesalius A. On the fabric of the human body: A TRANSLATION of De Humani Corporis Fabrica Libri Septem. Volume II: The Ligaments and Muscles. Translated by William Frank Richardson in collaboration with John Burd Carman. San Francisco: Jeremy Norman; 1998–2009:323–351
16. Vesalius, A. On the fabric of the human body: a translation of De Humani Corporis Fabrica Libri Septem. Volume IV: The Nerves. Translated by William Frank Richardson in collaboration with John Burd Carman. San Francisco: Jeremy Norman;1998–2009:237–251
17. Heckscher WS. Rembrandt's anatomy of Dr. Nicolaes Tulp. Washington Square: New York University Press; 1958
18. Ijpma F, van de Graaf R, Nicolae J, Meek M. The anatomy lesson of Dr. Nicolaes Tulp by Rembrandt (1632): a comparison of the painting with a dissected left forearm of a Dutch 52
19. Rifkin B, Ackerman M. Human anatomy: from the Renaissance to the digital age. New York: Abrams;2006
20. Winslow JB: Exposition anatomique de la structure du corps humain. volumes, Paris, Guillaume Desprez et Jean Desseartz, 1732
21. Ijpma FFA, van de Graaf RC, van Gulik TM. Petrus Camper's work on the anatomy and pathology of the arm and hand in the 18th century. J Hand Surg Am 2010;35A(8):1382–1387
22. Bartoníček J, Naňka O. Josias Weitbrecht, the founder of syndesmology, and the history of the retinacula of Weitbrecht. Surg Radiol Anat 2019;41(10):1103–1111
23. Kaplan EB. Weitbrecht's syndesmology. Philadelphia PA: WB Saunders; 1969
24. Bell C. The hand: its mechanism and vital endowments as evincing design. New York: Classics of Surgery Library, Gryphon Editions; 1985
25. Moore W. The knife man. New York: Broadway Books; 2005
26. Brenner P, Rayan G. Dupuytren's disease: a concept of surgical treatment. Wien, New York: Springer Verlag; 2003
27. Wylock P. The life and times of Guillaume Dupuytren. Brussels University; 2010
28. Richardson R. The making of Mr. Gray's anatomy. Oxford; 2008
29. Gray H, Carter HV. Anatomy, descriptive and surgical. 1858, JW Parker and Son, London, England. Reprinted by the Classics of Medicine Library; 1981
30. Acland R. Practice manual for microvascular surgery. 2nd ed. St Louis, MO: CV Mosby; 1989
31. Federative International Programme on Anatomical Terminologies (FIPAT): Terminologica Anatomica. International Anatomical Terminology. Stuttgart, Germany: Thieme;2011
32. Davis L. J.B. Murphy: stormy petrel of surgery. Putnam;1938
33. McMurrich JP. The nomenclature of the carpal bones. Anat Rec 1914;8(3):173–183
34. Johnson RP. The evolution of carpal nomenclature: a short review. J Hand Surg Am 1990;15(5):834–838
35. Nuland SB. Crawford Long of Georgia. In: The origins of anesthesia. Birminghan AL: Classics of Medicine Library;1983
36. Nuland SB. Announcement and controversy. In: The origins of anesthesia. , Birminghan AL: Classics of Medicine Library;1983
37. Crowe SJ. Halsted of Johns Hopkins. Springfield, IL: Charles C. Thomas; 1957

38. Lancet. 1867, vol I, pp. 326, 357, 387, 507; vol II, p. 95. Reprinted in The Collected Papers of Joseph, Baron Lister. Volume 2: Classics of Surgery Library, Birmingham, AL; 1979

39. Mallon W. Ernest Amory Codman: the end result of a life in surgery. Philadelphia, PA: Saunders; 2000

40. Fulton JF. Harvey Cushing: a biography. Springfield, IL: Charles C Thomas; 1946

41. Halsted WS. Surgical papers, in 2 volumes. Volume 2, pp. 3–88, pp. 220–223, 427–476. Reprinted 1984. , Birmingham, AL: Classics of Medicine Library, Gryphon Editions

42. Nuland SB. Doctors: the illustrated history of medical pioneers. New York: Black Dog and Leventhal Publishers; 2008

43. Gedeon A. Wilhelm Conrad Roentgen. In: Science and technology in medicine. Stuttgart, Germany: Springer; 2006

44. Peltier L. The classic: injuries of the wrist, by E. Destot. Clin Orth Rel Res 1986;202:3–11

45. Destot E. Injuries of the wrist. New York: Paul B. Hoeber; 1926:72–73

46. Pacyga D. Chicago: a biography. University of Chicago Press; 2009

47. Kanavel AB. Infections of the hand. Philadelphia, PA: Lea and Febiger; 1912

48. Manchot C. The cutaneous arteries of the human skin. Translated by Jovanka Ristic and William Morain. Berlin: Springer-Verlag; 1983

49. Salmon M. Book 1: Arteries of the muscles of the extremities and the trunk, Book 2: Arterial anastamotic pathways of the extremities In: Ian Taylor G, Razaboni Rosa M, eds. St. Louis, MO: Quality Medical Publishing; 1994

50. Daniel RK, Taylor GI. Distant transfer of an island flap by microvascular anastomoses: a clinical technique. Plast Reconstr Surg 1973;52(2):111–117

51. Taylor GI, Gianoutsos MP, Morris SF. The neurovascular territories of the skin and muscles: anatomic study and clinical implications. Plast Reconstr Surg 1994;94(1):1–36

52. Koman LA, et al. Vascular disorders. In: Green's operative hand surgery. 6th ed. Wolfe SW, editor in chief. New York: Elsevier; 2011: 2197–2240

53. Bilderback KK, Rayan GM. The septa of Legueu and Juvara: an anatomic study. J Hand Surg Am 2004;29(3):494–499

54. Guyon F. Note on the anatomical condition affecting the underside of the wrist not previously reported. J Hand Surg 2006;31B:147–148, originally in Bulletins de La Socieitie Anatomique de Paris, 1861, second series 6, 184–186

55. Maroukis BL, Ogawa T, Rehim SA, Chung KC. Guyon canal: the evolution of clinical anatomy. J Hand Surg Am 2015; 40(3, 40A)560–565

56. Lanz U. Anatomical variations of the median nerve in the carpal tunnel. J Hand Surg Am 1977; 2(1, 2A)44–53

57. Green DP, Morgan JP. Correlation between muscle morphology of the transverse carpal ligament and branching pattern of the motor branch of median nerve. J Hand Surg Am 2008; 33(9, 33A)1505–1511

58. Galzio RJ, Magliani V, Lucantoni D, D'Arrigo C. Bilateral anomalous course of the ulnar nerve at the wrist causing ulnar and median nerve compression syndrome: case report. J Neurosurg 1987;67(5):754–756

59. Tinel J. Nerve wounds. New York: William Wood; 1918

60. Pietrzak K, Grzybowski A, Kaczmarczyk J. Jules Tinel (1879-1952). J Neurol 2016;263(7):1471–1472

61. Westfall R. Never at rest: a biography of Isaac Newton. Cambridge, England: Cambridge University Press; 1980

62. Glickel SZ, Seiler JG III. The Littler legacy. ASSH Publication; 2019

63. Littler JW. On making a thumb: one hundred years of surgical effort. J Hand Surg Am 1976;1:35–51

64. Taghinia AH, Littler JW, Upton J. Refinements in pollicization: a 30-year experience. Plast Reconstr Surg 2012;130(3):423e–433e

65. Brand P, Yancey P. Pain: the gift nobody wants. Harper Perennial; 1995

66. Brand PW, Hollister AM. Clinical mechanics of the hand. 3rd ed. St Louis, MO: CV Mosby; 1999

67. Sunderland S. The intraneural topography of the radial, median and ulnar nerves. Brain 1945;68(68):243–299

68. Learmonth J. A technique for transplanting the ulnar nerve. Surg Gynecol Obstet 1942;75:792–793

69. McGowan AJ. The results of transposition of the ulnar nerve for traumatic ulnar neuritis. J Bone Joint Surg Br 1950; 32-B(3, 32B)293–301

70. Osborne G. The surgical treatment of tardy ulnar neuritis. J Bone Joint Surg 1957; (39):782

71. Phalen GS, Gardner WJ, La Londe AA. Neuropathy of the median nerve due to compression beneath the transverse carpal ligament. J Bone Joint Surg Am 1950;32A(1): 109–112

72. Phalen GS. The carpal tunnel syndrome: seventeen years' experience in diagnosis and treatment of 654 hands. J Bone Joint Surg 1966;48:211–228

73. Gelberman RH, Szabo RM, Mortensen WW. Carpal tunnel pressures and wrist position in patients with colles' fractures. J Trauma 1984;24(8):747–749

74. Green JR Jr, Rayan GM. The cubital tunnel: anatomic, histologic, and biomechanical study. J Shoulder Elbow Surg 1999;8(5):466–470

75. Bunnell S. Surgery of the hand. Philadelphia, PA: JB Lippincott; 1944

76. Bunnell S, Ed. Surgery in World War 2: hand surgery. Washington, DC: Office of the Surgeon General, Department of the Army; 1955

77. Newmeyer WL. The Second World War to 1971: the founding. In: American Society for Surgery of the Hand: the first fifty years. New York: Churchill Livingstone; 1995:1–17

78. Kleinert HE, Kutz JE, Ashbell TS. Primary repair of lacerated flexor tendons in no man's land. In: Proceedings, American Society for Surgery of the Hand. J Bone Joint Surg 1967;49A: 574–584

79. Breidenbach WC. Personal communication. Louisville, KY; 1995

80. Kleinert HE. Personal communication. Louisville, KY; 1998

81. Kleinert J. Personal communication. Louisville, KY; 1997

82. Kleinert HE, Kasdan ML. Anastamosis of digital vessels. J Ky Med Assoc 1965;63(63):106–108

83. Scheker LR, Kleinert HE, Hanel DP. Lateral arm composite tissue transfer to ipsilateral hand defects. J Hand Surg Am 1987;12(5 Pt 1):665–672

84. Kleinert HE, Jablon M, Tsai TM. An overview of replantation and results of 347 replants in 245 patients. J Trauma 1980;20(5):390–398

85. Lister GD, Kleinert HE, Kutz JE, Atasoy E. Primary flexor tendon repair followed by immediate controlled mobilization. J Hand Surg Am 1977;2(6):441–451

86. Acland RD. Modified needleholder for microsurgery. BMJ 1969;1(5644):635

87. Acland RD. Practice manual for microvascular surgery. 2nd ed. St Louis, MO: CV Mosby; 1989.

88. Acland R. Acland's video atlas of human anatomy. AclandAnatomy.com

89. Kleinert HE, Verdan C. Report of the Committee on Tendon Injuries (International Federation of Societies for Surgery of the Hand). J Hand Surg Am 1983;8(5 Pt 2):794–798

90. Verdan C. Syndrome of the quadriga. Surg Clin North Am 1960;40:425–426

91. Linschied RL, Dobyns JH, Beabout JW, Bryan RS. Traumatic instability of the wrist: diagnosis, classification, and pathomechanics. J Bone Joint Surg 1972;54-A(8):1612–1632

92. Dobyns J, Linscheid R. Carpal instability classification and historical perspective. In: Cooney W, ed. The wrist. 2nd ed. Wolters Kluwer; 2010:608–616

93. Taleisnik J. The ligaments of the wrist. J Hand Surg Am 1976;1(2):110–118

94. Berger RA, Linscheid RL, Berquist TH. Magnetic resonance imaging of the anterior radiocarpal ligaments. J Hand Surg Am 1994;19(2, 19A)295–303

95. Berger RA. The gross and histologic anatomy of the scapholunate interosseous ligament. J Hand Surg Am 1996;21(2):170–178

96. Ritt MJPF, Bishop AT, Berger RA, Linscheid RL, Berglund LJ, An KN. Lunotriquetral ligament properties: a comparison of three anatomic subregions. J Hand Surg Am 1998;23(3):425–431

97. Chase RA, Hentz VR, Apfelberg D. A dynamic myocutaneous flap for hand reconstruction. J Hand Surg Am 1980;5(6, 5A)594–599

98. Chase RA. The development of tissue transfer in hand surgery. J Hand Surg Am 1984; 9(4, 9A)463–477

99. Zancolli E. Structural and dynamic bases of hand surgery. Philadelphia, PA: JB Lippincott; 1968

100. Zancolli E. Structural and dynamic bases of hand surgery. 2nd ed. Philadelphia, PA: JB Lippincott; 1979

101. Zancolli E, Cozzi E. Atlas of surgical anatomy of the hand. Edinburgh, Scotland: Churchill Livingstone; 1991

102. Milford L. Retaining ligaments of the digits of the hand. Philadelphia, PA: WB Sauders; 1968

103. von Schroeder HP, Botte MJ. The functional significance of the long extensors and juncturae tendinum in finger extension. J Hand Surg Am 1993;18(4):641–647

104. von Schroeder HP, Botte M. Anatomy of the extensor tendons of the fingers: variations and multiplicity. J Hand Surg 1995;20:27–34

105. Sherrington C. The integrative action of the nervous system. Yale University Press. Reprinted 1986. Birmingham, AL: Classics of Medicine Library; 1906

106. Penfield W, Jasper H. Epilepsy and the functional anatomy of the human brain. Boston, MA: Little, Brown; 1954

107. Lundborg G. Nerve injury and repair: regeneration, reconstruction, and cortical remodeling. 2nd ed. Philadelphia, PA: Elsevier/Churchill Livingstone; 2004:219

108. Ethier C, Oby ER, Bauman MJ, Miller LE. Restoration of grasp following paralysis through brain-controlled stimulation of muscles. Nature 2012;485(7398):368–371

109. Yanagisawa T, Hirata M, Saitoh Y, et al. Real-time control of a prosthetic hand using human electrocorticography signals. J Neurosurg 2011;114(6):1715–1722

110. Yadav AP, Li D, Nicolelis MAL. A brain to spine interface for transferring artificial sensory information. Sci Rep 2020;10(1):900

Section II

Structural and Functional Fundamentals

Source: Leonardo on the Human Body.

2 Structural and Functional Anatomy of the Hand

Amit Gupta

*"To understand deformity and abnormality requires an apprecia-
tion of the normal function in the hand. To study normal function
requires an appreciation of anatomy."*

—Richard J. Smith, MD[1]

2.1 Introduction

The human hand is the unique instrument that executes the
commands of the brain and expresses the nuances of the mind. In
performing these tasks it has to adopt an infinite variety of postures (▶Fig. 2.1). Some of these postures are purely expressive
(▶Fig. 2.2), some are associated with varying degrees of touch
(▶Fig. 2.3), and others involve manipulating objects to gather
information (▶Fig. 2.4)—and then there are those that involve
applying forces to an object (▶Fig. 2.5). In order to achieve these
myriad of tasks, the hand has to be an adaptable device, a cha-
meleon of all instruments that is able to assume multitudes of
postures.

Sir Charles Bell (1833) wrote in *The Bridgewater Treatises,*
"attention to our most common actions will show us, how the
division into fingers, by combining motion with the sense of
touch adapts the hand to grasp, to feel and to compare."[2]

The shoulder joint functions as the attachment point of the
upper extremity to the torso and has a circular arc of motion
that keeps the hand in a circular cone within the visual field. It
is amazing that the extent of the visual field mimics the limits
of the shoulder's ability to place the hand in space. However,
with a combination of movements of all the joints of the upper
extremity, the hand can be placed in positions that the eye
cannot see. Thus, even in a normal sighted individual, the hand
can act as a surrogate of the eye, exploring and gathering tactile
information about objects and bodies beyond the visual field.[3]

The essential function of the elbow and forearm motion
acting in synchrony is to position the hand in space.

2.2 Prehension

In 1956, John Napier defined prehensile movements of the
human hand as those motions in which "the object is seized
and held within the compass of the hand." He went on to
further classify prehension into (1) power grip and (2) precision grip.[4]

In *power grip*, the object is held in a clamp formed by the
partly flexed fingers and the palm, with counter pressure
applied by the thumb ray in the plane of the palm (▶Fig. 2.6). In
precision grip, the object is pinched between the flexor aspects
of the fingers and the opposing thumb (▶Fig. 2.7).

The factors that influence the posture of the hand during
function include (a) the shape of the object; (b) the size of the
object; (c) physical factors such as the weight, temperature, and

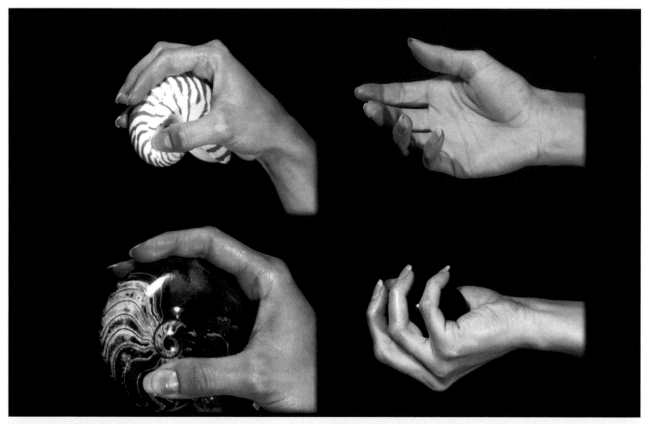

Fig. 2.1 The hand can adopt a wide variety of postures.

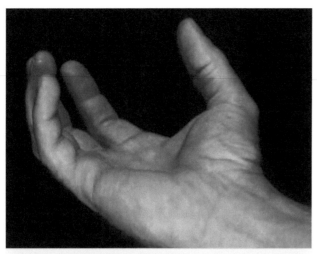

Fig. 2.2 Expressive posture of the hand.

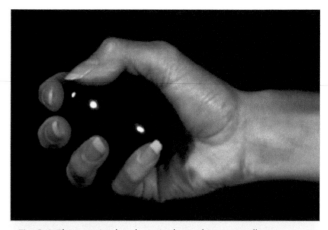

Fig. 2.4 The grasping hand manipulates objects to collect information.

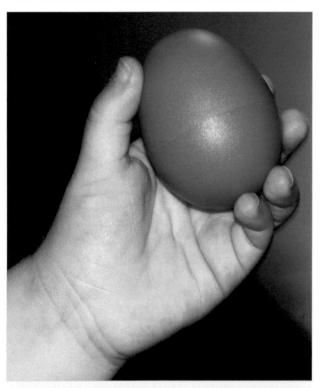

Fig. 2.3 Grasp with touch brings the sensate elements of the hand in contact with the object.

wetness or dryness of the object; and (d) motivational factors such as fear or hunger.

John Napier in 1956 further outlined *prehension* as comprising the following:

- Power grip: ability to apply forces and resist arbitrary forces that may be applied to the object (▶ Fig. 2.8).
- Precision handling: small adjustments of posture to control the direction in which the force is being applied (▶ Fig. 2.9).

Biomechanically, prehension can be defined as the application of *functionally effective forces* by the hand to an object given numerous constraints.[5]

Functionally effective forces are able to match the anticipated forces in the task for a stable grasp, are able to impart

motion to the object (i.e., manipulate it) or transport the object, and help in gathering sensory information about the state of interaction with the object during the task in order to ensure grasping and manipulative stability.

2.3 Surface Anatomy

Knowledge of surface anatomy is vital for the hand surgeon, as it is very important in the examination of the hand[3,6,7] (▶ Fig. 2.10).

The tendon of the flexor carpi ulnaris (FCU) can be readily palpated on the distal portion of the forearm on the ulnar side. As one goes distally palpating the FCU, one reaches a bony prominence that is the pisiform. The ulnar neurovascular bundle is located just on the radial side of the FCU tendon, the ulnar nerve being closer to the tendon and the ulnar artery located more radially. The hook of the hamate is located a fingerbreadth distal and radial to the pisiform and corresponds to the intersection of a line drawn from the center of the ring finger base to the distal wrist crease and a second line from the center of the base of the index finger to the pisiform. The deep motor branch of the ulnar nerve passes between the pisiform and the hamate hook and quickly runs deep to supply the interosseous muscles. The digital nerve to the small finger closely follows a line drawn from the hook of the hamate to the small finger palmar digital crease.

On the radial side one can easily palpate the tendon of the flexor carpi radialis (FCR). As one follows the tendon of the FCR, the first bony point that is palpable at the level of the wrist crease is the tubercle of the scaphoid. Distal to the tubercle of the scaphoid, the trapezial ridge can be palpated as can the mobile first carpometacarpal joint. The distal edge of the transverse carpal ligament spans the palm between the trapezial ridge and the hook of the hamate. The distal wrist crease marks the proximal border of the pisiform and hence the start of the transverse carpal ligament and the carpal tunnel. Kaplan's cardinal line is a line extended on the palm along the ulnar border of the fully abducted thumb. This marks the distal aspect of the tunnel. The superficial palmar arch is located 1 cm distal to this line. The radial digital nerve to the index finger lies deep to a line connecting the trapezial ridge to the radial border of the proximal digital crease of the index finger.

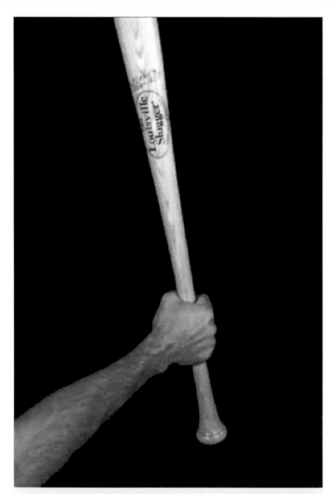

Fig. 2.5 Grip applying force to an object.

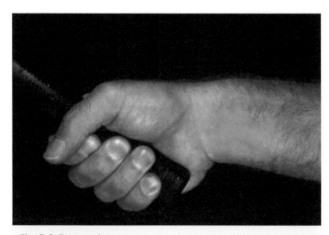

Fig. 2.6 Power grip.

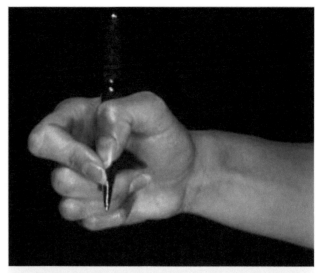

Fig. 2.7 Precision grip.

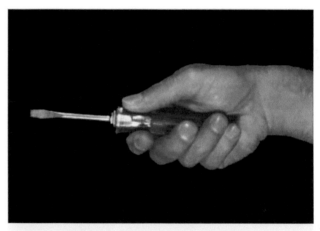

Fig. 2.8 Combined power grip and precision handling.

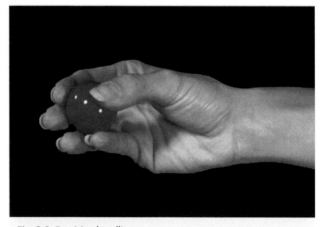

Fig. 2.9 Precision handling.

The surface markings of the index, long, and ring finger metacarpophalangeal joints are along the distal palmar crease, whereas the index metacarpal head lies deep to the proximal palmar crease.

On the dorsum of the wrist, the Lister's tubercle is a readily palpable bony marking. There is a soft spot just distal to the Lister's tubercle. This marks the gap between the third and fourth dorsal compartments and is the site for the 3/4 arthroscopic portal. This area also marks the point that corresponds to the scapholunate joint.

On the ulnar side of the wrist, the ulnar head and the ulnar styloid are easily palpable, as is the extensor carpi ulnaris

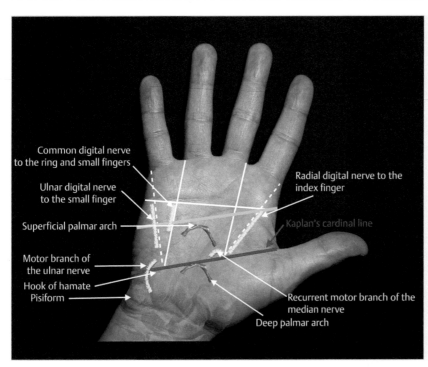

Fig. 2.10 Surface markings of the palm. Kaplan's cardinal line runs from the first web space in line with the abducted thumb parallel to the proximal palmar crease. The hook of the hamate lies on this line and is easily palpable. The motor branch of the ulnar nerve runs between the pisiform and the hook of the hamate then curves around the hook of the hamate. The superficial palmar arch lies 1 to 1.5 cm distal to the Kaplan's cardinal line. The deep palmar arch lies just proximal to the Kaplan's cardinal line. The radial digital nerve to the index finger lies on a line connecting the radial end of the basal crease of the index finger to the Kaplan's line. The motor branch of the median nerve lies at the junction of a line from the radial border of the middle finger to the Kaplan's line parallel to the digit. On a line from the ulnar border of the ring finger to the Kaplan's line parallel to the digit lies the common digital nerve to the ring and small fingers. The ulnar digital nerve to the small finger lies on a line from the ulnar border of the small finger basal digital crease to the Kaplan's line. The last two lines intersect the Kaplan's line at the hook of the hamate.

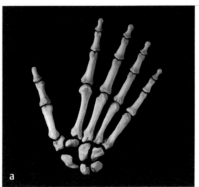
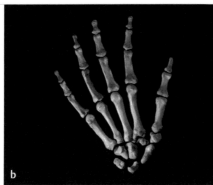

Fig. 2.11 (a) Dorsal and (b) palmar views of the hand skeleton.

(ECU) tendon. The fourth and the fifth carpometacarpal joints are quite mobile and are easily palpable, as are the more stable second and third carpometacarpal joints.

2.4 Structure

The skeletal structure of the hand consists of 27 bones, of which 19 are long bones (▶ Figs. 2.11a and 2.11b), 17 articulations, and 19 muscles.[3,7]

The hand skeleton can be studied in the following manner:

2.4.1 The Rays of the Hand

The thumb is a highly mobile component of the hand. Special structures like the saddle-shaped trapeziometacarpal joint and the special arrangements of the intrinsic and extrinsic muscles of the thumb allow a great deal of freedom to this ray and the ability to place the thumb in a plane at 45° to the digits and move across them. Together with the index and middle fingers, the thumb is useful in the precision manipulation of objects by the hand.

The ulnar digits are mainly used in power grasp. All the four digits of the hand from index to small fingers converge toward the tubercle of the scaphoid in flexion. In extension, generally the middle finger is the longest, whereas in flexion the ring finger becomes the longest, thus exposing it to injuries. The ring finger flexor digitorum profundus (FDP) is commonly ruptured in "jersey finger" injuries due to this anatomical peculiarity.

The transverse axis of the palm corresponds to the metacarpophalangeal joints and is at 75° to the long axis of the palm (▶ Fig. 2.12). This anatomical fact has design implications for glove design as well as during cast applications, allowing for appropriate movement of the metacarpophalangeal joints when the wrist is immobilized in a cast.

2.4.2 The Fixed and Mobile Elements

Littler in 1960 described the fixed and mobile elements of the hand[8] (▶ Fig. 2.13). The fixed elements of the hand consist of the distal carpal row and the second and the third metacarpals. The carpometacarpal joints of the index and long fingers have very thick and strong ligaments, allowing little movement between the components.

The thumb is the most mobile component in the hand, as it is able to assume a wide variety of positions and can be made to touch each digit due to its peculiar anatomic arrangement.

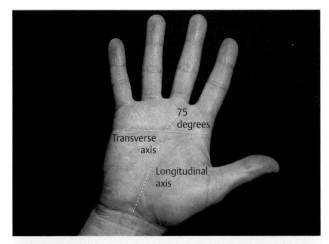

Fig. 2.12 The transverse axis of the hand is at 75° to the long axis of the hand.

The ulnar two metacarpal are very mobile due to rather lax carpometacarpal joints. The fourth carpometacarpal joint can move 20° while the fifth carpometacarpal joint can move about 44°[7,9,10] (▶Fig. 2.14).

2.4.3 The Arches of the Hand (▶Fig. 2.15)

The arches of the hand consists of multiple longitudinal (one for each digit) (▶Fig. 2.16, ▶Fig. 2.17) and two transverse arches[3,7] (▶Fig. 2.18, ▶Fig. 2.19).

The metacarpophalangeal joint is the main joint of the longitudinal arch of the digit. It has very important ligaments that span across the joint and control its stability. The anatomy of this key joint is discussed in great detail in Chapter 35.

The carpal arch (▶Fig. 2.18) has a deep palmar concavity and is formed by the osseous masses of the proximal and distal carpal rows bounded on the dorsal and palmar side by thick ligaments. The spanning transverse carpal ligaments also maintain the arch. The capitate forms the keystone of this arch.

The transverse metacarpal arch is formed by the metacarpal heads, which are arranged in a curved configuration maintained by the arrangement of the interpalmar plate ligaments (IPPL) and the fibrous structures (▶Fig. 2.19). The second and the third metacarpal heads are very stable, whereas the fourth and the fifth metacarpals can move and increase the concavity of this arch by virtue of their mobility at the carpometacarpal joints.[3,7,9]

2.4.4 The Fibrous Skeleton

The fibrous skeleton of the hand is very important for function and provides the following:
• Stability
• Mobility
• Fixation of the skin
• Containment
• Partition
• Protection and padding
• Connection

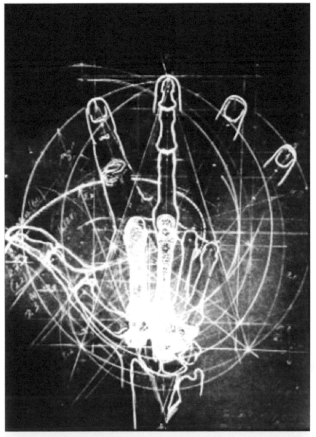

Fig. 2.13 The fixed elements of the hand.

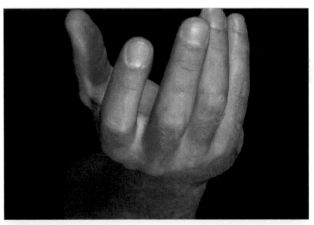

Fig. 2.14 The 4th and 5th metacarpals can move to cup the hand.

• Nourishment
• Tendon guidance
• Restraint

The shape of the joints (the PIP joints have bicondylar shape with inherent stability; the MP joints have great lateral stability in flexion as the joint surfaces are wider at the anterior aspect), the eccentric arrangement of the collateral ligaments, and the volar plates and joint capsule all provide *stability* to the finger joints.

Amazingly, the same components also provide *mobility* to the joints. The metacarpophalangeal joints are so shaped that on extension the narrow portion of the metacarpal head is in

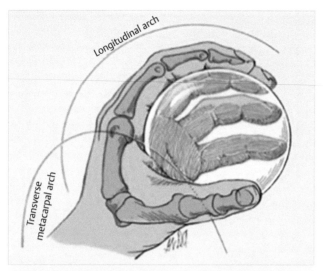

Fig. 2.15 Arches of the hand. (Copyright Kleinert Institute, Louisville, KY.)

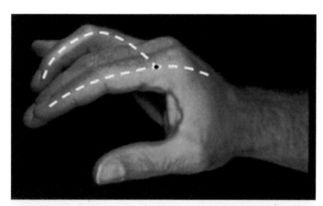

Fig. 2.16 Each digit represents a longitudinal arch.

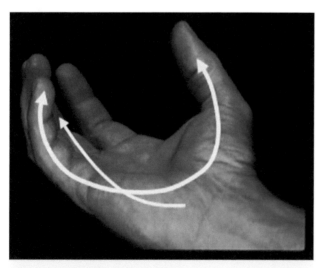

Fig. 2.17 Longitudinal arches of the hand.

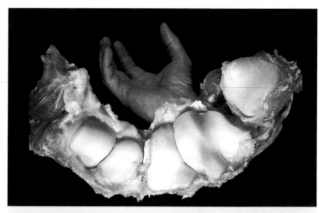

Fig. 2.18 The carpal arch at the CMC joint.

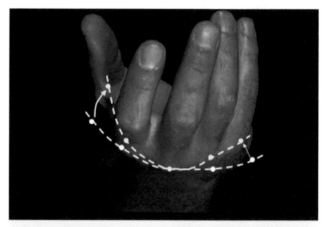

Fig. 2.19 The transverse metacarpal arch at the MC heads.

head comes in contact with the base of the proximal phalanx, locking the joint and making it more stable and less mobile. Similarly, the eccentric arrangement of the collateral ligaments results in these ligaments' being tighter in flexion of the joint, enhancing stability, but lax in extension, providing mobility. The volar plates are thick cartilaginous structures that increase the joint surface yet are able to get out of the way in flexion of the joint.[3,7]

The carpometacarpal joint of the thumb is structurally unstable and very mobile due to the lax arrangement of the ligaments and the unique saddle shape of the joint surfaces. The detailed anatomy of this joint is discussed in Chapter 34.

The retinacular ligaments of the hand anchor the glabrous skin of the hand to the hand skeleton. The superficial layer of the palmar aponeurosis is directly responsible for the tethering of the hand skin (►Fig. 2.20). The skin creases represent attachment of the palmar aponeurosis with their vertical fibers to the skin without the intervention of adipose tissue. The septae of Legueu and Juvara are fibrous bands that anchor the palmar skin to the palmar plate of the metacarpophalangeal joint in the sagittal plane.[11] They also provide *containment* and *partition* for the flexor tendons, as there are two septae on either side of each digital flexor tendon. (►Fig. 2.21).

The natatory ligament part of the palmar fascia holds the web spaces in their fascinating three-dimensional configuration (►Fig. 2.22). Further distally in the finger, on the lateral sides, Grayson's ligaments on the palmar side and Cleland's

contact with the base of the proximal phalanx, thus providing great lateral mobility in extension. The situation changes when the joint flexes and the wider part of the metacarpal ligaments on the dorsal side of the neurovascular bundles anchor the skin to the digital skeleton[12] (▶Fig. 2.23 and ▶Fig. 2.24).

The dorsal hand skin is very lax due to loose areolar tissue and the lack of any firm attachment to the underlying skeleton. The mobility of the dorsal skin in both longitudinal and transverse directions is essential for full digital flexion. Since there is a lot of loose areolar tissue in this region, edema fluid can easily collect here, hyperextending the metacarpophalangeal joints and secondarily flexing the proximal interphalangeal joints. One of the ways to minimize this effect is to keep the metacarpophalangeal joints flexed in a splint. This stretches the dorsal skin and decreases any dead space. The mobility, space and compliance of the dorsal skin must be addressed if the surgeon wants good movement of the digits following correction of hand stiffness.

The compartments of the hand *contain* the structures[12]. There are six hand compartments:

- Thenar (flexor pollicis brevis, abductor pollicis brevis, and opponens pollicis)
- Hypothenar (abductor digiti minimi, opponens digiti minimi, and flexor digiti minimi)
- Adductor (adductor pollicis)
- Interosseous: a. dorsal; b. palmar
- Carpal tunnel
- Digital

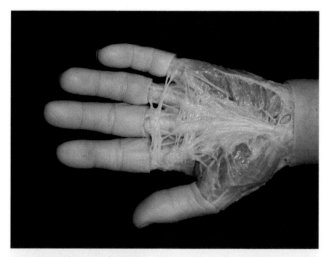

Fig. 2.20 The superficial layer of the palmar aponeurosis.

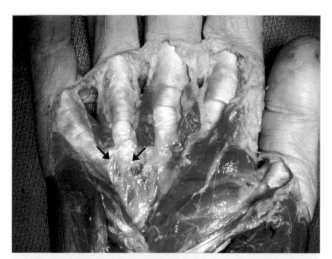

Fig. 2.21 Septa of Legueu and Juvara.

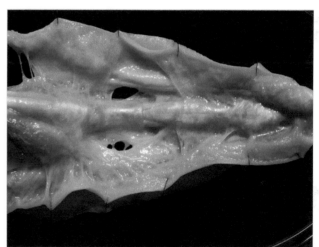

Fig. 2.23 Grayson's and Cleland's ligaments.

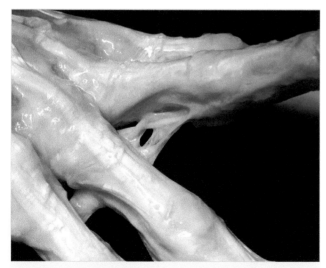

Fig. 2.22 The natatory ligaments.

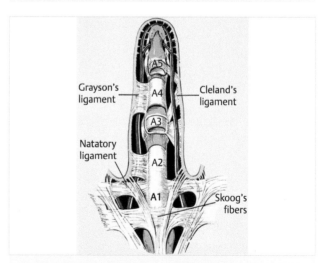

Fig. 2.24 Natatory, Grayson's, and Cleland's ligaments. (Copyright Kleinert Institute, Louisville, KY.)

The flexor tendon pulley system[13] also acts as *containment* structure and is discussed in detail in Chapter 28.

Dorsally, around the extensor tendons, there are infratendinous and supratendinous fascia that form a sharp falx between each of the metacarpal heads proximal to the interdigital webs.

The very special glabrous skin of the palm provides *protection* and *padding* and is stabilized by deep fibrous connections of the palmar fascia especially in the mid palmar area. Fibrous septae contain the special fat in the thenar and hypothenar areas, over the metacarpophalangeal joints and over each phalanx.[3] This structural arrangement allows the hand to apply considerable grip forces to the object without the direct contact of the skeletal structures and the object. The palmaris brevis, palmaris longus, flexor carpi ulnaris, and abductor pollicis brevis inserting onto the skin also assist in this function.

The dorsal retinaculum and transverse carpal ligament in the wrist region, and the palmar pulleys in the digits allow *connection, nourishment, tendon guidance,* and *restraint* while at the same time providing mechanical advantage and a fulcrum to change direction.

In the wrist area, the dorsal retinaculum is a thick fibrous layer divided into compartments (▶Fig. 2.25) that contain the dorsal tendons, termination of the posterior interosseous nerve, and vascular bundles either inside the compartments or on its surface (intercompartmental supraretinacular vessels). From anatomy books that are based on diagrams, one gets the impression that the dorsal retinaculum is a flat and two-dimensional structure. On the contrary, careful and detailed dissection has shown that the dorsal retinaculum is a beautiful three-dimensional layered structure (▶Fig. 2.26). The ulnar attachment of the dorsal retinaculum is to the pisiform to which the flexor retinaculum is also attached (▶Fig. 2.27). The dorsal and palmar ligaments thus form a tight "watchband"-like structure around the wrist, with the pisiform being the anchor point (▶Fig. 2.28). The dorsal compartments guide the extensor tendons and keep them restrained.

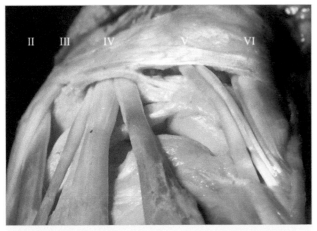

Fig. 2.25 The dorsal retinaculum, showing II, III, IV, V and VI compartment tendons.

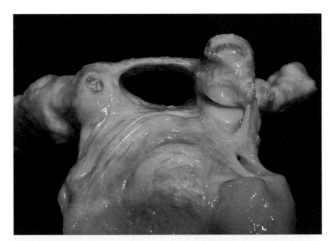

Fig. 2.27 Palmar carpal ligament and the carpal tunnel.

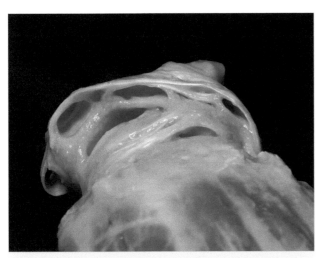

Fig. 2.26 The beautiful 3D layered structure of the dorsal retinaculum.

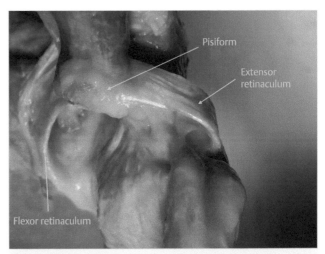

Fig. 2.28 The extensor and flexor retinaculum are both attached to the pisiform.

In the digits, the palmar pulleys perform a similar function for the finger tendons[13] (▶ Fig. 2.29). They guide the digital tendons to their osseous attachment, keep them restrained, provide mechanical advantage for the flexors, and also provide nourishment by virtue of their collagen structure.[14] The dorsal third of the tendons are nourished by direct blood supply through the vincula longum and vincula breve (the long and short vincula) (▶ Fig. 2.30). The palmar part, being mostly avascular, is nourished by diffusion of synovial fluid from the flexor tendon sheath. The collagen fibers of the flexor tendons are longitudinally orientated, while those of the dorsal surface of the annular pulleys are transversely oriented. On movement of the tendons in the pulley system, a latticework of longitudinal and transverse fibers traps and pumps the synovial fluid into the palmar third of the flexor tendons (the synovial pump) (▶ Fig. 2.31).

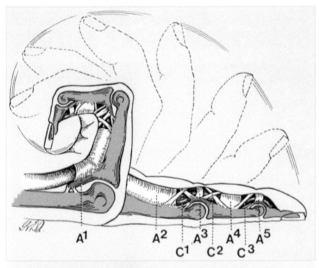

Fig. 2.29 The Palmar pulley system in the digit. (Copyright Kleinert Institute, Louisville, KY.)

2.5 Muscles and Tendons

2.5.1 Extensor Tendons

After passing through the 4th compartment, the four-extensor digitorum communis (EDC) tendons travel toward each digit (▶ Fig. 2.32). The extensor indices (EI) tendon is located deeper and ulnar to the extensor communis to the index finger. The extensor digiti minimi (EDM) tendon travels in a separate (5th) compartment, as does the extensor pollicis longus (EPL) tendon (3rd compartment).[17,18,19]

Proximal to the metacarpal head, strong intertendinous connections (*juncturae tendinum*) originate from the ring finger EDC and join the middle finger EDC and small finger EDC distally (▶ Fig. 2.33). These juncturae limit the independent extension of the ulnar three digits.[20] On flexing the metacarpophalangeal (MP) joint of the middle finger and/or small finger, the ring finger cannot be actively extended, as the individual extensor tendons

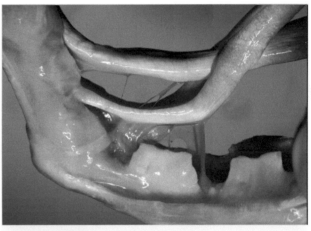

Fig. 2.30 Vincula longum and vincula breve.

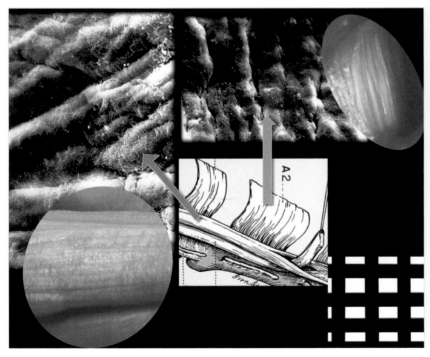

Fig. 2.31 The longitudinal collagen fibers of the flexor tendons and the transverse collagen fibers of the deep surface of the pulleys form a latticework and trap synovial fluid droplets that are then forced onto the palmar surface of the flexor tendons on movement of the digit.

pull the ring finger extensor distally through the juncturae, making it lax and thereby preventing active extension of that digit.

With a completely lacerated EDC to the middle or small finger proximal to the juncturae tendinum, the patient may still be able to actively extend the digit with the help of the juncturae from the ring finger EDC.

Over the MP joints, the EDCs to the middle and ring finger are located in the midline, while in the index finger the EDC is on the radial side and the EI is on the ulnar side. In the small finger, the EDC is on the radial side and the EDM is on the ulnar side.

At the metacarpophalangeal (MP) joint level, a sheet of tissue surrounds each extensor tendon (▶ Fig. 2.34a and ▶ Fig. 2.34b). This sheet of tissue, the sagittal band, passes palmarly to attach to the palmar periosteum of the proximal phalanx and the volar plate of the MP joint. As it goes palmarly, it runs between the deep and the superficial parts of the intrinsic tendons (the deep part inserting to the base of the proximal phalanx and the superficial portion inserting into the dorsal expansion). The

sagittal band or the dorsal hood thus forms a sling that helps lift the base of the proximal phalanx and thereby extends the MP joint. The sagittal band also stabilizes the extensor tendon over the MP joint, keeping the tendon centrally located.[1]

The fibers of the sagittal band lie perpendicular to the long axis of the proximal phalanx. In hyperextension of the MP joint, the band migrates proximally, and in flexion of the MP joint, it translates distally (▶ Fig. 2.35 and ▶ Fig. 2.59).

The extrinsic extensor continues over the proximal phalanx, dividing and reuniting, receiving contributions from the interossei and lumbricals, forming a latticework of transverse and oblique fibers over the proximal phalanx, called the dorsal digital expansion or the interosseous hood. The continuous system of interlaced fascia of the sagittal bands and the dorsal digital expansion is also known as metacarpophalangeal extensor hood.

If the MP joint is hyperextended, the distal extensor is lax and is no longer able to extend the PIP joint. In the absence

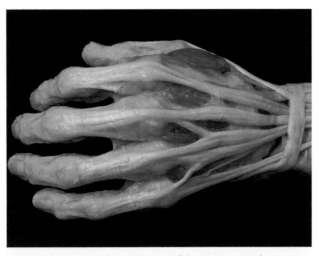

Fig. 2.32 Anatomical arrangement of the extensors in the dorsum of the wrist, hand, and digits.

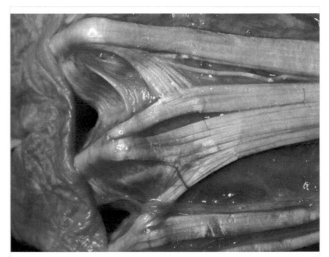

Fig. 2.33 Anatomy of the juncturae tendinum.

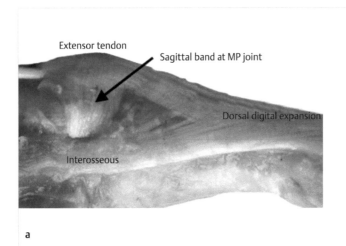

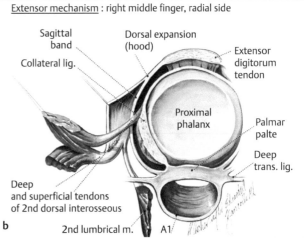

Fig. 2.34 (a) Sagittal band, dorsal digital expansion and interosseous contribution at the MP Joint. (b) Detailed anatomy at the MCP joint with the MC head removed, showing the sagittal band passing between the superficial and deep interossei to insert into the palmar plate of the MP joint. (Copyright Kleinert Institute, Louisville, KY.)

of a PIP joint extender like the interosseous or the lumbrical, and especially if both the flexors (FDS and FDP) are functioning (as happens in low ulnar nerve palsy), the finger assumes a significant claw posture. In these situations, if clinical examination demonstrates that the patient can actively extend the PIP joint on passive flexion of the MP joint (Bouvier positive), the clawing can be mitigated by a procedure that can keep the MP joint in flexion (MP volar capsulodesis or Zancolli lasso procedure).

Distal to the MP joint, the extensor tendon divides into three, one central slip and two lateral bands (▶ Fig. 2.36). The central slip continues distally to insert onto the base of the middle phalanx (▶ Fig. 2.37). The two lateral bands receive contributions from the interossei and on the radial side from the lumbrical (▶ Fig. 2.38). The lateral bands unite to form the terminal extensor tendon inserting onto the base of the distal phalanx at the dorsal lip (▶ Fig. 2.39).[21]

The triangular ligament is bounded proximally by the distal insertion of the central slip, laterally by the lateral bands, and distally by the terminal extensor tendon. The triangular ligament holds the lateral bands in place, restraining them from translating volarly.

Additionally, there are two retinacular ligaments described by Landsmeer[22] that add to the functionality of the extensor mechanism. The oblique retinacular ligament of Landsmeer, arising from the distal third of the proximal phalanx and the A2 pulley, travels distally to join the lateral band (▶ Fig. 2.40). It acts as a dynamic tenodesis helping coordinate the motion

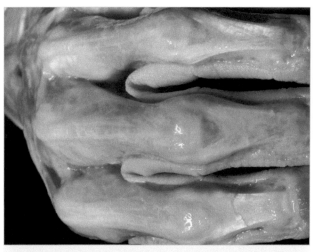

Fig. 2.37 Detailed dissection of the extensor mechanism in the digit.

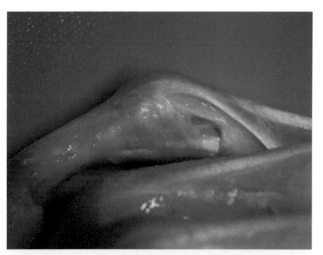

Fig. 2.38 The interosseous contribution to the extensor.

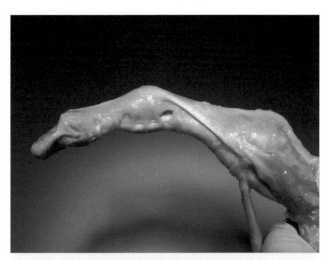

Fig. 2.35 The sagittal band and the interosseous hood.

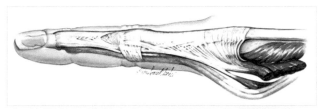

Fig. 2.36 Anatomy of the extensor mechanism in the finger. (Copyright Kleinert Institute, Louisville, KY.)

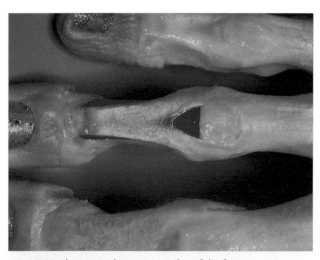

Fig. 2.39 The terminal extensor tendon of the finger.

of the proximal and distal interphalangeal joints. Extension of the proximal interphalangeal joint places the ligament in tension and extends the distal interphalangeal joint. It is possible to fully flex the distal interphalangeal joint actively only when the proximal interphalangeal joint is flexed. The transverse retinacular ligament of Landsmeer originates from the edge of the flexor sheath at the PIP joint and attaches to the lateral extensor band. The transverse retinacular ligament prevents excessive dorsal translation of the lateral bands on PIP extension and pulls the lateral bands over the PIP joint with PIP flexion.

2.5.2 Flexor Tendons

The muscle belly of the flexor digitorum profundus (FDP) originates from the palmar and medial aspect of the proximal part of the ulna and from the ulnar side of the interosseous membrane. The four tendons of the FDP pass under the transverse carpal ligament and enter the palm where, at the level of the metacarpal, the lumbrical muscle originates from the radial side of

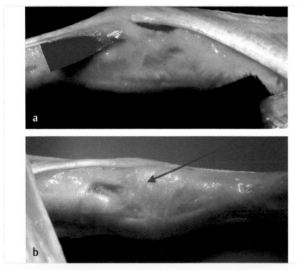

Fig. 2.40 (a) The oblique and (b) transverse retinacular ligaments of Landsmeer.

the tendon. Throughout the FDP's course from the muscle to the palm, there are several intertendinous fibers that tether the tendons to each other.

The muscle belly and tendon of the FDP to the index finger may be completely separate from the rest of the muscle and tendons, allowing it to act independently.

The muscle belly of the flexor digitorum superficialis (FDS) is palmar and superficial to the FDP muscle belly. The FDS muscle arises from the medial epicondyle, the coronoid process, and the volar aspect of the proximal radius. At the distal forearm, four broad and flat tendons arise from the muscle. Approaching the carpal tunnel, the FDS tendons to the middle and ring finger lie more superficial than the FDS tendons to the index and small fingers (▶ Fig. 2.41). Occasionally, the FDS to the small finger may be absent.

The FDS and the FDP enter the fibrous sheath just proximal to the metacarpophalangeal joints (▶ Fig. 2.42). Just after entering the fibrous sheath, at the proximal part of the proximal phalanx, the FDS tendon becomes flatter and splits into two parts (▶ Fig. 2.43) through which the FDP tendon passes (▶ Fig. 2.44). This area of separation of the FDS tendons is known as the *bifurca*. Each flat slip of the FDS encircles the FDP tendon, rotating 180° in the process.[16] The two slips then interdigitate and unite with each other to form *Camper's Chiasma*[23] (▶ Fig. 2.45).

The internal fibrous structure of the FDS from the bifurca to the chiasma is quite complex. At the bifurca, the tendon divides into two, each slip rotating 90° and passing dorsal to the FDP. As it does so, each slip divides into two. The lateral slips continue rotating another 90° and then insert onto the middle phalanx in a broad insertion distal to the palmar plate of the PIP joint. The medial slips interdigitate with each other, forming the *Camper's Chiasma* dorsal to the FDP tendon, after which each of the medial slips joins the contralateral lateral slip to reach its insertion into the base of the middle phalanx (▶ Fig. 2.43 and ▶ Fig. 2.45).[16]

The area of Camper's Chiasma has rich dorsal vascular supply through the vincula brevia (short vincula). The vincula longae (long vincula) may also penetrate through to the FDS tendon in this region (▶ Fig. 2.46).

The tendon of the FDP passes through the area of the Camper's Chiasma and exits the fibrous sheath distal to the

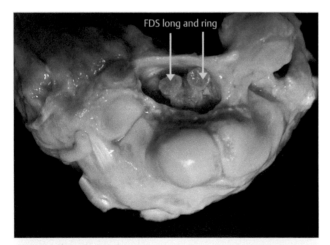

Fig. 2.41 The tendons of the FDS to the long and ring fingers superficial in the carpal tunnel.

FDS long and ring

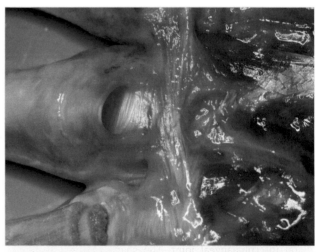

Fig. 2.42 The entrance to the fibrous pulley in the digit at A1.

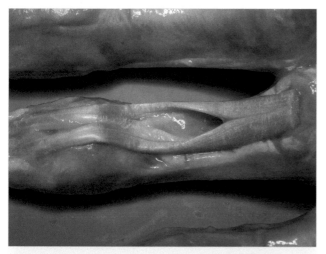

Fig. 2.43 The bifurca and the Camper's Chiasma of the FDS.

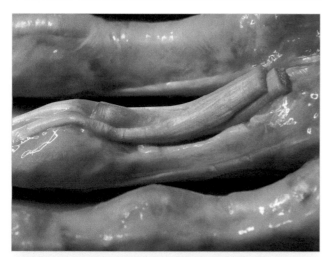

Fig. 2.44 The relationship of the FDS to the FDP at the bifurca and Chiasma.

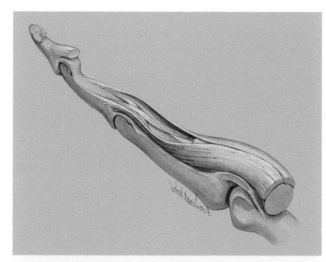

Fig. 2.45 Detailed anatomy of the FDS and the FDP at the bifurca and Chiasma. (Copyright Kleinert Institute, Louisville, KY.)

distal interphalangeal joint. The shape of the FDP tendon changes throughout. At the level where the FDS passes around

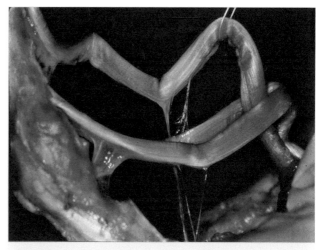

Fig. 2.46 Vincula longae and breve. (Courtesy of Dr Pathmanathan.)

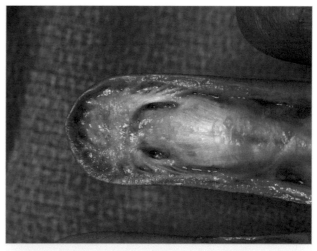

Fig. 2.47 The terminal insertion of the FDP into the distal phalanx.

the FDP, the tendon narrows. On reaching the PIP joint, the tendon widens again. The tendon narrows to pass through the A4 pulley and then fans out on reaching its insertion at the terminal phalanx. There is a groove on the palmar part of the central portion of the FDP tendon. This groove seems to start at a random point on the tendon and deepens as the tendon goes distally. Nearing its insertion, the tendon almost splits into two halves (▶ Fig. 2.47).

There is considerable morphological difference between a loaded and unloaded palmar portion of the FDP tendon. The fiber direction changes from wider treads in the unloaded position to narrower treads in the loaded position. This change in fiber configuration has been compared to treads on modern vehicle tires, helping channel synovial fluid toward the edges[16] (▶ Fig. 2.48).

This arrangement, along with the general collagen arrangement on the palmar aspect of the FDP and the dorsal surface of the annular pulleys, has led to the postulation of a "synovial pump" that helps push synovial fluid into the volar aspect of the tendon, thus nourishing it. Scanning electron microscopy has shown that the collagen arrangement on the palmar aspect of the FDP is longitudinal whereas the collagen arrangement

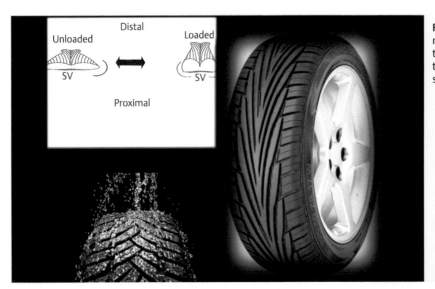

Fig. 2.48 The collagen fibers have different morphology in the unloaded and loaded FDP tendon. The collagen arrangements resemble treads of modern rain tires that channel the synovial fluid toward the edges.

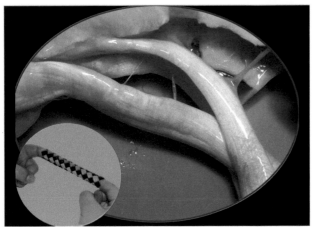

Fig. 2.49 "Chinese finger trap" action of the FDS at the bifurca and Chiasma on the FDP tendon.

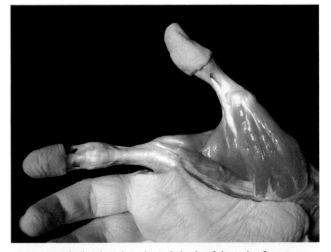

Fig. 2.50 The lumbrical on the radial side of the index finger.

on the deeper surface of the annular pulley is transverse. In the loaded finger, when the two surfaces interact closely, they form a crisscross latticework that traps synovial fluid and forces that fluid onto the palmar surface of the tendon (▶ Fig. 2.31).

For many years, considerable conjecture has been expanded on the relationship between the FDS and the FDP tendons and the role of the bifurcation and coming together of the FDS around the FDP. One of the oldest hypotheses is that the bifurca forms a pulleylike sling to constrain the FDP to the proximal phalanx, thus increasing its efficiency. The other hypothesis is that the bifurca and chiasma form a frictionless tunnel for the FDP. There is an argument based on the fiber arrangement of the chiasma that the FDS at the bifurca and chiasma acts like a "Chinese finger trap" on the FDP tendon. It may add to the FDP pull, or it may play a role in synovial fluid circulation and tendon nutrition[16] (▶ Fig. 2.49).

2.5.3 Interosseous Muscles

The interosseous muscles are part of the intrinsic musculature of the hand or the muscles that originate and insert in the hand territory.

There are seven interossei: four dorsal and three palmar interossei. The dorsal interossei have two parts: palmar and dorsal. The palmar portion of the dorsal interossei and the palmar interossei have similar insertions by aponeurosis into the lateral bands of the extensor tendon on both radial and ulnar side through oblique and transverse fibers. As they are palmar to the MP joints, they flex the MP joints. The interossei can, through their insertion into the lateral bands of the extensor, extend the proximal and distal interphalangeal joints.[1,21]

The dorsal parts of the dorsal interossei insert by tendinous insertion deep to the extensor sagittal band into the base of the proximal phalanx. The second and third dorsal interossei move the middle finger from side to side (▶ Fig. 2.34). The first and third dorsal interossei move the index and ring finger away (abduct) from the central axis of the middle finger.

The interossei are all supplied by the deep motor branch of the ulnar nerve.

2.5.4 Lumbrical Muscles

These special muscles are the only muscles to arise from a tendon and insert into another tendon. The radial two lumbricals originate from the radial side of the FDP tendon whereas the ulnar two lumbricals are bipennate with origin from contiguous sides of the FDPs to the middle, ring and small fingers (▶ Fig. 2.50). They course palmar to the deep transverse metacarpal ligaments

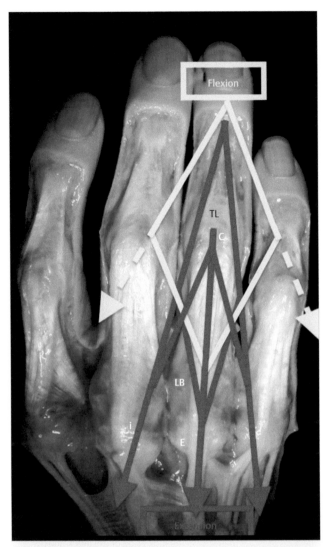

Fig. 2.51 The rhombus of Winslow.

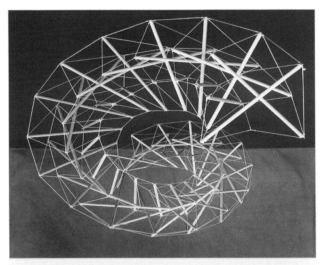

Fig. 2.52 A tensegrity structure. (Used with permission from Marcelo Pars at www.tensegriteit.nl.)

The Rhombus of Winslow

In 1732 Danish born French anatomist Jacob Benignus (name later changed to Jacques-Benigne Winslow) Winslow (1669–1760) proposed a general topological approximation of the extensor mechanism and the intrinsic attachments. This model has been popularized by Dr. Eduardo Zancolli[11] and has also been studied by computer models.[24] Garcia-Elias[21] confirmed that the geometry changes in the extensor mechanism are due not to changes in length of its different bundles but rather to changes in their orientation. The study also supported the view of Van Zwieten,[25] who compared the intercrossing fibers to a Chinese finger trap, where crisscrossing stiff fibers form a system which, if pulled longitudinally, becomes longer and at the same time narrower. The system changes from a wide to a narrow perspective depending on the position of the digit and the forces acting on the system (▶ Fig. 2.51).

Tensegrity

Buckminster Fuller introduced the theory of tensegrity or the concept of tension providing structural integrity (▶ Fig. 2.52). Various systems of the body are examples of tension's providing structural integrity.[26] The extensor mechanism as related to the digit could be a good model of a tensegrity system, as the system is stabilized by soft tissue forces in tension.

2.6 Movements of the Hand

The hand is a versatile structure, able to adapt to a wide variety of objects, gathering information from those objects and imparting forces to them. To exert the optimal forces to the objects and to present the most sensitive parts of the fingers to the objects, the movements of the hand follow a very definite and intricate geometrical pattern in grasp and release–the equiangular spiral (▶ Fig. 2.53).

William J. Littler (▶ Fig. 2.54) in his "On the adaptability of man's hand," posed a fundamental question: "Does the motion path of the digit in flexion and extension follow a specific

on the radial side of the MP joints, and insert into the radial lateral band of the extensor tendon (▶ Fig. 2.34).

The lumbricals have very little effect on the flexion of the MP joint. They help extend the interphalangeal joints with the MP joint in flexion. They are also a controlling mechanism between the extensor and flexor system.

The radial two lumbricals are supplied by the median nerve through the common digital sensory nerves. The ulnar two lumbricals are supplied by the deep motor branch of the ulnar nerve.

2.5.5 The Intrinsic Muscles of the Thumb

The intrinsic muscles of the thumb are grouped into a lateral group: the abductor pollicis brevis, the opponens pollicis, and the flexor pollicis brevis. The medial group consists of the adductor pollicis.

2.5.6 Hypothenar muscles

The hypothenar muscles consist of the flexor digiti minimi and the abductor digiti minimi, both supplied by the ulnar nerve.

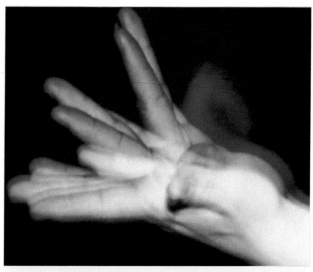

Fig. 2.53 The motion path of digits follows an equiangular spiral.

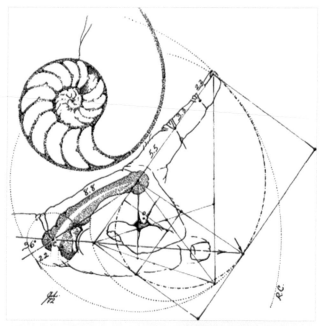

Fig. 2.55 The motion segments of the digits are arranged according to the Fibonacci sequence; the motion path of the digits follows the equiangular spiral. Reproduced with Permission from Littler, J.W. On the adaptability of man's hand (with reference to the equiangular curve). Hand 1973;5:187–191. Littler's original drawing showing the length relationships in the digit.

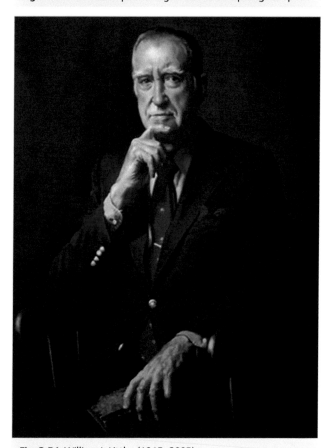

Fig. 2.54 William J. Littler (1915–2005).

numbers is that the third number in the sequence is the sum of the preceding two numbers ($F_n = F_{n-1} + F_{n-2}$). The other important characteristic is that the higher of the two consecutive numbers divided by the lower number is a constant, 1.618039, or the *Golden Mean*.

Although Fibonacci is generally given credit in the Western literature for these number sequences, there is considerable evidence that these number sequences were well known and studied in India long before Fibonacci by Pingala (450 BC), Virhanka (6th century AD), Gopala (1135), and Hemchandra (1150).[30]

The equiangular spiral is a pattern often repeated in nature (▶Fig. 2.56) and is seen in the petal arrangement of flowers, seed arrangements (as in the sunflower), spiderwebs, whirlpools, galaxies, and hurricanes. It is a pattern that optimizes space and force in nature. It is used in the hand to optimize grip force in a constrained space. It gives the hand its adaptability and also presents the most sensate parts of the hand to the object being manipulated (▶Fig. 2.57). This pattern in the human hand remains constant throughout life, as the bones increase in length proportionately with growth (▶Fig. 2.58).

The movements of the fingers depend on the dynamic balance of the extrinsic and intrinsic muscles and tendons as well as the viscoelastic forces that are the conglomerate of forces that resist the lengthening of a muscle tendon unit. Muscle cells, perimysium, fascia, tendon sheath, ligaments, and joint inertia all contribute to the viscoelastic forces.

The flexor digitorum profundus (FDP) and the "Chinese finger trap" action of the flexor digitorum superficialis (FDS) acting on the FDP, and also its independent contraction, initiate flexion of the proximal interphalangeal (PIP) joint. This activity, combined with relaxation of the viscoelastic force of the extensor tendon, helps in flexion of the

mathematical pattern?" (▶Fig. 2.55). He suggested that the bones of the finger and hand are arranged according to the Fibonacci sequence and thus are able to outline the equiangular spiral in grasp and release.[27] We conducted experiments in our lab and mathematically answered Dr. Littler's question.[28] The motion path of the digits in flexion and extension follows the equiangular spiral.[29]

The Fibonacci sequence is a series of numbers described by Leonardo Di Pisa, or Fibonacci, in his book *Liber Abaci*, published in 1202. One of the characteristics of the Fibonacci sequence of

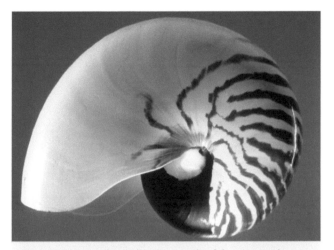

Fig. 2.56 The nautilus shell is an example of the equiangular spiral.

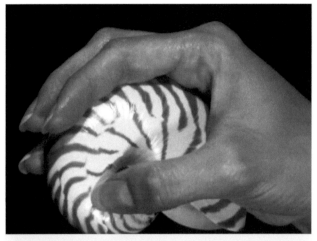

Fig. 2.57 The hand has the ability to adapt and present the most sensate part to the object.

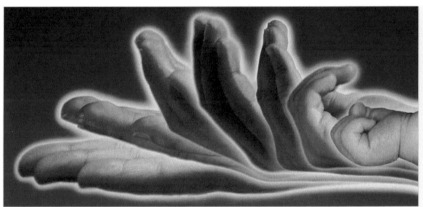

Fig. 2.58 The pattern of grasp and release following the equiangular spiral remains constant throughout life. The anatomical structures increase in size proportionally with growth, maintaining the Fibonacci relationship of the motion segments and the equiangular spiral motion in grasp and release. (The cover photograph of The Growing Hand: Diagnosis and Management of the Upper Extremity in Children. Gupta A, Kay SPJ, Scheker L (Eds)Mosby; 2000.)

metacarpophalangeal (MP) joint. On the distal interphalangeal (DIP) joint, the oblique retinacular ligament provides a viscoelastic extension force that is relaxed as the PIP joint flexes, and thus the DIP also flexes concurrently with the PIP joint (▶Fig. 2.59 a–n).

Extension starts at the MP joint by the action of the sagittal band on the base of the proximal phalanx. Hyperextension of the MP joint is prevented by the recruitment of the interossei through their insertion into the extensor hood. When the central slip of the extensor tightens, largely by the action of the intrinsic insertion into lateral band and the contribution that the central slip receives from the lateral band, it results in the extension of the PIP joint.

The motion of the PIP and DIP joints are interlinked by the oblique retinacular ligament (ORL) of Landsmeer that passes volar to the axis of the PIP joint. Extension of the PIP joint produces a concomitant extension of the DIP joint by viscoelastic force of the ORL. Once mechanical advantage is gained, active extension of the PIP and DIP joints are possible through the combined action of the extensor tendon and the intrinsics.

We conducted motion analysis with dynamic electromyography[31] (▶Fig. 2.60). Summary of our studies show the following: (1) The extensor digitorum and extensor indices are pure extensors of the fingers; (2) the FDP is the pure digital flexor; (3) the FDS acts in a biphasic manner and is recruited in power grip; (4) the intrinsics act in a biphasic manner and provide controlling torque to MP and IP joints; (5) the

lumbricals are very special. In the past they were regarded as major MP joint flexors. However, we found that the lumbricals are silent during finger flexion phase and do not contribute to MP flexion. They act as accessory digital extensors. Acting with the contracting digital extensor, the lumbrical pulls the FDP distally, relaxes the FDP, thus removing the viscoelastic constraint to extension of the digit. They are essentially controlling muscles. High concentration of sensory receptors have been found in the lumbricals supporting this "control" role.

Opposition

Opposition is a very special motion and is controlled by muscles that are supplied by all major nerves in the forearm and hand. The movement starts with extension/abduction to get the thumb away from the plane of the hand. The motion is controlled by abductor pollicis longus (APL), extensor pollicis brevis (EPB), and extensor pollicis longus (EPL). These extrinsic muscles are supplied by the posterior interosseous nerve from the radial nerve. The next motion is palmar abduction and pronation controlled by the abductor pollicis brevis (APB) and opponens pollicis (OP), supplied by the recurrent branch of the median nerve. Following this, are flexion and adduction, controlled by the flexor pollicis brevis (FPB), supplied by the median and the ulnar nerves and adductor pollicis (AP), supplied by the ulnar nerve. Finally, force is exerted through

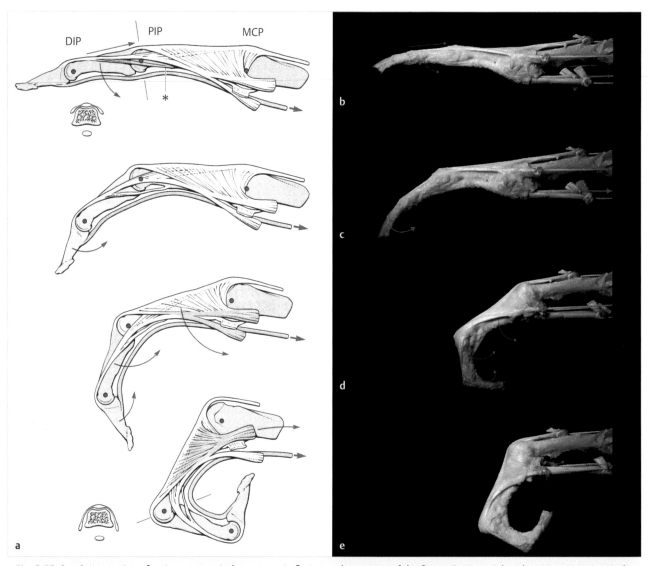

Fig. 2.59 (**a–e**) Interaction of various anatomical structures in flexion and extension of the finger. (a: From Schmidt H-M, Lanz U. Surgical Anatomy of the Hand. Thieme, Stuttgart; 2004.)

(Continued)

the flexor pollicis longus (FPL), innervated by the anterior interosseous nerve, a branch of the median nerve.[3]

Sequence of flexion of the digit. Flexion is initiated by the FDP and starts at the PIP joint. Viscoelastic tightness of the oblique retinacular ligament simultaneously flexes the DIP joint. Flexion of the PIP joint also initiates and increases the flexion of the MP joint by putting tension on the lumbrical and intrinsic tendons and by a distal shift of the extensor hood.

The radial nerve lifts the thumb out of the plane of the palm in preparation for opposition (retropulsion), the median nerve controls the attitude of opposition, and the ulnar nerve adds power to opposition.

2.7 Sensation and Proprioception

Glabrous skin has four types of mechanoreceptors: Meissener's corpuscles, located in the dermal papillae; Merkel's disks, at the papillae or ridges; Ruffini corpuscles, located in the deeper reticular layers of the dermis; and Pacinian corpuscles, in the subcutaneus tissue (▶Fig. 2.61). The Meissener's (FA I) and

Pacinian (along with Golgi bodies) (FA II) are fast-acting (FA), whereas the Merkel (SA I) and Ruffini (SA II) are slow-acting (SA) receptors.[5]

These mechanoreceptors have been extensively studied using microneurography, where recordings were made after inserting tungsten microelectrodes into the median nerve. The studies of Roland Johansson, Ake Vallbo, and Johan Wessberg are summarized.[32,33]

The fast-adapting (FA I & II) fibers demonstrate fast action with no static response. The FA I (Meissner's corpuscles) and the SA I (Merkel disks) are edge-sensitive; have small, well defined cutaneous fields; and have high innervation densities, especially at the fingertips. There is less innervation density of these fibers in the palm of the hand. The FA II (Pacinian corpuscles and Golgi-Mazzoni bodies) and the SA II (Ruffini endings) have large, obscure borders of their receptive fields and are distributed in the palm. They innervate deeper receptors. The FA receptors respond to changes in skin deformation, whereas the SA receptors show a static response that is dependent on the strength of the maintained skin deformation (▶Fig. 2.62).

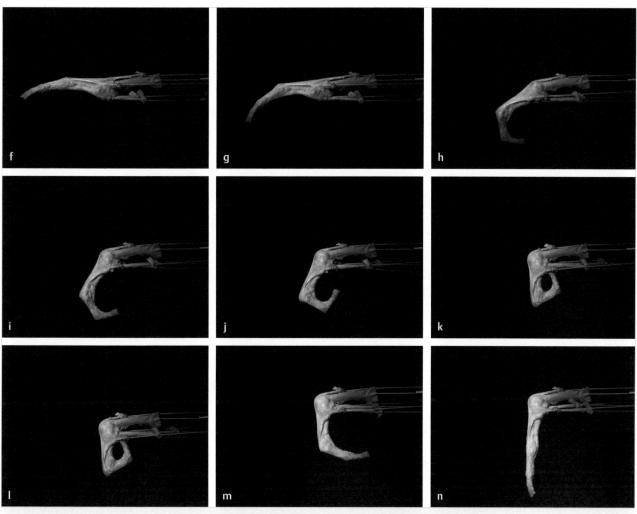

Fig. 2.59 (*Continued*) (**f–n**) Interaction of various anatomical structures in flexion and extension of the finger.

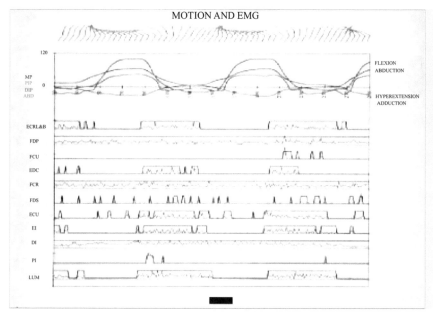

Fig. 2.60 Results of motion analysis in grasp and release with concurrent EMGs: (1) Extensor digitorum and extensor indices are pure extensors of the fingers; (2) FDP is the pure digital flexor; (3) FDS acts in a biphasic manner and is recruited in power grip; (4) the intrinsics act in biphasic manner and provide controlling torque to MP and IP joints; (5) the lumbricals act as accessory digital extensors.

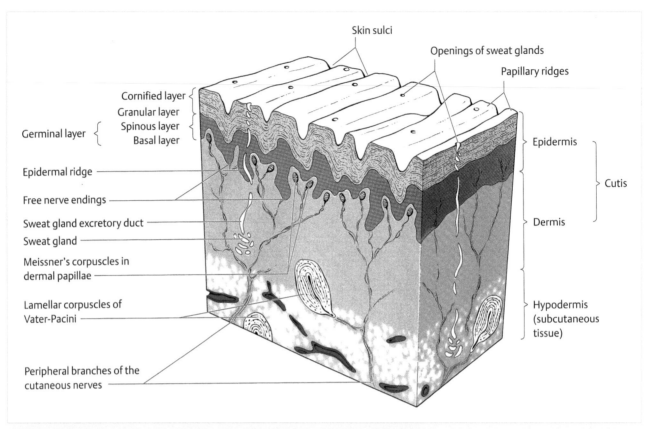

Fig. 2.61 The mechanoreceptors of the glabrous skin. (From Schmidt H-M, Lanz U: Surgical Anatomy of the Hand. Thieme. Stuttgart 2004.)

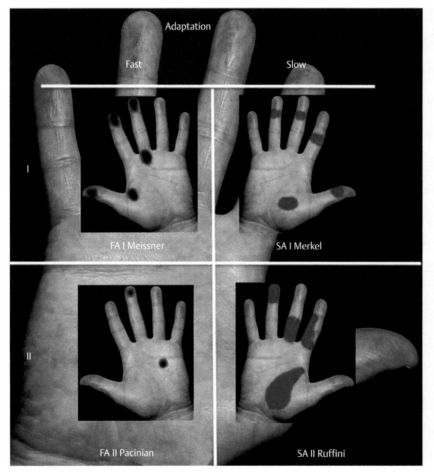

Fig. 2.62 The distribution of different mechanoreceptors in the palm and fingers.

Proprioception

Sir Charles Sherrington coined the term *proprioception* for the collective position sense stemming from sensors in the muscles, joint, and tendons. It is defined as the sense of the relative position of neighboring parts of the body and the strength of the effort being employed in movement.

Touch

Sir Charles Bell[2] in his *Bridgewater Treatise on the Hand,* wrote in 1833, "Attention to our most common actions will show us, how the division into fingers, by combining motion with sense of touch adapts the hand to grasp, to feel and to compare."

One of the fundamental functions of the hand and especially the fingertips is to sense and gather information from the object it is grasping. Sensation and proprioception are also important in holding and manipulating objects. It is therefore not surprising that the fingertips have been compared to the somesthetic macula of the eye. It is estimated that there are 17,000 cutaneous mechanoreceptors in each hand.

According to Goran Lundborg,[33] the hand is a sensory organ as important as the eye or the ear. The sense of touch is essential for hand function, as the hand can explore and obtain information from the environment and objects.

The tactile property of the hand is the ability to perceive touch (passive tactile perception or *passive touch*).

More important is the function of the hand that combines motor and sensory abilities to feel the object and move the hand around the object (active tactile perception or *active touch* or *haptics*).

Active Touch or Haptics

"Grasp to feel; feel to grasp."

The sensory and motor functions of the hand are interlinked and combine in exploring the object it is grasping, constantly gathering information from the object as it imparts forces to the object. This ability, where the hand is moving to grasp, feeling to grasp, grasping to feel, and grasping to move objects, is called active touch or human haptics.[34]

Lederman and Klatsky[36] outlined a set of procedures that they called exploratory procedures (EP) whereby the hand obtains information about the physical characteristics of the object. Lateral motion (▶Fig. 2.63) extracts information about texture; *pressure* (▶Fig. 2.64) determines the hardness of the object; *static contact* gives information about temperature; enclosing the object (▶Fig. 2.65) shows the volume and global shape; *unsupported holding* reveals approximation of weight and finally, *contour following* reveals fine spatial details about the object (▶Fig. 2.66).

Dr. Mandayam Srinivasan and his colleagues have done tremendous work at the Touch Lab at Massachusetts Institute of Technology, Cambridge, MA, on the sensory, kinesthetic, and motor aspects of human touch (Srinivasan M. Personal communication) (▶Table 2.1, 2.2 and 2.3). Their findings are summarized:

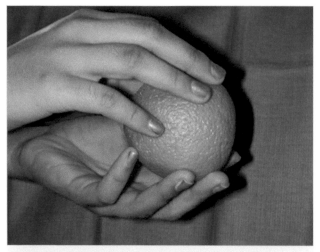

Fig. 2.63 Lateral motion reveals the texture of the object.

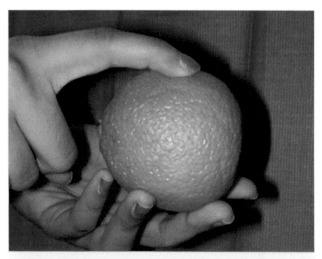

Fig. 2.64 Pressure determines the hardness of the object.

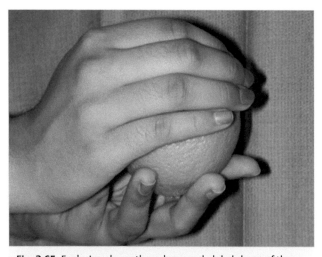

Fig. 2.65 Enclosing shows the volume and global shape of the object.

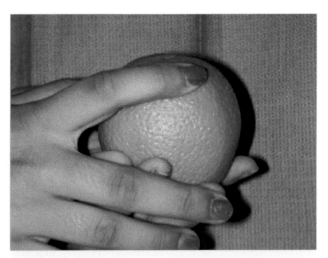

Fig. 2.66 Contour following reveals the spatial details of the object.

Table 2.1 Tactile Sensory System

(Data mainly for the fingertip)	
Absolute detection threshold	20 µm @ static
	10 µm @ 10 Hz
	0.1 µm @ 250 Hz
Pressure threshold	0.3 mN/mm²
Feature detection	0.1 µm for texture
	2 µm for single dot
Temporal resolution	10 ms between two taps
Frequency range	1 kHz
Frequency resolution	10% to 80%
Spatial resolution Localization 2-point limen	0.15 mm 1 mm

(*Limen:* the point at which a stimulus is strong enough to produce a physiological response.)

Table 2.2 Kinesthetic Sensory System

Position resolution	1°–2° at joints
	0.5 mm at fingertip
Position reproduction	5°–10°
Bandwidth	–20 to 30 Hz
Motor System	
Motion:	
Range of motion Velocity	20°–100°
	0.1 m/s at fingertip
	1 m/s at wrist
Bandwidth unexpected signals	1–2 Hz
periodic signals	2–5 Hz
reflex action	10 Hz
Forces:	
Single finger Typical range Controllable range Control resolution Grasp force range	1–10 N up to 100 N 0.05–0.5 N 50–100 N

Table 2.3 Active touch, including tactile, kinesthetic, and motor systems

Resolution	
Length	10% or less
Velocity	10%
Acceleration	20%
Force	7%
Compliance	
Rigid surface (e.g., piano key)	8%
Deformable surface (e.g., rubber)	3%
Viscosity	14%
Mass	21%
Rigidity perception	25 N/mm or greater

2.8 Control of Digital Motion

Control is defined biomechanically as the mastery of redundancies of motion.

Control of digital motion is complex. The hand muscles have strong influence from glabrous skin and the very strong direct cortical motor neural connections define their prominent role in the control of hand muscles. Additionally, there are sensorimotor and proprioceptive controls that function in tandem to control digital motion. The important factors that affect digital motion control are the following:[5,34,37,38]

1. Sensorimotor systems
   a. Muscle and tendon systems
   b. Proprioception (including skin, muscle spindles, and tendon
   c. Spinal reflexes
   d. Corticospinal pathways
   e. Thalamic relays
   f. Cerebellum
   g. Basal ganglia
   h. Brainstem motor control
   i. Posterior parietal cortex
   j. Corticomotor neural connections
   k. Premotor cortex
   l. Motor cortex
   m. Somatosensory cortex
2. Other sensory inputs: visual, auditory, olfactory, somatosensory, and vestibular.
3. Limbic structures, emotion, bimanual coordination, learning, and memory.
4. Cognition, creativity and motivation
5. Social interactions, language, art and music, religion and spirituality.

2.9 Grasp

As we have seen, the human hand is made up of a conglomerate of bones, muscles, tendons, fascia, ligaments, nerves and blood vessels enclosed by loose dorsal skin, and a very special palmar glabrous skin. This complex structure also represents several million years of evolution. The use of tools and the grasping abilities of the hand have shaped human destiny.

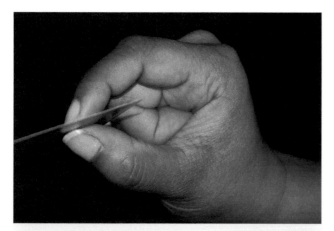

Fig. 2.67 Precision pinch.

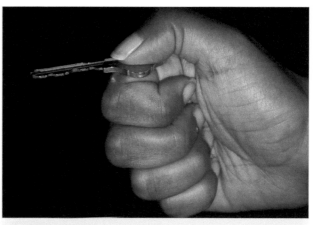

Fig. 2.69 Key pinch.

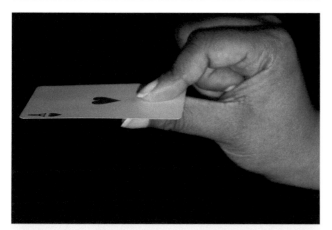

Fig. 2.68 Opposition pinch.

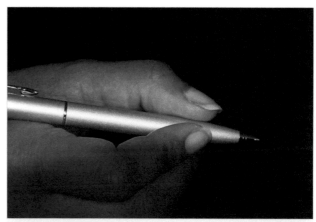

Fig. 2.70 Precision handling.

The human hand itself is a very uniquely unspecialized structure in that it is supremely adaptable to the object and the task in front of it. The ability to grasp and manipulate objects is fundamental to the progress of the human race.

Prehension is the application of functionally effective forces by the hand to an object for a task, given numerous constraints.[5] The prehensile grasping hand has power grip as well as the ability for precision handling. Prehension depends largely on the posture that the hand adapts: cylindrical grip, tip pinch, hook grip, palmar pinch, spherical grip or lateral pinch, and many others.

The prehensile posture of the hand depends on the object and the task to be performed. To achieve the task, the hand must apply forces to the object to match the anticipated forces and impart motion as necessary (manipulate) or transport the object while gathering sensory and spatial information about the object so that forces can be modulated to ensure grasping and manipulative stability.

There are seven types of "grip" that make up the grasp of the human hand:[3,4,39]

1. **Precision pinch** (▶ Fig. 2.67): Terminal or tip to tip pinch. The DIP joint of the index finger and the IP joint of the thumb are flexed at the tips and brought together to pinch an object between them. The function of the FDP to the index and FPL must be intact for this pinch. The tip of the thumb and index must also be sensate and have a good distal phalanx and nail for this pinch to work. This type of grip is essential for picking up small objects.

2. **Opposition pinch** (▶ Fig. 2.68): This pinch brings the pulp of the thumb and the index finger together, with the IP joint of the thumb and the DIP joint of the index finger coming together in forceful extension. In this type of pinch, it is important for good activity of the first dorsal interosseous as well as the FDP of the index and the thenar musculature.

3. **Key pinch** (▶ Fig. 2.69): This pinch is like holding a key between the thumb and the middle phalanx of the index finger. The tip of the thumb exerts pressure on it, and the object is held between them. The muscles acting in this pinch are the FDS of the index, the first dorsal interosseous, and the adductor pollicis. The first dorsal interosseous resists the force of the adducting thumb.

4. **Precision handling** (▶ Fig. 2.70): This is also called the three-point chuck. In this precision mode, the object is manipulated by the thumb, index, and middle finger tips.

5. **Hook grip** (▶ Fig. 2.71): This grip is involved when picking up an object with the four fingers, which are flexed at the IP, joins around the object, with the MP joints in extension.

6. **Power grasp** (▶ Fig. 2.72): The fingers and the thumb are flexed around the object with the wrist in extension exerting power, as if gripping a bat or a racket.

7. **Span grasp** (▶ Fig. 2.73): This grasp is used when gripping a ball in which the MP and the IP joints of the fingers are flexed while holding the object and the thumb is stabilizing the object on the opposite side.

47

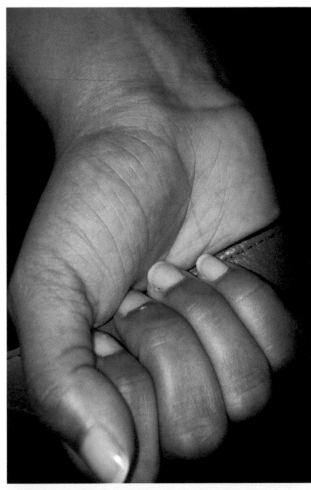

Fig. 2.71 Hook grip.

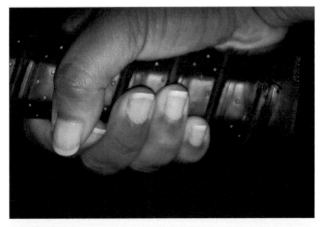

Fig. 2.72 Power grasp.

Prehension involves a number of phases: precontact, contact, and release.[5]

Precontact

To perform a grasping task, a series of preparatory steps and planning occur in the central nervous system prior to execution of the motion.

The grasping hand must first be transported to the object by the arm (*transport component*), followed by the actual grasping

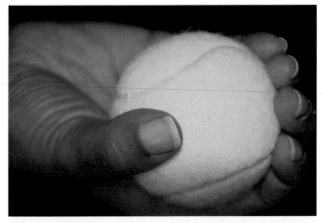

Fig. 2.73 Span grasp.

by the hand (*manipulation or grasp component*). These acts are temporally linked for a coordinated prehensile motion. The transport component is a fast or high-velocity ("ballistic") phase, while the grasping phase is a low-velocity ("adjustment") phase.

Visual input helps in the recognition of object location, recognition, and orientation, allowing a ballistic transport component that takes the hand to the object, to be followed by the actual grasping. All these activities are occurring simultaneously while the hand is also adopting the posture for grasp.

There are planning processes to be executed for a successful grasp and completion of tasks. The planning process prior to object contact involves three aspects:
• perceiving task-specific object properties
• selecting a grasp strategy, and
• planning a hand location and orientation.

Visual information about the object's properties like size, weight, and shape, helps in choosing an opposition space for the hand. Moreover, prior experience and memory tell us how the objects that we see will behave. So vision and memory or experience helps in precontact postural planning of the grasping hand.

The length, radius of curvature and spatial density of the opposable surfaces of the object; the anticipated forces, such as weight, inertial forces, and torques; the opposition vector's magnitude and orientation; and the degrees of freedom determined by the direction of movement, range of movement, and resolution of movement all define the approach vector and precontact posture of the grasping hand.

Contact

During contact, the grasping hand comes into contact with the object and gathers information about the object and the task to be performed through the sensory system, described earlier in the chapter.

Active touch is involved in this process, and exploratory motions of the grasping hand include wielding, jiggling, holding, lateral motion, pressure, contact, enclosing, and contour following. During the contact phase of grasp, active touch or haptics is more important than visual clues. The grasping hand is able to gather information about the grasped object that includes the following: roughness, hardness, temperature, weight, size, shape, moment of inertia, and mass distribution in the object.

The glabrous skin is very important in this phase as it forms our contact with the object. Montagna and Parakkal stated, "the largest sense organ of the body, interposed between the organism, and its environment, the skin must maintain that organism in a constant state of awareness of all environmental changes."[40] Elden[41] described the skin as an organ of functional contact, manipulation, and adaptation with objects in the environment.

The glabrous skin's papillary ridges are externally protruding projections or folds of the stratum corneum that provide resistance to shearing forces. Their function is similar to that of automobile tires in increasing grip on the contact surface. On the finger pads and the palm, the skin has properties that are important for force generation and friction.

The eccrine glands of the glabrous skin are important in thermoregulation of the body, especially on mental and sensory stimulation. They also provide, through micro-sweating, a thin lubrication film of molecular proportion that is important for boundary lubrication between the hand and the object during grasp, reducing friction between the surfaces. Just the right amount of sweat through the autonomically innervated seat glands results in good grip through boundary lubrication. If there is too little sweat, as happens in denervation situations, the skin will be dry and there will be slipping between the hand and the object. Alternatively, if there is too much sweating, as happens in emotional stimulation, again there will be slip due to too much lubrication.

The mechanoreceptors show varied activity during the different phases of grasp. At the start of contact, the FAI (Meissener's) are very active and are especially affected by friction; the FAII (Pacinian) have weaker response. During holding phase, the SAII (Ruffini)) show strong activity, especially to shearing forces. During slippage, there is strong activity in FAI (Meissner's), FAII (Pacinian) and SAI (Merkel) but no response in SAII (Ruffini). During release phase, there are distinct bursts of activity in the FAI, FAII, and SAI receptors, with no response from SAII.

The other proprioceptive receptors, like the muscle spindles and the Golgi tendon organs, are active during various phases of grasp, controlling different aspects of the grasping and release process.

The extrinsic and the intrinsic muscles are active in different phases, as has already been discussed. The lumbrical muscles play a special role in control of grasp, as they constantly help in the adjustment of the tension of the extensor digitorum and the FDP. The extensor mechanism, arranged in a rhombus of Winslow fashion, lengthens and contracts with grasp and release. The joints of the fingers are affected by the muscular activity and respond by motion and torque production.

Release

In the release phase, the hand relaxes into the position of rest, or the position of the function in which the muscles and tendons are at equilibrium.

2.10 Conclusion

The hand is an extension of the brain. The conglomerate of bones, joints, muscles, tendons, ligaments, fascia, nerves, and blood vessels are arranged in a structural order that helps the hand act as a functional unit. A detailed study of the structural and functional anatomy of the hand is essential to understand the pathological conditions and deformities and the surgical principles and techniques in correcting them. A thorough appreciation of the functional anatomy of the hand is important to understand the function of the hand and to design devices with which to measure hand function.[42]

References

1. Smith JR. Balance and kinetics of the fingers under normal and pathological conditions. Clin Orthop Relat Res 1974; 104:98–111
2. Bell, C. The Hand: Its Mechanism and Vital Endowments as Evincing Design. London, England: William Pickering; 1833
3. Belliappa PP. Scheker L: Functional anatomy of the hand. Emerg Med Clin North Am 1993;11(3):557–583
4. Napier J. The prehensile movements of the human hand. J Bone Jt Surg–Br Vol 1956;38B(4):902–913
5. MacKenzie CL, Iberall T. The Grasping Hand, 1st ed. Amsterdam: North-Holland, 1994. (Advances in Psychology; Vol. 104)
6. Kaplan, EB: Functional and Surgical Anatomy of the Hand. 2nd ed. Philadelphia, PA: J. B. Lippincott Co; 1965
7. Hentz VR. Functional anatomy of the hand and arm. Emerg Med Clin North Am 1985;3(2):197–220
8. Littler JW. The physiology and dynamic function of the Hand. Surg Clin North A 1960 Apr,40:259–266
9. Chase RA. Atlas of Hand Surgery. Philadelphia, PA: W.B. Saunders Co; 1973
10. Littler JW. Symposium on Reconstructive Hand Surgery Vol. 9. St. Louis, MO: C.V. Mosby; 1974
11. Zancolli E. Structural and Dynamic Basis of Hand Surgery Philadelphia, Lippincott, Williams and Wilkins, 1979
12. Bojsen-Moller F, Schmidt L. The palmar aponeurosis and the central spaces of the hand. J Anat 1974;117(Pt 1):55–68
13. Doyle JR. Anatomy of the flexor tendon sheath and pulley system: a current review. J Hand Surg Am 1989;14:349–351
14. Bogumill GP. Functional anatomy of the flexor tendon system of the hand. Hand Surg 2002;7(1):33–46
15. Amis AA, Jones M. The interior of the flexor tendon sheath of the finger. JBJS(B) 1988;70-B:583–587
16. Walbeehm ET, McGrouther DA. An anatomical study of the mechanical interactions of flexor digitorum superficialis and profundus and the flexor tendon sheath in zone 2. J Hand Surg Am 1995;20(3):269–280
17. Taleisnik J, Gelberman RH, Miller BW, Szabo RM. The extensor retinaculum of the wrist. J Hand Surg Am 1984;9(4):495–501
18. von Schroeder HP, Botte MJ. Anatomy and functional significance of the long extensors to the fingers and thumb. Clin Orthop Relat Res 2001;(383):74–83
19. Iwamoto A, Morris RP, Andersen C, Patterson RM, Viegas SF. An anatomic and biomechanic study of the wrist extensor retinaculum septa and tendon compartments. J Hand Surg Am 2006;31(6):896–903
20. Wehbe, M. Junctura anatomy. J Hand Surg Am 1992; 17(6):1124–1129
21. Garcia-Elias M, An K-N, Berglund L, Linscheid RL, Cooney WP, Chao EYS. Extensor mechanism of the fingers. I. A quantitative geometric study. J Hand Surg Am 1991;16(6):1130–1136
22. Landsmeer JMF. The anatomy of the dorsal aponeurosis of the finger and its functional significance. Anat Ret 1949; 104:31–44
23. Ijpma FFA, Van De Graaf RC, Van Gulik TM. Petrus Camper's work on the anatomy and pathology of the arm and hand in the 18th century. J Hand Surg Am 2010;35(8):1382–1387

24. Saxena A, Lipson H, Valero-Cuevas FJ. Functional inference of complex anatomical tendinous networks at a macroscopic scale via sparse experimentation. PLoS Comput Biol 2012;8(11):20–27

25. Van Zwieten KJ. The extensor assembly of the fingers in man and non-human primates: a morphological, functional and comparative anatomical study, PhD Thesis, University of Leiden, 1980, J. J. Groen en Zoon, Leiden

26. Levin SM. Putting the shoulder to the wheel: a new biomechanical model for the shoulder girdle. Biomed Sci Instrum 1997;33:412–417

27. Littler JW. On the adaptability of man's hand (with reference to the equiangular curve). Hand 1973;5:187–191

28. Rash GS, Belliappa PP, Wachowiak MP, Somia NN, Gupta A. A demonstration of the validity of a 3-D video motion analysis method for measuring finger flexion and extension. J Biomech 1999;32(12)

29. Gupta A, Rash GS, Somia NN, Wachowiak MP, Jones J, Desoky A. The motion path of the digits. J Hand Surg Am 1998;23(6):1038–1042

30. Singh P. The so-called Fibonacci numbers in ancient and medieval India. Historia Mathematica 1985;12: 229–244

31. Somia N, Rash G, Wacowaik M, Gupta A. The initiation and sequence of digital joint motion: a three-dimensional motion analysis. J Hand Surg J Br Soc Surg Hand 1998;23(6):792–795

32. Johansson RS, Vallbo AB. Tactile sensory coding in the glabrous skin of the human hand. Trends in Neuroscience 1983;6(1): 27–32

33. Valbo AB, Wessberg J. Proprioceptive mechanisms and the control of finger movements. In: Wing AM, Haggard P, Flanagan (Eds.), Hand and Brain. The Neurophysiology and Psychology of Hand Movements. San Diego, CA: Academic Press; 1996

34. Lundborg G. The Hand and the Brain. From Lucy's Thumb to the Thought Controlled Robotic Hand. London, England: Springer-Verlag; 2014

35. Gordon G (Ed). Active Touch. The Mechanism of Recognition of Objects by Manipulation. A Multi-disciplinary Approach. Oxford, England: Pergamon Press; 1978

36. Lederman SJ, Klatzky RL. Hand movements: a window into haptic object recognition. CP 1985;19: 342–368

37. Gorniak SL, Zatsiorsky VM, Latash ML. Hierarchical control of static prehension: I. Biomechanics. Exp Brain Res 2009;193(4):615–631

38. Smith AM. Finger movements: control. Encycl Neurosci 2010:221–225

39. Duncan SFM, Saracevic CE. Biomechanics of the hand. Hand Clin 2013;29(4):483–492

40. Montagna DF, Parakkal PF. The Structure and Function of Skin, 3rd ed. New York: Academic Press; 1974

41. Elden HR. Biophysical Properties of Skin. New York: John Wiley and Sons; 1971

42. Wilson B, Graham J, Quesada P, Gupta A. Preliminary evaluation of global hand function measurement device. In: Proceedings of the IEEE International Conference on Systems, Man and Cybernetics. Vol 3. 2000

3 Sense and Proprioception

Vasudeva G. Iyer

Movements with precision and dexterity are essential for achieving the multitude of functions demanded of the human hand; although it is the cerebral motor cortex that sends commands to the hand to produce well-coordinated movements, without adequate sensory input this cannot be achieved. Great advances have been made in our understanding of the mechanics of sensory input in the past two decades using information gathered through three techniques: behavioral methods (psychophysics), electrophysiological methods (microneurography, nerve conduction studies, and evoked potential recordings), and functional magnetic resonance imaging (fMRI). In this chapter, we review the structural and functional anatomy of sensory receptors of the hand in general and thereafter focus on proprioception.

3.1 Sensations

Detection of a stimulus and recognition that an event has occurred constitute sensation, whereas interpretation and appreciation of that event constitute perception.[1] The major categories of stimuli are visual, auditory, gustatory (taste), olfactory (smell), mechanical, thermal, and nociceptive (pain). From the various stimuli reaching the brain, an image of the body and of the external world is constructed and updated continuously, a process essential for generating prompt and appropriate responses to changes within and outside the body.

To deal with different varieties of stimuli, it is necessary to have a variety of sensors (receptors) and separate populations of neurons to transmit them to the brain. It is crucial not only to sense and discriminate between different types of stimuli but also to acquire information regarding the intensity, topography, and frequency of the stimuli. These needs have led to the evolution of receptors with unique characteristics, a variety of neurotransmitters, and axons with differing conduction velocities.

3.1.1 The Somatosensory Unit

Each somatosensory unit consists of the dorsal root ganglion (DRG) cell, its axon, and all the receptors it innervates. The DRGs are pseudounipolar cells (▶ Fig. 3.1), with the peripheral portion of the axon terminating in receptors (either as bare nerve ending or in an encapsulated structure) and the proximal portion in the dorsal horn or more proximally in the central nervous system. ▶ Table 3.1 shows the various sensory units and the receptors.

Somatosensory Receptors

General Principles

Receptors are akin to transducers and generate electrical discharges in response to specific stimuli. Appropriate stimulus

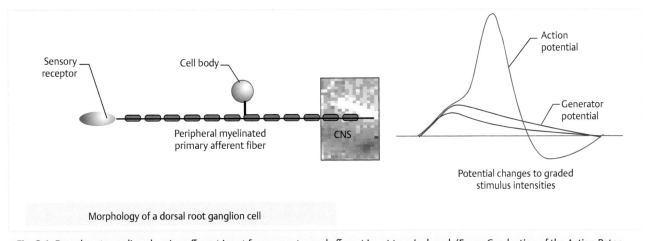

Fig. 3.1 Dorsal root ganglion showing afferent input from receptor and efferent input to spinal cord. (From: Conduction of the Action Potential in Greenstein B, Greenstein A, ed. Color Atlas of Neuroscience. 1st Edition. Thieme; 1999.)

Table 3.1 Innervation pattern of somatosensory receptors

Receptor	Nerve fiber type	Nerve fiber diameter (µM)	Conduction velocity (m/s)
Free nerve endings	C	0.2–1.5	0.5–2
Free nerve endings	A delta	1–6	5–30
Merkel's disc	A beta	6–12	40–70
Meissner's, pacinian corpuscles	A beta	6–12	40–70
Ruffini's endings	A beta	6–12	40–70
Muscle spindle type 1 afferents	A alpha	12–20	70–120
Muscle spindle type 2 afferents	A beta	6–12	40–70
Golgi tendon organ	A alpha	12–20	70–120

induces a change in the transmembrane potential (receptor potential) by changing the permeability of the ion channels of the cell membrane; this may be triggered by mechanical deformation of the membrane causing opening of ion channels, by change in temperature altering permeability of the membrane, or by release of a chemical which may open the channels. The usual change in the membrane is opening of the sodium channels, causing influx of positively charged sodium ions. This in turn leads to migration of sodium ions from the surrounding tissues, eventually leading to change in the membrane potential of the adjacent node of Ranvier. When the receptor potential is large enough to cause depolarization of the nerve fiber terminating in the receptor, an action potential is triggered, which propagates along the axon toward the DRG (▶ Fig. 3.2).

Determination of stimulus strength is crucial for meaningful sensory perception. As the stimulus strength increases, the amplitude of the receptor potential increases in proportion initially, along with an increase in the frequency of the action potential; however, with an intense stimulation, after the initial increase, there is progressively less and less additional increase in frequency of action potential. This general characteristic of receptors bestows an important attribute of being able to respond to an extreme range of stimuli, from very weak to very intense.[2]

Spatial resolution is essential for perception and recognition of complex stimuli. Two techniques are used to modulate spatial resolution: divergence and convergence. When a single receptor sends input to more than one ganglion cell, divergence occurs; on the other hand, when a single ganglion cell receives input from several receptors, convergence occurs, leading to poor spatial resolution but allowing detection of relatively weak stimuli.

Information regarding intensity of stimuli is transmitted by change in the rate and temporal codes. From the firing rate of individual neurons and the number of neurons responding, the intensity of the stimulus is derived.

Surround inhibition of receptor field serves to increase contrast. Tactile receptors show a central area of high sensitivity with surround or lateral inhibition, so that each receptor responds to stimulus occurring in one specific area.

Sensory pathways and their destinations adhere to strict topographic representation at each step to facilitate accurate generation of body schema.

Anatomy of Somatosensory Receptors (▶ Fig. 3.3)

Nociceptors

Free nerve endings (FNEs) sense pain and are ubiquitous in the skin. They often penetrate the epidermis and end in stratum granulosum; there are FNEs that surround the hair follicles as well. They are also present in connective tissue, bones, and joints. They are unencapsulated and exhibit little structural specialization. FNEs may be terminals of C fibers or A delta fibers; the C fiber terminals lack Schwann cell investment and are intimately associated with the epithelium, unlike the A delta terminals.

A variety of stimuli may be perceived as pain, including chemicals related to tissue damage, pH alterations, and heat above 45°C. Noxious stimuli can activate C and/or A delta FNEs. The A delta terminals respond to intense mechanical stimuli and the C terminals respond to noxious mechanical, noxious heat, and chemical stimuli. The *first pain* is rapidly perceived and is discriminative (location and source). The *second pain* is of longer duration and is characterized as severe and often described as of agonizing quality. The first pain results from stimuli carried through the A delta and the second pain through the C fibers.

Certain C terminals contain two neuroactive peptides: calcitonin gene-related peptides (CGRPs) and substance P. Tissue damage leads to release of prostaglandin, bradykinin, and serotonin, which can initiate action potential in the nociceptor; branches of the stimulated axon can release substance P and CGRP through local axon reflex, which can lead to histamine release from mast cells and capillary dilation, leading to inflammatory response.

Some FNEs can serve as multimodal receptors; an example is the nerve ending containing certain ion channels. Thus nerve terminals with a subfamily of transient receptor potential vanilloid, a cation channel that opens when the temperature increases, generally serve as thermal receptors; high concentration of prostaglandin or bradykinin can lower the threshold at which these channels open, thus transforming the terminal into nociceptors.[3]

Thermoceptors

Some FNEs in the epidermis and dermis serve as thermoceptors; these slowly adapting receptors may respond to cold, warmth, or temperature-sensitive nociception. The cold and warm receptors occur separately as distinct spots. Cold receptors respond to decrease in temperature over a range of 5 to 43°C and are more numerous than warm receptors; the latter respond to increasing temperature of up to 45°C.[4] When temperature goes over 45°C or falls below 13°C, the sensation of pain occurs. Warm receptors are innervated by unmyelinated C fibers and cold receptors by thinly myelinated A delta fibers.

Mechanoreceptors

Mechanoreceptors respond to physical deformation of skin or subcutaneous structures, from touch, pressure, stretch, or vibration. A delta FNEs in the skin, muscles, tendons, ligaments, and joint capsules as well as A beta terminals around hair follicles (peritrichial nerve endings), along with more specialized receptors such as Meissner's and pacinian corpuscles, constitute mechanoreceptors. Based on microneurographic studies, four categories of mechanoreceptors can be identified (▶ Table 3.2): fast-adapting (phasic) FA I and FA II and slow-adapting (tonic) SA I and SA II. The FA I and FA II receptors respond promptly to mechanical stimuli such as skin indentation but adapt quickly; the slow-adapting receptors show regular and sustained response. FA I afferents connect to Meissner's corpuscles and FA II to pacinian corpuscles.[5] The SA I afferents connect to Merkel's cell neurite complexes and SA II to Ruffini's endings. The FA I and SA I units are quite dense at the fingertips.

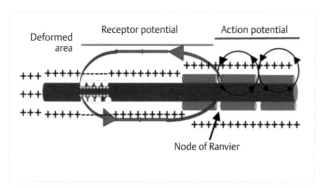

Fig. 3.2 Development of receptor potential and subsequently action potential in the nerve terminal in a mechanoreceptor.

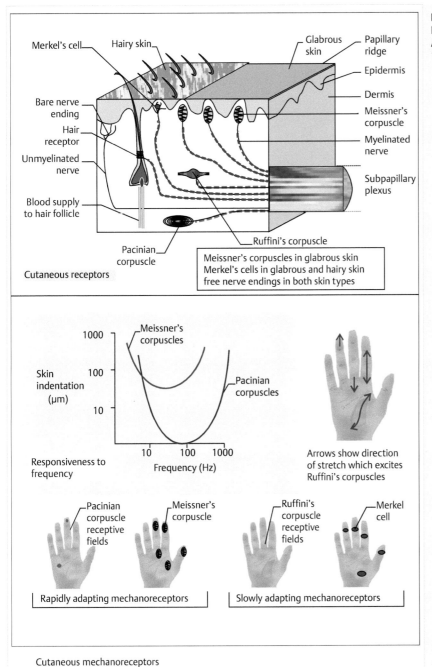

Fig. 3.3 Somatosensory receptors. (From: Proprioceptors I in Green stein B, Greenstein A, ed. Color Atlas of Neuroscience. Thieme; 1999.)

Merkel's Nerve Endings

Merkel's nerve endings are seen in the basal layers (stratum basalis) of hairy and glabrous skin. Iggo and Muir[6] used the term *touch corpuscle* to describe the clusters of Merkel's cells and the nerve endings, which form dome-shaped elevation of the epidermis (▶ Fig. 3.4). They are abundant at the fingertips, contributing to the formation of the ridges. A single large myelinated A beta axon branches and ends in close proximity to an entire group of specialized epithelial cells called the Merkel's cells (Merkel's cell neurite complex, Merkel's discs). They generate action potentials as the stimulus intensity is increased and go into a tonic phase of firing, which may continue for several minutes. They are slowly adapting mechanoreceptors, are considered to be highly sensitive to touch, and are believed to be important in the recognition of texture, shape, and edges of objects.

Meissner's Corpuscles

Also known as tactile corpuscles, they are located in the dermal papillae at the dermoepidermal junction. They consist of cells arranged as horizontal lamellae surrounded by connective tissue. One single A beta axon travels between the lamellae after losing its myelin sheath. They are fast-adapting mechanical receptors sensitive to light touch and vibration at low frequency. They are believed to be important for tactile two-point discrimination.

Ruffini's End Organs

Also known as bulbous corpuscles, they are found in the deeper layers of glabrous skin and also the joint capsules. Hagert et al[7] reported that they are the predominant mechanoreceptor type found in the ligaments of the wrist joint. They consist

Table 3.2 Location and function of somatosensory receptors

Receptor	Location	Adaptation rate	Function
FNE C	Epidermis, dermis, muscle, joint capsule	Slow	Pain, temperature
FNE A delta	Epidermis, dermis, muscle, joint capsule	Slow	Pain, temperature, crude touch, pressure
Merkel's disc	Basal epidermis	Slow	Discriminatory touch
Meissner's corpuscle	Papillae of dermis	Rapid	Touch, two-point discrimination
Pacinian corpuscle	Dermis, hypodermis, ligaments, joint capsules	Rapid	Deep pressure, vibration
Ruffini's endings	Dermis, hypodermis, joint capsule	Slow	Stretch
Peritrichial	Nerve terminal around the hair follicle	Rapid	Touch, hair movement
Muscle spindles NB intrafusal	Skeletal muscle	Rapid and slow	Muscle length and velocity
Muscle spindle NC intrafusal	Skeletal muscle	Rapid and slow	Muscle length
Golgi tendon organ	Myotendinous junction	Rapid and slow	Muscle tension

Abbreviations: FNE, fine nerve endings; NB, nuclear bag; NC, nuclear chain.

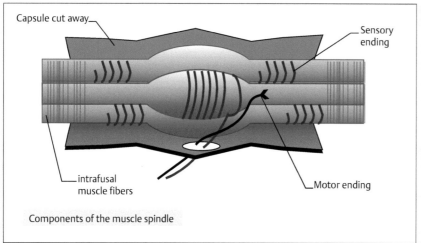

Components of the muscle spindle

Fig. 3.4 Structure of muscle spindle (From: Proprioceptors I in Green stein B, Greenstein A, ed. Color Atlas of Neuroscience. Thieme; 1999.)

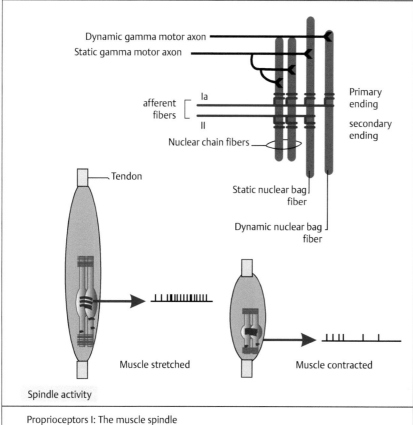

Spindle activity

Proprioceptors I: The muscle spindle

of multibranched encapsulated A beta nerve endings and are elongated and spindle-shaped.[8] The long axis of the capsule is parallel to the stretch lines of skin. They are slow-adapting low-threshold mechanoreceptors responding to stretching of the collagen bundles in the joint capsule and skin. Such receptors located in the joint capsules detect changes in the angle of the joint, providing information regarding joint position and rotation.

Pacinian Corpuscles

Also known as lamellated sensory capsules, they are the largest of the mechanoreceptors. They are located in the dermis, ligaments, joint capsules, and the subcutaneous tissue. They are oval structures with 20 to 60 concentric lamellae separated by gelatinous material. The lamellae are thin, modified Schwann cells and in the center is the inner bulb, a fluid-filled cavity with a thin A beta nerve ending. They are fast-adapting high-threshold mechanoreceptors responding to pressure and vibration.

Muscle Spindles

These are spindle-shaped encapsulated structures, with each end attached to connective tissue sheath of the skeletal muscle fibers (extrafusal fibers). Each spindle (▶ Fig. 3.4) contains 3 to 12 small muscle fibers (intrafusal fibers), which are of two types: larger nuclear bag (NB) and smaller nuclear chain (NC) fibers. The central portion of intrafusal fibers has very little actomyosin and consequentially less contractile; this area is encircled by type A alpha nerve endings (primary/annulospiral ending) in the case of NB fibers and by type A beta nerve endings (secondary/flower-spray ending) in the case of NC fibers. The peripheral contractile portions of intrafusal fibers are innervated by gamma motor neurons (fusimotor neurons).

Muscle spindles are dynamic stretch receptors that monitor the muscle length. Stretch of extrafusal muscle fibers will cause stretch of the intrafusal fibers also due to their parallel position. This will lead to stimulation of the intrafusal nerve endings and generation of action potentials. During slow stretch, the afferent input from both primary and secondary endings increase in proportion to the stretch (static response) and continue for several minutes, leading to steady afferent input.[9] A sudden stretch will lead to an outburst of discharge from the primary endings, lasting only as long as the length is increasing (dynamic response). During contraction of the muscle, the intrafusal fibers also shorten, which in turn will reduce the afferent output.

The reactivity of the spindle can be altered by the gamma motor neuron activity (▶ Fig. 3.5); in the resting muscle, there is some gamma excitation, leading to continuous afferent input. This can be increased by enhanced gamma discharge leading to a contracted state of intrafusal fibers. The gamma motor neuron output is controlled by brainstem (bulboreticular facilitatory system), along with the cerebellum, basal ganglia, and motor cortex.

During volitional muscle contraction, there is simultaneous firing of the alpha motor neuron and the gamma motor neuron, so that the sensitivity of the intrafusal fibers is maintained and readapted dynamically based on the changing muscle length.

The spindles have a large presence in antigravity muscles, and they most likely play an important role to stabilize the body and different joints. Their input is crucial for both the conscious and subconscious components of proprioception (see hereafter).

Golgi Tendon Organ (GTO)

These receptors are located at the myotendinous junction. They consist of collagen bundles enclosed within a connective tissue capsule. Unlike muscle spindles, which are placed parallel to the muscle fibers, the GTO is placed in series; they do not receive motor innervation. Afferent input is through Ib nerve fibers, which show multiple delicate terminals between the collagen bundles of the GTO (▶ Fig. 3.6).

Contraction or stretching of the muscle fibers increases the tension on the tendon, resulting in stimulation of the GTO. Like the spindle, it also shows dynamic or tonic response depending on how quickly the tension increases. The input can also cause stimulation of interneurons at the spinal cord level, causing inhibition of anterior horn cell. This in turn prevents excessive tension of the muscle and facilitates rapid relaxation.

The muscle spindles are stimulated by mild stretch of muscle, but the GTOs are simulated only when the stretch is sufficient to increase the tension in the tendon; muscle spindles sense the muscle fiber length and rate of change, while GTOs sense the tension generated by muscle stretch or contraction.

Sensory Pathways

Although DRGs constitute the common pathway (first-order neuron) for all somatosensory receptors, the central pathways differ depending on the specific sensory input (▶ Fig. 3.7). There are three major ascending sensory systems: the anterolateral system (pain, temperature, nondiscriminatory touch), the dorsal column–medial lemniscal system (fine touch, pressure, vibration, joint position, and movement sense), and the spinocerebellar system (subconscious proprioception).

C and alpha delta DRGs (pain, temperature, and crude touch) → dorsal horn → second-order neurons arise from Rexed lamina II, IV, and V and cross the midline to form anterior and lateral spinothalamic tracts → third-order neurons originate in the thalamus (VPL) and form thalamocortical projections → S1 and S2 areas of cortex and rostral insula and anterior cingulate (some of the second-order neurons form spinoreticular tract, terminating in the reticular formation and making further connections to the intralaminar nuclei of thalamus, which in turn connects to hypothalamus, limbic system, and sensory cortex).

A beta DRGs (touch, pressure, vibration, and joint position and movement sense) → ipsilateral dorsal columns → second-order neurons arise in nucleus gracilis and cuneatus and cross midline to form medial lemniscus → third-order neurons originate in the thalamus (VPL) and form thalamocortical projections → S1 and S2 areas of cortex, A alpha and A beta DRGs → second-order neurons originate from nucleus dorsalis (Clark's column, lamina VII) and form dorsal spinocerebellar tract→ ipsilateral cerebellum.

3.2 Biomechanics of Proprioception

Ever since Charles Sherrington introduced the term *proprioception* ("proprius" meaning self and "ception" for perception), there has been longstanding debate regarding the underlying

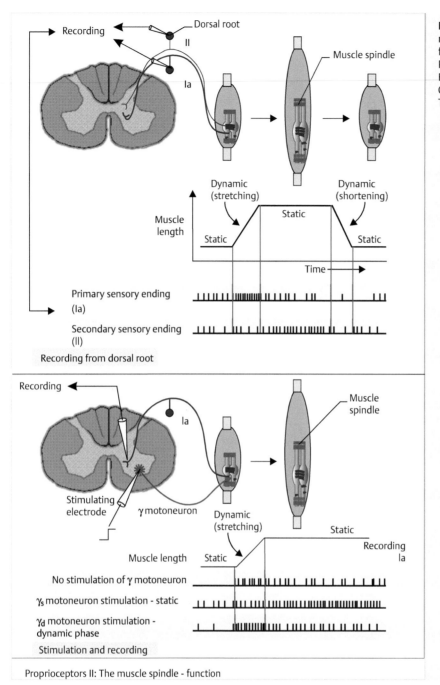

Fig. 3.5 Role of gamma motor neuron in modulating the discharge from intrafusal fibers during muscle contraction. (From: Proprioceptors II: The Muscle Spindle - Function in Greenstein B, Greenstein A, ed. Color Atlas of Neuroscience. 1st Edition. Thieme; 1999.)

sensations and mechanisms involved in this process. Previously, Charles Bell had used the term *muscle sense* and considered it a sixth sense.[10] Henry Bastian had coined the term *kinesthesia*, referring to the sensations arising from receptors not only in the muscles but also in the tendons and joints and skin.[11]

Proprioception is currently used to describe the sense of position and movement of the limbs and the body in the absence of visual input. This concept forms the basis of the bedside assessment, in which the patient (with eyes closed) is asked to indicate the direction of a perceived movement at a joint, when the joint is passively moved by the examiner. The movement detection threshold can vary depending on the velocity of movement and the particular joint.

Although, in the past, the general thinking has been that the neural basis for joint position and movement sense is the same, Proske[12] considers them as sensations processed separately within the central nervous system; this is supported by the observation that muscle vibration at 100 Hz leads to sensation of limb movement and position, presumably by stimulation of

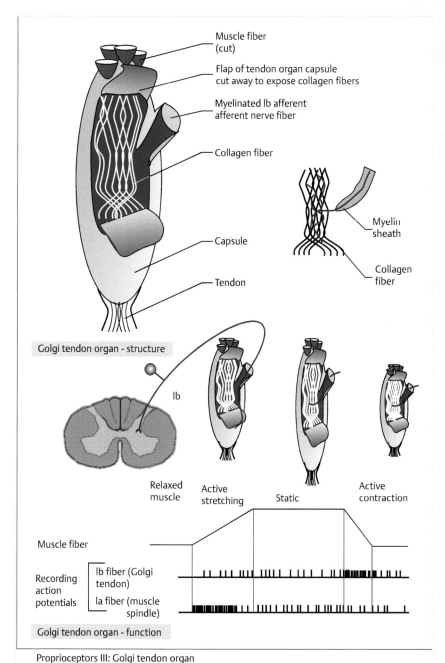

Fig. 3.6 Structure of Golgi tendon organ. (From: Proprioceptors III: The Golgi Tendon Organ in Greenstein B, Greenstein A, ed. Color Atlas of Neuroscience. 1st Edition. Thieme; 1999.)

Ia afferents of muscle spindles, whereas on stimulation at 50 Hz the illusion of movement faded, while position illusion persisted. He believes that positional cue is derived from the effort required to hold a limb against gravity. Rosker and Sarabon,[13] in their review of existing literature on kinesthesia, comment on three subsenses that contribute to the position and movement sense: orientation and position of individual limbs and body, limb movements, and the sensation of effort/the muscle force used to effect the movement.

Proprioception is a form mechanoception, based on input from muscle spindles, GTOs, and receptors in the joint capsule and adjacent tissues. There are two types of spindle afferents: primary (Ia) and secondary (II). They are responsive to alterations in muscle length. The primary afferents are highly responsive to changes in the velocity of muscle contraction, whereas the secondary afferents are less sensitive to dynamic changes and discharge at a regular rate. Thus it is believed that the primary afferents provide information regarding limb movement, whereas the secondary afferents provide information regarding the position. GTOs provide information regarding the tension generated during muscle contraction. Joint receptors important for proprioception include Ruffini's endings, Golgi endings, and

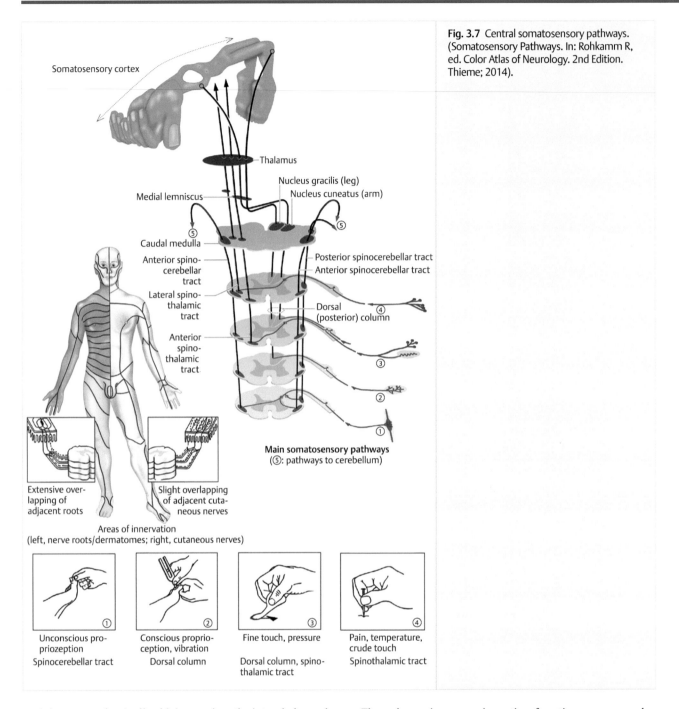

Fig. 3.7 Central somatosensory pathways. (Somatosensory Pathways. In: Rohkamm R, ed. Color Atlas of Neurology. 2nd Edition. Thieme; 2014).

Somatosensory cortex

Thalamus

Nucleus gracilis (leg)
Nucleus cuneatus (arm)

Medial lemniscus

Caudal medulla

Anterior spino-cerebellar tract

Posterior spinocerebellar tract
Anterior spinocerebellar tract

Lateral spino-thalamic tract

Dorsal (posterior) column

Anterior spino-thalamic tract

Main somatosensory pathways
(⑤: pathways to cerebellum)

Extensive over-lapping of adjacent roots

Slight overlapping of adjacent cuta-neous nerves

Areas of innervation
(left, nerve roots/dermatomes; right, cutaneous nerves)

① Unconscious pro-priozeption
Spinocerebellar tract

② Conscious proprio-ception, vibration
Dorsal column

③ Fine touch, pressure
Dorsal column, spino-thalamic tract

④ Pain, temperature, crude touch
Spinothalamic tract

pacinian corpuscles. In distal joints such as the interphalangeal joints, the input from cutaneous receptors are considered to be more important,[14] whereas in larger joints many different proprioceptors may come into play.

Proprioception involves conscious as well as subconscious sensory input. *Conscious* input results in joint position and kinesthetic perception. The central pathways that carry these signals to the sensory cortex were described earlier. Conduction in these pathways can be studied by recording somatosensory evoked potentials in response to electric stimulation of the median or ulnar nerve at the wrist; the average conduction time to the sensory cortex is about 20 ms.

The *subconscious* proprioception functions as a complex system of neuromuscular control, which involves stabilizing joints and regulating input of motor neurons supplying the agonist and antagonist muscles. The major proprioceptive input in this system is destined to the cerebellum through the spinocerebellar tracts. The cerebellum plays a major role in achieving coordinated activity of different muscles to produce smooth joint movements. The presumed functions include integration of afferent information from the periphery with the information from the cortex (through the corticopontocerebellar tract input) to coordinate and plan movements.

There are also spinal reflexes that control activity of muscles involved in the movements of the joints. The most well-known monosynaptic reflex, which lends itself to bedside evaluation, is the muscle stretch reflex; a sudden tap on the tendon causes excitation of the muscle spindles leading to reflex contraction of the muscle. In the upper extremity, the biceps, triceps, and brachioradialis reflexes are easy to elicit and are used clinically to assess the intactness of the reflex pathway.

This can also be tested electrophysiologically by recording the H reflex. It is unclear whether the actual physiological function of this reflex is protection of joint.

Polysynaptic reflexes have one or more interneurons between the DRG axon terminal and the anterior horn cell. These reflexes may be modified by intraspinal (e.g., Renshaw's cell) and supraspinal systems. Feed-forward inhibition is achieved through cortical control and may be important in controlling the specificity of arm and hand movements.[15] Feedback inhibition is achieved by the effect of peripheral input from muscle spindles. Reciprocal inhibition of antagonist muscle during voluntary movement is through activity of inhibitory interneurons in the spinal cord. Another example of polysynaptic reflex is the recurrent inhibition to control activity of synergistic motor neurons of agonist muscles through excitation of Renshaw's cells. These reflex activities are important in the stabilization of the joints so that precise volitional movements can be achieved.

Evaluation of kinesthetic sense uses techniques which can be simple and useful at the bedside or quite complex for research purposes. Most common tests evaluate the ability to perceive joint position by active and passive repositioning techniques, as well as movement sense under differing speed, range, and direction of movement. One could use devices such as goniometers and isokinetic dynamometers to make the tests more quantitative. More complex methods to assess joint position and movement, force, effort, and tracking are used in rehabilitation of patients with problems such as stroke.[16]

The recent insights into the biomechanics of proprioception have led to several applications in clinical medicine, especially in areas such as sports and rehabilitation medicine.[17] Incorrect perception of body alignment and posture may lead to injuries in sports.[18] Partial deafferentation of joints may occur after surgical procedures and in certain neurological disorders; such patients will need proprioceptive training including training to compensate by visual input. Fatigue leads to decreased joint position acuity, based on studies of shoulder and knee joints;[19] training protocols may be modified taking into consideration how long it takes for kinesthesia to recover after fatigue sets in. Another observation is that to increase in sensory input from stimulation of receptors by bracing and taping, a common practice in sports, may prevent injuries or even improve performance.[20] In addition to modifying peripheral kinesthetic sensory input, there have been studies on influencing the process of central adaptation; activity of the cerebral cortex increases with novel activity but becomes less on repeated movements.[21] Further understanding of proprioceptive mechanisms has the potential to make significant contributions to improving physical training, avoiding sports injuries, and developing more effective rehabilitation techniques.

References

1. Hendry SH and Hsiao SS. Fundamentals of sensory systems. In: Squire L, Bloom F, Dulac S, Ghosh A, Spitzer N, eds. Fundamental Neuroscience. Boston, MA: Academic Press; 2008:535–659

2. Hall JE. Sensory receptors, neuronal circuits for processing information. In: Hall JE, ed. Guyton and Hall Textbook of Medical Physiology. Philadelphia, PA: Saunders; 2011:559–570

3. Hendry SH and Hsiao SS. Somatosensory system. In: Squire L, Bloom F, Dulac S, Ghosh A, Spitzer N, eds. Fundamental Neuroscience. Boston, MA: Academic Press; 2008:581–608

4. Stevens JC. Thermal sensibility. In: Heller M, Schiff W, eds. The Psychology of Touch. Hillsdale, NJ: Erlbaum; 1991:61–90

5. Jones LA and Lederman SJ. Neurophysiology of hand function. In: Jones LA, Lederman SJ, eds. Human Hand Function. New York, NY: Oxford University Press; 2006:24–43

6. Iggo A, Muir AR. The structure and function of a slowly adapting touch corpuscle in hairy skin. J Physiol 1969;200(3):763–796

7. Hagert E, Garcia-Elias M, Forsgren S, Ljung BO. Immunohistochemical analysis of wrist ligament innervation in relation to their structural composition. J Hand Surg Am 2007;32(1):30–36

8. Munger BL, Ide C. The structure and function of cutaneous sensory receptors. Arch Histol Cytol 1988;51(1):1–34

9. Prochazka A, Hullinger M. Muscle afferent function and its significance for motor control mechanisms during voluntary movements in cat, monkey and man. In: Desmedt JE, ed. Motor Control Mechanisms in Health and Disease. New York, NY: Raven; 1983:93–132

10. McCloskey DI. Kinesthetic sensibility. Physiol Rev 1978;58(4):763–820

11. Clarac F. Some historical reflections on the neural control of locomotion. Brain Res Brain Res Rev 2008;57(1):13–21

12. Proske U. Kinesthesia: the role of muscle receptors. Muscle Nerve 2006;34(5):545–558

13. Rosker J, Sarabon N. Kinaesthesia and methods for its assessment: literature review. Sport Sci Rev 2012;19(5–6):165–208

14. Collins DF, Refshauge KM, Todd G, Gandevia SC. Cutaneous receptors contribute to kinesthesia at the index finger, elbow, and knee. J Neurophysiol 2005;94(3):1699–1706

15. Hagert E. Proprioception of the wrist joint: a review of current concepts and possible implications on the rehabilitation of the wrist. J Hand Ther 2010;23(1):2–16, quiz 17

16. Chung YJ, Cho SH, Lee YH. Effect of the knee joint tracking training in closed kinetic chain condition for stroke patients. Restor Neurol Neurosci 2006;24(3):173–180

17. Myers JB, Oyama S. Sensorimotor factors affecting outcome following shoulder injury. Clin Sports Med 2008;27(3):481–490, x

18. Lephart SM. Reestablishing proprioception, kinesthesia, joint position sense and neuromuscular control in rehabilitation. In: Coryell P, ed. Rehabilitation Techniques in Sports Medicine. St Louis, MO: Times Mirror Mosby College Publishing; 1993

19. Tripp BL, Yochem EM, Uhl TL. Functional fatigue and upper extremity sensorimotor system acuity in baseball athletes. J Athl Train 2007;42(1):90–98

20. Ulkar B, Kunduracioglu B, Cetin C, Güner RS. Effect of positioning and bracing on passive position sense of shoulder joint. Br J Sports Med 2004;38(5):549–552

21. Taube W, Gruber M, Gollhofer A. Spinal and supraspinal adaptations associated with balance training and their functional relevance. Acta Physiol (Oxf) 2008;193(2):101–116

4 Joint Senses and Proprioception

Elisabet Hagert and Susanne Rein

"The experience of hands is tactile …
They live in the land of feeling where touch is everything
And where the mystery of touch is the bridge between
nerve and soul."

—Harry Martinsson, *Human Hands*[1]

4.1 Introduction

Martinsson's poem about the human hand[1] and its intimate role in bridging the outer world with our innermost perceptions is an eloquent description of the role of proprioception and joint sense in allowing us conscious and unconscious interaction with the world around us. Although *tactility* pertains to the sensory role of the skin, this sensory function originates from fine nerve endings and mechanoreceptors located primarily in the pulp of the fingertips. These mechanoreceptors are also present in the joints of the human hand, indicating that joints, in addition to their mechanical function, have a sensory function. In this chapter, we briefly describe the known sensory innervation of joints

in the human hand, the different joint senses, and their respective function in hand proprioception.

4.2 Innervation of Joints in the Human Hand

Sensory nerve endings, so-called mechanoreceptors, are the primary focus of innervation studies in joints. They are able to detect mechanical stimuli, such as changes in joint position and velocity, transform them into neural excitations, and signal this information from the joint via afferent nerves and dorsal root ganglia to the spinal cord. Sensory nerve endings in ligaments are classified according to Freeman and Wyke[2] into four types, based on their typical shape (▶ Fig. 4.1) and neurophysiological traits (▶ Table 4.1). Sensory nerve endings are found mostly close to ligament insertions into bone as well as in the epiligamentous region of ligaments,[3–6] where they can act as monitors of tension and force applied to the ligament.[7]

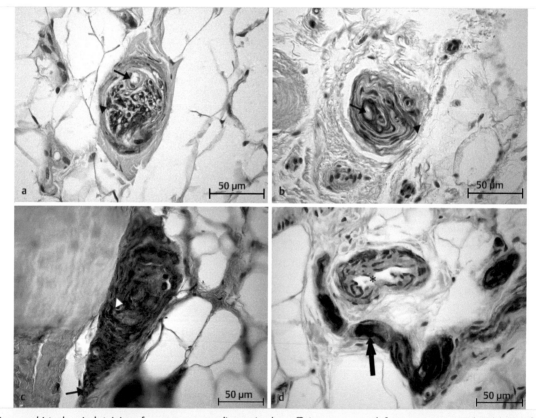

Fig. 4.1 Immunohistochemical staining of sensory nerve endings using low-affinity nerve growth factor receptor p75 (p75) (magnification × 400). **(a)** A Ruffini ending characterized by p75 immunoreactive (IR) dendritic nerve endings (*arrowhead*), a clearly visible central axon without IR (*arrow*), and a thin, at times partial, encapsulation of the corpuscle. **(b)** In contrast, the Pacini corpuscle has an onion-layered p75 IR capsule (*arrowhead*) and central axon (*arrow*). **(c)** The Golgi-like ending is larger, with an afferent nerve fascicle (*arrow*) coursing to the center of the corpuscle. Typically smaller corpuscles within the Golgi-like ending are seen (*arrowhead*). **(d)** Finally, free nerve endings (*arrow*) are p75 IR and often located close to vessels (*star*).

Table 4.1 Classification of mechanoreceptors in ligaments based on Freeman and Wyke,[2] modified by Hagert,[8] outlining the morphology and function of the various sensory nerve endings found in the human hand

Type	Eponym/Name (descriptive)	Characteristics	Neurophysiological trait	Role in joint function	IR patterns in mechanoreceptors
I	Ruffini (dendritic)	Coil-shaped. Partial encapsulation. Arborizing nerve branches with bulbous terminals. 50–100 μm.	Slowly adapting Low-threshold	Static joint position Changes in velocity/amplitude	Central axon – *PGP9.5, S100* Terminal nerve branches – *PGP9.5, trkB* Incomplete capsule – *p75*
II	Pacini (lamellated)	Rounded, ovular corpuscle. Thick lamellar capsule. 20–50 μm.	Rapidly adapting Low-threshold	Joint acceleration/deceleration	Central axon – *PGP9.5, S100* Thick capsule – *p75*
III	Golgi-like (grouped dendritic)	Large, spherical. Partial encapsulation. Groups of arborizing and terminal nerve endings. >150 μm.	Rapidly adapting High-threshold	Extreme ranges of joint motion	Terminal nerve branches – *PGP9.5, S100, trkB* Incomplete capsule – *p75*
IV	Free nerve endings	Varicose appearance, often close to arterioles. Groups or single fibers	Aδ fibers - fast C fibers - slow	Noxious, nociceptive, inflammatory	Axon – *PGP9.5, trkB*
V	Unclassifiable	Variable size, appearance, and degree of encapsulation.	Unknown	Unknown	Incomplete capsule – *p75* Variable IR pattern

Abbreviations: Protein Gene Product 9.5 (PGP9.5); S-100 protein (S100); tyrosine kinase receptor B (trkB); low-affinity neurotrophic receptor p75 (p75); immunoreactions (IR).
Source: Reprinted from Hagert.[8]

4.2.1 Wrist

The innervation of wrist ligaments has been intensively studied.[3,5,6,9–12] Its pattern was found to vary distinctly, with a pronounced innervation in the dorsal ligaments and in the entire scapholunate interosseous ligament (SLIL),[10,11] an intermediate innervation in the volar triquetral ligaments, and only limited to occasional innervation of the volar radial ligaments.[3,9] Based on this, the dorsal ligaments and the SLIL are considered sensory important ligaments in wrist proprioception, with the Ruffini ending (▶Fig. 4.1a) being the predominant mechanoreceptor type.[5]

The triangular fibrocartilage complex also represents a richly innervated region with a homogenous distribution of Ruffini endings, but also free nerve endings (▶Fig. 4.1d) in the ulnar and dorsal areas, Pacini corpuscles (▶Fig. 4.1b) in the radial and dorsal areas, and Golgi-like endings (Fig. 4.1c) in the ulnar and ventral areas.[13]

4.2.2 Finger Joints

Ruffini endings and Pacini corpuscles have been identified in the proximal interphalangeal joint (PIP), with a greater density of innervation in the proximal region as compared to midsubstance/distal joint.[14] In addition, Ruffini endings have been mainly found in the proximal volar plate, where they are particularly able to monitor joint position changes. Pacini corpuscles, on the other hand, were primarily seen in association with the C1 pulley, suggesting that they sense acceleration and deceleration of the finger.[14] The density of free nerve endings and Pacini corpuscles were consistently greater in palmar areas than in dorsal or lateral parts of the PIP and metacarpophalangeal joint capsules.[15]

4.2.3 Thumb Trapeziometacarpal Joint

The dorsal ligaments of the thumb trapeziometacarpal joint (TMJ) have an abundance of sensory nerve endings, mainly close to the metacarpal insertion, whereas the ulnar collateral showed little, and the anterior oblique ligament no, innervation. As with the wrist ligaments, Ruffini endings were the predominant receptor type in the TMJ, indicating a function in providing information regarding thumb position and velocity.[4]

4.3 The Joint Senses and Proprioception

The term *proprioception* is derived from Latin, *proprius*, belonging to one's own, and *-ception*, to perceive. The term was first established by the 1932 Nobel Laureate in Physiology or Medicine, Sir Charles Scott Sherrington, who in 1906[16] defined proprioception as sensations arising in the deep areas of the body, contributing to conscious sensations (*muscle sense*), total posture (*postural equilibrium*), and segmental posture (*joint stability*). To delineate the proprioceptive role of joints, the term *sensorimotor function* was adapted in 1997, meaning the "total integration of sensory, motor and central processes pertaining to joint stability."[17] Based on this, the joints senses can be divided into three specific senses (▶Fig. 4.2):

- *Kinesthesia*: the conscious sense of joint motion
- *Joint position sense*: the conscious appreciation of joint position/angle
- *Neuromuscular*: the unconscious control of joints, joint reflexes

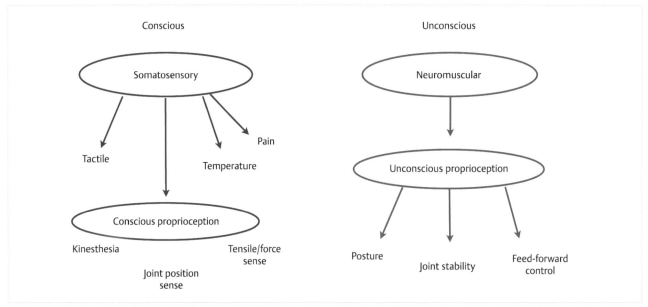

Fig. 4.2 A schematic presentation of the different proprioception senses. The somatosensory senses are conscious appreciations of proprioception, whereas the neuromuscular senses reflect the unconscious control in joint proprioception. (Reproduced with permission from Hagert.[31])

4.4 Conscious Joint Senses

The conscious joint senses—kinesthesia and joint position sense—were first recognized by Bastian in the 19th century.[18] Although these senses are of great importance in our conscious appreciation of joint motion and position, thorough investigations have concluded that these senses are primarily influenced by the action of muscle spindles,[19-22] with some afference from skin receptors[23] and minor afference from joint receptors. Skin receptors are primarily of importance in the kinesthesia of finger joints,[24] since the muscles controlling the fingers are located at a distance, in the forearm and hand. Joint receptors are similarly thought to be of importance whenever a muscle traverses more than one major joint,[25] thus limiting the sensitivity of the muscle spindle in detecting motion.[1]

In the human hand, the dependency on cutaneous sensation for finger kinesthesia and joint position sense is readily appreciated in patients with sensory loss following nerve injury.[26]

Similarly, the kinesthesia and joint position sense of the wrist is primarily influenced by muscle receptors and not joint sensation. This has been recently described in studies on patients who have undergone partial wrist denervation, where the conscious joint senses remained intact despite the surgical removing or anesthetizing the anterior and/or posterior interosseous nerves (AIN/PIN).[27,28] In instances of partial joint denervation, a joint sense influenced by muscles spindles will naturally be retained, as well as the afference of nerves still innervating the joint, but the unconscious proprioception of the wrist may regardless still be disturbed,[29] as discussed hereafter.

4.5 Unconscious Joint Sense

The unconscious proprioception sense is equivalent to joint neuromuscular sense. This sense includes the anticipatory control of muscles around a joint through so-called feed-forward control, as well as the ability to unconsciously maintain joint stability and equilibrium.[17,30] The neuromuscular sense is greatly influenced by spinal reflexes for immediate joint control, as well as integrations in the cerebellum for planning, anticipating, and executing joint control. Hence, while the neuromuscular control of a joint is the hardest to objectively quantify or assess, it is likely of greatest importance in maintaining joint stability.

Conscious assessment techniques (i.e., joint position sense) used to measure conscious proprioception cannot be applied to the unconscious proprioception sense. Rather, this sense demands techniques assessing reflex muscle activation,[31] such as through the use of electromyography (EMG) or sensory activation potential (SAP) in determining muscle control.

Studies on in vivo wrist joint proprioception using EMG[32] and SAP[33] have shown that the wrist has distinct patterns of reflex activation following disturbance of the SLIL (▶ Fig. 4.3a). Within 20 ms of joint perturbation, antagonist muscles are activated, indicating fast joint protective reflexes through monosynaptic spinal control.[32] Deafferentation of the SLIL by anesthetizing the PIN resulted in significant loss of these joint protective reflexes (▶ Fig. 4.3b).[34] Similarly, sectioning of the SLIL significantly reduced the afferent signals through primarily the median and radial nerves.[33] These findings show that denervation of the AIN and/or PIN, while resulting in no alteration of conscious wrist proprioception,[27,28] will have adverse effects on the unconscious

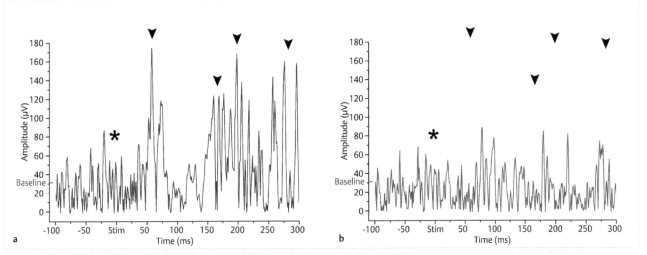

Fig. 4.3 Rectified EMG from a flexor carpi ulnaris muscle illustrating the EMG excitations (*arrowheads*) seen following stimulation (*) of the scapholunate interosseous ligament (**a**) and the loss of excitatory reactions following desensitization of the posterior interosseous nerve (**b**).

neuromuscular control of the wrist joint. Hence denervation procedures should be advocated, carefully, only in wrists where the proprioceptive function may already be considered inferior, such as in cases of advanced wrist osteoarthritis, and not as a routine in minor procedures, such as removal of ganglion cysts, as these patients may suffer disturbances in their joint proprioceptive functions.

References

1. Martinsson H. Människans händer [Man's hands]. Dikter om ljus och mörker [Poems of light and darkness]. Vol 1. Sweden: Bonnier; 1971:41
2. Freeman MA, Wyke B. The innervation of the knee joint. An anatomical and histological study in the cat. J Anat 1967;101(Pt 3):505–532
3. Hagert E, Garcia-Elias M, Forsgren S, Ljung BO. Immunohistochemical analysis of wrist ligament innervation in relation to their structural composition. J Hand Surg Am 2007;32(1):30–36
4. Hagert E, Lee J, Ladd AL. Innervation patterns of thumb trapeziometacarpal joint ligaments. J Hand Surg Am 2012;37(4):706–714.e1
5. Lin YT, Berger RA, Berger EJ, et al. Nerve endings of the wrist joint: a preliminary report of the dorsal radiocarpal ligament. J Orthop Res 2006;24(6):1225–1230
6. Tomita K, Berger EJ, Berger RA, Kraisarin J, An KN. Distribution of nerve endings in the human dorsal radiocarpal ligament. J Hand Surg Am 2007;32(4):466–473
7. Takebayashi T, Yamashita T, Minaki Y, Ishii S. Mechanosensitive afferent units in the lateral ligament of the ankle. J Bone Joint Surg Br 1997;79(3):490–493
8. Hagert E. Wrist Ligaments—Innervation Patterns and Ligamento-Muscular Reflexes [PhD thesis]. Stockholm: Department of Clinical Science and Education, Section of Hand Surgery, Karolinska Institutet; 2008
9. Hagert E, Forsgren S, Ljung BO. Differences in the presence of mechanoreceptors and nerve structures between wrist ligaments may imply differential roles in wrist stabilization. J Orthop Res 2005;23(4):757–763
10. Hagert E, Ljung BO, Forsgren S. General innervation pattern and sensory corpuscles in the scapholunate interosseous ligament. Cells Tissues Organs 2004;177(1):47–54
11. Mataliotakis G, Doukas M, Kostas I, Lykissas M, Batistatou A, Beris A. Sensory innervation of the subregions of the scapholunate interosseous ligament in relation to their structural composition. J Hand Surg Am 2009;34(8):1413–1421
12. Petrie S, Collins J, Solomonow M, Wink C, Chuinard R. Mechanoreceptors in the palmar wrist ligaments. J Bone Joint Surg Br 1997;79(3):494–496
13. Cavalcante ML, Rodrigues CJ, Mattar R Jr. Mechanoreceptors and nerve endings of the triangular fibrocartilage in the human wrist. J Hand Surg Am 2004;29(3):432–435, discussion 436–438
14. Chikenji T, Suzuki D, Fujimiya M, Moriya T, Tsubota S. Distribution of nerve endings in the human proximal interphalangeal joint and surrounding structures. J Hand Surg Am 2010;35(8):1286–1293
15. Chen YG, McClinton MA, DaSilva MF, Shaw Wilgis EF. Innervation of the metacarpophalangeal and interphalangeal joints: a microanatomic and histologic study of the nerve endings. J Hand Surg Am 2000;25(1):128–133
16. Sherrington CS. The Integrative Action of the Nervous System. New Haven, CT: Yale University Press; 1906
17. Lephart SM, Riemann BL, Fu FH. Introduction to the sensorimotor system. In: Lephart SM, Fu FH, eds. Proprioception and Neuromuscular Control in Joint Stability. Champaign, IL: Human Kinetics; 2000:xvii–xxiv
18. Bastian HC. The "muscular sense"; its nature and cortical localisation. Brain 1888;10:1–137
19. Gandevia SC, Refshauge KM, Collins DF. Proprioception: peripheral inputs and perceptual interactions. Adv Exp Med Biol 2002;508:61–68
20. Gandevia SC, Smith JL, Crawford M, Proske U, Taylor JL. Motor commands contribute to human position sense. J Physiol 2006;571(Pt 3):703–710
21. Proske U, Wise AK, Gregory JE. The role of muscle receptors in the detection of movements. Prog Neurobiol 2000;60(1):85–96
22. Proske U. Kinesthesia: the role of muscle receptors. Muscle Nerve 2006;34(5):545–558
23. Edin BB. Quantitative analysis of static strain sensitivity in human mechanoreceptors from hairy skin. J Neurophysiol 1992;67(5):1105–1113
24. Collins DF, Refshauge KM, Todd G, Gandevia SC. Cutaneous receptors contribute to kinesthesia at the index finger, elbow, and knee. J Neurophysiol 2005;94(3):1699–1706
25. Sturnieks DL, Wright JR, Fitzpatrick RC. Detection of simultaneous movement at two human arm joints. J Physiol 2007;585 (Pt 3):833–842

26. Moberg E. The role of cutaneous afferents in position sense, kinaesthesia, and motor function of the hand. Brain 1983;106 (Pt 1):1–19

27. Patterson RW, Van Niel M, Shimko P, Pace C, Seitz WH Jr. Proprioception of the wrist following posterior interosseous sensory neurectomy. J Hand Surg Am 2010;35(1):52–56

28. Gay A, Harbst K, Hansen DK, Laskowski ER, Berger RA, Kaufman KR. Effect of partial wrist denervation on wrist kinesthesia: wrist denervation does not impair proprioception. J Hand Surg Am 2011;36(11):1774–1779

29. Hagert E. Proprioception of the wrist following posterior interosseous sensory neurectomy. J Hand Surg Am 2010;35(4): 690–691

30. Sjölander P, Johansson H, Djupsjöbacka M. Spinal and supraspinal effects of activity in ligament afferents. J Electromyogr Kinesiol 2002;12(3):167–176

31. Hagert E. Proprioception of the wrist joint: a review of current concepts and possible implications on the rehabilitation of the wrist. J Hand Ther 2010;23(1):2–16, quiz 17

32. Hagert E, Persson JK, Werner M, Ljung BO. Evidence of wrist proprioceptive reflexes elicited after stimulation of the scapholunate interosseous ligament. J Hand Surg Am 2009;34(4):642–651

33. Vekris MD, Mataliotakis GI, Beris AE. The scapholunate interosseous ligament afferent proprioceptive pathway: a human in vivo experimental study. J Hand Surg Am 2011;36(1):37–46

34. Hagert E, Persson JK. Desensitizing the posterior interosseous nerve alters wrist proprioceptive reflexes. J Hand Surg Am 2010;35(7):1059–1066

5 The Hand and the Brain

Anders Björkman

5.1 Introduction

The everyday use of hands is highly dependent on the interaction between the sensory and motor systems in the central nervous system (CNS). The interaction of sensory systems, such as those for vision, hearing, and somatosensory function, can help in identifying external objects and the body's relationship to them and thereby create an internal representation of the external world in the brain. This internal representation is the framework used by the motor system in the CNS to plan, coordinate, and execute motor programs used to guide purposeful movement of different body parts, such as the hand.[1-3] Furthermore, it is through the moving hand that a large diversity of tactile experience is unveiled; hence, the moving hand is a facilitating agent for more complex tactile experiences. Because many motor and sensory acts of daily life are unconscious, we are often unaware of their complexity. However, this complexity becomes apparent when a person sustains an injury to the nervous system, such as a median or ulnar nerve injury in the forearm, often resulting in a permanently impaired somatosensory function as well as decreased motor function in the hand.[4]

The CNS in general and the brain in particular have a tremendous motor- and sensory-related capacity, controlling some 640 different muscles in the body and somatosensory information from these muscles and the skin. This is made possible by the large amount of interacting nerve cells and nerve tracts in the brain (▶Fig. 5.1).

Anatomically, the brain is composed of macroscopically symmetric regions: prosencephalon (diencephalon and telencephalon), mesencephalon, and rhombencephalon (medulla oblongata, pons, and cerebellum). The most caudal and in many respects the simplest part of the CNS, the spinal cord extends from the base of the skull to the first lumbar vertebra (▶Fig. 5.2). The spinal cord is divided into a central core of gray matter, containing the nerve cell bodies, and an outer layer of white matter, containing ascending and descending tracts of myelinated axons.

Nerve tracts in the CNS representing motor and sensory control are bilaterally symmetrical and, if connecting the brain to the spinal cord, cross to the contralateral side of the spinal cord or brain. Thus, motor and sensory control of one hand is mediated mainly by the contralateral brain hemisphere. Although the CNS is often described in anatomical terms, its functional organization is much more complex and different anatomical brain areas contribute to various functional systems. The primary motor cortex, located in the precentral gyrus of the frontal lobe, and the primary somatosensory cortex, located in the postcentral gyrus of the parietal lobe (▶Fig. 5.3), contain large numbers of different highly specialized neurons processing information before sending it on to other areas inside the brain or to the spinal cord and on to the muscles. Already in the end of the 19th century and in the first half of the 20th century, cerebral somatosensory and motor maps

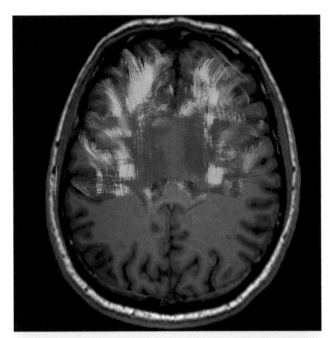

Fig. 5.1 Axial T1-weighted MRI at a supraventricular level with overlaid fiber tracking to the anterior part of the brain, generated from MR diffusion tensor images (DTI). Color coding corresponds to fiber orientation (*red* represents right–left, *blue* craniocaudal, and *green* anteroposterior orientation).

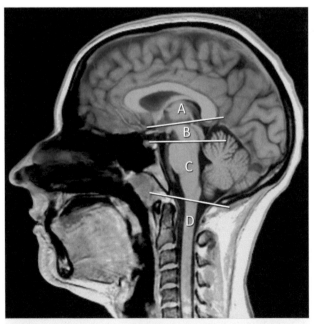

Fig. 5.2 The central nervous system (CNS). Sagittal T1-weighted MRI of the brain showing borders between the prosencephalon (A), mesencephalon (B), and the lowest part of the brain, the rhombencephalon (C). Below the base of the skull, the CNS continues as the spinal cord (D) embedded in the spinal canal.

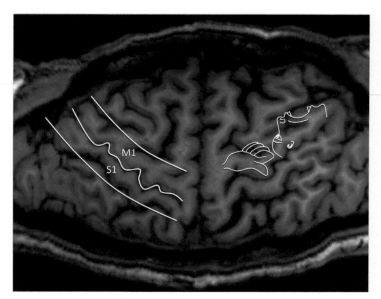

Fig. 5.3 Curved multiplanar MR reconstruction of the brain surface with the precentral and postcentral gyri outlined, representing the primary motor cortex (M1) and primary somatosensory cortex (S1), respectively (right hemisphere). Overlaid on the left hemisphere, a schematic illustrates the large presentation of body areas with high motor and somatosensory complexity, such as the hand and face, in the primary motor cortex.

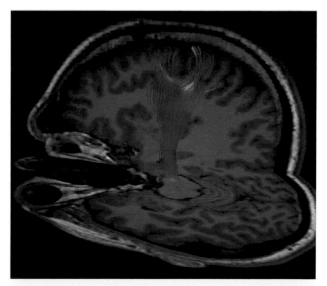

Fig. 5.4 MRI with overlaid fiber tracking of the corticospinal and spinocortical tracts from and to the hand areas in the primary motor (anterior) and somatosensory cortex (posterior), respectively. Fiber tracking generated from MR diffusion tensor images (DTI).

were characterized in great detail by several scientists, including Charles Sherrington and Wilder Penfield.[5] They showed that the hand and face, including the tongue, are represented in sensory and motor cortex by very large areas, reflecting the large number of nerve cells needed for fine motor control and somatosensory processing in these body parts compared to, for example, the legs or torso (▶ Fig. 5.3).

Furthermore, tremendous advances in neurobiology and in functional neuroimaging have shown that both the motor and the somatosensory systems are much more complex than first assumed. A seemingly simple task such as grasping a glass of water for drinking involves a complex network of several different cerebral areas working together in a highly orchestrated manner to achieve the goal. A key issue in understanding the working hand is knowledge of how the motor and somatosensory systems interact and how information from sensory receptors in the skin, joints, and muscles is used for appropriate

motor control. Understanding this is not only fundamental in its own but also of importance in understanding disorders in these systems and their treatment.

5.2 Motor System

The anatomy of the muscles controlling the human hand places special needs on the system responsible for control of voluntary movement. Many muscles controlling hand and finger movement are located in the forearm or proximal hand, and they have long, sometimes multiple, tendons crossing several joints and sometimes acting on multiple fingers. Thus, control of hand and individual finger movements requires a complex pattern of neural activation and inhibition of several muscles.

Movement in the upper extremity is generated by stimulation of skeletal muscle fibers by lower motor neurons, with their cell bodies located in the anterior horn of the spinal cord. Activity in the lower motor neurons is coordinated by interneurons forming local circuits in the spinal cord. The activity in these local circuits is in turn governed by input from descending projections from upper motor neurons located in the cerebral cortex and brainstem[1,2] and also by feedback from somatosensory nerves.

The primary motor cortex has a distinct order, somatotopy, where neurons controlling the different body parts and patterns of movement are located together. However, the neurons are not equally divided between the different body parts; instead, a disproportionally large area, which is to say a large amount of nerve cells of the primary motor cortex, is devoted to muscular control of the hand compared to the lower extremity (▶ Fig. 5.3). In fact, monosynaptic projections from the primary motor cortex onto spinal motor neurons are most dense for muscles controlling hand and finger movement. This results in a greatly enhanced capacity to perform fine hand and finger movement (▶ Fig. 5.4).

It is important to understand that the primary motor cortex does not contain a map of nerve cells controlling individual muscles; instead, patterns of movement are represented in the motor map of the primary motor cortex.[6] Neurons controlling hand and finger movement are located mainly within the hand area of the primary motor cortex; however, they also overlap

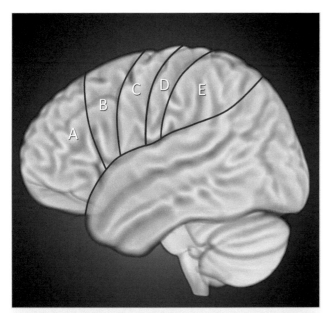

Fig. 5.5 Lateral view of the brain with the main areas of cortical motor control outlined. Purpose: prefrontal cortex (**A**); planning: premotor areas (**B**); and execution: primary motor cortex (**C**). Main cortical areas of sensory guidance are the primary somatosensory cortex (**D**) and posterior parietal areas (**E**).

areas [BA] 5, 7, 39, and 40) play an important role in sensory guidance of movement. Neurons in area 5 receive central and peripheral nerve signals, allowing these neurons to integrate central motor commands with peripheral sensory information during reaching and grasping and thus making it possible to moderate and correct the motor plan and commands.[3] Furthermore, the parietal cortex is critical for the integration of visual data necessary for coordination of eye and hand movements.[8] Premotor areas also have a cognitive function. Specific neurons, known as mirror neurons, are activated during motor acts but also when a person simply watches another person perform a motor act.[9] These neurons are thought to be important for our understanding of the intentions and acts of other people as well as for learning new motor skills.

Somatosensory and visual cortex and cerebellum are also important in the formation of a motor plan, as they mediate information on the current state of the body to the premotor areas, such as the position, posture, and movement of the arms and hands and their interaction with the environment.[10,11]

Information from the somatosensory and visual cortex to the motor system can play at least three functional roles: (1) feedback control of ongoing movements, such as to help adjust the output signal from the neurons controlling muscles acting on the hand to ensure that a person applies adequate force to an object to grasp it and to be able to manipulate it, but not to crush it or let it slip; (2) feed-forward control of intended movement, such as by positioning the hands appropriately while awaiting an approaching object, such as a ball; and (3) motor learning. The importance of somatosensory and visual information for movement of the hand becomes obvious after an injury to these systems. Such injuries not only cause impairment of object identification but also result in a severe impairment of the ability to move the hand and arm, especially when the movement includes interactions with objects.

After the complex process of motor planning comes the last stage in the control of voluntary movement, the coordination of muscle contractions needed to perform the planned movement. This is done by the primary motor cortex, brainstem, and spinal cord (▶Fig. 5.6).

The motor network is not completely hierarchical, sending information in a specific sequence between different brain areas where the primary motor cortex is the final common path. Although the primary motor cortex has the most direct access to the lower motor neurons, the premotor and parietal cortical areas can also influence spinal motor function through their own corticospinal projections. Furthermore, all areas in the motor network are heavily interconnected (▶Fig. 5.7).

As mentioned earlier, the motor output signal is monitored by neurons in the premotor areas and also by visual and tactile information. Furthermore, the motor network is monitored and modulated by the basal ganglia and the cerebellum. The cerebellum is well connected to the motor network (▶Fig. 5.7) and acts, for example, to correct errors in ongoing movements. Specialized neurons in the cerebellum assess the difference between the ongoing motor commands as issued by the motor network and the actual movement being performed. Furthermore, the cerebellum is important for learning new motor skills. The basal ganglia gate motor commands from the motor network, a function of great importance for the initiation of movement and the design of movement sequences. Diseases

extensively with neurons controlling more proximal muscles of the arm. This highly dynamic organization of the finger, hand, and arm motor maps in the primary motor cortex makes complex and well-coordinated movement possible in the upper extremity. This dynamic organization stands in striking contrast to the primary somatosensory cortex, where sensory information from the hand and fingers is sent to and processed in specific areas.

Although the primary motor cortex has the most direct access to the spinal interneurons and motor neurons, it does not solely control voluntary movement. Instead, it has been shown that the motor system is organized in a functional hierarchy including several different cerebral areas forming a motor network, where each level is concerned with a different decision. Cerebral control of movement is generally divided into three sequential stages—goal setting, planning, and coordination of muscle contracture—during which intentions are transformed into actions.[2,7] Most voluntary motor acts have a specific goal, so the first stage of the network is concerned with deciding the purpose or goal of the movement, which requires the prefrontal cortex (the anterior part of the frontal lobes lying in front of the motor and premotor areas) (▶Fig. 5.5).

At the next level, a motor plan is formed, involving interactions between the premotor areas (located anteriorly to the precentral gyrus or primary motor cortex) and somatosensory areas of the cerebral cortex. Normal behavior does not include a single movement of the hand and fingers; instead, it normally constitutes a sequence of movements that together form a behavior satisfying a specific aim. Movement design is mainly attributed to premotor areas. Neurons in premotor areas that control hand movements are strongly influenced by tactile stimuli on the glabrous surface of the palm and digits.[2] Furthermore, posterior parietal regions in the brain (Brodmann's

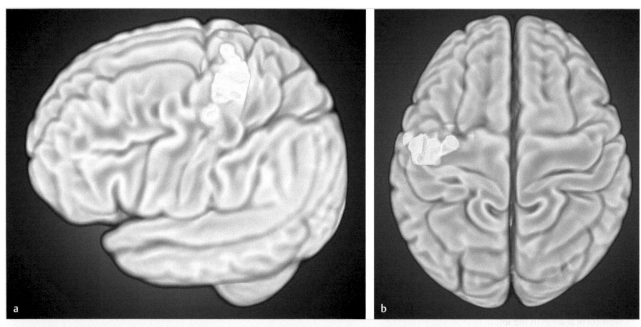

Fig. 5.6 (a,b) Activation of the primary motor cortex in the left hemisphere as visualized by fMRI during tapping of the fingers on the right hand (lateral view, left; view from above, right).

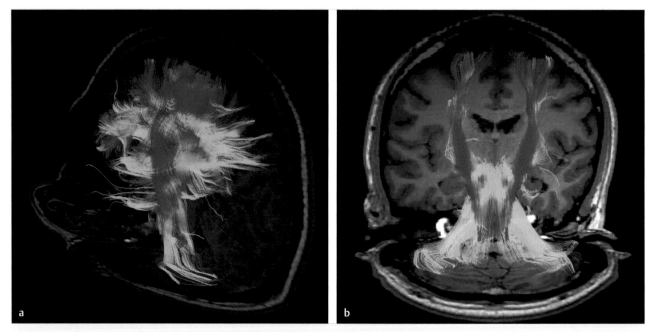

Fig. 5.7 MR fiber tracking illustrating the corticospinal and spinocortical tracts and intrahemispheric connectivity (a) and corticospinal and spinocortical tracts and connections through the basal ganglia, mesencephalon, and pons via the cerebellar peduncles to the cerebellum (b) (color coding: *blue* for craniocaudal directions, *green* for anteroposterior directions).

in the basal ganglia such as Parkinson's disease, in which dopaminergic neurons in the basal ganglia are destroyed, cause difficulties both in initiating movement and in terminating movement once initiated.

5.3 Somatosensory System

The somatosensory system of the brain has the daunting task of processing information from thousands of receptors in the fingers and hands into cognitive information about the external world and for the purpose of fine motor control.[3]

Perception of touch on the hand begins when cutaneous mechanoreceptors are stimulated. Following stimulation, the afferent nerve signals are conveyed to the sensory neuron located in the dorsal root ganglion. The axons of the neurons located in the dorsal root ganglion are of the pseudounipolar type, having two branches—a distal process projecting to the periphery and a proximal process projecting to the CNS.[1,2]

Several different specialized receptors provide information about stimuli acting on the fingers and hand.[12,13] For example, the median nerve contains more than 20 different afferent types of nerve fibers conveying information from different cutaneous

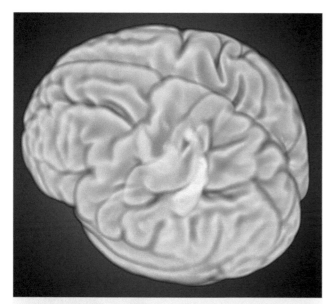

Fig. 5.8 Activation of the primary somatosensory cortex and adjacent cortical areas in the left hemisphere as visualized by fMRI during tactile stimulation of the right-hand fingers.

mechanoreceptors, proprioceptors, thermoreceptors, and nociceptors.

How precisely mechanical stimulation is perceived in different regions of the body varies. Mechanoreceptors are much more densely distributed in the fingertips than in the palm, which in turn is more densely populated than the forearm. The receptive fields, which is to say the skin area supplied by a single neuron, are much smaller in the fingertips (1–2 mm), compared with 5 to 10 mm in the palm and several centimeters on the forearm. This difference is mirrored in the capacity to detect fine sensory stimuli, which is far better in the fingertip compared to the forearm.

Sensory information is sent to the ventral posterior nuclear complex of the thalamus and cerebral cortex by two main ascending pathways. Tactile and proprioceptive information is sent in the dorsal column–medial lemniscal system, and pain and temperature information is sent in the spinothalamic tract. The thalamus is not simply a relay station; instead, the incoming afferent signals from peripheral receptors are processed in the thalamus. After an afferent nerve signal is processed, it is sent on to the primary somatosensory cortex located in the postcentral gyrus (▶Fig. 5.8). Interestingly, many nerve tracts send signals from cortical areas, such as the primary somatosensory cortex, to the thalamus. These tracts likely assist in the thalamic processing of afferent information from peripheral receptors. The primary somatosensory cortex comprises four cytoarchitectural different areas (BA): 1, 2, 3a, and 3b. Nerve cells in areas 1 and 3b receive information from receptors in the skin, whereas those in area 3a receive information primarily from muscle stretch receptors, and nerve cells in area 2 are responsible for assessing information about the size and shape of objects. Studies in humans and animals have shown that each of the four different areas in the primary somatosensory cortex contains a separate and complete neuronal representation of the body surface forming an orderly somatotopic map of the body surface. As in the motor system, the somatosensory map of the body surface does not reflect the actual size of the different body parts. Instead, each body part is represented in

relation to the importance of the sensory information from that body part. Thus, a disproportionally large cerebral area, which is to say number of neurons, in both hemispheres is devoted to the fingers and hands; in fact, more neurons are devoted to somatosensory information from the fingers than to the entire trunk. The neurons processing sensory input from the fingers are organized in sequential, partly overlapping areas. The thumb and index finger, which most often operate independently, have distinct, slightly larger, cortical territories compared with digits 3 to 5, which most often are used together and thus have slightly smaller and more overlapping neuronal representations in the primary somatosensory cortex.[14] The different areas in the primary somatosensory cortex are extensively interconnected within the ipsilateral hemisphere as well as between the two hemispheres (▶Fig. 5.8).[15,16]

Following cutaneous stimulation of the fingers in healthy persons, the neurons in the contralateral primary somatosensory cortex are activated; interestingly, at the same time neurons in area 2 of the ipsilateral primary somatosensory cortex are inhibited (▶Fig. 5.9). During unilateral cutaneous finger stimulation, this is clinically reflected as an increase in the perception threshold in contralateral, nonstimulated, fingers.[17] However, the physiological meaning and the exact mechanisms of this ipsilateral inhibition are not completely understood. The dynamics between the primary somatosensory cortices in the two brain hemispheres, and especially the process of maintaining symmetric neuronal representations in the hemispheres, may be of importance for the control of symmetric bilateral motor activity.[15]

Following processing of the sensory information in the different areas of primary somatosensory cortex, the information is sent on to higher-order centers in the cerebral cortex, such as the secondary somatosensory cortex, where it forms the basis for object identification. Information is also sent to the primary motor cortex, where it forms the basis for object manipulation. Whereas the receptive fields in the primary somatosensory cortex are unilateral, the receptive fields in the secondary somatosensory cortex are often bilateral, including symmetric positions of the ipsilateral and contralateral hands. Furthermore, while the neurons in the primary somatosensory cortex respond exclusively to input from peripheral receptors, the secondary somatosensory cortex receives information from peripheral receptors, via the primary somatosensory cortex, and also from other higher-order areas such as those responsible for attention and goal setting.

5.4 Plasticity in the Somatosensory and Motor Systems

The brain has been seen as a rather static organ; until a few decades ago, it was widely believed by neuroscientists that no new neural connections could be formed in the adult brain. This picture has changed radically in the last decades. One of the most interesting questions in neuroscience today concerns the brain's ability to modify its organization and ultimately its function based on sensory input, experience, learning, and injury, a phenomenon often referred to as brain plasticity.[2,7]

The effectiveness of synaptic connections in somatosensory and motor systems is continuously adopted in response to functional demands—that is, activity-dependent plasticity. Synaptic transmission is facilitated in pathways that are frequently used, while those less used atrophy. In this way, repeated practice of a

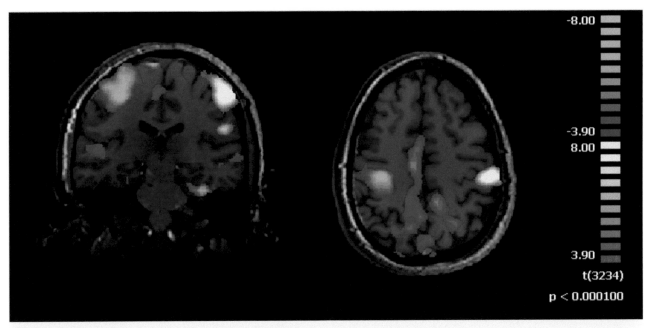

Fig. 5.9 MRI shows activation (color coding: *yellow* to *red*) in the contralateral primary somatosensory cortex following cutaneous stimulation of median nerve-innervated fingers. Simultaneous inhibition (color coding: *blue* to *green*) of primary somatosensory cortex ipsilateral to the stimulation.

task leads to increased speed and accuracy of performance; this is called long-term potentiation. These effects persist for some time after the initial stimulus and subsequently show gradual declines. Long-term potentiation is probably one of the major mechanisms by which somatosensory and motor learning and memory consolidation take place in the brain. For example, the "reading fingers" in blind humans who read Braille improve in accuracy, which is to say its sensibility, and more neurons are activated in the brain when they read or use their reading fingers for other tactile tasks.[18] Another example involves string players who manipulate the strings individually with their left hand and handle the bow with the right-hand, using all fingers together as a unit. The nerve cell representation of the right hand fingers in the motor cortex is identical to that of nonmusicians, whereas representation of the left-hand fingers is larger than in nonmusicians.[19,20] Inactivity of one hand, such as when placed in a cast, results in brain plasticity characterized by an increased cerebral representation of the nonimmobilized hand and decreased representation of the immobilized hand.[21]

An injury to the nervous system, involving the CNS or peripheral nervous system (PNS), also results in plasticity.[22–24] Following amputation of a finger, the neurons in the primary somatosensory cortex that process tactile information from the amputated finger start to respond to tactile stimulation from adjacent fingers instead.[25] Following amputation of an arm, primary somatosensory cortex areas representing the amputated hand and arm may start to respond to tactile stimulation of the face, the body area located next to the hand area in the primary somatosensory cortex. A surprising consequence of this is that these patients also may find that touching the face on the same side as the amputation causes tactile sensations corresponding to the amputated fingers.[26]

Several factors are of importance for the possibility of plasticity; most important is age, which diminishes the brain's capacity for plasticity. However, the capacity for plasticity is never lost.[27] Injuries to the CNS and PNS show a substantially better outcome in children compared to adults. A median nerve injury sustained before age 12 results, in general, in a very good clinical outcome, while the same injury sustained after age 12 results, in general, in a substantial somatosensory deficit; this difference in outcome has partly been attributed to greater plasticity in the young brain.[28,29]

Plasticity also opens possibilities for treating patients who have injuries in the CNS and PNS. The dynamic capacity of the brain can be guided using specific training programs or drugs to substitute for or improve functions that have been damaged or lost due to injuries.[30,31] In stroke patients with motor deficiencies of one hand, it has been shown that an injection of an anesthetic agent around the shoulder on the same side as the motor deficit hand, anesthetizing part of the brachial plexus that supplies the muscles around the shoulder, results in rapid improvement, within minutes after anesthesia, of motor function in the ipsilateral hand.[31] Furthermore, application of an anesthetic cream to the forearm in healthy persons as well as in patients with median nerve injuries results in a rapidly improved somatosensory function in the ipsilateral hand. In these cases, sensory stimulation of the hand during forearm anesthesia has been shown to activate the cortical hand and forearm areas; thus, the neurons—normally responding to tactile input from the forearm—start, after forearm anesthesia, to respond to tactile stimulation from the hand.[32]

Further knowledge of the cerebral mechanisms controlling somatosensory and motor functions in the hands and upper extremity and of how injury to nerves in the upper extremity affects the brain will present new possibilities for treating such injuries by targeting plasticity mechanisms in order to improve function.

Acknowledgments

I thank J. Lätt, P. Mannfolk, T. O. Strandberg, Á. Löve, and I. M. Björkman-Burtscher for providing illustrations; Skåne University Hospital; Center for Medical Imaging and Physiology; and Lund University, Sweden.

References

1. Purves D, Augustine GJ, Fitzpatrick D, Hall WC, LaMantia AS, White LE. Neuroscience. 5th ed. Sunderland, MA: Sinauer Associates Inc; 2012

2. Kandel ER, Schwartz JH, Jessel TM, Siegelbaum SA, Hudspeth AJ. Principles of Neural Science. 5th ed. New York, NY: McGraw Hill; 2013

3. Mountcastle V. The Sensory Hand. Cambridge, MA: Harvard University Press; 2005

4. Lundborg G. Nerve Injury and Repair. Regeneration, Reconstruction and Cortical Re-modelling. 2nd ed. Philadelphia, PA: Elsevier; 2004

5. Penfield W, Rasmussen T. The Cerebral Cortex of Man: A Clinical Study of Localization of Function. New York, NY: MacMillan; 1950

6. Graziano MS. Progress in understanding spatial coordinate systems in the primate brain. Neuron 2006;51(1):7–9

7. Purves D, Cabeza R, Huettel SA, LaBar KS, Platt ML, Woldorff MG. Principles of Cognitive Science. 2nd ed. Sunderland, MA: Sinauer Associates Inc; 2013

8. Goodale MA, Westwood DA, Milner AD. Two distinct modes of control for object-directed action. Prog Brain Res 2004;144: 131–144

9. Rizzolatti G, Craighero L. The mirror-neuron system. Annu Rev Neurosci 2004;27:169–192

10. Rizzolatti G, Luppino G. The cortical motor system. Neuron 2001;31(6):889–901

11. Rizzolatti G, Matelli M. Two different streams form the dorsal visual system: anatomy and functions. Exp Brain Res 2003;153(2): 146–157

12. Johnson KO. The roles and functions of cutaneous mechanoreceptors. Curr Opin Neurobiol 2001;11(4):455–461

13. Johansson R, Vallbo Å. Tactile sensory coding in the glabrous skin of the human hand. Trends Neurosci 1983;6:27–32

14. Shoham D, Grinvald A. The cortical representation of the hand in macaque and human area S-I: high resolution optical imaging. J Neurosci 2001;21(17):6820–6835

15. Calford MB, Tweedale R. Interhemispheric transfer of plasticity in the cerebral cortex. Science 1990;249(4970):805–807

16. Iwamura Y. Bilateral receptive field neurons and callosal connections in the somatosensory cortex. Philos Trans R Soc Lond B Biol Sci 2000;355(1394):267–273

17. Schäfer K, Blankenburg F, Kupers R, et al. Negative BOLD signal changes in ipsilateral primary somatosensory cortex are associated with perfusion decreases and behavioral evidence for functional inhibition. Neuroimage 2012;59(4):3119–3127

18. Barnes SJ, Finnerty GT. Sensory experience and cortical rewiring. Neuroscientist 2010;16(2):186–198

19. Elbert T, Rockstroh B. Reorganization of human cerebral cortex: the range of changes following use and injury. Neuroscientist 2004;10(2):129–141

20. Elbert T, Pantev C, Wienbruch C, Rockstroh B, Taub E. Increased cortical representation of the fingers of the left hand in string players. Science 1995;270(5234):305–307

21. Weibull A, Flondell M, Rosén B, Björkman A. Cerebral and clinical effects of short-term hand immobilisation. Eur J Neurosci 2011;33(4):699–704

22. Taylor KS, Anastakis DJ, Davis KD. Cutting your nerve changes your brain. Brain 2009;132(Pt 11):3122–3133

23. Chen R, Cohen LG, Hallett M. Nervous system reorganization following injury. Neuroscience 2002;111(4):761–773

24. Wall JT, Xu J, Wang X. Human brain plasticity: an emerging view of the multiple substrates and mechanisms that cause cortical changes and related sensory dysfunctions after injuries of sensory inputs from the body. Brain Res Brain Res Rev 2002;39(2–3): 181–215

25. Merzenich MM, Nelson RJ, Stryker MP, Cynader MS, Schoppmann A, Zook JM. Somatosensory cortical map changes following digit amputation in adult monkeys. J Comp Neurol 1984;224(4): 591–605

26. Ramachandran VS, Rogers-Ramachandran D. Phantom limbs and neural plasticity. Arch Neurol 2000;57(3):317–320

27. Pascual-Leone A, Freitas C, Oberman L, et al. Characterizing brain cortical plasticity and network dynamics across the age-span in health and disease with TMS-EEG and TMS-fMRI. Brain Topogr 2011;24(3–4):302–315

28. Chemnitz A, Andersson G, Rosén B, Dahlin LB, Björkman A. Poor electroneurography but excellent hand function 31 years after nerve repair in childhood. Neuroreport 2013;24(1):6–9

29. Chemnitz A, Björkman A, Dahlin LB, Rosén B. Functional outcome thirty years after median and ulnar nerve repair in childhood and adolescence. J Bone Joint Surg Am 2013;95(4):329–337

30. Duffau H. Brain plasticity: from pathophysiological mechanisms to therapeutic applications. J Clin Neurosci 2006;13(9): 885–897

31. Muellbacher W, Richards C, Ziemann U, et al. Improving hand function in chronic stroke. Arch Neurol 2002;59(8):1278–1282

32. Björkman A, Rosén B, Lundborg G. Acute improvement of hand sensibility after selective ipsilateral cutaneous forearm anaesthesia. Eur J Neurosci 2004;20(10):2733–2736

6 Structure and Function of Muscles

Richard L. Lieber and Jan Fridén

6.1 Overview

The functional abilities of the hand and upper extremity occur by the integration of several systems. Movement is accomplished by contraction of muscles that interact with the skeletal system to achieve a vast array of motions and joint configurations. The astounding dexterity of the hand is the result of the great diversity of skeletal muscles. In this chapter, macroscopic and microscopic aspects of muscle structure are discussed, with emphasis on their relationships to muscle function and their clinical significance.

6.2 Muscle Architecture

Gross examination reveals that most skeletal muscles have a common thematic arrangement: the bulk of the muscle is composed of fibers that project from proximal to distal tendons, which in turn arise from and insert onto bony structures. However, the manner in which these fibers are organized is hugely variable and has profound effects on the physiological properties of muscles.[1,2] This arrangement of muscle fibers, relative to the axis of force generation, is referred to as "muscle architecture."

The categories of muscle architecture are numerous. For simplicity, it is easiest to consider broad organization of muscle fibers in one of three categories. Muscles with fibers arranged parallel to the axis of motion are termed "longitudinal." Longitudinal muscles make up a relatively small proportion of the muscle in the body; many muscles have fibers that are oriented obliquely to the muscle's line of action. The angle between this line of action and the muscle fibers is termed the "pennation angle," and these muscles are classified as "unipennate" and "multipennate" depending on whether their fibers have single or variable pennation angles, respectively.

Based on geometric considerations, it is easy to understand why differences in fiber pennation affect force production capacity between muscles. Consider a simple longitudinal muscle in which every fiber can produce the same amount of force. Adding more fibers in parallel would result in greater force production capacity. However, anatomic space limitations prevent the unlimited addition of fibers in parallel. By placing fibers at an angle, it becomes possible to increase the number of fibers without changing the total volume occupied by the muscle. Modulation of pennation angle allows the placement of muscles in a way that best fits within the anatomic constraints that arise due to the bony skeleton.

6.2.1 PCSA and Fiber Length

Although changing pennation angle increases fiber number while maintaining a constant volume, these fibers do not contract in a line that is parallel with the line of action of the muscle, and they will also necessarily be shorter than the original fibers. These two alterations have physiologic consequences. To summarize the overall effects of muscle fiber arrangement,

two important architectural parameters are used: physiological cross-sectional area (PCSA) and fiber length (L_f). These are considered the most important parameters because they are the most predictive of muscle biomechanical function.

L_f determines the excursion of a muscle. Muscle fibers are composed of many repeating subunits (sarcomeres) that can expand or contract in length. Placing more sarcomeres in series (i.e., having a longer muscle fiber) changes its total excursion capability because excursion of the fiber may be calculated as the sum of the excursions of the individual sarcomeres in series.

PCSA is an important determinant of muscle function because it is the only architectural parameter that is directly related to the maximum force capacity of a muscle.[3] PCSA cannot be measured directly—it is a conceptual "cross-sectional area" that represents the total functional cross-sectional area of all the muscle fibers. It is calculated using the equation

$$PCSA = \frac{muscle\ mass \times \cos(\theta)}{\rho \times L_f}$$

which has been validated in a guinea pig hindlimb model.[3] In this equation, ρ represents muscle density[4] and θ represents pennation angle. Inspection of this equation reveals the basis for its form. Mass/density gives muscle volume, and dividing the volume by fiber length yields a cross-sectional area. However, due to pennation angle, fibers do not pull strictly in line with the axis of force generation, so not all of the force produced is transmitted to the tendons and into joint movement. To estimate the percentage of total force that contributes to functional motion, the term is scaled by the factor of the cosine of the pennation angle. This term arises from a geometric consideration of fiber pennation and standard trigonometric relationships.

By considering these two factors simultaneously, it is possible to compare architectural organization among muscles. Presentation in graphical form (▶ Fig. 6.1) makes it possible to visualize groupings and differences among upper-extremity muscles. While many variables may be considered when comparing skeletal muscles, it has been determined that PCSA and L_f are the two strongest discriminating factors—that is, that plotting muscle data on the PCSA–L_f plane will provide the greatest spread between the data.[5] As part of this analysis, a "score" for quantitatively describing the difference between two muscles was developed and is termed the architectural difference index (ADI). To reconstruct lost muscle function (secondary to trauma, nervous system injury, tendon rupture, etc.), a functional donor muscle is transferred to recapitulate the function that has been lost. Donor selection is a key surgical choice, and ADI may be a reasonable benchmark for selecting potential donor muscles or deciding between two potential transfers (ADI for potential upper extremity pairings are summarized in Table 6.1). It would be unwise to transfer a donor muscle whose force production potential or excursion is vastly different from that of the target muscle. In fact, architectural mismatch has been blamed for the poor clinical results observed in the flexor carpi ulnaris to extensor digitorum communis tendon transfer.[6]

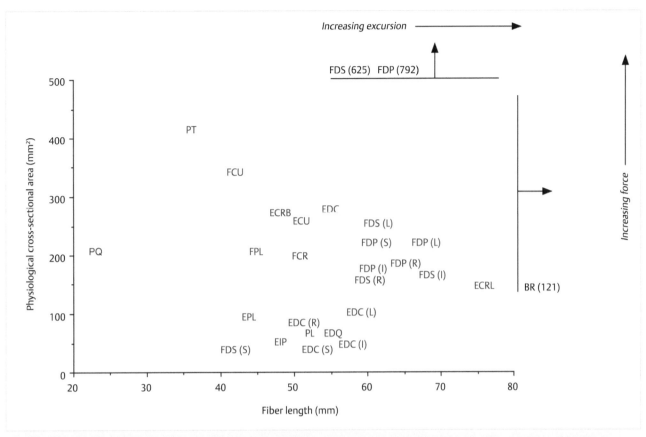

Fig. 6.1 Scatter graph of PCSA and L_f for muscles of the human hand and forearm. L_f is proportional to muscle excursion, and PCSA is proportional to maximum tetanic force. The architectural similarity between two muscles can be quantified via the ADI. Data collated from several studies.[7–9] BR, brachioradialis; EDC (I), extensor digitorum communis to the index; EDC (L), extensor digitorum communis long; EDC (R), extensor digitorum communis ring; and EDC (S), extensor digitorum small fingers, respectively; EDC, combined properties of the individual EDC bellies, considered as a single muscle; ECRB, extensor carpi radialis brevis; ECRL, extensor carpi radialis longus; ECU, extensor carpi ulnaris; EDQ, extensor digiti quinti; EIP, extensor indicis proprius; EPL, extensor pollicis longus; FCR, flexor carpi radialis; FCU, flexor carpi ulnaris; FDP (I), FDP (L), FDP (R), and FDP (S), flexor digitorum profundus muscles; FDP, combined properties of FDP bellies; FDS (I), FDS (L), FDS (R), and FDS (S), flexor digitorum superficialis muscles; FDS, combined properties of FDS bellies; FPL, flexor pollicis longus; PQ, pronator quadratus; PL, palmaris longus; PT, pronator teres.

6.2.2 Mechanics of Joint Motion

While muscle architecture yields important information about how muscles produce force and over what distance, this information by itself is not sufficient to provide an understanding of how muscle contraction corresponds to joint movement. This is because joint movement must be considered in the context of rotational physics—how the muscle traverses its joint(s) determines how linear contraction of muscle fibers translates into rotational joint motion. The moment arm is defined as the distance between the muscle and the center of rotation of the joint that it crosses; the joint torque is the product of the muscle force and the moment arm (▶ Fig. 6.2). Increasing moment arm, therefore, enables greater torque production for a given force. However, increasing moment arm often occurs at the expense of range of motion; greater linear muscle excursion is needed to obtain the same angular motion.

One set of structures that help illustrate the interplay among moment arm, force, and range of motion are the pulleys found on flexor side of the fingers. The pulleys keep the flexor tendons in close apposition to the bone surface—the moment arms at the joints are therefore small (in the 7- to 17-mm range),[10] allowing full finger closure through the actions of flexor digitorum superficialis and flexor digitorum profundus. In the setting of a flexor tendon injury to this region that needs surgical repair, it is sometimes necessary to release a pulley for surgical access. The general surgical dogma is that the A2 and A4 pulleys should be repaired if release was necessary[11,12]; the increase in moment arm means that the muscle excursion may not be sufficient to fully close the finger into a tight fist after pulley release.[13] However, recent work suggests that reconstruction of A4 may not be necessary after repair of a flexor tendon injury in this region, since the skin itself is a fairly effective pulley.[14]

6.3 Molecular Anatomy

Physiological parameters observed in muscle arise due to molecular interactions. Several key proteins, actin and myosin, are responsible for force development through active contraction. The force that arises from active muscle contraction is termed active tension, while passive tension is the force associated with passive muscle stretch without contraction. Like a rubber band, muscles produce a restoring force when stretched beyond a slack length, and the proteins thought to be associated

Table 6.1 Architectural difference index values for muscles of the human forearm

	FCR	FCU	PL	ECRB	ECRL	ECU	FDS (I)	FDS (L)	FDS (R)	FDS (S)	FDP (I)	FDP (L)	FDP (R)	FDP (S)	FPL	EDC (I)	EDC (L)	EDC (R)	EDC (S)	EDQ	EIP	EPL	PT	PQ
FCR																								
FCU	0.63																							
PL	0.63	1.23																						
ECRB	0.36	0.65	0.87																					
ECRL	0.94	1.40	0.94	0.86																				
ECU	0.27	0.39	0.90	0.33	1.06																			
FDS (I)	0.31	0.62	0.78	0.56	0.99	0.34																		
FDS (L)	0.42	0.46	1.02	0.38	1.00	0.23	0.37																	
FDS (R)	0.20	0.80	0.52	0.43	0.78	0.43	0.34	0.51																
FDS (S)	0.84	1.44	0.25	1.03	1.03	1.10	1.01	1.23	0.73															
FDP (I)	0.22	0.77	0.62	0.35	0.73	0.39	0.34	0.43	0.12	0.82														
FDP (L)	0.46	0.51	1.02	0.49	1.02	0.31	0.30	0.14	0.52	1.25	0.45													
FDP (R)	0.24	0.63	0.71	0.50	0.95	0.32	0.08	0.38	0.26	0.95	0.27	0.33												
FDP (S)	0.27	0.66	0.79	0.23	0.78	0.29	0.37	0.28	0.29	0.99	0.18	0.34	0.32											
FPL	0.15	0.61	0.65	0.44	1.07	0.30	0.39	0.50	0.32	0.84	0.36	0.54	0.32	0.40										
EDC (I)	0.77	1.38	0.20	0.96	0.86	1.03	0.91	1.13	0.63	0.21	0.71	1.14	0.84	0.88	0.81									
EDC (L)	0.59	1.21	0.28	0.73	0.68	0.84	0.74	0.92	0.43	0.40	0.49	0.93	0.67	0.65	0.65	0.25								
EDC (R)	0.58	1.20	0.10	0.80	0.87	0.85	0.75	0.97	0.46	0.27	0.56	0.98	0.68	0.73	0.61	0.20	0.20							
EDC (S)	0.78	1.39	0.16	1.01	0.98	1.05	0.92	1.17	0.66	0.15	0.76	1.17	0.86	0.93	0.80	0.13	0.34	0.21						
EDQ	0.61	1.19	0.12	0.89	1.01	0.87	0.72	1.00	0.51	0.34	0.62	0.99	0.67	0.79	0.62	0.30	0.36	0.20	0.24					
EIP	0.77	1.39	0.20	0.96	0.91	1.04	0.94	1.15	0.65	0.12	0.74	1.17	0.87	0.90	0.80	0.11	0.28	0.20	0.12	0.31				
EPL	0.53	1.11	0.19	0.79	1.04	0.79	0.72	0.95	0.48	0.35	0.58	0.96	0.65	0.74	0.51	0.38	0.38	0.21	0.32	0.19	0.34			
PT	0.71	0.57	1.26	0.45	1.24	0.54	0.87	0.58	0.84	1.41	0.77	0.72	0.83	0.63	0.72	1.36	1.15	1.19	1.39	1.27	1.34	1.15		
PQ	0.92	1.42	0.75	0.87	0.86	1.01	1.18	1.20	0.86	0.69	0.87	1.28	1.11	0.95	0.95	0.70	0.26	0.68	0.76	0.86	0.64	0.77	1.14	
BR	10.3	1.30	1.24	1.02	0.74	1.05	0.86	0.89	0.91	1.43	0.84	0.82	0.88	0.84	1.16	1.23	1.06	1.19	1.32	1.23	1.31	1.30	1.34	1.48

Abbreviations: BR, brachioradialis; EDC (I), extensor digitorum communis to the index; EDC (L), extensor digitorum communis long; EDC (R), extensor digitorum communis ring and; EDC (S), extensor digitorum communis small fingers, respectively; EDC, combined properties of the individual EDC bellies, considered as a single muscle; ECRB, extensor carpi radialis brevis; ECRL, extensor carpi radialis longus; ECU, extensor carpi ulnaris; EDQ, extensor digiti quinti; EIP, extensor indicis proprius; EPL, extensor pollicis longus; FCR, flexor carpi radialis; FCU, flexor carpi ulnaris; FDP (I), FDP (L), FDP (R), and FDP (S), flexor digitorum profundus muscles; FDP, combined properties of FDP bellies; FDS (I), FDS (L), FDS (R), and FDS (S), flexor digitorum superficialis muscles; FDS, combined properties of FDS bellies; FPL, flexor pollicis longus; PQ, pronator quadratus; PL, palmaris longus; PT, pronator teres.

Source: Adapted from Lieber and Brown.[5]

Note: Values range from about 0.1 to 1.8, with a mean value of 0.74.

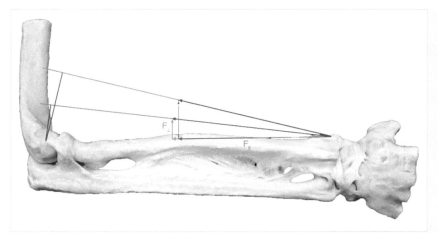

Fig. 6.2 Force diagram illustrating the effect of different moment arms. The force path of two muscles with different moment arms are illustrated in *blue* and *green*, and the moment arms are noted in *red*. Parallel ($F_{||}$) and perpendicular ($F_\perp$) force vectors associated with active contraction of these muscles are shown in *purple*, with their component forces illustrated in *gray*. Note that the muscle with the longer moment arm has the larger perpendicular component force vector, meaning that it can generate more torque.

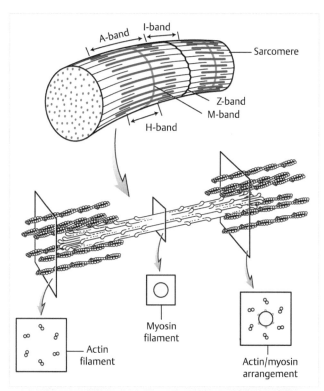

Fig. 6.3 Schematic diagram of a sarcomere. The two primary components responsible for active tension are actin and myosin. Note that myosin filaments have a bare region in the middle that is devoid of myosin heads. The main intracellular component that plays a role in passive tension is titin, which extends the length of a half-sarcomere.

with passive tension are titin and collagen. These proteins and their respective locations within the sarcomere are summarized in ▶ Fig. 6.3.

6.3.1 Active Tension

During active tension production, myosin and actin interact to produce force. The overlap of the two myofilaments is the key determinant of force production capability,[15] as summarized for isometric contractions of a single sarcomere in ▶ Fig. 6.4.

The shape of this sarcomere length–tension relationship is best understood through a consideration of the organization of myosin filaments. Myosin filaments are composed of bundles of myosin molecules, each of which has a head domain (responsible for interaction with actin filaments) and a long tail domain, which are connected through a neck domain. The myosin molecules assemble in an antiparallel fashion; a myosin filament therefore has a region of myosin heads at each end and an area in its middle in which myosin heads are absent.

This structural motif is responsible for the plateau and descending regions in ▶ Fig. 6.4. The plateau represents complete overlap by actin of the region of the myosin filament that contains the heads; changing sarcomere length in this region does not change force production, because there is no change in the number of cross-bridges between actin and myosin filaments due to the middle region of the filament, where heads are absent. However, stretch beyond the plateau results in a linear decrease in force production, as the actin filaments pass through the area of the myosin filament that contains the head domains. Overlap between actin and myosin continues to decrease with increasing sarcomere length and force production capacity disappears when myosin and actin filaments no longer overlap. The exact sarcomere length at which this occurs depends on the length of the filaments—myosin filaments are 1.65 µm long and actin filaments vary from 1 to 1.4 µm, with some dependence on fiber type.[16]

Shortening the sarcomere from the plateau region also causes a decrease in force. At short sarcomere lengths, actin from one half of a sarcomere slides into the region typically occupied by actin from the other half. While this overlap of actin filaments is possible, it is not optimal; actin from one side may interfere with actin–myosin cross-bridge formation. Accordingly, force continues to decrease with sarcomere shortening.

Muscle models are often predicated upon the assumption that muscles are optimized for efficiency and thereby assume minimization of performance criteria (such as mechanical work, energy expenditure, and tracking error),[17] with muscles thought likely to operate primarily on the plateau region of their length–tension curves. However, few data support this conclusion. In fact, past experiments involving wrist movers have demonstrated unexpected sarcomere length ranges.[18–20] Understanding the normal sarcomere length operating range may be critical for any surgical procedure that changes muscle length, such as tendon transfers.

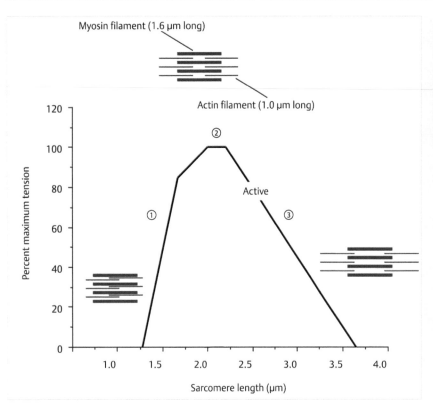

Myosin filament (1.6 µm long)

Actin filament (1.0 µm long)

Fig. 6.4 Relationship between sarcomere length and predicted isometric force. The ascending limb (region 1) represents interference in actin–myosin cross-bridge formation by actin from the other half of the sarcomere. The plateau (region 2) reflects optimal actin–myosin overlap, which decreases as the sarcomere extends into the descending limb (region 3), producing correspondingly less force.

Another strong determinant of active tension physiology is muscle fiber type. There are a variety of methods for classifying muscle fibers based on parameters, such as metabolic pathway, immunohistochemistry, and myosin heavy-chain (MHC) isoform. While they differ slightly in exact classification, the three broad categories of fibers are slow oxidative, fast oxidative/glycolytic, and fast glycolytic, which describe maximum contraction speed as well as metabolic mechanism. These categories correspond broadly to the presence of MHC-1, MHC-2A, and MHC-2X isoforms in the muscle fibers. Despite the difference in fiber-shortening speed, this likely has little applicability to muscle performance or physiology. However, muscle fibers do exhibit differential fatigue patterns and are associated with differing motor unit sizes. Slow oxidative fibers generally are the most fatigue-resistant and are associated with small motor neurons that innervate few fibers. Conversely, fast glycolytic fibers have poor endurance capacity and are found in motor units with large neurons that innervate many fibers. Fast oxidative/glycolytic fibers are intermediates, in terms of both fatigue resistance and motor unit innervation number.

When compared with the rest of the upper extremity, intrinsic muscles of the hand have significantly more slow myosin than muscles of the arm or forearm. It has been suggested that this may reflect the importance of precise manual dexterity.[21] The need for dexterity to be augmented by good range of motion and force production capability is reflected by the composition of extrinsic muscles of the hand, found in the forearm. The size of the forearm allows placement of muscles with fiber lengths and PCSAs large enough to provide sufficient excursion and force at the digital and carpal joints, thereby enhancing the intrinsic dexterity of the hand. The lower amounts of slow myosin found in these forearm muscles imply that force production

is prioritized over fatigue resistance and that motor control of forearm muscles does not need to be as precisely regulated as that of the hand.

6.3.2 Passive Tension

Stretched muscle produces a restoring force without active contraction. This force is termed "passive tension," and the exact nature of its origin is of interest to both basic scientists and clinicians. Understanding the components that contribute to passive tension may help better define the molecular pathology of spasticity seen in cerebral palsy (or other upper motor neuron injury) or decreased range of motion observed in muscle injury. Clinicians also have interest in passive tension; during tendon transfers, surgeons choose donor muscle length based on muscle "feel"—specifically, they use passive tension to guide their intraoperative decisions. This practice is supported and advocated for in current surgical texts.[12,22] However, no clear relationship has been established between whole muscle passive and active tension production systems, so it is unclear whether using passive tension as a tool for surgical decision making is the optimal strategy. In fact, one study examined the sarcomere length of donor muscles after tendon transfer and found that donor muscles were transferred at long sarcomere lengths and were predicted to generate less than 30% of their maximal force.[23]

The two main proteins currently thought to bear passive load in muscle are titin[24,25] and extracellular collagen. Titin is a giant protein that extends half the length of the sarcomere and has been clearly implicated in passive load bearing within the sarcomere.[26] Furthermore, it has been shown that the molecular weight of titin may vary between muscles, and it has been suggested that this may account for variations in passive tension between muscles.[27] However, when tested at larger size scales that included extracellular matrix material, muscle stiffness was found to be much greater in fiber bundles, which include the extracellular matrix, than in single fibers.[28] This finding suggests that extracellular collagen may be the primary contributor to passive tension at scales beyond single fibers. Furthermore, in whole muscle preparations, it was found that passive tension experimental behavior correlated poorly with theoretical predictions.[29] These findings support the idea that when considering whole muscles, titin may not be a major determinant of passive tension.

A recent study showed that hand muscles have more collagen and larger titins than skeletal muscle from all regions of the body that were studied, making the muscles of the hand very unique in their biochemical makeup.[21] The exact interpretation of these findings is not yet precisely defined. It is known that titin has a role in mechanotransduction,[30] so it has been suggested that modulation of titin size may serve to modify this protein's mechanotransduction capability.

It is also important that clinicians are aware of the role that collagen plays in passive tension; the high amounts of collagen found in hand muscles may have clinically relevant correlations in hand surgery and rehabilitation. There still is much to be learned about passive tension; the specific roles of titin and collagen remain active questions of scientific study.

References

1. Burkholder TJ, Fingado B, Baron S, Lieber RL. Relationship between muscle fiber types and sizes and muscle architectural properties in the mouse hindlimb. J Morphol 1994;221(2):177–190

2. Lieber RL, Fridén J. Functional and clinical significance of skeletal muscle architecture. Muscle Nerve 2000;23(11):1647–1666

3. Powell PL, Roy RR, Kanim P, Bello MA, Edgerton VR. Predictability of skeletal muscle tension from architectural determinations in guinea pig hindlimbs. J Appl Physiol 1984;57(6):1715–1721

4. Ward SR, Lieber RL. Density and hydration of fresh and fixed human skeletal muscle. J Biomech 2005;38(11):2317–2320

5. Lieber RL, Brown CC. Quantitative method for comparison of skeletal muscle architectural properties. J Biomech 1992;25(5):557–560

6. Lieber RL, Pontén E, Burkholder TJ, Fridén J. Sarcomere length changes after flexor carpi ulnaris to extensor digitorum communis tendon transfer. J Hand Surg Am 1996;21(4):612–618

7. Fridén J, Lieber RL. Quantitative evaluation of the posterior deltoid to triceps tendon transfer based on muscle architectural properties. J Hand Surg Am 2001;26(1):147–155

8. Lieber RL, Fazeli BM, Botte MJ. Architecture of selected wrist flexor and extensor muscles. J Hand Surg Am 1990;15(2):244–250

9. Lieber RL, Jacobson MD, Fazeli BM, Abrams RA, Botte MJ. Architecture of selected muscles of the arm and forearm: anatomy and implications for tendon transfer. J Hand Surg Am 1992;17(5):787–798

10. Franko OI, Winters TM, Tirrell TF, Hentzen ER, Lieber RL. Moment arms of the human digital flexors. J Biomech 2011;44(10):1987–1990

11. Lister GD. Incision and closure of the flexor sheath during primary tendon repair. Hand 1983;15(2):123–135

12. Wolfe SW, Hotchkiss RN, Pederson WC, Kozin SH, eds. Greene's Operative Hand Surgery. 6th ed. Philadelphia, PA: Elsevier; 2011

13. Doyle WB. The finger flexor tendon sheath and pulleys: anatomy and reconstruction. Paper presented at: the AAOS Symposium on Tendon Surgery; 1975; St. Louis, MO

14. Franko OI, Lee NM, Finneran JJ, et al. Quantification of partial or complete A4 pulley release with FDP repair in cadaveric tendons. J Hand Surg Am 2011;36(3):439–445

15. Gordon AM, Huxley AF, Julian FJ. The variation in isometric tension with sarcomere length in vertebrate muscle fibres. J Physiol 1966;184(1):170–192

16. Gokhin DS, Kim NE, Lewis SA, Hoenecke HR, D'Lima DD, Fowler VM. Thin filament length correlates with fiber type in human skeletal muscle. Am J Physiol Cell Physiol 2012;302(3):

17. Kaufman KR, An KW, Litchy WJ, Chao EY. Physiological prediction of muscle forces—I. Theoretical formulation. Neuroscience 1991;40(3):781–792

18. Lieber RL, Fridén J. Intraoperative measurement and biomechanical modeling of the flexor carpi ulnaris-to-extensor carpi radialis longus tendon transfer. J Biomech Eng 1997;119(4):386–391

19. Lieber RL, Ljung BO, Fridén J. Sarcomere length in wrist extensor muscles. Changes may provide insights into the etiology of chronic lateral epicondylitis. Acta Orthop Scand 1997;68(3):249–254

20. Lieber RL, Loren GJ, Fridén J. In vivo measurement of human wrist extensor muscle sarcomere length changes. J Neurophysiol 1994;71(3):874–881

21. Tirrell TF, Cook MS, Carr JA, Lin E, Ward SR, Lieber RL. Human skeletal muscle biochemical diversity. J Exp Biol 2012;215(Pt 15):2551–2559

22. Berger RA, Weiss A-PC. Hand Surgery. Philadelphia, PA: Lippincott Williams & Wilkins; 2004

23. Fridén J, Lieber RL. Evidence for muscle attachment at relatively long lengths in tendon transfer surgery. J Hand Surg Am 1998;23(1):105–110

24. Magid A, Law DJ. Myofibrils bear most of the resting tension in frog skeletal muscle. Science 1985;230(4731):1280–1282

25. Wang K, McCarter R, Wright J, Beverly J, Ramirez-Mitchell R. Viscoelasticity of the sarcomere matrix of skeletal muscles. The titin-myosin composite filament is a dual-stage molecular spring. Biophys J 1993;64(4):1161–1177

26. Labeit S, Kolmerer B. Titins: giant proteins in charge of muscle ultrastructure and elasticity. Science 1995;270(5234):293–296

27. Prado LG, Makarenko I, Andresen C, Krüger M, Opitz CA, Linke WA. Isoform diversity of giant proteins in relation to passive and active contractile properties of rabbit skeletal muscles. J Gen Physiol 2005;126(5):461–480

28. Meyer GA, Lieber RL. Elucidation of extracellular matrix mechanics from muscle fibers and fiber bundles. J Biomech 2011;44(4):771–773

29. Winters TM, Takahashi M, Lieber RL, Ward SR. Whole muscle length-tension relationships are accurately modeled as scaled sarcomeres in rabbit hindlimb muscles. J Biomech 2011;44(1):109–115

30. Krüger M, Linke WA. The giant protein titin: a regulatory node that integrates myocyte signaling pathways. J Biol Chem 2011;286(12):9905–9912

7 Ultrastructure of Bones and Joints

Gregory I. Bain, Duncan McGuire, and Quentin Fogg

7.1 Bone

7.1.1 Subchondral Bone Plate

The subchondral bone plate underlies the articular cartilage and is composed of three to five layers of bone. The layers are bridged by trabecular struts and, in some cases, plates of bone, thus separating the layers with small spherical voids (▶Figs. 7.1 and 7.2). This arrangement is referred to as the subchondral multilaminar plate. The thickness of the subchondral multilaminar plate and the number of laminations increase in the zones of highest stress. Typically, in the center of the joint there are up to five laminations, while away from the center of the joint there are often two or three laminations.

Immediately below the subchondral bone plate is the metaphysis. This area consists of trabecular bone with a complex arrangement that takes the physiological loads from the articular surface and spreads them down to the metaphyseal and diaphyseal regions of the bone. The subchondral bone has spherical voids between the trabeculae; however, further away from the subchondral bone plate, the voids become ellipsoid.

The structure of the cortical and trabecular bone is determined by genetic factors and by Wolff's law. As can be seen in ▶Fig. 7.3, thick struts of bone extend down from the volar aspect of the lunate facet to the volar cortex of the distal radius.

7.1.2 Corner Zones

There is a concentration of cancellous bone at the corner areas of the distal radial metaphysis. These are located at the dorsal, radiopalmar, and ulnopalmar corners and consist mainly of platelike trabeculae. On serial sectioning, an appreciation can be gained for this distribution (▶Fig. 7.4). We propose that these concentrations of trabeculae merge and reinforce the cortical pillars.

7.1.3 Physeal Scar

There is an axially oriented condensation of trabeculae spanning the entire width of the distal radius. This is the physeal scar, the remnant of the epiphyseal growth plate. The trabeculae of the transition zone merge with this layer distally and with the trabecular vault proximally (▶Fig. 7.5).

7.1.4 Trabecular Vault

The metaphyseal region of the distal radius has a relatively thin cortex and contains a concentration of cancellous bone arranged in a series of arches. We have called this structure the trabecular vault. The apex of the arch lies deep to the physeal scar and extends down toward the thicker cortex of the metaphyseal–diaphyseal junction (▶Figs. 7.5 and 7.6). This arrangement is very similar to that seen in the arches of a gothic cathedral.

The cancellous bone in this region consists principally of platelike trabeculae in a longitudinal arrangement. The

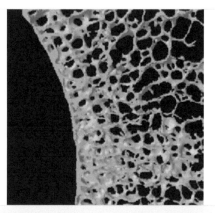

Fig. 7.1 The subchondral multilaminar plate comprises three to five layers of bone separated by small spherical voids.[1]

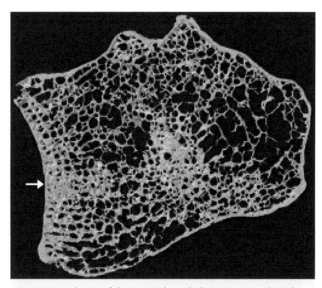

Fig. 7.2 Axial view of the sigmoid notch demonstrating the subchondral multilaminar plate (*arrow*).[1]

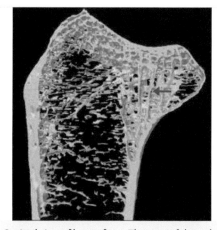

Fig. 7.3 Sagittal view of lunate facet. The apex of the trabecular vault is eccentrically located, toward the volar lip of the distal radius. There is trabecular reinforcement of the volar aspect of the lunate facet (*arrow*).[1]

plates of trabeculae are interconnected by smaller struts (or rods) of cancellous bone, features that have been previously described.[2]

The trabecular vault underlying the lunate facet typically has its apex located eccentrically toward the volar lip of the distal radius to accommodate the volar projection of the lunate facet (▶ Fig. 7.6). There is typically trabecular reinforcement of the volar aspect of the lunate facet (▶ Fig. 7.3). The apex of the trabecular vault underlying the scaphoid facet is centrally rather than eccentrically located (▶ Fig. 7.5).

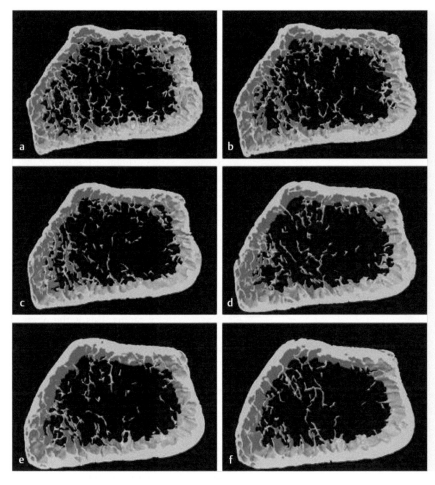

Fig. 7.4 (a–f) Serial sections of the distal radial metaphysis. There are concentrations of trabeculae at the dorsal, radiopalmar, and ulnopalmar corners. Image (a) is most distal and (f) is most proximal.[1]

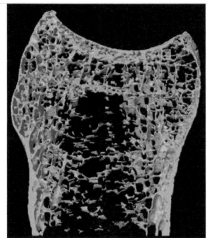

Fig. 7.5 Sagittal view of the distal radius through the scaphoid facet. The distal radius comprises a thin metaphyseal cortex and a thicker diaphyseal cortex. The metaphyseal region contains a concentration of cancellous bone arranged in a series of arches and is called the trabecular vault. The physeal scar abuts the apex of the trabecular vault. There is a subchondral bone plate underlying the articular surface; this structure is called the subchondral multilaminar plate.[1]

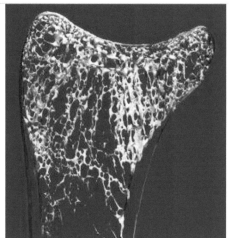

Fig. 7.6 Sagittal view of the lunate facet demonstrating the trabecular vault. The trabecular vault's apex is eccentrically located toward the volar lip of the distal radius.[1]

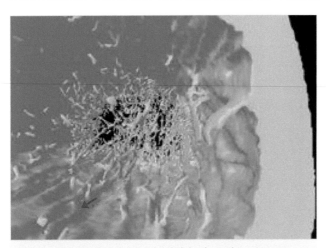

Fig. 7.7 Axial view of the distal radial diaphysis demonstrating the trabeculae as they contribute to the formation of the longitudinal subcortical ridges of bone (*arrow*).[1]

7.1.5 Pillars

We identified the presence of three cortical thickenings representing the three pillars of the distal radius. These are located on the radiopalmar, ulnopalmar, and dorsal aspects of the metaphyseal–diaphyseal junction of the distal radius. It can be clearly seen that the relative density of the cortex is greater at the three pillars of the metaphyseal–diaphyseal junction. It is our belief that these pillars are the principal areas of force transmission from the articular surface, through the trabecular vault to the shaft of the radius.

7.1.6 Diaphysis

The endosteal surface of the metaphyseal–diaphyseal junction and the diaphysis are lined by longitudinally arranged ridges of bone (▶ Fig. 7.7). Individual trabeculae of the trabecular vault can be seen to insert into the endosteal surface of the bone, contributing to the formation of these longitudinal ridges. The longitudinal ridges then continue into the diaphyseal region.

Cartilage

The articular cartilage of the joint is an important anatomical structure. It reduces friction and allows smooth, painless movement between joint surfaces. The chondrocyte is a highly specialized cell and is the only cell type found in cartilage. It is found within the matrix, which also consists of collagen, proteoglycans, and noncollagenous proteins. In hyaline cartilage, 95% of the collagen is type II collagen, which is very stable and has a half-life of 25 years. Collagen arcades are important for resisting tensile forces within the cartilage. The chondral matrix has a high water content (up to 80% of cartilage weight), which is important because the hydrostatic pressures within the cartilage can absorb stresses that are placed onto it. Proteoglycans are produced by the chondrocytes and are made up of glycosaminoglycans, of which chondroitin sulfate and keratin sulfate are the predominant types. Proteoglycans retain and regulate the water content in cartilage and so play an important role in the age-related degeneration of articular cartilage.[3] The chondrocytes within the articular cartilage have a low metabolic rate, and it is for this reason that they are able to

survive only on the oxygenation from the synovial fluid. The articular surface is covered with synovial fluid. Due to the hydrophobic chains, a barrier layer is created that is important for minimizing friction at the articular surface. There are no blood vessels, lymphatic vessels, or nerves in cartilage.[4]

The ability of cartilage to heal is limited by a lack of vascularity and undifferentiated cells that can migrate to, and participate in, the repair process. Superficial cartilage injuries have a very limited inflammatory response due the avascularity of the area and do not heal. Deeper injuries that penetrate the subchondral bone incite a classic inflammatory reaction, with cells entering the defect from the bone marrow space.[5] Mesenchymal cells then differentiate to form fibrocartilage and repair the defect. However, this type of cartilage is inferior to the native hyaline cartilage and is only half as thick.

Immobilization of a joint has a profound effect on cartilage. It has been shown in animal and human studies that there is significant cartilage thinning in response to immobilization and lack of weight bearing.[6] It has also been shown that cartilage's biochemical and biomechanical properties do not return to normal levels even after long-term follow-up, although the clinical significance of this is uncertain.[7]

Within the joint, structures such as the synovial fringes or plicae are common. These assist in distribution of the synovial fluid throughout the joint. Capsular tissues that take a load will tend to form fibrocartilage or even bone. Good examples of this are the patella, the volar plate with the sesamoids, and the dorsal plate of the proximal interphalangeal (PIP) joint.

Ligaments

Composition

Ligaments consist of 60 to 70% water. Eighty percent of their dry weight is made up of collagen (mostly type I collagen with smaller amounts of the other types, appearing mainly around the insertions to bone). Proteoglycans make up about 1% of the dry weight and are responsible for binding water and growth factors.[8]

Ligaments are extremely resilient structures, and they are loaded cyclically more than virtually any other structure in the body. Like bone, ligaments adjust their mechanical properties in response to load. This has been shown by the deterioration of ligament properties in response to immobilization.[9] With exercise-related loading, they then improve their properties, but at a much slower rate.

Function

The ligaments are primarily responsible for providing stability of the individual joint. There are always six degrees of freedom for any joint. The congruency of the joint intrinsically provides stability to the joint. The ligaments are the primary stabilizer of the joint and are increasingly important, particularly in joints where there is less congruency.

The joint will usually have a primary plane of motion, such as PIP joint flexion–extension plane. It therefore requires restraints in the other degrees of freedom, which are radial deviation, ulnar deviation, supination, and pronation. Each ligament will have a primary function; for example, the ulnar collateral ligament prevents radial deviation. Idealistically, the orientation of each

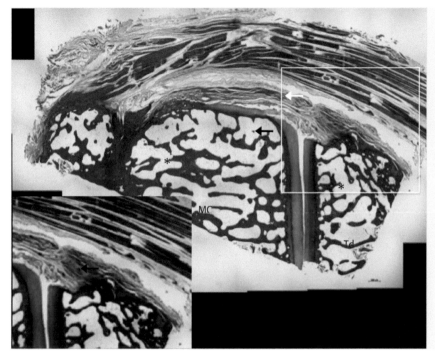

Fig. 7.8 Attachment of tendon and capsule. This longitudinal section of the second carpometacarpal joint demonstrates the distal attachment of the extensor carpi radialis longus tendon (*white arrow*) and the carpometacarpal joint capsule (*black arrow*). The entheses of both soft tissues can be compared; notice, in particular, the thickening of bone at each attachment (*). The white rectangular is the area of the zoomed-in picture on the bottom left. This enables the detail of the capsular attachment to be more clearly visualized. The thickened core of the capsule (*black arrow*) may be considered ligamentous, with a thin epiligamentous layer of disorganized tissue providing passage and support for other tissues. Modified Masson's Trichrome, ×20.[10]

ligament complex will be orthogonal to the other ligament complexes. Due to the variety of functions that are required of the various joints, this rule angle approximates 90°.

The ligament functions as an organ of tension, and on the opposite side of the joint will be an articulation that acts in compression. For example, the ulnar collateral ligament at the PIP joint when placed under strain will lead to loading of the radial condyle of the PIP joint.

Ligament Insertion to Bone

The attachment of ligament to bone is a complex structure designed to dissipate forces over the transition area. There are two types of insertions: direct and indirect. The direct insertion is more common, with the transition occurring through four zones, from tendon substance to fibrocartilage to calcified fibrocartilage and then merging into the bone.[11] The indirect insertion is more complex and consists of distinct superficial and deep fibers that merge with the periosteum. The ligament is attached firmly to the bone by structures called Sharpey's fibres.[12] Bone is often thickened at the site of a ligament insertion (▶Fig. 7.8).

Ligament Injuries

When the joint is taken past its physiological load, the bone will fracture, or the ligament will be torn from the bone, or the ligament will rupture midsubstance. Because of the orientation of the individual ligaments within a joint, the ligamentous injury that occurs often tears in a **Z** configuration. Once the ligament gives way, the line of tension will be to the edge of the ligament and often the line of weakness between one ligament and the other. With further rotation of the joint, it is common for the next ligament to then be under tension, and that ligament will often fail at the opposite end of the articulation to produce a Z-type tear.

If the magnitude of force is greater, then multiple ligaments may be avulsed from the same bone. This is seen on the medial epicondyle during elbow dislocations and also in ulnar translocation of the carpus.

The ligament insertion is important in the development of intra-articular fractures. There is a strong association between the location of the fractures and the ligament insertions.[13] There is an inverse relationship between the location of the ligaments and the location of the fracture. It is likely that when the joint reaches the extreme of physiological motion, the tension within the ligament complex causes a localized area of compression and ultimate fracture.

The insertion site is also known as an enthesis, and stress concentrations at this transition site make it vulnerable to acute or overuse injuries, especially in sport. Ligaments tolerate forces parallel to their fibers and insertion sites well. However, they do not tolerate shear forces well and fail at a much lower load when forces are perpendicular to their insertions.[14] They are also the primary targets in the inflammatory spondyloarthropathies, most commonly ankylosing spondylitis and rheumatoid arthritis.[15] All fibrocartilage associated with normal entheses is avascular, which contributes to a poor healing response at and near attachment sites.[16]

7.1.7 Capsule

The joint capsule is similar in structure to ligaments. It consists of dense fibrous connective tissue and is lined by synovium (▶Fig. 7.9). Similar to bone, the capsule's thickness and fiber orientation vary depending on the stresses it endures in different regions. The capsule is often supported by tendons which attach to it, such as the rotator cuff and distal radius (▶Fig. 7.10). Nerve supply to the capsule and synovium is usually from the nerves that innervate the muscles acting on the joint, which supply pain and proprioceptive fibers. Capsular tissue may be modified to form part of the actual joint; for example, the meniscus in the knee joint is modified capsular tissue with type II collagen which has formed fibrocartilage.[17] The attachment to bone is through the same insertional transition zone as ligaments.

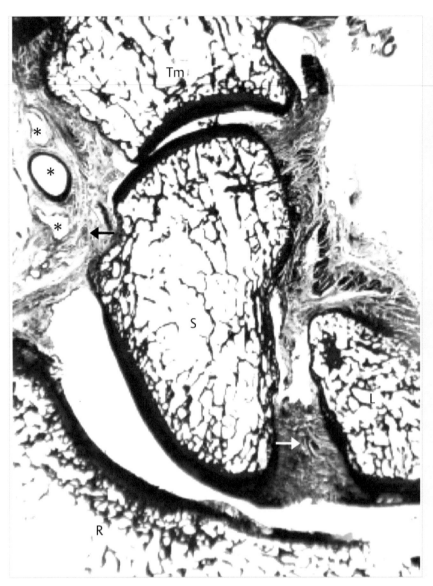

Fig. 7.9 This coronal section of the wrist demonstrates the thick, organized fibers of an interosseous ligament (scapholunate ligament, *white arrow*) and the bony attachment of disorganized capsular tissue (*black arrow*). This section emphasizes the importance of the capsular tissue in supporting vasculature (*), in this case the radial artery and its venae comitantes. L, lunate; R, radius; S, scaphoid; Tm, trapezium. Modified Masson's trichrome, ×20.[9]

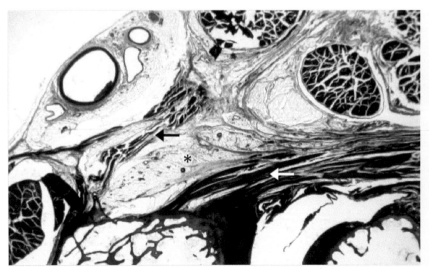

Fig. 7.10 Ligament versus joint capsule. The radial wrist capsule demonstrates well-organized (regular) bands of dense (red-staining) fibers; these may be described as distinct ligaments, such as the radiocarpal ligament demonstrated (*white arrow*) or the thickened band (*black arrow*) connected to the sheath of the flexor carpi radialis tendon. The tissue between these bands (*) is composed of thin, disorganized (irregular) fibers and neurovascular structures. MC, metacarpal; Td, trapezoid; Modified Masson's trichrome, ×100.[9]

References

1. Gregory Ian Bain, Simon Bruce Murdoch MacLean, Tom McNaughton, Ruth Williams. Microstructure of the Distal Radius and Its Relevance to Distal Radius Fractures, Wrist Surg 2017; 06(04):30–315

2. Kinney JH, Ladd AJ. The relationship between three-dimensional connectivity and the elastic properties of trabecular bone. J Bone Miner Res 1998;13(5):839–845

3. Karvonen RL, Negendank WG, Teitge RA, Reed AH, Miller PR, Fernandez-Madrid F. Factors affecting articular cartilage thickness in osteoarthritis and aging. J Rheumatol 1994;21(7):1310–1318

4. Mankin HJ, Grodzinsky AJ, Buckwater JA. Articular cartilage and ostcoarthritis. In: Einhorn TA, O'Keefe RJ, Buckwalter JA, eds. Orthopaedic Basic Science: Foundations of Clinical Practice. 3rd ed. Rosemont, IL: American Academy of Orthopaedic Surgeons; 2007:191–222

5. Frisbie DD, Oxford JT, Southwood L, et al. Early events in cartilage repair after subchondral bone microfracture. Clin Orthop Relat Res 2003;(407):215–227

6. Hinterwimmer S, Krammer M, Krötz M, et al. Cartilage atrophy in the knees of patients after seven weeks of partial load bearing. Arthritis Rheum 2004;50(8):2516–2520

7. Hudelmaier M, Glaser C, Hohe J, et al. Age-related changes in the morphology and deformational behavior of knee joint cartilage. Arthritis Rheum 2001;44(11):2556–2561

8. Frank CB, Shrive NG, Lo IKY, Hart DA. Form and function of tendon and ligament. In: Einhorn TA, O'Keefe RJ, Buckwalter JA, eds. Orthopaedic Basic Science: Foundations of Clinical Practice. 3rd ed. Rosemont, IL: American Academy of Orthopaedic Surgeons; 2007:191–222

9. Yasuda K, Hayashi K. Changes in biomechanical properties of tendons and ligaments from joint disuse. Osteoarthritis Cartilage 1999;7(1):122–129

10. Fogg QA. Scaphoid Variation and an Anatomical Basis for Variable Carpal Mechanics (thesis). Adelaide: University of Adelaide, Department of Anatomical Sciences; 2004:161–221.

11. Clark J, Stechschulte DJ Jr. The interface between bone and tendon at an insertion site: a study of the quadriceps tendon insertion. J Anat 1998;192(Pt 4):605–616

12. Raspanti M, Cesari C, De Pasquale V, et al. A histological and electron-microscopic study of the architecture and ultrastructure of human periodontal tissues. Arch Oral Biol 2000;45(3):185–192

13. Mandziak DG, Watts AC, Bain GI. Ligament contribution to patterns of articular fractures of the distal radius. J Hand Surg Am 2011;36(10):1621–1625

14. Woo SL, Smith DW, Hildebrand KA, Zeminski JA, Johnson LA. Engineering the healing of the rabbit medial collateral ligament. Med Biol Eng Comput 1998;36(3):359–364

15. Benjamin M, McGonagle D. The anatomical basis for disease localisation in seronegative spondyloarthropathy at entheses and related sites. J Anat 2001;199(Pt 5):03–526

16. Benjamin M, Toumi H, Ralphs JR, Bydder G, Best TM, Milz S. Where tendons and ligaments meet bone: attachment sites ('entheses') in relation to exercise and/or mechanical load. J Anat 2006;208(4):471–490

17. Ralphs JR, Benjamin M. The joint capsule: structure, composition, ageing and disease. J Anat 1994;184(Pt 3):503–509

8 The Blood Vessels and Microcirculation

Maria Siemionow, Jacek Szopinski, and Krzysztof Kusza

8.1 Vascular Supply to the Hand from the Base to the Fingertips

With the advancement of hand surgery and techniques of vascular imaging, knowledge of vascular anatomy of the hand is mandatory. During the early embryonic period, the axial artery arises initially and then develops into the brachial artery in the upper arm and the interosseous artery in the forearm, providing the main supply of blood to the upper extremity. Next, the median (MA), ulnar, and radial (RA) arteries appear as sprouts of the arterial trunk. In the beginning, the MA, together with the interosseous artery, is involved in the majority of the blood supply to the forearm and hand; however, it dwindles after the second embryonic month and is replaced by the ulnar and radial arteries. Finally, the RA and UA provide most of the blood supply to the hand and are supported by the MA and interosseous arterial system.

The blood vessels in the hand communicate via four major arches: the anterior and posterior carpal arch at the level of carpal bones and the superficial and deep palmar arch (SPA and DPA) at the midpalmar level. These arches form three circuits on the palmar side and one circuit on the dorsal side of the hand. The dorsal arch is the source vessel for the anatomically diverse dorsal metacarpal artery system. The SPA and DPA are the most important, because they provide the blood supply to all of the fingers. The SPA represents the last segment of the ulnar artery and runs in the volar aspect of the midpalm, dorsal to the palmar aponeurosis and volar to the flexor tendons and the lumbrical muscles. Despite statements indicating that the variations in the SPA are so numerous that it is difficult to establish a specific type, a wide variety of classification systems can be found in classical anatomy textbooks and the literature. The SPA is classified between complete and incomplete types. Either the existence of an anastomosis with a contributing artery or the situation when the UA alone reaches the index finger is defined as complete arch (85%) (▶ Fig. 8.1). When no

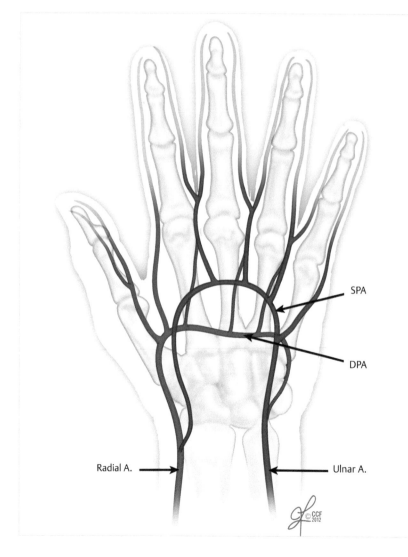

SPA

DPA

Radial A.   Ulnar A.

Fig. 8.1 Schematic drawing of the complete types of the superficial and deep palmar arches (SPA and DPA). (Reprinted with permission, Cleveland Clinic Center for Medical Art & Photography © 2012. All Rights Reserved.)

presence of such anastomosis can be seen, the SPA is defined as incomplete (15%) (►Fig. 8.2). Bilateralism of the complete SPA can be detected in 80% of patients, and the same type of arch can be found in 60% of cases. Bilateralism of incomplete SPA can be detected less frequently (4%).[1]

At the adult stage, the MA sometime remains (0.9–20% of cases) as a thin artery that runs along the median nerve, frequently arising from the common or anterior interosseous artery.[2] It may terminate at the wrist, anastomose with the SPA (►Fig. 8.3), or give off branches to the index finger and thumb at the palmar side without anastomosing with the RA or UA.

The DPA is formed mainly by the RA that passes to the dorsal side of the hand under the abductor pollicis longus and extensor pollicis brevis tendons. It then pierces the first (or, rarely, second) interosseous space and forms the DPA with the deep palmar branch of the UA (►Fig. 8.1). The DPA does not have as many variations as the SPA but may be incomplete as well (►Fig. 8.4) and is a source of three to four palmar metacarpal arteries.

Arterial vascularization of the palmar subcutaneous tissue is supported by palmar branches (4–12, average 7) arising from the main digital arteries. The branches anastomose with their counterparts on the opposite side within the subcutaneous tissue. There are three anatomical patterns: I-shaped (64%), with a single vessel, narrow V-shaped (23%) with a bifurcation starting at the origin of the vessel, and Y-shaped (13%), branching off beyond the origin of the vessel.[3] The small vein or veins accompanying the palmar branches drain either into the superficial longitudinal venous network or into the deep venous network accompanying the main digital artery.

Recent studies on vascular anatomy of the upper extremity demonstrate a great deal of variability in the first web space as the source of vessels for blood supply to the thumb and index finger, as well as in their communications with the ulnar-sided vessels.

At the level of fingertips, the microcirculatory network of the nail folds is accessible for in vivo examination (capillaroscopy). Capillaroscopy gives remarkable information from both clinical and diagnostic points of view. In healthy adults, the capillaroscopic pattern consists of parallel capillary loops disposed in rows and formed by an arteriolar afferent branch, a reflexion apex, and a venular efferent branch. The capillary arteriolar branch usually has a diameter inferior to the venular one. The arteriovenous ratio is about 1:5 to 1:2.

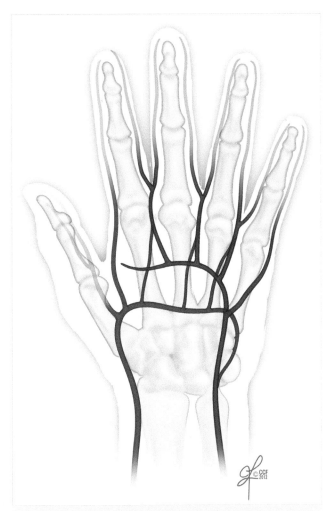

Fig. 8.2 Schematic drawing of an incomplete SPA. (Reprinted with permission, Cleveland Clinic Center for Medical Art & Photography © 2012. All Rights Reserved.)

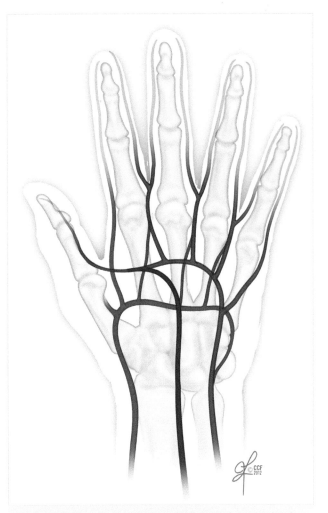

Fig. 8.3 Median artery contributing to the SPA. (Reprinted with permission, Cleveland Clinic Center for Medical Art & Photography © 2012. All Rights Reserved.)

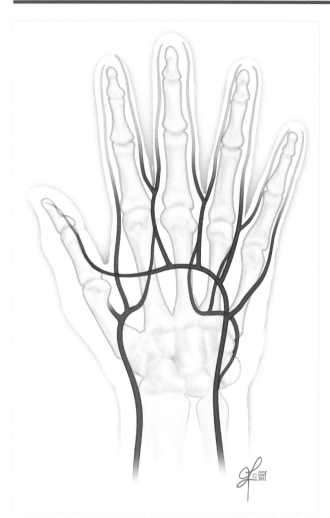

Fig. 8.4 Schematic drawing of an incomplete DPA. (Reprinted with permission, Cleveland Clinic Center for Medical Art & Photography © 2012. All Rights Reserved.)

8.2 Differences between Large, Medium-Sized, and Small Arteries and Veins and the Vascular Network of the Microcirculation

The wall composition of vessels has been described as consisting of three structurally distinct layers: the intima (endothelium), media, and adventitia (▶ Fig. 8.5). The structure and the thickness of each separate layer depend on the size and function of the vessel in the vascular system (▶ Table 8.1). Moreover, evidence suggests that the cellular and extracellular components of these three layers are interconnected in multiple ways; thus, their traditionally distinct boundaries are blurred.

The *intima*, a physiological barrier between blood components and extravascular tissues, consists of endothelial cells and a basement membrane. The endothelial cells are arranged longitudinally in the direction of flow with an overall thickness of 0.2 to 0.5 µm, except the location of cell nucleus. In feeding arterioles, the endothelial cells are approximately 100 µm in length

by 10 µm in width, and this 10:1 ratio is reduced as downstream arterioles diminish in diameter. The endothelial cells functionally participate in controlling vessel tone via production and release of vasoactive cytokines that influence the neighboring smooth muscle cells. Recently, the intracellular cytoskeletal components were intensively studied and it was found that they participate in the signaling pathways, causing the synthesis and release of the vasoactive factors that ultimately fine-tune the contractile state of vessels' smooth muscle cells in response to blood flow or pressure stimuli. The shear forces caused by blood flow induce the stress fiber formation and the stabilization of microtubules, allowing the polarization of the endothelial cells, with the microtubule-organizing center redistributed to the downstream side of the nucleus. The endothelial cells within the intima may vary phenotypically. Between the typical endothelial cells, the endothelial progenitor cells can be found; they are able to transdifferentiate into mesenchymal cells with smooth muscle phenotype.

The basement membrane under endothelial cells is approximately 0.1 µm in thickness and consists primarily of collagen type IV, laminin, and heparan sulfate proteoglycans. Additional components include collagens type I, III, and V, and fibronectin. Besides its primary function, which is to provide anchoring support for the endothelium, basement membrane exposed to blood components after injury provides signals for the recruitment and migration of cells across the vessel wall.[4]

The *media* consists of cells and the extracellular matrix (ECM). The ECM consists of lamellae of elastic material with intervening layers of vascular smooth muscle (VSM) cells, collagen fibers, and ground substance. The ECM is responsible for the passive mechanical properties of the arteries. In the proximal aorta, elastin is the dominant component of the ECM, whereas in the distal aorta and its branches the collagen-to-elastin ratio is reversed, with a predominance of collagen in peripheral muscular arteries. The proportion of elastin and collagen type I and type III differs markedly between species and has a substantially differential mechanical effect on the stiffness and distensibility of the vessel wall. Additionally, since the structure of ECM is determined at a very young developmental stage and thereafter remains quite stable, several neurohormonal factors as well as chemical modifications (i.e., glycation, cross-linking) may modulate the properties of the ECM during the subject's life. The morphology supports the main role of the very proximal part of vascular system (i.e., aorta and its major branches), which is to serve as a temporal buffer for the blood during the ejection phase of the heart.

In the distal arteries and at the level of microcirculation, VSM cells largely predominate within the media, forming one or more cell layers (i.e., one or two layers in feed arterioles). The VSM cells control vascular diameter via cell contraction and relaxation processes. The VSC cells are spindle-shaped, with an average length of approximately 100 µm, arranged perpendicular to the longitudinal axis of the vessel in a circumferential fashion. The cells wrap around the vascular circumference and maintain their position but sometimes overlap each other transversally to the longitudinal axis of the vessel wall. The population of VSM cells is not homogenous. They may have different mixtures of phenotypes, not only with contractile and synthetic but also with proliferative and apoptotic behavior. The occurrence of

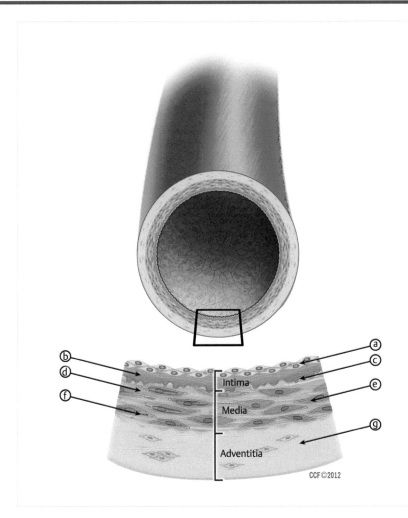

Fig. 8.5 Schematic representation of an arteriole. The arteriolar wall consists of three layers: the intima, media, and adventitia. Endothelial cells **(a)** run parallel to the longitudinal axis and sit on a basement membrane **(b)** apposed by an internal elastic lamina **(c)**. Extracellular matrix (ECM) **(d)** with vascular smooth muscle cells (VSM) **(e)** creates the media. Cytoskeletal stress fibers **(f)** within the VSM cells play an important role in vessel's response to pressure. The adventitia is predominantly created by the fibroblasts and ECM **(g)**. (Reprinted with permission, Cleveland Clinic Center for Medical Art & Photography © 2012. All Rights Reserved.)

Table 8.1 Function and histological compartments of vessels within the vascular system

	Large arteries	Medium-sized arteries	Arterioles	Capillaries	Venules
Diameter	>2 mm	150 µm to 2 mm	8–150 µm	<8 µm	>15 µm
Wall thickness	1 mm	1 mm	6 µm	0.5 µm	1 µm
Intima	+	++	+++	+++	+
Media	++	++	+	0	+
Function	Conduit; compliance	Compliance; resistance	Resistance	Exchange	Collection

each of the phenotypes depends not only on age but also on location in the vascular tree and prevailing conditions. Moreover, the embryonic origin of the different VSM cells is different in various parts of the vascular tree. In the avian abdominal aorta and small muscular arteries, the VSM cells are of mesodermal origin, whereas those of the aortic arch and thoracic aorta are mainly derived from the ectodermal cardiac neural crest—essential in the formation and organization of elastic laminae and tensoreceptors in the great vessels.[5] In the microcirculation network, the VSM cells are created during embryogenesis, as a result of complex angiogenesis in hypoxic conditions.

In arterioles, besides the VSM cells, an internal elastic lamina can be found. The internal elastic lamina is a sheet of approximately 0.3 µm in thickness consisting primarily of degradation-resistant elastin molecules. The lamina is not present in all arterioles but is supposed to provide the recoil properties of the vessel wall that are important in dealing with pulsatile blood pressure. Interestingly, the internal elastic lamina appears wavy with evenly distributed ridges, which suggests that under physiological conditions it does not contribute significantly to the viscoelastic characteristics of the vessel wall. Additionally, on scanning micrographs, small fenestrae can be observed within the solid structure of the internal elastic lamina. The fenestrae grow in size and number during development, enable the transport of molecules from the blood to the media and extravascular tissues, and allow for direct contact between endothelial and VSM cells.[6] Importantly, the size and number of these holes have been shown to change in response to different stimuli, which potentially makes the structure able to remodel rapidly.

The *adventitia* consist of some fibroblasts, not surrounded by the basement membrane, embedded in an ECM made of thick bundles of collagen fibers oriented along the longitudinal axis of the vessel. Some cells in the adventitia considered as the fibroblasts are probably stem mesenchymal progenitor cells. Within adventitia of the arterioles, the nonmyelinated nerve endings are also present at a distance of approximately 5 µm from the outermost VSM.[7] Additionally, the elastic fibers arranged with a longitudinal pitch are also present, especially in the expandable tissues such as skeletal muscles. Historically, the adventitia was considered as a structural support for the vessel and a scaffold for the anchoring of nerve endings. Currently, it is suggested that the fibroblasts contribute to the plasticity of the arteriolar wall (modulation of VSM activity), participate in production and remodeling of the ECM compounds (TGF-β, endothelin-1, α-actin), generate inflammatory signals, and potentially contribute to the generation of tensile force. In response to injury, the fibroblasts can transform to myofibroblasts and perhaps into smooth muscle cells, which play crucial role in the vascular repair.

8.3 Outline of Anatomy and Physiology of Microcirculation for Metabolite Exchange

The microcirculatory network represents the most distal segment of the vascular tree and is characterized by arteriolar diameters equal to or below 150 µm. The microcirculatory network consists of arterioles, venules, and capillaries. The terminal arteriolar branching patterns not only vary between tissues and organs but also may change during the subject's life (▶ Fig. 8.6). Several physiological mechanisms, such as gas and metabolite exchange, as well as heat exchange, take place at the microcirculatory level.[8]

The macrocirculation and the microcirculation are integrally and functionally dependent segments of the blood circulation and cannot be discussed separately. Due to cyclical activity of the cardiac pump and the properties of the aorta, the proximal part of the arterial tree corresponds to vascular territory with the presence of pulsatile pressure and flow. The pulsatility is progressively attenuated (▶ Fig. 8.7). In the static model, arterial pressure is the mean arterial pressure, which depends on cardiac output (CO) and peripheral vascular resistance (PVR). The CO is a function of heart rate and stroke volume. The PVR is influenced by blood viscosity, vessel diameter, and vessel length, according to Poiseuille's law. Since microcirculation represents a distal part of the vascular tree, the pulsatile function has almost completely disappeared and the resistance for a single vessel can be calculated as the mean pressure divided by the blood flow.[9] However, pulsatile pressure

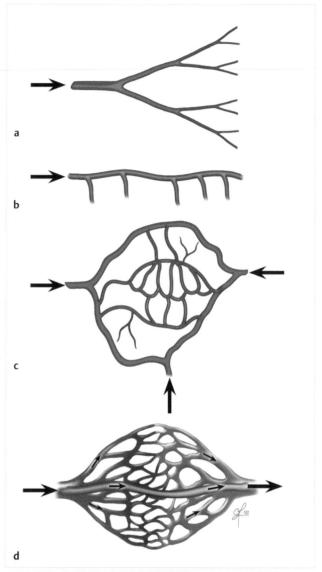

Fig. 8.6 Schematic representations of the terminal arteriolar branching patterns within the microcirculation: **(a)** a symmetrical tree; **(b)** asymmetrical tree; **(c)** arteriolar–arteriolar connections; **(d)** symmetrical tree with metarteriole (arteriovenous shunt). (Reprinted with permission, Cleveland Clinic Center for Medical Art & Photography © 2012. All Rights Reserved.)

generated by heart penetrates deeply into the microcirculation. By contrast, reflected waves that originate in the microcirculation influence pressure pulse in the macrocirculation (Fig. 8.7). Pressure registered in the capillaries of the extremities ranges from 10 to 20 mm Hg. Pressure and flow within the microcirculation are under acute and long-term control systems.[10] Acute control includes nervous mechanisms, myogenic response, flow-dependent dilation, and vasomotion. Long-term regulation includes structural changes (smooth muscle hypertrophy/hyperplasia and radial growth of lumen), which are determined by shear and circumferential stress and functional changes (regulation of vascular tone by circulation vasoactive hormones).

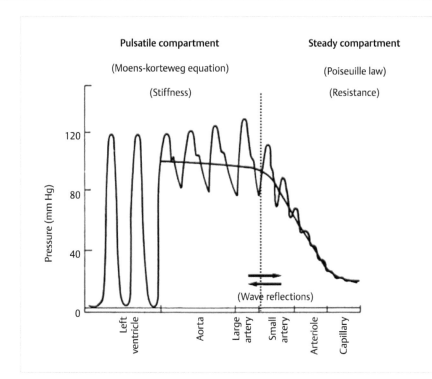

Fig. 8.7 Blood pressure along the arterial tree. The systolic blood pressure and pulsatile pressure are amplificated from the proximal to the distal part of the macrocirculation. The pulsatile pressure is attenuated till arterioles and almost disappears at the level of capillaries. (Reproduced with permission from Safar ME, Boudier HS. Vascular development, pulse pressure, and the mechanism of hypertension. Hypertension 2005;46:206.)

Oxygen delivery to tissues has traditionally been considered to take place almost exclusively at the capillary level. Currently, there is strong evidence that a substantial amount of oxygen is exchanged through the arterioles (sometimes to greater degree than in capillaries) and in postcapillary venules. Moreover, the gas exchange is not just a simple process of one-way diffusion (O_2 transport to tissues and CO_2 from tissues), but the gas diffusive transfer between microvessels may also play an important role in tissue oxygenation. The parallel arrangement of small arteries and veins results in relatively easy oxygen transfer from arterial to venous vessels and may result in diffusion shunting of oxygen. The gas transfer from arterioles to capillaries and among capillaries contributes to homogenous tissue oxygenation. CO_2 diffusion from venules to arterioles reduces pH in arterial blood and thus increases O_2 release from hemoglobin. In this regard, it has been shown that diffusion shunting of O_2 from arterioles to the postcapillary venules is enhanced during hyperoxia, while during hypoxia CO_2 accumulates in the peripheral vessels.[11] Longitudinal O_2 gradients and spatial heterogeneity are only weakly dependent on mean systemic blood pressure, supporting the hypothesis that venules play an important role in oxygen delivery. Fluid, electrolytes, gases, and small and large molecular weight substances can transverse the capillary endothelium by several different mechanisms: diffusion, bulk flow, vesicular transport, and active transport. The input of the microcirculation after hand trauma, ischemia–reperfusion injury, and no-reflow phenomenon should be always considered and assessed.

References

1. Bilge O, Pinar Y, Ozer MA, Gövsa F. A morphometric study on the superficial palmar arch of the hand. Surg Radiol Anat 2006;28(4): 343–350
2. Tsuruo Y, Ueyama T, Ito T, et al. Persistent median artery in the hand: a report with a brief review of the literature. Anat Sci Int 2006;81(4): 242–252
3. Voche P, Merle M. Vascular supply of the palmar subcutaneous tissue of fingers. Br J Plast Surg 1996;49(5):315–318
4. Siemionow M, Wang WZ, Anderson G, Firrell J. Leukocyte--endothelial interaction and capillary perfusion in ischemia/reperfusion of the rat cremaster muscle. Microcirc Endothelium Lymphatics 1991;7(4–6):183–197
5. Rosenquist TH, Beall AC, Módis L, Fishman R. Impaired elastic matrix development in the great arteries after ablation of the cardiac neural crest. Anat Rec 1990;226(3):347–359
6. Martinez-Lemus LA. The dynamic structure of arterioles. Basic Clin Pharmacol Toxicol 2012;110(1):5–11
7. Rhodin JA. The ultrastructure of mammalian arterioles and precapillary sphincters. J Ultrastruct Res 1967;18(1):181–223
8. Szopinski J, Kusza K, Semionow M. Microcirculatory responses to hypovolemic shock. J Trauma 2011;71(6):1779–1788
9. Safar ME, Struijker-Boudier HA. Cross-talk between macro-and micro-circulation. Acta Physiol (Oxf) 2010;198(4):417–430
10. Siemionow M, Arslan E. Ischemia/reperfusion injury: a review in relation to free tissue transfers. Microsurgery 2004;24(6): 468–475
11. Tritto I, Ambrosio G. Spotlight on microcirculation: an update. Cardiovasc Res 1999;42(3):600–606

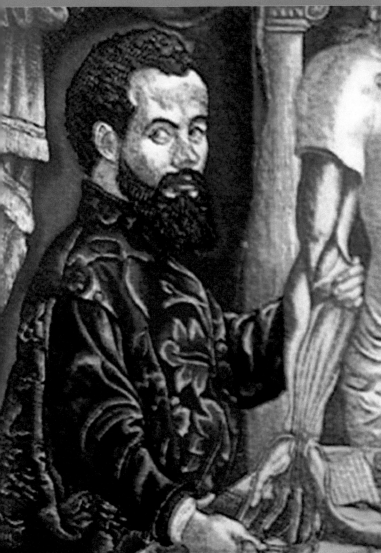

Section III

General Anatomy and Function

Vesalius

9 Nerves of the Upper Extremity

Peter Hahn and Ranjan Gupta

The great German philosopher Immanuel Kant once stated, *"The hand is the visible part of the brain."* With our hands, we have the ability to build, fabricate, and manifest our creativity. Without them, humanity ceases to evolve. Our hands, *the active agents of the cerebral system, and by extension, the human soul* (taken from the *Karma Indriya*), are in turn controlled by the complex neural network of the upper extremity. This network of nerves is named the brachial plexus and bridges the gap between the cerebrum and the hand, thereby allowing the translation of thought into gestures and meaningful function.

The brachial plexus is regularly formed by ventral rami from C5–T1, with contributions from C4 and T2 nerve roots intermittently,[1,5] and is responsible for the innervation of the entire upper limb. The plexus formation begins at the level of the scalene muscles, continues under the clavicle, and ends at the level of the axilla. The portion of the plexus within the posterior triangle of the neck is referred to as the supraclavicular region (▶Fig. 9.1), whereas the portion distal to the axilla is known as the infraclavicular region (▶Fig. 9.2). The brachial plexus is divided into roots, trunks, divisions, cords, and terminal branches (▶Fig. 9.3).[1,5] These roots are derived from the five ventral rami of the spinal nerves from C5–T1, after they have given off segmental supply to the muscles of the neck. They emerge from the interval between the anterior and middle scalene muscles. Near the posterior portion of the first rib, the ventral rami merge to form trunks. C5 and C6 rami unite to from the superior trunk, C7 rami continue to form the middle trunk, and C8 and T1 rami unite to form the inferior trunk. Near the lateral region of the first rib, each trunk splits into an anterior and a posterior division, giving rise to three anterior divisions and three posterior divisions. Ultimately, the anterior divisions give rise to nerves that innervate the anterior compartments of the upper limb, whereas the posterior divisions innervate the posterior parts of the limb.

At the level of the proximal third of the clavicle, the six divisions regroup to form three cords. The anterior divisions of the superior and middle trunks unite to form the lateral cord. The anterior division of the inferior trunk continues as the medial cord, while the three posterior divisions of each trunk join to form the posterior cord. These cords traverse with and span the first and second parts of the axillary artery; their names indicate their position with respect to the axillary artery. At the level of the axilla, the cords recombine and divide to form terminal branches. The lateral cord gives rise to the musculocutaneous nerve. The medial cord gives off the ulnar nerve and medial cord of the median nerve. The remaining portions of the

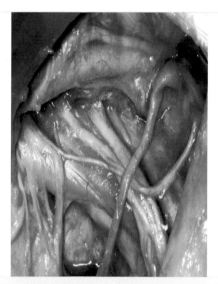

Fig. 9.1 Supraclavicular branches of the brachial plexus are located in the posterior triangle of the neck.

Fig. 9.2 Infraclavicular branches of brachial plexus are located in the axilla.

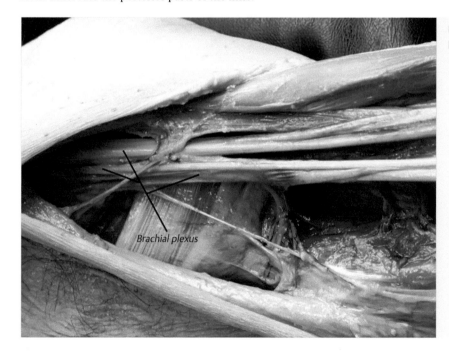

Brachial plexus

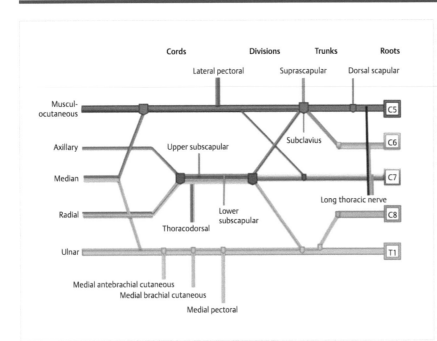

Fig. 9.3 Distribution of the brachial plexus.

medial and lateral cords then combine to form the median nerve, whereas the posterior cord ultimately branches into the axillary and radial nerves.

Branches of the Brachial Plexus

Several branches stem throughout the brachial plexus. They are divided into the *supraclavicular* and *infraclavicular* branches.

9.1 Supraclavicular Branches of the Brachial Plexus

At the posterior triangle of the neck, the supraclavicular nerves of the brachial plexus arise from the rami and trunks of the brachial plexus (▶ Fig. 9.1).

The first nerve from the brachial plexus that arises proximally is the *dorsal scapular nerve*,[2] and it originates from the fifth cervical ventral ramus in the majority (75%) of cases within the posterior cervical triangle deep to the prevertebral fascia. It courses through the middle scalene muscle and travels posteriorly between the posterior scalene muscle and the serratus posterior superior and levator scapulae muscles to innervate the rhomboid major and minor muscles and, occasionally, the levator scapulae muscles.

The *long thoracic nerve*[3] innervates the serratus anterior muscle; arises from the posterior aspect of the ventral rami of C5, C6, and C7; and travels through the apex of the axilla posterior to the brachial plexus. The first two roots (C5 and C6) pierce the substance of the scalenus medius muscle and then unite and join the C7 root on the surface of the scalenus medius muscle. It then travels beneath the posterior aspect of the trunks of the brachial plexus and stays within the fascia. After its supraclavicular course, the long thoracic nerve approaches the superior margin of the first rib at the middle axillary line, and continues obliquely in an anterosuperior to posteroinferior

direction in the axilla. At the posterior angle of the second rib, the nerve becomes embedded in the fascia of the serratus anterior muscle and descends inferiorly between the middle and posterior axillary lines, giving off two or three branches to each digitation of the muscle as it progresses.

The *suprascapular nerve*[4,5] (▶ Fig. 9.4) is a mixed motor and sensory nerve originating from the ventral rami of spinal nerves C4, C5, and C6 or at the upper trunk of the brachial plexus. It innervates the supraspinatus and infraspinatus muscles as well as the glenohumeral joint. The *suprascapular nerve* initially passes through the scapular notch inferior to the transverse scapular ligament. From there, it courses obliquely and laterally in the supraspinous fossa along the inferior surface of the supraspinatus muscle to the base of the scapular spine. It then curves medially to innervate the infraspinatus muscle. The muscular branch to the supraspinatus muscle arises behind the transverse scapular ligament. The sensory branch of the suprascapular nerve comes off immediately after passing the suprascapular notch, turns laterally along the base of the coracoid process, and eventually innervates the acromioclavicular joint and the superior aspect of the subacromial bursa. Additionally, just before entering the infraspinous fossa, a branch of the suprascapular nerve runs laterally and enters the posterior inferior aspect of the capsule deep to the tendons of the infraspinatus muscle.

The *nerve to the subclavius muscle*[1] arises anterior from the superior trunk of the brachial plexus. With contributions primarily from C5 and occasionally from C4 and C6, it descends posterior to the clavicle but in front of the brachial plexus and supplies the subclavius muscle.

Branches of Cords of Brachial Plexus

The infraclavicular branches of the brachial plexus arise from the cords of the brachial plexus at the level of the clavicle (▶ Fig. 9.2).

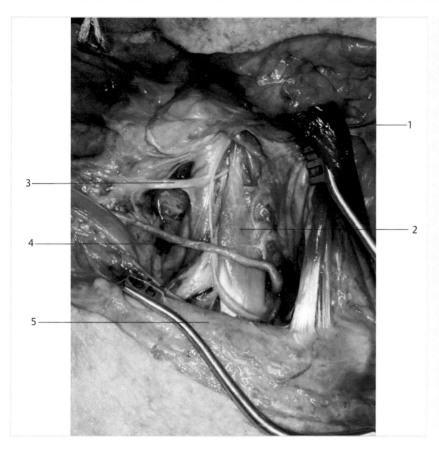

Fig. 9.4 Suprascapular nerve. 1, sterno-cleidomastoid muscle; 2, anterior scalenus; 3, suprascapular nerve; 4, suprascapular vessels; 5, clavicle.

Table 9.1 Branches of the lateral cord

Nerve	Contributing spinal nerves	Course	Innervated structures	Surgical note
Lateral pectoral	C5/C6/C7	Pierces clavipectoral fascia; sends branch to medial pectoral nerve	Pectoralis major	
Lateral antebrachial cutaneous	C5/C6/C7; continuation of musculocutaneous nerve	Pierces brachial fascia proximal to lateral epicondyle and closely associates with cephalic vein	Sensation to lateral forearm	At risk during invasive procedures involving access to cubital fossa; particularly when cephalic vein is punctured just lateral to biceps tendon and crossed by nerve
Lateral cord of median	C6/C7	See medial cord	See medial cord	See medial cord
Musculocutaneous	C5/C6/C7	Runs anterior and lateral to axillary artery and exits axilla after piercing coracobrachialis and travels in between biceps and brachialis; continues as **lateral antebrachial cutaneous nerve**	Coracobrachialis, biceps brachii, brachialis	Not commonly injured, but may become entrapped with relocation of tendon of long head of biceps

Source: Data from Zhang et al.[24]

Branches of the Lateral Cord

The lateral cord is formed from the anterior divisions from the upper and middle trunks with contributions from C5 to C7. It gives rise to the *lateral pectoral nerve*; *the musculocutaneous nerve*, which continues as the *lateral antebrachial cutaneous nerve* in the forearm; and the *lateral root of the median nerve* (Table 9.1).

The *lateral pectoral nerve*[1] derives its name from its origin in the lateral cord of the brachial plexus. It contains nerve fibers from the anterior divisions of C5 to C7 and pierces the clavipectoral fascia to supply the pectoralis major muscle. It also sends a branch to the medial pectoral nerve, which supplies the pectoral minor muscle.

The *musculocutaneous nerve* (▶ Fig. 9.5, 9.6)[5–7] is one of the two terminal branches of the lateral cord and is composed of

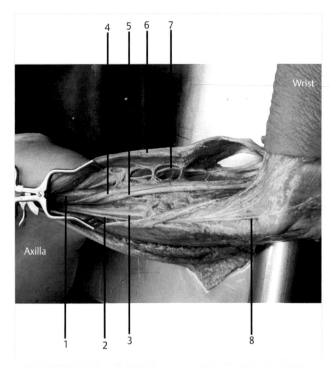

Fig. 9.5 Branches of the brachial plexus through the course of the arm. 1, coracobrachialis; 2, medial cutaneous nerve of arm; 3, ulnar nerve; 4, brachial artery; 5, median nerve; 6, biceps; 7, musculocutaneous nerve; 8, medial antebrachial cutaneous nerve.

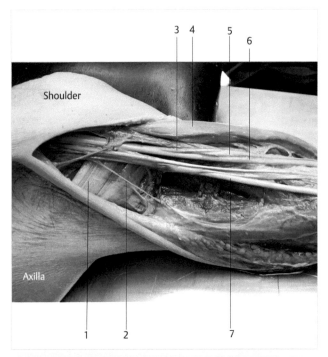

Fig. 9.6 Medial brachial cutaneous nerve. 1, latissimus dorsi; 2, medial brachial cutaneous nerve; 3, musculocutaneous; 4, biceps; 5, brachial artery; 6, median nerve; 7, ulnar nerve.

fibers derived from C5, C6, and C7. The main nerve trunk arises from the lateral cord of the brachial plexus at the lower border of the pectoralis minor muscle and runs anterior and lateral to

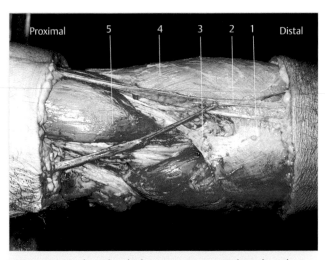

Fig. 9.7 Lateral antebrachial cutaneous nerve. 1, lateral antebrachial cutaneous nerve; 2, cephlic vein; 3, lacertus fibrosus; 4, extensor muscles; 5, biceps.

the axillary artery. As it runs laterally, it sends a primary branch 6 cm distal to the coracoid process and enters the deep surface of the coracobrachialis muscle. The primary motor branch for the biceps muscles branches 10 to 13 cm distal to the coracoid process and bifurcates into two secondary branches. The proximal branch innervates the short head of the biceps, and the distal branch innervates the long head of the biceps. The motor branch innervating the brachialis muscle exits from the main trunk of the musculocutaneous nerve 14 to 18 cm distal to the coracoid process, with a single or two primary branches supplying the brachialis. As the musculocutaneous nerve continues toward the elbow joint, it emerges from beneath the biceps muscle and becomes the *lateral antebrachial cutaneous nerve* (Fig. 9.6).

The *lateral antebrachial cutaneous nerve* (▶ Fig. 9.7)[8,9] provides sensory innervation to the lateral aspect of the forearm and is a continuation of the musculocutaneous nerve. It pierces the brachial fascia 3 cm proximal to the lateral epicondyle and emerges from the subcutaneous fat distal to the lateral border of the biceps tendon and is closely associated with the cephalic vein. At the elbow, it is located medial to the lateral epicondyle as it crosses the interepicondylar line and travels parallel and volar to the cephalic vein. It is never farther than 1 cm from cephalic vein proximal to the crossover of the abductor pollicis longus and extensor pollicis brevis with the extensor carpi radialis longus and extensor carpi radialis brevis.

The other terminal branch of the lateral cord is the *lateral root of the median nerve*. It joins the *medial root of the median nerve* off of the medial cord, lateral to the axillary artery, to form the *median nerve* (see median nerve hereafter).

Branches of the Medial Cord

The medial cord is a continuation of the anterior division of the lower trunk with contributions from C8 and T1. It gives rise to the **medial pectoral nerve**, **medial antebrachial cutaneous nerve**, and **medial brachial cutaneous nerve**. After the medial cord gives off the **medial root of the median nerve**, it continues distally as the **ulnar nerve** (see ulnar nerve hereafter; Table 9.2).

Table 9.2 Branches of the medial cord

Nerve	Contributing spinal nerves	Course	Innervated structures	Surgical note
Medial pectoral	C8–T1	Runs through deep surface of pectoralis minor and lies lateral to lateral pectoral nerve	Pectoralis major	
Medial brachial cutaneous	C8–T1	Runs along medial side of axillary and brachial veins	Medial surface of arm and proximal part of forearm	Susceptible to injury during cubital tunnel surgery
Medial antebrachial cutaneous	C8–T1	Initially runs with ulnar nerve, pierces brachial fascia with basilic vein, and enters subcutaneous tissue, dividing into ulnar and volar branches	Medial surface of forearm	Nerve divides into two main branches anterior and posterior to medial epicondyle; posterior branch susceptible to injury during cubital tunnel surgery and anterior branch susceptible during venipuncture
Ulnar	C8–T1; occasionally C7	Descends medially in the arm posterior to the medial epicondyle of humerus onto the ulnar aspect of forearm; passes through Guyon's canal in hand prior to branching into superficial and deep branches in hand	Flexor carpi ulnaris, medial half of flexor digitorum profundus, intrinsic muscles of hand except for radial two lumbricals and thenar eminence, skin of hand medial to ulnar side of ring finger to little finger	Closed reduction and K-wiring of displaced supracondylar fractures frequently cause iatrogenic injury; medial pin can damage ulnar nerve during insertion or after insertion by constricting the cubital tunnel
Medial root of median	C8–T1; contribution from lateral root of median (C6–C7)	Lateral and medial roots merge lateral to axillary artery to form the median nerve; descends with brachial artery in arm; **anterior interosseous nerve** branches off of median nerve deep to pronator teres prior to passing in between two heads of pronator teres; median nerve continues on deep surface of flexor digitorum superficiales; gives off superficial palmar branch prior to entering carpal tunnel under the flexor retinaculum	Muscles of anterior forearm compartment (except for flexor carpi ulnaris, and ulnar half of flexor digitorum profundus, 5 intrinsic muscles of hand and the ulnar two lumbricals), palmar skin from radial side of ring finger to thumb. The median nerve supplies the radial two lumbricals through the common digital branches.	Median nerve especially vulnerable to injury during carpal tunnel release, during both open and endoscopic procedures; variant anatomy may increase risk of iatrogenic injury

Source: Data from Zhang et al.[24]

The *medial pectoral nerve*[1] supplies the deep portion of the pectoralis major. It runs through the deep surface of the pectoralis minor muscle and lies lateral to the lateral pectoral nerve.

The *medial brachial cutaneous nerve* (▶ Figs. 9.5, 9.6)[10,11] is a tenuous nerve that supplies skin over the medial surface of the arm and the proximal part of the forearm. It comes off the medial cord of the brachial plexus and courses with the basilic vein and medial to the brachial artery. At the midportion of the arm, there is an arborization of several cutaneous branches through the muscular fascia across the ulnar nerve to become subcutaneous to the skin of the medial arm.

The *medial antebrachial cutaneous nerve* (▶ Figs. 9.5, 9.8)[12] supplies the skin over the medial surface of the forearm. It runs

in between the axillary artery and vein and then runs distally anterior and medial to the brachial artery. At the midforearm level, it emerges from under brachial fascia adjacent to the basilic vein and divides into a volar and ulnar branch. The volar branch passes in front of the median basilic vein and descends on the ulnar side of the forearm. The ulnar branch passes obliquely downward on the medial side of the basilic vein in front of the medial epicondyle and descends on the ulnar side of the medial forearm.

The Median Nerve

The *median nerve* (▶ Fig. 9.3) is formed by two terminal branches, one from the medial cord (C8, T1) and the other from

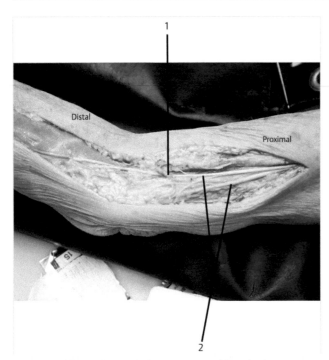

Fig. 9.8 Medial antebrachial cutaneous nerve. 1, basilic vein; 2, medial antebrachial cutaneous nerve.

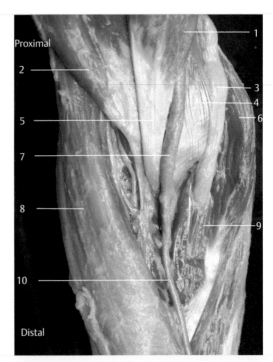

Fig. 9.9 Median nerve in the proximal forearm.1, biceps muscle; 2, brachialis muscle; 3, median nerve; 4, brachialis tendon; 5, biceps tendon; 6, felxor carpi radialis; 7, brachial artery; 8, brachioradialis; 9, two heads of pronator teres; 10, radial artery.

the lateral cord (C5, C6, C7). These two branches travel around the axillary artery and unite either anterior or lateral to the artery so as to form the median nerve.

Median Nerve in Arm

In the upper arm, the median nerve does not give off any branches. It can be identified proximally posterior to coracobrachialis and distally in the groove between the belly of the biceps and brachialis. In the proximal half of the arm, the median nerve lies lateral to the brachial artery and its accompanying veins. In the distal half of the arm, the nerve crosses anterior to the artery and veins and assumes a medial position in relation to these structures. The median nerve lies entirely anterior to the medial intermuscular septum (▶Fig. 9.5, 9.7).[7,12,13]

Median Nerve at the Elbow

The median nerve is anterior to the intermuscular septum in the proximal part of the arm but pierces the septum in the midarm and then lies immediately posterior to the intermuscular septum within the epimysium of the triceps. The median nerve can subsequently be isolated proximal to pronator teres on the anterior aspect of the elbow. It can then be seen passing between the humeral and ulnar heads of the pronator teres and can be traced distally after sending branches to the pronator teres. The median nerve can be seen running vertically across the interval between the humeral head of pronator teres and flexor carpi radialis before passing deep to the proximal border of the flexor digitorum superficialis (▶Fig. 9.9).[14]

Median Nerve in Forearm

In the proximal forearm, the median nerve passes between the humeral and ulnar heads of pronator teres (82%), whereas the

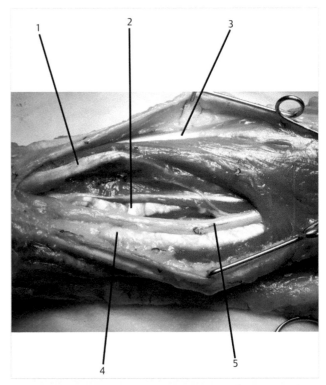

Fig. 9.10 Median nerve in the distal forearm. 1, flexor carpi radialis; 2, flexor pollicis longus; 3, brachioradialis; 4, FDS; 5, median nerve.

ulnar artery passes deep to both the heads (▶Fig. 9.9, 9.10).[9,15] In about 9% of cases, the deep head of pronator teres is absent and the median nerve and ulnar artery travel deep to the superficial head. In around 7%, the median nerve travels deep to both heads of pronator teres. In around 2%, the median nerve travels through the substance of the superficial head of the pronator teres.[44] Distal to the pronator teres, the median nerve joins the ulnar artery. It passes deep to the proximal fibrous arch of flexor digitorum superficialis and runs distally in the midline of the forearm, closely attached by the bicipital aponeurosis in the cubital fossa to the deep surface of flexor digitorum superficialis, which it supplies. Deep to the humeral head of pronator teres, the *anterior interosseous nerve* arises from the posterior aspect of the median nerve and runs along the interosseous membrane between the flexor digitorum profundus and flexor pollicis longus. Approximately 5 cm proximal to the flexor retinaculum, the median nerve emerges from the lateral border of flexor digitorum superficialis to become more superficial and gives off the **superficial palmar branch** before passing into the hand through the carpal tunnel.

Anterior interosseous nerve[5,16] (▶ Fig. 9.11) is the major branch of the median nerve to supply the deep compartment of the forearm. It typically branches immediately distal to the flexor digitorum superficialis arch and innervates the flexor digitorum profundus (index and long fingers), flexor pollicis longus, and pronator quadratus. The anterior interosseous nerve courses distally on the interosseous membrane, often radial to the anterior interosseous artery (80%), and passes dorsal to and innervating the pronator quadratus muscle. It also sends sensory branches to the distal radioulnar, radiocarpal, intercarpal, and middle and ring finger carpometacarpal joints.

Palmar cutaneous nerve of median nerve[17–19] (▶ Fig. 9.12) arises from the radial side of the median nerve 5 to 7 cm proximal to the wrist joint and runs parallel with the parent nerve down along the ulnar side of the tendon of the flexor carpi radialis and crosses the base of the thenar eminence over the prominence of the tubercle of the scaphoid. It pierces the flexor retinaculum and divides into a lateral and medial branch. The lateral branch supplies the ball of the thumb, and the medial branch supplies the skin of the palm.

Median Nerve at Wrist and Hand

As the median nerve crosses the distal forearm deep to the flexor digitorum superficialis to the wrist crease, it becomes superficial and lies between the tendons of palmaris longus and flexor carpi radialis. It then traverses the carpal tunnel, where it lies superficial to the tendons of flexor digitorum profundus and flexor pollicis longus, and divides into two branches at the distal border of the flexor retinaculum: the ulnar and radial divisions (▶ Fig. 9.13). The ulnar division divides into the common digital nerves to the second and third web spaces. The radial division branches into the common digital nerve to the thumb and the proper digital nerve to the radial index finger. Two branches arising from common digital nerves (▶ Fig. 9.17b) supply the first and second lumbrical muscles. Before reaching the base of the fingers, the nerve lies between the long flexor tendons with their associated lumbricals. As the nerve proceeds from the hand into the digits, its relationship with the blood vessels reverses: the common digital nerves are initially dorsal to the superficial palmar arch and palmar to the flexor tendons in the palm (▶ Fig 9.17). After branching in the distal palm, the proper digital nerves become palmar to the digital arteries. All digital nerves proceed into the digit just palmar to the artery and lie along the side of the flexor tendons. Both nerve and artery

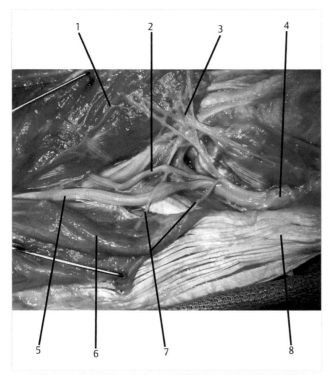

Fig. 9.11 Anterior interosseous nerve branches from median nerve. 1, flexor digitorum superficialis; 2, anterior interosseous nerve; 3, branches to flexor digitorum superficialis from median nerve; 4, median nerve; 5, continuation of median nerve after bifurcation; 6, pronator teres (superficial head); 7, branches to pronator teres from anterior interosseous nerve; 8, common flexor tendon.

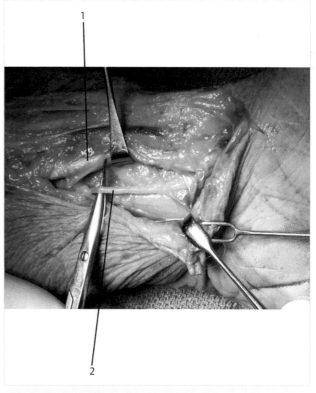

Fig. 9.12 Palmar cutaneous nerve of median nerve. 1, flexor carpi radialis tendon (retracted); 2, palmar cutaneous nerve of median nerve.

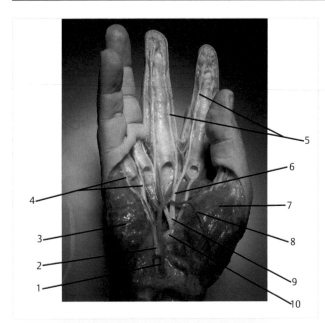

Fig. 9.13 Median and ulnar nerve distribution in the hand. 1, ulnar artery; 2, ulnar nerve; 3, hypothenar eminence; 4, digital nerves of ulnar nerve; 5, digital nerves of median nerve; 6, common digital nerve from median nerve; 7, thenar eminence; 8, superficial radial artery; 9, median nerve; 10, flexor retinaculum.

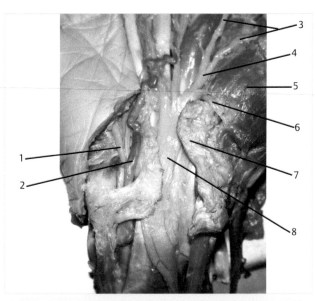

Fig. 9.14 Motor branch of the median nerve in the hand. 1, ulnar nerve; 2, ulnar artery; 3, digital nerves; 4, common digital nerve; 5, thenar eminence; 6, motor branch of median nerve; 7, flexor retinaculum (cut); 8, median nerve.

pass between the Cleland and Grayson ligaments while giving off numerous branches to the digit. These digital nerves provide sensory innervation to half of the palmar skin, dorsal skin up to the midportion of the middle phalanx for the index, the middle and radial sides of the ring finger, and the subungual region of the tip of the thumb.[18,19]

The motor branch to the thenar musculature typically originates from the radial aspect of the median nerve; however, four variations in the branching pattern have been described.[27] In the extraligamentous type (56%), the thenar motor branch arises distal to the transverse carpal ligament (TCL) and then runs a retrograde course to reach the thenar muscles (▶Fig. 9.14).[18,19] In the subligamentous type (34%), the branch arises within the carpal tunnel and remains deep to the TCL until it reaches the thenar muscles. In the transligamentous type (9%), the branch arises within the carpal tunnel and then pierces the TCL to reach the thenar muscles. In the preligamentous type (1%), the thenar branch arises proximal to the carpal tunnel and then pierces the antebrachial fascia to run superficial to the TCL.[29] Upon exiting the TCL, the motor branch then penetrates the septum between the central palmar compartment and thenar muscles before it enters the thenar muscle group between flexor pollicis brevis and abductor pollicis brevis muscles and terminates in the opponens pollicis. However, variations of the motor branch innervation are common, such as having two terminal branches to abductor pollicis brevis and flexor pollicis brevis (30%) or having independent branches to abductor pollicis brevis and opponens pollicis (40%). Additionally, up to 75% of the population has an accessory thenar nerve arising from either the first common digital nerve (25%) or the radial proper digital nerve to the thumb (50%).[28]

The Ulnar Nerve

The *ulnar nerve* (C8 and T1) arises from the medial cord of the brachial plexus and does not have any branches in the arm but continues distally, lying medial to the axillary artery.

Ulnar Nerve in Arm

In the proximal arm, the ulnar nerve lies anterior to the medial intermuscular septum but posterior to the brachial artery and median nerve (▶Fig. 9.5, 9.7).[7,12] In the midarm, it pierces the septum to lie deep to the medial intermuscular septum in a groove in the triceps, where it is accompanied by the superior ulnar collateral artery. It is easily mobilized within the upper arm, because it has no branches in this region of the arm. The arcade of Struthers is present in 20 to 70% of individuals. This thick fascial band is formed by the medial intermuscular septum, internal brachial ligament, and triceps fascia so as to span from the medial head of the triceps muscle to the medial intermuscular septum, and it may be a site of nerve compression.[28]

Ulnar Nerve in Elbow

The ulnar nerve and the ulnar collateral artery are found posterior to the intermuscular septum. The nerve then passes distally posterior to the medial epicondyle in the cubital tunnel before entering between the two heads of flexor carpi ulnaris (FCU). The cubital tunnel is a fibro-osseous structure bordered by the ulnar groove of the medial epicondyle, a fascial arcade or arcuate ligament, and the FCU muscle bellies. The posterior and oblique bands of the ulnar collateral ligament comprise a portion of the cubital tunnel floor. Articular branches to the elbow joint arise from within the cubital tunnel (▶Fig. 9.15).[14]

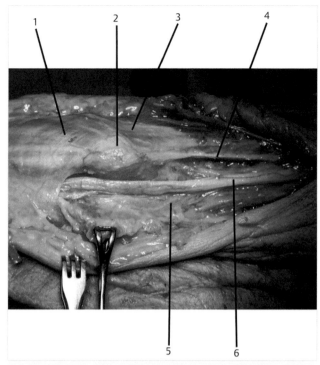

Fig. 9.15 Ulnar nerve at the level of the elbow. 1, common flexor tendon; 2, medial epicondyle; 3, pronator teres; 4, medial intermuscular septum; 5, branch of ulnar nerve to elbow joint; 6, ulnar nerve.

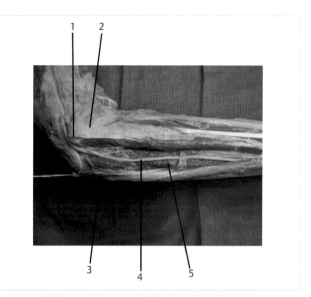

Fig. 9.16 Ulnar nerve at the level of the forearm. 1, medial epicondyle; 2, common flexor tendon; 3, flexor carpi ulnaris (retracted and detached from common flexor tendon); 4, ulnar nerve; 5, flexor digitorum profundus.

Ulnar Nerve in Forearm

At the proximal forearm, the ulnar nerve enters the anterior compartment of the forearm and can then be readily traced between the two heads of FCU, which it supplies. It then travels down the forearm on the anterior surface of the flexor digitorum profundus and provides motor branches to supply the medial half of this muscle (ring + small digits). Motor branches to FCU may arise 4 cm proximal to the elbow joint, from within the cubital tunnel, or from up to 10 cm distal to the medial epicondyle. Most commonly, there are one to two motor branches to FCU. The proximal FCU branch may divide to innervate the flexor digitorum profundus muscle. Typically, there is a single branch to flexor digitorum profundus (80%) that arises approximately 3 cm distal to the medial epicondyle and runs distally for about 2.5 cm before entering the interval between the FCU and flexor digitorum superficialis in the forearm (▶ Fig. 9.16).[9,15]

Ulnar Nerve in Wrist and Hand

Just proximal to the wrist crease, the ulnar nerve, accompanied by the ulnar artery on its radial side, emerges from under the FCU to pass over the flexor retinaculum of the wrist (▶ Fig. 9.17).[18,19] The **dorsal sensory branch of the ulnar nerve** branches approximately 6 cm proximal to the ulnar head and courses distally and dorsally to supply the dorsal ulnar wrist and hand, the dorsal and proximal ring, and small fingers. The ulnar artery remains dorsal and radial to the

ulnar nerve as it enters the distal ulnar tunnel at the leading edge of the volar carpal ligament. As the ulnar nerve crosses the flexor retinaculum, it travels through the Guyon canal. This 4-cm–long tunnel is divided into three zones. Zone 1 begins at the proximal edge of volar carpal ligament approximately 2 cm proximal to pisiform. The floor of zone 1 is the TCL. Zone 1 ends with a nerve bifurcation, approximately 1 cm distal to pisiform. The palmaris brevis muscle is the transversely orientated muscle that serves as the roof of the distal ulnar tunnel in zone 2. At the level of the pisiform, the ulnar nerve divides into two branches: The deep branch becomes the motor branch, divides in Guyon's canal to send a branch to the abductor digiti minimi, and then courses around the hook of the hamate to innervate the flexor digiti minimi and opponens digiti minimi. It then courses across the midpalmar space dorsal to the flexor tendons to supply the third and fourth lumbricals, the adductor pollicis, the flexor pollicis brevis, and all the interossei. It penetrates the interval between the two heads of the adductor pollicis before reaching and innervating the first dorsal interosseous. Zone 3 consists of the superficial branch, which remains superficial and innervates the palmaris brevis muscle, continues into the palm, and provides a proper digital branch to the ulnar side of the little finger and a common digital branch to the radial and ulnar side of the ring finger (▶ Fig. 9.17b).

Dorsal cutaneous nerve of ulnar nerve (▶ Fig. 9.18)[5,18,19] supplies the skin over the ulnar half of the wrist, the ulnar side of the dorsum of the hand, the dorsum of the little finger, and the adjacent border of the ring finger as far distally as the distal interphalangeal joints. It emerges from deep to FCU approximately 5 to 8 cm proximal to the ulnar styloid and travels around the ulnar border of the wrist superficial to the extensor

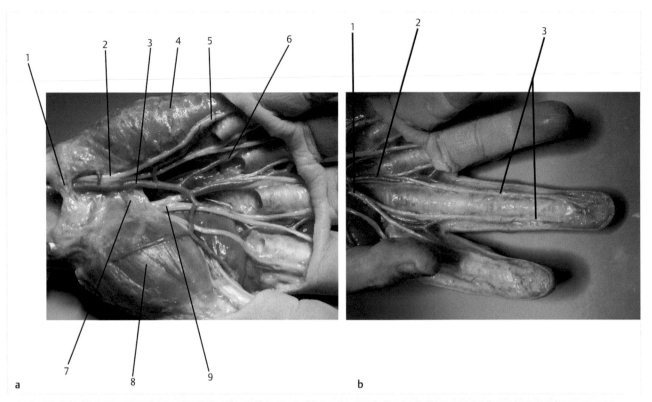

Fig. 9.17 (a) Ulnar nerve distribution in the hand. 1, palmar carpal ligament (roof of tunnel of Guyon); 2, ulnar nerve; 3, ulnar artery; 4, hypothenar eminence; 5, digital nerve; 6, digital artery; 7, flexor retinaculum; 8, thenar eminence; 9, median nerve. **(b)** Common digital nerve. 1, common digital nerve; 2, digital artery; 3, digital nerve.

retinaculum and extensor carpi ulnaris tendon. At this point, its branches spread and fan out to supply sensory innervation to the ulnar side of the dorsal hand, the dorsum of the little finger, and the dorsum of the radial side of the ring finger.

Branches of the Posterior Cord

The posterior cord is formed from the posterior divisions of all three trunks with contributions from C5 to T1 and subsequently gives rise to five nerves (*upper and lower subscapular*, *thoracodorsal*, *axillary*, and *radial nerves*). These nerves innervate the extensors of the upper limb and supply cutaneous innervation to the extensor surface of the upper limb (Table 9.3).

The first branch off the posterior cord is the *upper subscapular nerve*[1,20] (C5 and C6) and passes directly into the upper part of the subscapularis muscle. The lower subscapular nerve1,20 (C5 and C6) divides into two branches itself. One of the branches enters into the lower part of the subscapularis muscle, and the other branch continues to supply the teres major. The *thoracodorsal nerve*[1,20] (C6, C7, C8) (or middle subscapular nerve) arises between the upper and lower subscapular nerves and runs inferolaterally to supply the apex of the latissimus dorsi muscle.

The *axillary nerve*[5,21] (▶ Fig. 9.19) is one of two terminal branches of the posterior cord with contributions from C5 and C6. It innervates the deltoid muscle and teres minor and provides sensory innervation to the shoulder joint and inferior region of the deltoid muscle by the *superior lateral cutaneous nerve*.[21] From the brachial plexus, it descends inferolaterally on the anterior surface of subscapularis muscle to enter the

quadrangular space in company with the posterior circumflex humeral vessels. As the axillary nerve trunk continues distally, it initially splits into anterior and posterior branches 4 to 5 cm from the origin of the brachial plexus. The anterior branch winds around the surgical neck of the humerus superior to the posterior circumflex artery, approximately 7 cm below the tip of the acromion, and pierces the anterior and middle part of the deltoid. The posterior branch is located more superficially than the anterior, and all its branches are directed posteriorly. It gives off a branch to the teres minor before it penetrates the posterior part of the deltoid muscle. The *superior lateral cutaneous nerve* also originates from the posterior branch and sweeps around the posterior border of the deltoid muscle, perforating the deep fascia to supply the skin overlying the posterior part of the deltoid and over the long head of the triceps brachii.

Radial Nerve

The other terminal branch of the posterior cord, the *radial nerve*, is made with contributions from C5 to T1. The radial nerve supplies the extensor muscles of the upper limb and provides cutaneous innervation to the skin of the extensor region.

Radial Nerve in Arm

The radial nerve first passes behind the axillary artery lying on subscapularis and the tendons of latissimus dorsi and teres major. After entering the triangular interval at the midshaft of the humerus, the radial nerve crosses the midline of the midshaft of the humerus 15 cm proximal to the distal articular

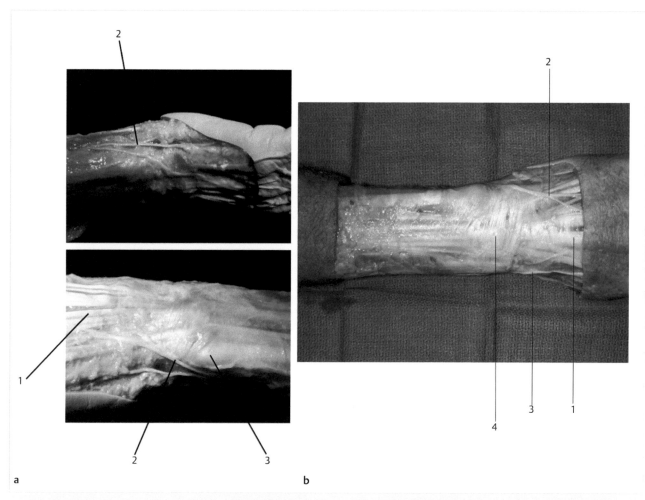

Fig. 9.18 **(a)** Dorsal branch of ulnar nerve. 1, tendons of extensor digitorum; 2, dorsal branch of ulnar nerve; 3, ulnar styloid. **(b)** View of both superficial branch of radial nerve and dorsal branch of ulnar nerve. 1, tendons of extensor digitorum; 2, superficial radial nerve; 3, dorsal branch of ulnar nerve; 4, extensor retinaculum.

Table 9.3 Branches of the posterior cord

Nerve	Contributing spinal nerves	Course	Innervated structures	Surgical note
Upper subscapular	C5	Passes posteriorly, entering subscapularis directly	Superior part of subscapularis	During routine anterior approach to shoulder, nerves to subscapularis are in surgical field and can lead to inadvertent neurologic damage; dissection should not be done on anterior surface of subscapularis muscle belly medial to glenohumeral joint
Lower subscapular	C6	Passes inferolaterally deep to subscapular artery and vein	Inferior portion of subscapularis	Closely associated with axillary nerve and can lead to inadvertent neurologic damage during routine anterior approach to shoulder; dissection should not be done on anterior surface of subscapularis muscle belly medial to glenohumeral joint
Thoracodorsal	C6/C7/C8	Runs inferolaterally along posterior axillary wall to apical part of latissimus dorsi	Latissimus dorsi	Thoracodorsal nerve injury can occur during thoracotomy or during axillary clearance for breast cancer. In brachial plexus injuries, this nerve may be spared and can act as a source of nerve transfer or for innervated latissimus dorsi transfer.

(Continued)

Table 9.3 (*Continued*) Branches of the posterior cord

Nerve	Contributing spinal nerves	Course	Innervated structures	Surgical note
Axillary	C5/C6	Descends inferolaterally on anterior surface of subscapularis to enter quadrangular space with posterior circumflex humeral vessels; gives rise to **superior lateral cutaneous nerve** and then winds around surgical neck of humerus deep to deltoid	Glenohumeral joint, deltoid, teres minor; skin over inferior part of deltoid	Since axillary nerve runs through quadrangular space where it touches surgical neck of humerus, it can be easily damaged by surgery, fractures of surgical neck of humerus, or anterior dislocation of shoulder; dissection carried out inferior to teres minor can damage axillary nerve, making it critical to identify muscular interval between infraspinatus and teres minor and to stay within interval
Radial	C5/C6/C7/C8/T1	Passes behind axillary artery lying on subscapularis; accompanied by profunda brachii artery, passes obliquely across back of humerus in spiral groove; then pierces lateral intermuscular septum and enters anterior compartment of arm between brachialis and brachioradialis; at level of lateral epicondyle, gives off posterior interosseous nerve and continues as superficial terminal branch	Triceps, anconeus, brachioradialis, extensor carpi radialis longus, and lateral part of brachialis; skin of posterior and inferolateral arm, posterior forearm, and dorsum of hand lateral to midline of ring finger	Radial nerve injured in 1 in 8 humeral fractures; posterior interosseous nerve is vulnerable to injury as it winds around neck of radius within substance of supinator muscle; superficial radial nerve may be damaged during operations near the radial styloid such as when inserting Kirschner wires to maintain reduction of a displaced radius fracture

Source: Data from Zhang et al.[24]

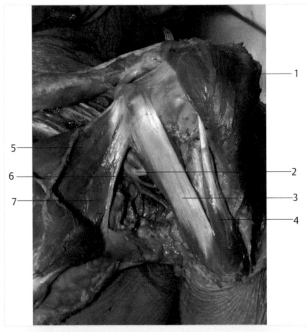

Fig. 9.19 Axillary nerve. 1, deltoid; 2, axillary nerve; 3, long head of triceps; 4, lateral head of triceps; 5, infraspinatus; 6, posterior circumflex humeral artery; 7, teres minor.

surface. It emerges from the inferior border of teres major after having passed through the triangular interval. In the posterior arm, it is joined by the profunda brachii, which originates from the brachial artery. The radial nerve and profunda brachii run obliquely downward from the medial to the lateral side, lying on the medial head of the triceps. At this point, it runs deep to the lateral head of the triceps closely associated with the humerus in the spiral groove. The radial nerve trifurcates as it comes into contact with the medial border of the humerus, where it provides a large branch to the medial head of the triceps and the *posterior antebrachial cutaneous nerve*. The branch to the medial head of the triceps courses distally to eventually supply the anconeus (▶ Fig. 9.20).[5,7,12,22]

The *posterior antebrachial cutaneous nerve*[23] supplies the posterior aspect of the forearm with sensory innervation, remains adjacent to the radial nerve as it courses along the posterior humerus, then continues posteriorly after it diverges from the radial nerve immediately proximal to the lateral intermuscular septum. Having curved around the lateral border of the humerus deep to the lateral head of triceps, the radial nerve continues to pierce the lateral intermuscular septum approximately 10 cm proximal to the olecranon fossa and runs distally in the anterior compartment of the arm between the lateral head of triceps and brachialis.

Radial Nerve at Elbow

The radial nerve at the elbow lies deep to brachioradialis, anterior to the humerus, and lateral to brachialis.[24] Just proximal to the supinator, the radial nerve bifurcates into two terminal branches, one superficial and one deep: the *superficial sensory branch* and the *posterior interosseous nerve*.[5,14]

Superficial branch of radial nerve[5,7,15] (▶ Fig. 9.18, 9.21) continues distally, lateral to the radial artery, in the flexor compartment of the forearm under cover of brachioradialis. In the forearm, it runs between brachioradialis and the extensor carpi radialis longus and then pierces the fascia between them 10 cm proximal to

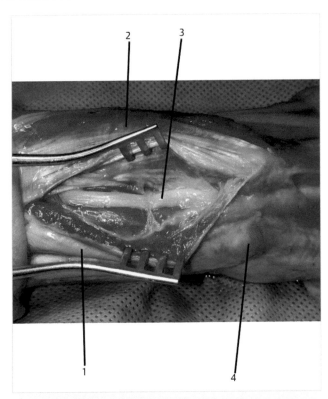

Fig. 9.20 Radial nerve in the arm. 1, long head of triceps (retracted); 2, medial (deep) head of triceps; 3, radial nerve; 4, lateral head of triceps (retracted).

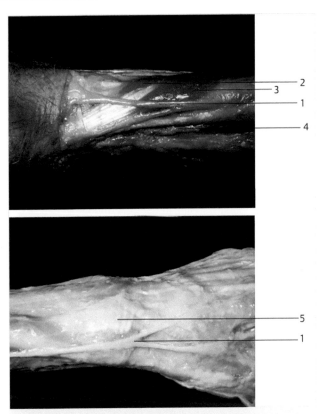

Fig. 9.21 Superficial branch of radial nerve. 1, superficial branch of radial nerve; 2, extensor pollicis longus; 3, abductor pollicis longus; 4, radial artery; 5, extensor retinaculum.

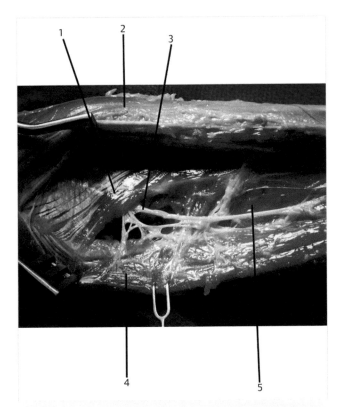

Fig. 9.22 Posterior interosseous nerve. 1, supinator; 2, extensor carpi radialis; 3, posterior interosseous nerve; 4, extensor digitorum communis; 5, abductor pollicis longus.

the radial styloid to emerge on the dorsum of the wrist. The nerve continues to run across the tendon sheaths of the abductor pollicis longus and extensor pollicis brevis, where it divides into two or three terminal branches, which supply the skin of the dorsum of the radial two and half digits, as far distally as the center of the middle phalanges. One branch may traverse the anatomical snuff box to cross the tendon of extensor pollicis longus.

Posterior interosseous nerve[5,7,15] (▶ Fig. 9.22) is the motor nerve for the posterior compartment of the forearm. It runs deep to the arcade of Frohse and then emerges from the posterior border of the supinator. It then enters and passes between the two heads of the supinator and may come in direct contact with the neck of the radius. At this point, it passes as one bundle, which subsequently divides into three main trunks and spreads into tiny branches to the extensor muscles of the forearm. Two main trunks curve medially and dorsally with very short branches. The other trunk courses distally as a single branch located at the lateral side. The posterior interosseous nerve supplies all of the wrist extensors (except for extensor carpi radialis longus which is innervated by radial nerve), including extensor carpi radialis brevis, extensor digitorum, extensor digiti minimi, extensor carpi ulnaris, supinator, abductor pollicis longus, extensor pollicis brevis, extensor pollicis longus, and extensor indicis.

Nerve of Henle

Although several anatomists have studied the sympathetic nerves of the upper extremity, the nerve of Henle (Fig. 9.23) also termed the *palmar cutaneous branch* of the ulnar nerve—has not received much specific attention considering its anatomic relationship and surgical importance. The nerve of Henle has far more responsibilities than palmar cutaneus sensation. This distinct branch of the ulnar nerve provides sympathetic innervation to the ulnar artery. Along the course of the ulnar nerve, it gives off inconsistent cutaneous branches, but it consistently sends fibers to the ulnar artery. This distribution pattern suggests that this nerve carries sensory fibers innervating the hypothenar area and sympathetic fibers innervating the ulnar artery. The variability observed in the course of the nerve of Henle can be a source of confusion.[25,26]

As a branch of the ulnar nerve, it primarily originates anywhere from 5 to 11 cm distal from the medial epicondyle. The nerve can be found traveling in the same fibrous sheath as the ulnar nerve 5 cm distally, where it turns radially as it courses in the vascular sheath of the ulnar artery and vein. As it continues distally posterior to the muscular branches of the ulnar artery, the main trunk of the nerve of Henle splits into its sensory terminal branches about 6.5 cm proximal to the wrist crease, whence it travels into one of four distinct distribution patterns (▶Fig. 9.24):

1. Ulnar type (▶Fig. 9.24a): The majority of distribution patterns follow the ulnar type. In this configuration, the nerve follows the ulnar artery distally through to the division of the superficial and deep branches of the ulnar artery. During this course, approximately four branches supply sensory innervation to the distal ulnar and palmar aspect of the forearm up to 3 cm distal to the wrist crease, outlined by the tendons of the FCU and the palmaris longus. One branch crosses to the site right before entering the distal ulnar tunnel.
2. Radioulnar type (▶Fig. 9.24b): In this configuration, the nerve also travels distally with the ulnar artery to the division of the superficial and deep branches of the ulnar artery. The nerve of Henle then divides, giving off one branch to supply the ulnar edge of the wrist crease, while

another branch crosses over to the subcutaneous tissue over the palmaris longus tendon.
3. Vessel type (▶Fig. 9.24c): In the vessel-typed pattern, as the ulnar nerve returns to the vascular sheath of the ulnar artery and vein, small branches to the ulnar nerve extend from the beginning of the ulnar nerve contained within the vascular sheath to the ulnar artery to the palmar arch.
4. Radial type (▶Fig. 9.24d): In the radial type, the main trunk travels distally with the ulnar artery down to the palmar arch but provides two branches to subcutaneous tissue overlying the palmaris longus tendon at the wrist crease.

Careful evaluation must be done as surgical dissection of the nerve of Henle can lead to sensory loss at the distal forearm. In

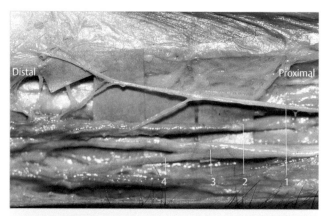

Fig. 9.23 Typical Nerve of Henle that arises 16cm. proximal to the ulnar styloid. 1,Nerve of Henle; 2, ulnar artery; 3, ulnar nerve; 4, Superficial branch of the ulnar nerve. (Reproduced with permission from McCabe SJ, Kleinert JM: The Nerve of Henle. J Hand Surg 1990: 15A(5) 784-788.)

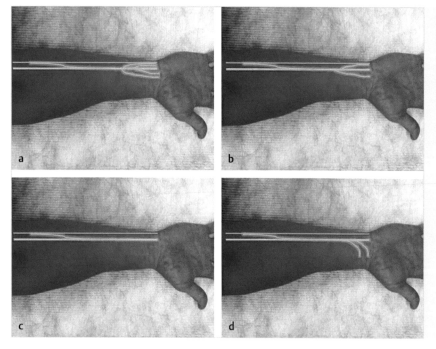

Fig. 9.24 Schematic drawing of the four distribution patterns of the nerve of Henle: (**a**) ulnar type, (**b**) radioulnar type, (**c**) vessel-related type, (**d**) radial type. The *blue line* indicates the ulnar nerve, the *red line* indicates the ulnar artery, and the *green line* indicates the nerve of Henle.

some common procedures at the distal forearm, such as carpal tunnel release, the location of the nerve of Henle has considerable bearing on the manner in which incisions are made. Since the distal, palmar sensory branch of the nerve of Henle is usually located medially to the axis of the ring finger, carpal tunnel incisions are best made in line with the midaxis of the ring finger.[26] Careful dissection is also warranted between the skin and palmar fascia to avoid sensory loss, as one may encounter branches of the nerve of Henle.

Anatomic Variations of the Nerves to the Upper Extremity

The classic description of the anatomy of the upper limb is an oversimplification. In actuality, many variant forms exist that can account for unexpected clinical signs and symptoms.

The two most common anatomic variations encountered in the upper limb are the communications seen between the median and ulnar nerve. In the forearm, median and ulnar communication was first documented by the Swedish anatomist Martin in 1763 and later by Gruber in 1890; hence this communication came to be known as the *Martin–Gruber anastomosis*.[30,31] In this anatomical variation, the median nerve contributes a motor connection to the ulnar nerve in two distinct patterns. This motor connection can stem either from the main trunk of the median nerve in the proximal forearm or from the anterior interosseous nerve (▶ Fig. 9.25a and ▶ Fig. 9.26a).[31] Before joining the main trunk of the ulnar nerve, it crosses obliquely in the proximal forearm and contributes to the innervation of the intrinsic muscles of the hand. This variation is classified into four types. Type I is classified by an anastomotic branch connection between the anterior interosseous and ulnar nerves. A connection between the median and ulnar nerve trunks is classified as type II. A connection between branches innervating the flexor digitorum profundus muscle is type III. And finally, an anastomotic branch from the median or anterior interosseous nerve to the ulnar nerve at two different points is labeled type IV.[32] Its reported incidence has ranged anywhere from 5 to 40% in the literature.[31] However, anatomic studies have reported a range closer to 11 to 24%.[32]

In contradistinction to the motor contribution seen from the median nerve to the ulnar nerve demonstrated with Martin–Gruber anastomosis, Riche and Cannieu in 1897 identified a neural connection in the hand between the deep branch of the ulnar nerve and the recurrent motor branch of the median nerve to the thenar eminence[33] (▶ Fig. 9.25b and ▶ Fig. 9.26b). It has been reported that this anatomic variation exists at a frequency ranging from 77 to 83.3% in the general population.[34] More important, these specific anastamoses in the setting of an ulnar or median nerve lesion can often complicate clinical and electrophysiologic findings.[35]

In the forearm, a reverse Martin-Gruber communication or Marinacci communication whereby a motor communication from the ulnar nerve travels to the median nerve distally in the forearm.[36]

In the palm, communication between the median and ulnar nerves can be seen in 81% cases. The branch, known as Berrettini communication (Fig. 9.26d) can be of four types: Group 1 (communication in an oblique course from the ulnar to the median nerve originating >4mm beyond the distal margin of the flexor retinaculum); Group 2 (communication parallel to the distal margin of the flexor retinaculum); Group 3 (an oblique course from the ulnar nerve to the third common digital nerve distal to the flexor retinaculum) and Group 4 (atypical communication).[37]

Communications between the musculocutaneous nerve and median nerve are another variation seen within the brachial plexus. Within the anterior plane, communications between musculocutaneous nerves and median nerves are the most frequent of all the variations observed in the brachial plexus.[36,37] There are four types of communications observed between the musculocutaneous nerve and the median nerves (Table 9.4).

Precise knowledge of variations in the nerve formations of the upper extremity can serve not only as a valuable resource with which to manage unexpected clinical signs and symptoms but also as an important tool during upper extremity surgical management. This knowledge may prove useful for the clinician in order to avoid major complications or harm.

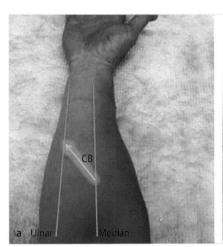 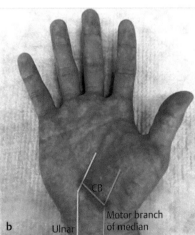

Fig. 9.25 Schematic diagram of the (a) Martin–Gruber anastomosis and the (b) Riche–Cannieu anastomosis. CB: communicating branch.

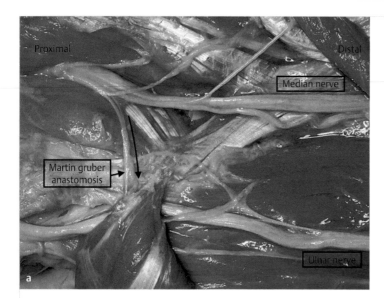

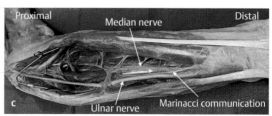

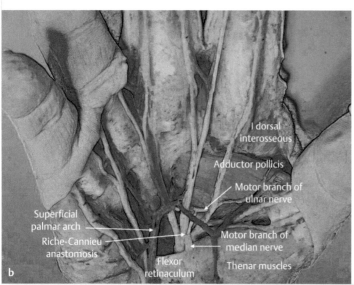

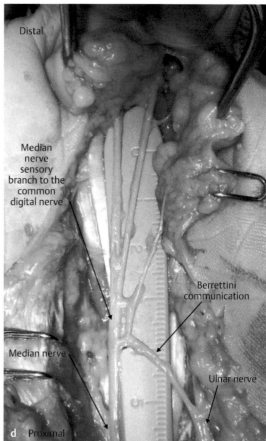

Fig. 9.26 (a) Dissection showing Martin-Gruber anastomosis between the median nerve and the ulnar nerve in the proximal forearm (Black arrow shows the direction of motor fibers from median to ulnar nerve). (b) Digitally enhanced drawing of dissection showing Riche-Cannieu anastomosis between the deep motor branch of the ulnar nerve and the thenar motor branch of the median nerve. (c) Dissection showing Marinacci communication between the ulnar nerve and the median nerve in the mid forearm (White arrow shows the direction of motor fibers from the ulnar nerve to the median nerve. (d) Dissection showing the Berrettini communication between the ulnar nerve to the median nerve.

Ultrastructure/Cross Section of Nerves

The peripheral nerve primarily consists of nerve fibers, fascicles, connective tissue, blood vessels, lymphatic and intercellular spaces, and nervi nervorum. Peripheral neural tissue is organized into fascicles, with groups of myelinated axons ensheathed with connective tissue. The fascicle is also the smallest unit of the nerve that can be surgically manipulated. It forms plexuses that are not simply parallel and that possess a high degree of variability. This structure changes rapidly; along the length of a major nerve, the maximal unaltered segment will be 15 to 20 mm.[38–43]

Peripheral nerves are further organized into three anatomic compartments by several different layers of connective tissue defined as the epineurium, perineurium, and endoneurium (Table 9.5).

The external epineurium (▶ Fig. 9.27, *square*) is the outermost layer of the peripheral nerve that provides a supportive and protective framework. The internal epineurium surrounds individual fascicles, cushions against external pressure, and allows longitudinal excursion. In addition to surrounding the perineurial ensheathment of the fascicles, it also contains type 1 collagen, fibroblasts, adipose cells, and lymphatics. It has well-developed vascular plexus with channels feeding endoneurial plexuses. The next layer, the perineurium (▶ Fig. 9.27, *arrow*), is a thick, dense sheath that surrounds each fascicle and acts as the blood–nerve barrier. It is composed of several layers of flat mesothelial cells covered by basement membrane and interspersed collagen fibrils and tenascin C. These cells are linked with tight junctions and act as a bidirectional barrier to diffusion so as to maintain osmotic milieu and fluid pressure. It also provides high tensile strength that resists up to 750 mm Hg. The deepest layer is the

Table 9.4 Nerve architecture

Layer	Structure	Function
Epineurium	Surrounds individual fascicles with inner and outer layer	Provides supportive and protective framework; cushions against external pressure; allows longitudinal excursion
Perineurium	Surrounds each fascicle; composed of up to 10 layers and has flattened mesothelial cells with tight junctions	Acts a blood–nerve barrier (extension of blood–brain barrier) and a bidirectional barrier to diffusion; provides high tensile strength
Endoneurium	Deepest and smallest unit; surrounds individual nerve fibers	Loose collagenous matrix which enables undulated course of nerve fibers inside fascicles; increases resistance to stretching; prevents electrical impulse interference

Source: Data from Einhorn et al.[38]

Table 9.5 Variations of communications between the musculocutaneous and median nerve

Type	Communication
1	Communications are *proximal* to the point of entry of the musculocutaneous nerve into the coracobrachialis
2	Communications are *distal* to the point of entry of the musculocutaneous nerve into the coracobrachialis
3	Musculocutaneous nerve does not pierce the coracobrachialis
4	Communications are *proximal* to the point of entry of the musculocutaneous nerve into the coracobrachialis and additional communication take place *distally*

Source: Data from Venieratos and Anagnostopoulou.[36]

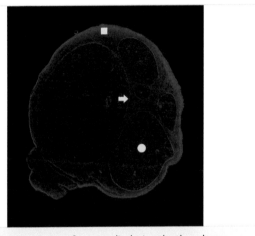

Fig. 9.27 Cross section of a nerve displaying the three layers that compose the peripheral nerve, including the epineurium (*square*), the perineurium (*arrow*), and the innermost layer, the endoneurium (*circle*), which surrounds individual nerve fibers.

endoneurium (▶Fig. 9.27, *circle*). The endoneurium surrounds individual myelinated axons along with blood vessels so as to fill all of the available spaces in the intrafascicular compartment that is enveloped by the perineurial sheaths. The endoneurium consists of a substantial amount of extracellular matrix and dispersed cells (fibroblasts, macrophages, mast cells). The endoneurial extracellular matrix molecules such as collagen are produced by Schwann cells and endoneurial fibroblasts and increase the nerve's resistance to mechanical forces.

Vascularity of Peripheral Nerves

The blood supply of the peripheral nerve is composed of a set of well-developed intraneural microvascular plexuses.[44–46] The blood vessels that supply a nerve terminate in a capillary plexus and are located in the perineurium. Peripheral nerves possess two distinct and functionally independent vascular systems: an extrinsic system and an intrinsic system. The extrinsic system is composed of regional nutritive vessels and epineurial vessels, whereas the intrinsic system is made up of longitudinally oriented microvessels in the endoneurium. Both intrinsic and extrinsic segmental longitudinal vessels run in loose connective tissue surrounding the nerve and communicate with the intraneural microvascular plexuses, offering considerable overlap and anastamoses between the two systems. Additionally, endoneurial capillary walls are composed of nonfenestrated endothelial cells that are joined by tight junctions and surrounded by continuous basal laminae. However, this barrier is much less efficient in dorsal root and autonomic ganglia and in distal parts of peripheral nerves. Combined with high basal nerve blood flow and moderate metabolic demands, this system offers a high degree of resistance to ischemia for peripheral nerves.

Summary

Safe and successful surgery requires knowledge of anatomy and technical skill. Both go hand in hand and are dependent upon one another. Although surgical proficiency can be learned only by practical experience, knowledge of anatomy must be continuously studied in books and through dissection. Anatomy has not changed in the past several years, but iatrogenic nerve injuries continue to occur. A greater visual understanding and knowledge of the anatomy and biology of nerves will help in avoiding these injuries.

References

1. Moore KL, Dalley AF, Agur A. Clinically Oriented Anatomy. 6th ed. Baltimore, MD: Williams & Wilkins Co; 1985
2. Tubbs RS, Tyler-Kabara EC, Aikens AC, et al. Surgical anatomy of the dorsal scapular nerve. J Neurosurg 2005;102(5):910–911
3. Ebraheim NA, Lu J, Porshinsky B, Heck BE, Yeasting RA. Vulnerability of long thoracic nerve: an anatomic study. J Shoulder Elbow Surg 1998;7(5):458–461
4. Ebraheim NA, Whitehead JL, Alla SR, et al. The suprascapular nerve and its articular branch to the acromioclavicular joint: an anatomic study. J Shoulder Elbow Surg 2011;20(2):e13–e17
5. Tubiana R, Masquelet A, McCullough C. Peripheral nerves of the upper extremity. In: Atlas of Surgical Exposures of the Upper and Lower Extremities. London: Martin Dunitz Ltd.; 2000:83–118

6. Flatow EL, Bigliani LU, April EW. An anatomic study of the musculocutaneous nerve and its relationship to the coracoid process. Clin Orthop Relat Res 1989;(244):166–171

7. Hoppenfeld S, deBoer P. The humerus. In: Surgical Exposures in Orthopaedics: The Anatomic Approach. Philadelphia, PA: Lippincott Williams & Wilkins; 2003:68–104

8. Wongkerdsook W, Agthong S, Amarase C, Yotnuengnit P, Huanmanop T, Chentanez V. Anatomy of the lateral antebrachial cutaneous nerve in relation to the lateral epicondyle and cephalic vein. Clin Anat 2011;24(1):56–61

9. Hoppenfeld S, deBoer P. The forearm. In: Surgical Exposures in Orthopaedics: The Anatomic Approach. Philadelphia, PA: Lippincott Williams & Wilkins; 2003:141–172

10. Chowdhry S, Elston JB, Lefkowitz T, Wilhelmi BJ. Avoiding the medial brachial cutaneous nerve in brachioplasty: an anatomical study. Eplasty 2010;10:e16

11. Masear VR, Meyer RD, Pichora DR. Surgical anatomy of the medial antebrachial cutaneous nerve. J Hand Surg Am 1989;14(2, Pt 1): 267–271

12. Reckling F, Reckling J, Mohn M. Arm. In: Orthopaedic Anatomy and Surgical Approaches. St. Louis, MO: Mosby-Year Book Inc; 1990:43–60

13. Hoppenfeld S, deBoer P. The shoulder. In: Surgical Exposures in Orthopaedics: The Anatomic Approach. Philadelphia, PA: Lippincott Williams & Wilkins; 2003:1–68

14. Hoppenfeld S, deBoer P. The elbow. In: Surgical Exposures in Orthopaedics: The Anatomic Approach. Philadelphia, PA: Lippincott Williams & Wilkins; 2003:105–140

15. Reckling F, Reckling J, Mohn M. Forearm. In: Orthopaedic Anatomy and Surgical Approaches. St. Louis, MO: Mosby-Year Book Inc; 1990:89–110

16. Svízenská I, Cizmár I, Visna P. An anatomical study of the anterior interosseous nerve and its innervation of the pronator quadratus muscle. J Hand Surg [Br] 2005;30(6):635–637

17. Chaynes P, Bécue J, Vaysse P, Laude M. Relationships of the palmar cutaneous branch of the median nerve: a morphometric study. Surg Radiol Anat 2004;26(4):275–280

18. Hoppenfeld S, deBoer P. The wrist and hand. In: Surgical Exposures in Orthopaedics: The Anatomic Approach. Philadelphia, PA: Lippincott Williams & Wilkins; 2003:173–246

19. Reckling F, Reckling J, Mohn M. Wrist and Hand. In: Orthopaedic Anatomy and Surgical Approaches. St. Louis, MO: Mosby-Year Book Inc; 1990:111–164

20. Kasper JC, Itamura JM, Tibone JE, Levin SL, Stevanovic MV. Human cadaveric study of subscapularis muscle innervation and guidelines to prevent denervation. J Shoulder Elbow Surg 2008;17(4):659–662

21. Loukas M, Grabska J, Tubbs RS, Apaydin N, Jordan R. Mapping the axillary nerve within the deltoid muscle. Surg Radiol Anat 2009;31(1):43–47

22. Carlan D, Pratt J, Patterson JM, Weiland AJ, Boyer MI, Gelberman RH. The radial nerve in the brachium: an anatomic study in human cadavers. J Hand Surg Am 2007;32(8):1177–1182

23. MacAvoy MC, Rust SS, Green DP. Anatomy of the posterior antebrachial cutaneous nerve: practical information for the surgeon operating on the lateral aspect of the elbow. J Hand Surg Am 2006;31(6):908–911

24. Zhang J, Moore AE, Stringer MD. Iatrogenic upper limb nerve injuries: a systematic review. ANZ J Surg 2011;81(4):227–236

25. Balogh B, Valencak J, Vesely M, Flammer M, Gruber H, Piza-Katzer H. The nerve of Henle: an anatomic and immunohistochemical study. J Hand Surg Am 1999;24(5):1103–1108

26. McCabe SJ, Kleinert JM. The nerve of Henlé. J Hand Surg Am 1990;15(5):784–788

27. Mannerfelt L, Hybrinette CH. Important anomaly of the thenar branch of the median nerve. Bull Hosp Jt Dis 1972;33:15

28. Leversedge FJ, Boyer MI, Goldfarb CA. A Pocketbook Manual of Hand and Upper Extremity Anatomy: Primus Manus. Philadelphia, PA: Lippincott; 2010

29. Al-Qattan MM. Variations in the course of the thenar motor branch of the median nerve and their relationship to the hypertrophic muscle overlying the transverse carpal ligament. J Hand Surg Am 2010;35(11):1820–1824

30. Sarikcioglu L, Demirel BM. Martin-Gruber and Marinacci communications--anatomic or physiologic consideration. J Hist Neurosci 2006;15(2):99–101

31. Erdem HR, Ergun S, Erturk C, Ozel S. Electrophysiological evaluation of the incidence of martin-gruber anastomosis in healthy subjects. Yonsei Med J 2002;43(3):291–295

32. Lee KS, Oh CS, Chung IH, Sunwoo IN. An anatomic study of the Martin-Gruber anastomosis: electrodiagnostic implications. Muscle Nerve 2005;31(1):95–97

33. Harness D, Sekeles E. The double anastomotic innervation of thenar muscles. J Anat 1971;109(Pt 3):461–466

34. Kimura I, Ayyar DR, Lippmann SM. Electrophysiological verification of the ulnar to median nerve communications in the hand and forearm. Tohoku J Exp Med 1983;141(3):269–274

35. Saperstein DS, King RB. Motor neuron presentation of an ulnar neuropathy and Riche-Cannieu anastomosis. Electromyogr Clin Neurophysiol 2000;40(2):119–122

36. Smith JL, Siddiqui SA, Ebraheim NA. Comprehensive Summary of Anastomoses between the median and ulnar nerves in the forearm and hand. J Hand Microsurg. 2019: 11(1):1–5

37. Stancic MF, Micovic V, Potocnjak M: The anatomy of Berrettini branch: implications for carpal tunnel release. J. Neurosurg.1999;91(6):1027–30

38. Venieratos D, Anagnostopoulou S. Classification of communications between the musculocutaneous and median nerves. Clin Anat 1998;11(5):327–331

39. Loukas M, Aqueelah H. Musculocutaneous and median nerve connections within, proximal and distal to the coracobrachialis muscle. Folia Morphol (Warsz) 2005;64(2):101–108

40. Einhorn T, O'Keefe R, Buckwalter J. Form and function of the peripheral nerves and spinal cord. In: Orthopaedic Basic Science. Rosemont, IL: American Academy of Orthopaedic Surgeons; 2008:245–258

41. Dyck PJ, Thomas PK, Lambert EH, et al. Peripheral Neuropathy. 2nd ed. London: WB Saunders Company; 1984

42. Drury R, Wallington EA. Carleton's Histological Techniques—Nerves and Nerve Injuries. 2nd ed. New York, NY: Churchill-Livingstone; 1980:35–49

43. Weller RO, Cervos-Navarro J. Pathology of Peripheral Nerves. London: Butterworths; 1977:5–67

44. Platt CI, Krekoski CA, Ward RV, Edwards DR, Gavrilovic J. Extracellular matrix and matrix metalloproteinases in sciatic nerve. J Neurosci Res 2003;74(3):417–429

45. Scherer SS, Arroyo EJ. Recent progress on the molecular organization of myelinated axons. J Peripher Nerv Syst 2002;7(1):1–12

46. Kandel ER, Schwartz JK. Principles of Neural Science. 4th ed. New York, NY: McGraw-Hill; 2000

47. Scherer SS, Arroyo EJ. Recent progress on the molecular organization of myelinated axons. J Peripher Nerv Syst 2002;7(1):1–12

48. Martin CH, Seiler JG III, Lesesne JS. The cutaneous innervation of the palm: an anatomic study of the ulnar and median nerves. J Hand Surg Am 1996;21(4):634–638

10 The Brachial Plexus

Joshua M. Abzug, Dan A. Zlotolow, and Scott H. Kozin

10.1 Introduction

The brachial plexus is a confluence of nerves that control all function, motor and sensory, for the entire upper extremity. Knowledge of this anatomy and the surrounding structures is crucial for anyone caring for the upper limb or performing surgeries in the neck and shoulder region. Understanding of which muscles are innervated by which nerves, and subsequently where those nerves come from, is needed to perform an appropriate physical examination or interpret electrodiagnostic studies. This chapter will describe the relevant anatomy and provide case examples.

10.2 Neural Anatomy

The brachial plexus is typically made up of the ventral rami of the C5–T1 nerve roots. This "normal" pattern occurs in 75% of the population.[1] In 20 to 25% of the population, there is an additional contribution from the C4 nerve root, termed a prefixed cord. Approximately 1% of the population has a postfixed cord, where there is an additional contribution from the T2 nerve root.[1]

The brachial plexus has five distinct components: the roots, trunks, divisions, cords, and terminal branches. As this branching pattern is somewhat complicated, the mnemonic "Randy Travis Drinks Cold Beer" (Roots Trunks Divisions Cords Branches) may be helpful for remembering the order of branching from proximal to distal. The five roots, C5–T1, combine to form the upper, middle, and lower trunks (▶ Fig. 10.1). C5 and C6 combine to form the upper trunk, C7 continues to form the middle trunk, and C8 and T1 combine to form the lower trunk.

Subsequently, each trunk divides into anterior and posterior divisions, for a total of three anterior divisions and three posterior divisions. The anterior divisions supply innervation to the flexor compartments of the arm and forearm, whereas the posterior divisions supply innervation to the extensor compartments.

The divisions combine to form three cords, termed the lateral, medial, and posterior cords, based on their relationship to the axillary artery (▶ Fig. 10.2). The lateral cord is formed by the combination of the anterior divisions from the upper and middle trunk, whereas the medial cord is a continuation of the anterior division of the lower trunk. All three posterior divisions combine to form the posterior cord.

The terminal branches of the brachial plexus are the major peripheral nerves of the upper extremity: the axillary nerve, the musculocutaneous nerve, the median nerve, the ulnar nerve, and the radial nerve. The musculocutaneous nerve is a terminal branch from the lateral cord, and the ulnar nerve is a terminal branch from the medial cord. Contributions from both the lateral and medial cords combine to form the median nerve terminal branch. The posterior cord terminal branches are the axillary and radial nerves.

Numerous smaller branches arise from the brachial plexus to provide motor and/or sensory innervation throughout the upper extremity. We think it best to segregate these branches based on the distinct components of the brachial plexus in order to make it easier to remember each one. There are three branches from the root level. The dorsal scapular nerve, which innervates the rhomboids, arises from the C5 nerve root. The phrenic nerve, which innervates the diaphragm, is composed of contributions from the C3, C4, and C5 nerve roots. Last, the long thoracic nerve, which innervates the serratus anterior, is composed of contributions from the C5, C6, and C7 nerve roots.

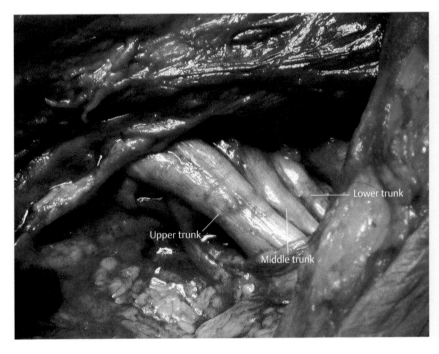

Fig. 10.1 Cadaveric exposure of the right brachial plexus demonstrating the upper, middle, and lower trunks. (The image is provided courtesy of Shriners Hospitals for Children, Philadelphia, PA.)

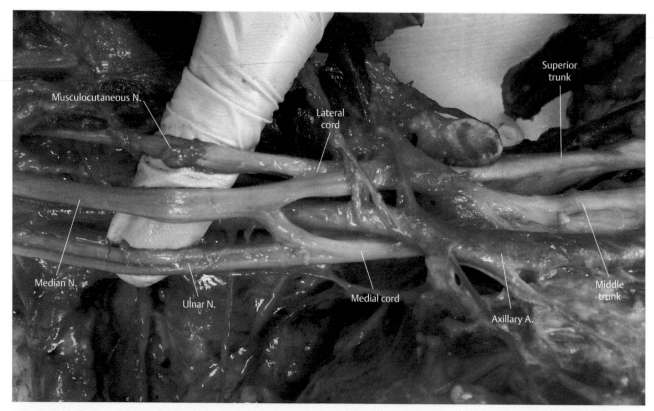

Fig. 10.2 Cadaveric exposure of the right brachial plexus with clavicle resected, demonstrating the cords and terminal branches. (The image is provided courtesy of Shriners Hospitals for Children, Philadelphia, PA.)

Only two branches arise from the level of the trunks, both of which come off the upper trunk. In the proximal portion of the upper trunk, the nerve to subclavius arises and travels along the anterior aspect of the plexus to innervate the subclavius muscle. The suprascapular nerve, which innervates the supraspinatus and infraspinatus muscles, has a very distal takeoff. We have noted that there is often a trifurcation of the upper trunk into the anterior and posterior divisions and suprascapular nerve (▶ Fig. 10.3). No branches arise from the level of the divisions.

Numerous smaller branches come off the level of the cords; however, these can be remembered by breaking things down into the individual cord branches. Only one branch arises from the lateral cord, the lateral pectoral nerve, which innervates the pectoralis major. The posterior and medial cords have three branches each. Arising from the medial cord from proximal to distal is the medial pectoral nerve, which innervates the pectoralis major and minor; the medial cutaneous nerve of the arm, which supplies sensation to the medial arm; and the medial cutaneous nerve of the forearm, which supplies sensation to the medial forearm. The branches of the posterior cord from proximal to distal are the upper subscapular nerve, which innervates the subscapularis; the thoracodorsal nerve, which innervates the latissimus dorsi; and the lower subscapular nerve, which innervates the subscapularis and teres major.

All of the aforementioned peripheral nerves are part of the parasympathetic nervous system. The sympathetic nervous system travels as the sympathetic chain and synapses in the inferior cervical and upper thoracic ganglia. Injury to the sympathetic fibers in the region of the brachial plexus, particularly affecting the superior cervical ganglion, can result in Horner's syndrome on the ipsilateral side.

10.3 Vascular Anatomy

The vessels about the brachial plexus include the subclavian artery and vein, which become the axillary artery and vein upon entering the axilla. Four branches arise from the subclavian artery medial to the anterior scalene: the vertebral artery, the thyrocervical trunk, the internal thoracic artery, and the costocervical trunk (▶ Fig. 10.4). The thyrocervical trunk gives off the transverse cervical artery, suprascapular artery, and inferior thyroid artery. Identification of the transverse cervical artery can be made by observing its course on the anterior aspect of the upper trunk. The dorsal scapular artery typically crosses the C7 root in a transverse direction. The suprascapular artery runs parallel but inferior to the transverse cervical artery and courses to join the suprascapular nerve. It is important to note that the suprascapular artery has been noted to arise directly from the subclavian artery in more than 20% of cases.

10.4 Lymphatic Anatomy

Knowledge of the drainage of the lymphatic system is important for those caring for brachial plexus injuries, as the main drainage for the majority of the body is via the thoracic duct. This structure runs on the left side of the body and ascends on

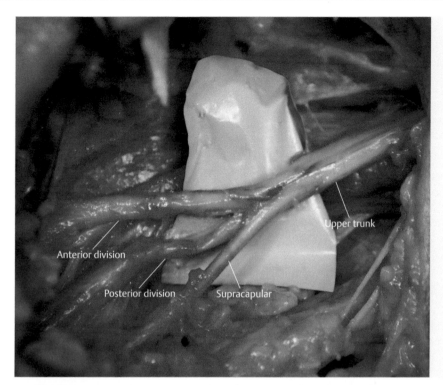

Fig. 10.3 Cadaveric exposure of the left brachial plexus from cephalad, showing a trifurcation of the upper trunk into the anterior and posterior divisions and the suprascapular nerve. (The image is provided courtesy of Shriners Hospitals for Children, Philadelphia, PA.)

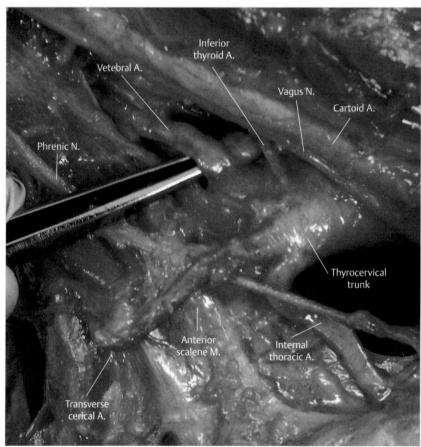

Fig. 10.4 Branches from the subclavian artery include the vertebral artery, the thyrocervical trunk, and the internal thoracic artery. (The image is provided courtesy of Shriners Hospitals for Children, Philadelphia, PA.)

the front of the vertebral bodies between the aorta and azygous veins. As the thoracic duct leaves the thorax, it travels behind the subclavian artery and ends at the confluence of the left subclavian and left internal jugular veins. Injury to the thoracic duct can occur during dissection of the brachial plexus or surrounding structures on the left side. The lymphatic fluid is clear, and injury to the thoracic duct can lead to deficiencies in the protein and salt content of the blood.

10.5 Posterior Triangle of the Neck

The roots and trunks of the brachial plexus lie within the posterior triangle of the neck. This region is bounded anteriorly by the posterior border of the sternocleidomastoid muscle and posteriorly by the anterior border of the trapezius muscle, whose intersection superiorly forms the apex of the triangle. The base of the triangle is the middle third of the clavicle.

Within the posterior triangle of the neck are the various structures that aid in localizing the brachial plexus when surgical procedures are performed. Particular examples of these structures include the omohyoid muscle, the phrenic nerve, the subclavian artery, the transverse cervical artery, the dorsal scapular artery, the external jugular vein, and the anterior and middle scalene muscles (▶ Fig. 10.5). As noted hereafter, all of these structures are integral in localizing the brachial plexus during surgical exploration.

10.6 Exposure of the Brachial Plexus

An incision is made in a skin crease of the neck, following Langer's lines, from the sternocleidomastoid to the anterior edge of the trapezius, thus paralleling the base of the posterior triangle of the neck.[2] Subcutaneous fat will be present, and dissection through this will reveal the platysma. In infants, no platysma will be visible, as it is underdeveloped. Once the fascia is identified and incised, the sternocleidomastoid should be identified and dissection begun from its posterior border in a lateral

direction. The external jugular vein will be visible and may need to be ligated. A fat pad superficial to the carotid sheath is now visible and will need to be elevated, ideally without entering the carotid sheath. On the left side, it is crucial to avoid injury to the thoracic duct as well.

Identification of the anterior and middle scalene muscles should now be performed. The phrenic nerve will be visualized lying on the anterior surface of the anterior scalene. In the inferior aspect of the wound, the omohyoid muscle should be visible. This is the "door" to the supraclavicular plexus. Deep to the omohyoid, the C5 and C6 nerve roots should be visible. The clavicle and subclavian vessels are at the inferior portion of the wound, marking the inferior extent of the posterior triangle of the neck. The C5 and C6 nerve roots can be traced distally to identify the upper trunk and trifurcation into the anterior and posterior divisions and suprascapular nerve. The transverse cervical artery crosses the upper trunk and requires ligation (▶ Fig. 10.6). At this trifurcation, the anterior division is medial, the posterior division is in the middle, and the suprascapular nerve is lateral. The C7 root can be identified by locating the dorsal scapular artery that runs across it in a transverse direction. Inferior exposure of C8 and T1 must identify and respect the subclavian artery just behind the clavicle and superficial to these roots.

Exposure of the infraclavicular plexus requires extending the incision toward the coracoid and then between the deltoid and pectoralis major muscles. The cephalic vein is isolated and mobilized. Identification of the deeper pectoralis minor muscle is the key to exposing the infraclavicular plexus. Release of the pectoralis minor from the coracoid will permit visualization of the infraclavicular plexus. An osteotomy of

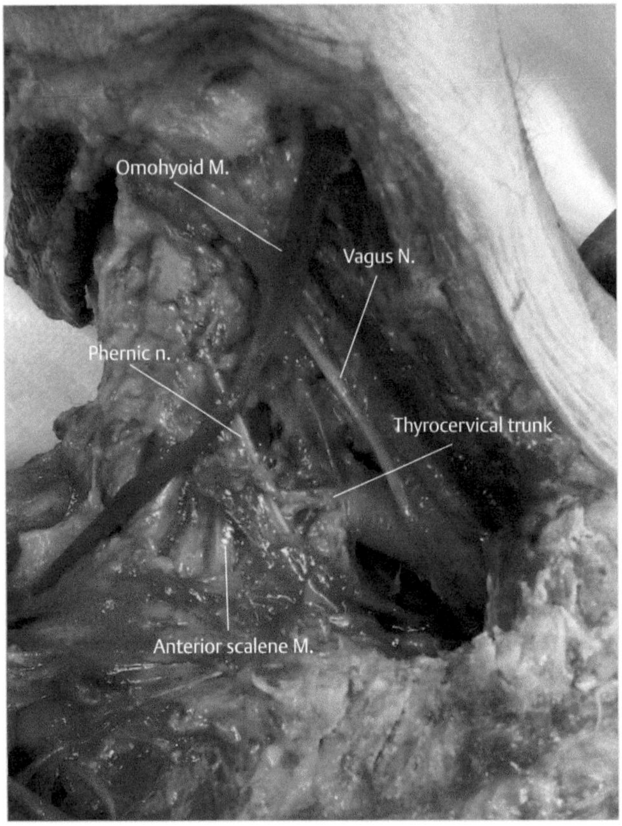

Fig. 10.5 Important structures within the posterior triangle of the neck include the omohyoid muscle and the phrenic nerve. The vagus nerve resides medial to the phrenic nerve and adjacent to the carotid sheath. (The image is provided courtesy of Shriners Hospitals for Children, Philadelphia, PA.)

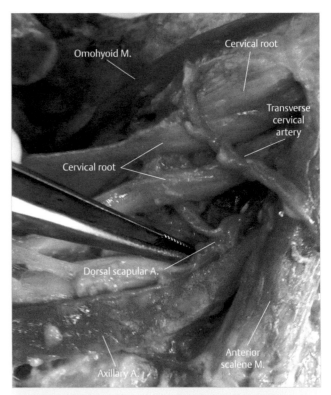

Fig. 10.6 The transverse cervical artery crosses the upper trunk and requires ligation during brachial plexus exposure. (The image is provided courtesy of Shriners Hospitals for Children, Philadelphia, PA.)

the clavicle may be necessary to allow extensile exposure of the plexus in cases with extensive scarring.

10.7 Case Example 1: Adult Injury

Christopher is a 16-year-old male who was riding a motorbike when he collided with his opponent. He sustained multiple fractures, including his right humerus, right hip, right distal femur, and right tibia. He also sustained a right subclavian artery laceration that required grafting and a concomitant brachial plexus injury. Ultimately, he required a right transfemoral amputation and ambulated with prosthesis. He had no return of upper trunk function and underwent exploration 6 months after injury (▶Fig. 10.7).

A supraclavicular approach was performed via an incision across the upper border of the clavicle (▶Fig. 10.7a). The omohyoid muscle was retracted in a cephalad direction to expose the underlying brachial plexus and upper trunk (▶Fig. 10.7b). The phrenic nerve was isolated and protected along the anterior scalene (▶Fig. 10.7c). There was a large neuroma of the upper trunk (▶Fig. 10.7d). The neuroma was sharply excised back to viable fascicles (▶Fig. 10.7e). There was a 3-cm defect after the neuroma was resected (▶Fig. 10.7f). Sural nerve interposition grafting was performed to bridge the defect (▶Fig. 10.7g). Ultimately, a total of six grafts were used between C5/C6 and upper trunk (suprascapular, posterior division, and anterior division).

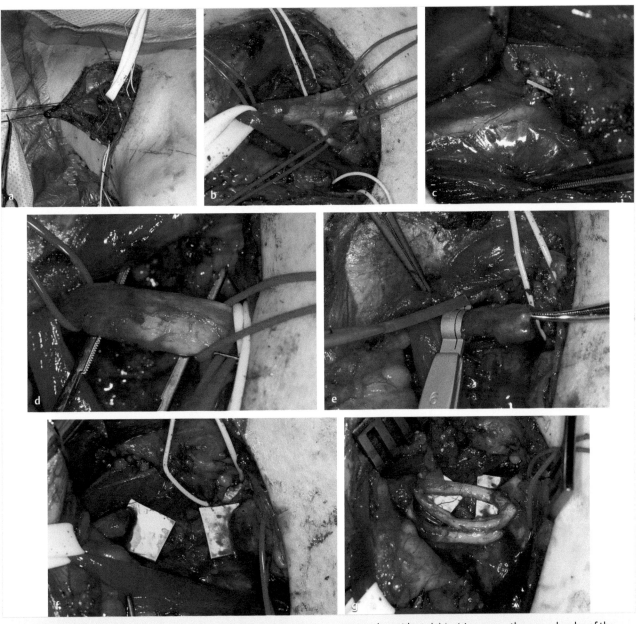

Fig. 10.7 A 16-year-old male sustained a right brachial plexus injury in a motorcycle accident. (a) Incision across the upper border of the clavicle. (b) The omohyoid muscle is retracted in a cephalad direction to expose the underlying brachial plexus. Note the trifurcation of the suprascapular nerve, posterior division, and anterior division. (c) Phrenic nerve isolated along the anterior scalene muscle. (d) Neuroma of upper trunk. (e) Sharp resection of neuroma back to normal-appearing fascicles. (f) Defect between C5/C6 and upper trunk (suprascapular, posterior division, and anterior division). (g) Sural nerve grafting from C5/C6 to upper trunk. (The images are provided courtesy of Shriners Hospital for Children, Philadelphia, PA.)

10.8 Case Example 2: Obstetrical Injury

Madison is a 6-month-old female born at 40 weeks of gestation, weighing 8 pounds 12 ounces. Vacuum-assisted delivery was performed, which was complicated by right shoulder dystocia requiring multiple maneuvers to effectuate delivery. Apgar scores were 1 at 1 minute and 7 at 5 minutes. There were no fractures detected.

Initial examination noted profound deficits in C5, C6, and C7. The C8 and T1 nerve roots appeared uninjured, as there was a positive grasp response and no Horner's syndrome. The C7 nerve root recovered over the first 3 months, with return of elbow extension, forearm pronation, and digital extension. Dense deficits remained in the C5 and C6 nerve roots, with absent shoulder movement, elbow flexion, and forearm supination. Exploration was performed at 6 months of age (▶ Fig. 10.8).

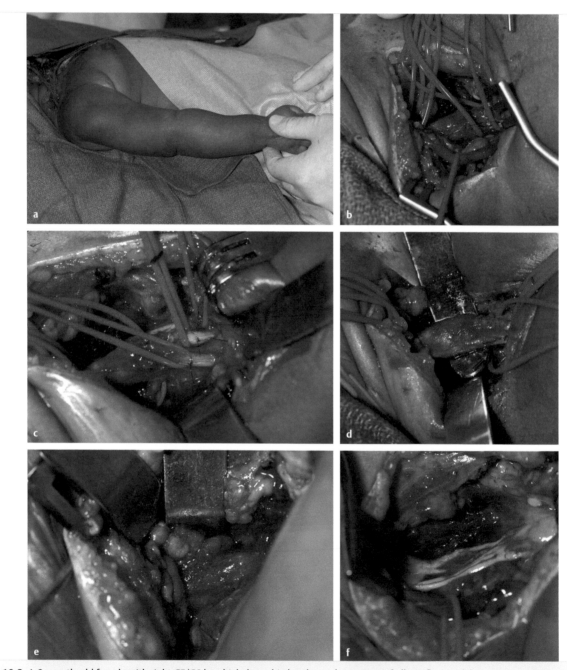

Fig. 10.8 A 6-month-old female with right C5/C6 brachial plexus birth palsy and no return of elbow flexion. (**a**) Operative positioning on operating room table. (**b**) Supraclavicular exposure with retraction of omohyoid. (**c**) Isolation of suprascapular nerve, posterior division of upper trunk, and anterior division of upper trunk distal to neuroma. (**d**) Large neuroma of upper trunk. (**e**) C5 nerve root after neuroma resection. (**f**) Sural nerve grafting from C5 and C6 to suprascapular nerve, posterior division of upper trunk, and anterior division of upper trunk. (The images are provided courtesy of Shriners Hospital for Children, Philadelphia, PA.)

A transverse incision was made along Langer's lines just above the clavicle (▶Fig. 10.8a). The omohyoid muscle was retracted and the C5 and C6 nerve roots identified along with the neuroma (▶Fig. 10.8b). Distal to the neuroma, the suprascapular nerve, posterior division of upper trunk, and anterior division of upper trunk were tagged. The large neuroma was isolated and resected (▶Fig. 10.8c). The nerve roots were cut back until viable fascicles were visualized (▶Fig. 10.8d). Sural nerve grafting was performed between the C5 and C6 roots and the suprascapular nerve, posterior division of upper trunk, and anterior division of upper trunk (▶Fig. 10.8e). The coaptation sites were secured with fibrin glue.

References

1. Lee HY, Chung IH, Sir WS, et al. Variations of the ventral rami of the brachial plexus. J Korean Med Sci 1992;7(1):19–24
2. Kozin SH. Injuries of the brachial plexus. In: Iannotti JP, Williams GR, eds. Disorders of the Shoulder: Diagnosis and Management. 2nd ed. Philadelphia, PA: Lippincott Williams & White; 2007:1087–1134

11 Vascular Anatomy of the Upper Extremity

Alejandro Maciel-Miranda and Steven F. Morris

11.1 Vascular Anatomy of the Upper Extremity

Knowledge of the vascular anatomy of the upper extremity is obviously crucial to the treatment of a wide variety of hand and upper limb conditions. This chapter is essentially organized from "top to bottom" in that we describe the anatomy sequentially throughout the upper limb. We highlight the anatomy of specific vessels important to the harvest of tissue transfers and show variations in the vascular anatomy of the upper limb. Additionally, we review the lymphatics and demonstrate anatomical applications of the anatomy.

11.2 Axillary Artery

The axillary artery provides the main vascular supply to the upper limb. It extends from the lateral border of the first rib to the inferior border of the teres major muscle. It is divided into three parts, based on its relationship to the pectoralis minor muscle (▶ Table 11.1).[1] In the first part of the axillary artery, one major branch, the **superior thoracic artery**, arises and supplies

the first to third intercostal spaces and upper portion of the serratus anterior muscle and may send a branch to the pectoralis major muscle (▶ Fig. 11.1).

The second part, posterior to the pectoralis minor muscle, provides two branches, the thoracoacromial and lateral thoracic arteries. The second part of the axillary artery is adjacent to the level of cords of the brachial plexus.

The **thoracoacromial** artery pierces the clavipectoral fascia and has four branches:
- **The clavicular branch** supplies the subclavius and sends a nutrient branch to the clavicle.
- **The pectoral branches** that course between pectoralis major and minor supply the muscles as well as the breast.
- **The deltoid branch** runs through the deltopectoral groove, supplying the deltoid and pectoralis major. The deltoid branch gives off a cutaneous branch to supply the skin of the anterior aspect of the shoulder. Manchot referred to this artery as the "anterior subcutaneous deltoid artery."[2] There are usually three perforators to the skin over the anterior deltoid, with an average diameter of 0.8 mm. Most are musculocutaneous arteries with an average pedicle length of 37 ± 18 mm.[2]

Table 11.1 Branches of the axillary artery

Artery	Source	Branches	Supply to	Comments
Superior thoracic	First part of axillary artery	Unnamed muscular branches	Muscles of intercostal spaces 1 and 2	Superior thoracic artery anastomoses with the intercostal artery for intercostal spaces 1 and 2
Lateral thoracic	Second part of axillary artery	Unnamed muscular branches	Serratus anterior muscle, parts of adjacent muscles, skin and fascia of the anterolateral thoracic wall	Lateral thoracic artery is a rare case in that it enters the serratus anterior from its superficial surface
Thoracoacromial	Second part of axillary artery	Pectoral branch, clavicular branch, acromial branch, deltoid branch	Pectoralis major muscle, pectoralis minor muscle, subclavius muscle, deltoid muscle, shoulder joint	Thoracoacromial trunk pierces the costocoracoid membrane
Anterior circumflex humeral	Third part of axillary artery	Unnamed muscular branches	Deltoid muscle; arm muscles near the surgical neck of the humerus	Anastomoses with the posterior circumflex humeral artery
Posterior circumflex humeral	Third part of axillary artery	Unnamed muscular branches	Deltoid; arm muscles near the surgical neck of the humerus	Anastomoses with the anterior circumflex humeral artery; it passes through the quadrangular space with the axillary nerve
Subscapular	Third part of axillary artery	Circumflex scapular artery, thoracodorsal artery	Subscapularis muscle, teres major muscle, teres minor muscle, infraspinatus muscle	The circumflex scapular branch of the subscapular artery anastomoses with the suprascapular artery and the dorsal scapular artery to form the scapular anastomosis
Circumflex scapular	Subscapular artery	Unnamed muscular branches	Teres major muscle, teres minor muscle, infraspinatus muscle	Anastomoses with the suprascapular artery and the dorsal scapular artery; passes through the triangular space
Thoracodorsal	Subscapular artery	Unnamed muscular branches	Latissimus dorsi muscle	Thoracodorsal artery accompanies the thoracodorsal nerve

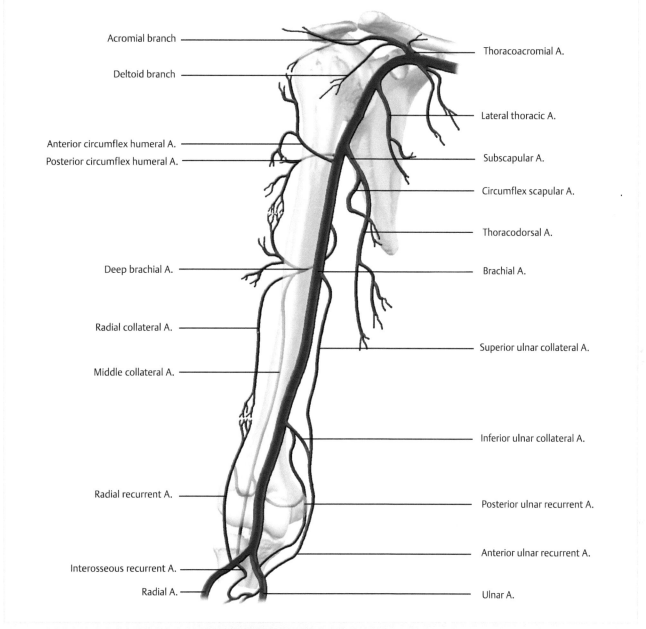

Acromial branch

Deltoid branch

Anterior circumflex humeral A.
Posterior circumflex humeral A.

Deep brachial A.

Radial collateral A.

Middle collateral A.

Radial recurrent A.

Interosseous recurrent A.

Radial A.

Thoracoacromial A.

Lateral thoracic A.

Subscapular A.

Circumflex scapular A.

Thoracodorsal A.

Brachial A.

Superior ulnar collateral A.

Inferior ulnar collateral A.

Posterior ulnar recurrent A.

Anterior ulnar recurrent A.

Ulnar A.

Fig. 11.1 Schematic view of the arteries of shoulder and upper arm.

- **The Acromial branch** supplies the medial border of the deltoid and reaches the acromion process, where it anastomoses with the suprascapular artery and forms the acromial network.

The **lateral thoracic artery** may arise from the second part of the axillary artery in about 50%, from a branch of the subscapular artery in 30%, from the first part of the axillary artery in 11%, or from the thoracoacromial artery in 7%.[3] It descends along the lateral border of the pectoralis minor and supplies the serratus anterior and pectoralis minor muscles; it also supplies branches to the lateral aspect of the breast and overlying skin.

Three major branches, the subscapular artery, anterior circumflex humeral artery, and posterior circumflex humeral artery, arise from the **third part of the axillary artery**. The

subscapular artery is the largest branch of the axillary artery; it courses caudally along the border of the subscapularis, under the latissimus dorsi muscle. It is accompanied by the lower subscapular and thoracodorsal nerves and supplies the subscapularis, teres major, latissimus dorsi, and serratus anterior muscles as well as the axillary lymph nodes. The subscapular artery divides into two secondary branches, the circumflex scapular and the thoracodorsal arteries.

The **circumflex scapular branch** passes dorsally through the triangular space (borders: subscapularis, teres major, and long head of triceps) to reach the infraspinatus fossa, where it anastomoses with the suprascapular and dorsal scapular arteries.

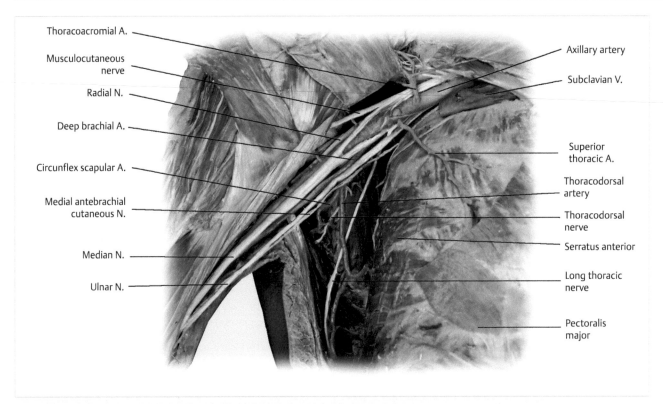

Thoracoacromial A.

Musculocutaneous nerve

Radial N.

Deep brachial A.

Circunflex scapular A.

Medial antebrachial cutaneous N.

Median N.

Ulnar N.

Axillary artery

Subclavian V.

Superior thoracic A.

Thoracodorsal artery

Thoracodorsal nerve

Serratus anterior

Long thoracic nerve

Pectoralis major

Fig. 11.2 Axillary artery and its branches in a cadaver dissection.

The **thoracodorsal branch** is the continuation of the subscapular artery, which travels along the deep surface of the latissimus dorsi muscle. This artery is accompanied by the thoracodorsal nerve and supplies the latissimus dorsi and subscapularis muscles. Branches of this vessel supply the serratus anterior, intercostal muscles, and pectoral muscles (▶ Fig. 11.2).

The **anterior circumflex humeral artery** may arise from a common stem with the posterior circumflex humeral artery. It runs deep to the coracobrachialis and the short and long heads of biceps, and it turns transversely around the anterior aspect of the surgical neck of the humerus. It anastomoses with the posterior circumflex humeral artery and branches of the thoracoacromial artery. The anterior circumflex humeral artery supplies small secondary branches: (1) **the bicipital branch** ascends the bicipital groove to enter and supply the tendon of the long head of the biceps, and (2) **the pectoral branch** descends along the tendon and supplies the pectoralis major muscle.

The **posterior circumflex humeral artery** passes dorsally through the quadrangular space (borders: teres minor, teres major, latissimus dorsi, and humerus) with the axillary nerve. It provides the primary vascular supply of the deltoid and teres major and minor muscles and gives off nutrient branches to the greater tubercle of the humerus, articular branches to the shoulder joint, acromial branches, and a descending muscular branch to the long and lateral heads of the triceps. The posterior circumflex humeral artery anastomoses with the ascending branch from the deep brachial artery. The deep brachial artery may arise from the posterior circumflex humeral artery in 7%, and the posterior circumflex artery is a branch of the deep brachial artery in 16%.[3]

The posterior subcutaneous deltoid artery supplies the skin of the posterior aspect of the shoulder[2,4] and gives off

two to three perforators which penetrate the marginal fibers of the deltoid muscle in 91%. The average diameter of the source vessel is 2.5 ± 0.3 mm, with an average pedicle length of 6 to 8 cm to the quadrangular space.[4] This vessel can provide the vascular supply of the "deltoid flap" (▶ Fig. 11.3).[5]

11.3 Brachial Artery

The **brachial artery** is the continuation of the axillary artery at the inferior border of the teres major muscle, and it ends in the antecubital fossa, where it divides into the radial and ulnar arteries. It lies medially in the neurovascular compartment of the arm, and as it courses distally, it gradually moves anterior to the humerus. At its termination, it lies midway between the two epicondyles of the humerus.[6] In the antecubital fossa, it lies medial to the bicipital tendon and passes deep to the bicipital aponeurosis. Throughout its course in the upper arm, the brachial artery is accompanied by the median nerve. The nerve crosses the artery and lies medial to it in the antecubital fossa. The artery is accompanied by one vein.[3] Bifurcation of the brachial artery around the antecubital fossa is considered an anatomical variation and may be present in around 5.75% of cases (▶ Fig. 11.4).[7]

In its course through the upper arm, the brachial artery sends an average of 6 cutaneous perforators (range, 2–10) which travel to the skin on either side of the biceps muscle. These arteries course between the biceps and the brachialis muscle to the skin over the lateral bicipital groove from the deltoid muscle insertion to the biceps tendon insertion. The vascular territory of the brachial artery is 162 ± 42 cm², the median diameter of the cutaneous perforators is 0.7 ± 0.4 mm, and the

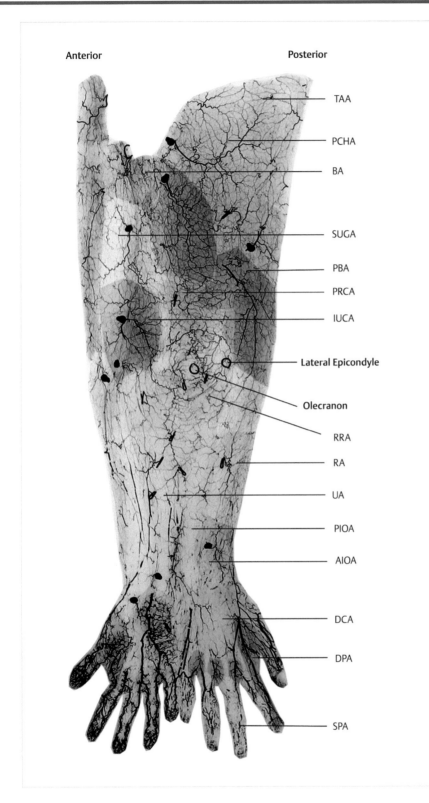

Fig. 11.3 Vascular territories of the skin of the upper limb. This represents the entire skin of the upper extremity of a human cadaver after lead oxide injection showing the distribution of cutaneous perforators to the skin. Vascular Territories:

TAA	Thoracoacromial artery
PCHA	Posterior circumflex humeral artery
BA	Brachial artery
SUCA	Superior Ulnar collateral artery
PBA	Profunda brachial artery
PRCA	Posterior radial collateral artery
IUCA	Inferior ulnar collateral artery
RRA	Radial recurrent artery
RA	Radial artery
UA	Ulnar artery
PIOA	Posterior interosseous artery
AIOA	Anterior interosseous artery
DCA	Dorsal carpal arch
DPA	Deep palmer arch
SPA	Superficial palmer arch

Labels on figure: Anterior, Posterior, TAA, PCHA, BA, SUGA, PBA, PRCA, IUCA, Lateral Epicondyle, Olecranon, RRA, RA, UA, PIOA, AIOA, DCA, DPA, SPA

superficial length of individual perforators is 30 ± 14 mm.[4] The **posterior brachial cutaneous artery** is a large, consistent, cutaneous branch of the brachial artery which has a mean diameter of 1.5 mm and pedicle length of 6.2 cm. This artery supplies the posterior brachial arm flap, which could be harvested as a osteocutaneous flap with the lateral aspect of the distal part of the humerus.[4,8,9]

The **branches of the brachial artery** are (1) the **profunda brachial artery**, (2) the **nutrient artery of the humerus**, (3) the **superior and inferior ulnar collateral arteries** and the terminal branches, and (4) the **radial and ulnar arteries**.

The **profunda brachial artery** arises from the brachial artery posteromedially, just distal to the teres major muscle. In 55%, it

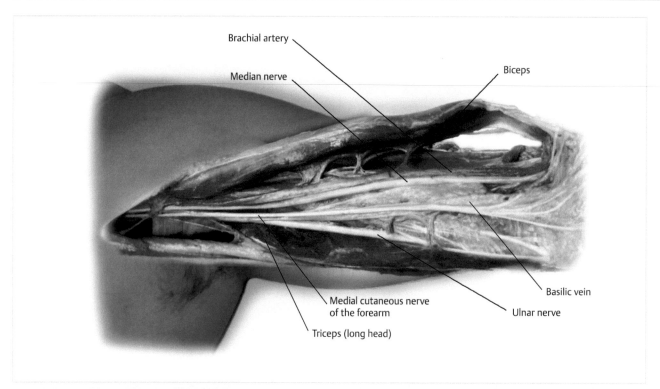

Fig. 11.4 Brachial artery in a cadaver dissection.

arises as a single trunk; it may also arise as a common trunk with the superior ulnar collateral artery in 22%, from the axillary in 16%, or as a branch of the posterior circumflex humeral artery in 7%.[3] The artery courses laterally between the medial and lateral heads of the triceps, through the spiral groove together with the radial nerve, before piercing the lateral intermuscular septum. A deltoid branch arises and divides into two terminal branches, the middle and radial collateral arteries on either side of the intermuscular septum. It anastomoses with the descending branch of the posterior circumflex humeral artery that may arise from the profunda brachial artery in 16% (▶ Fig. 11.5).[2]

Some perforators of the profunda brachial artery follow the posterior antebrachial cutaneous nerve to the skin of the lateral aspect of the arm via direct branches distal to the deltoid muscle insertion. It contributes two to six perforators to a vascular territory of 131 ± 30 cm².[4]

The **middle collateral branch** supplies the triceps entering through the medial head. It continues to the elbow, where it terminates at the olecranon articular network.

The **radial collateral branch** continues accompanying the radial nerve and supplies muscular branches to the lateral head of the triceps; it also supplies the skin over the lateral and distal half of the arm through septocutaneous perforators.

There are usually two perforators of the radial collateral branch which supply an average area of 64 ± 31 cm² along the lateral aspect of the distal arm. The mean diameter of the perforators is 1.6 ± 0.2 mm with an average length of 5.8 cm. There is a musculocutaneous/septocutaneous perforator ratio of 3:2.[4] The posterior radial collateral artery supplies the lateral arm flap which can be harvested as an osteocutaneous free flap including the lateral aspect of the distal humerus[10,11] or as a distally based flap for elbow coverage based on the radial recurrent artery.

The profunda brachial artery descends between the brachioradialis and brachialis muscles to the region of the lateral epicondyle, where it anastomoses with the **radial recurrent artery**.

The **nutrient humeral artery** arises near the origin of the superior ulnar collateral artery, crosses the brachialis, and enters a foramen near or distal to the middle of the humerus.

The **superior ulnar collateral artery** arises from the ulnar side of the brachial artery at the level of the insertion of the coracobrachialis. In 22% of cases, it may have a common trunk with the profunda brachial.[3] This artery accompanies the ulnar nerve posterior to the medial epicondyle and anastomoses with the posterior ulnar recurrent artery.

In 30% of dissections, the superior ulnar collateral artery supplied the skin as a direct cutaneous branch from the brachial artery. In the remaining dissections, it supplied the skin through septocutaneous (95%) or musculocutaneous (5%) perforators. There are usually one to two perforators with a mean vascular territory of 94 ± 29 cm². The superficial pedicle length is 56 ± 34 mm and the diameter was 0.9 ± 2 mm.[4] The medial arm flap can be based on this vessel[12,13]; however, the pedicle length is fairly short and the anatomy is quite variable.

The **inferior ulnar collateral artery** arises from the medial side of the brachial artery 5 cm proximal to the elbow and runs between the median nerve and the brachialis muscle and divides into anterior and posterior branches.

The inferior ulnar collateral artery and the ulnar recurrent artery together supply the medial aspect of the elbow, in an inverse relationship. An average of 2 ± 1 perforators were found in this territory, with a mean vessel diameter of 0.8 ± 0.2 mm, and a superficial length of 35 ± 12 mm.[4]

A **superficial brachial artery** may arise from the axillary artery or from the proximal end of the brachial artery. This

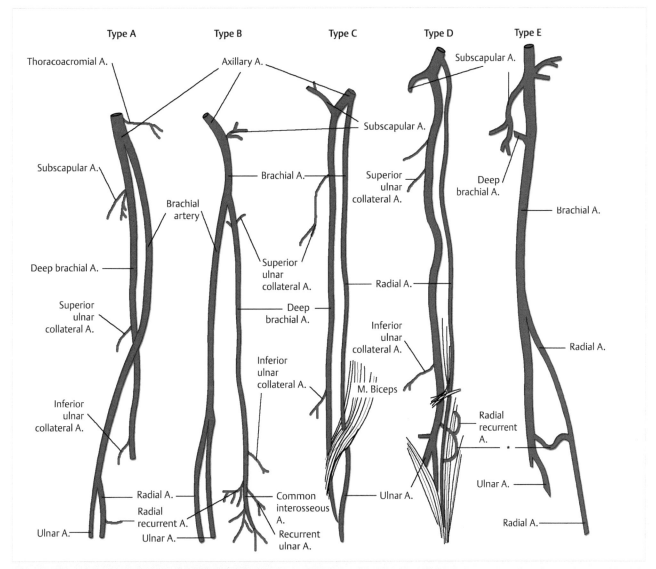

Fig. 11.5 Variations in the deep brachial artery anatomy.

artery runs superficially in the arm, slightly more lateral than the brachial artery. When this artery is present, it divides into ulnar and radial arteries, and the usual brachial artery may be absent or provide deep brachial and common interosseous artery branches. When the ulnar artery arises from the superficial brachial, the first runs superficially to the forearm flexors.

A high origin of the radial artery occurs in 14.27% of cases, being the most frequent anatomical variation in 107 specimens in a series of 750 extremities,[7] and may be as proximal as the axillary artery or from the brachial artery. It usually lies medially and then anterior to the median nerve and medial to the biceps muscle, and runs in its usual position in the forearm. Uniting vessels that course deep to the biceps tendon were constant, as are referred to as a sling connection.

A high origin of the ulnar artery occurs in 2.26% of cases.[7] It may arise from the axillary or brachial arteries, usually lying anterior to the brachial and median nerves and superficial in the antecubital fossa. When derived from the axillary artery, it arises from its anterior aspect and courses between the lateral and medial cords of the median nerve.

A variant division of the brachial artery into ulnar and radial arteries as far as 8 cm distal to the antecubital fossa may lead to difficulties raising a standard radial forearm flap.[14]

There are 15 cutaneous vascular territories in the upper arm, and each source artery provides a variable number of cutaneous perforators. An average of 48 ± 19 perforators (≥ 0.5-mm diameter) in 15 vascular territories supply the integument of the upper extremity.[4]

11.4 Ulnar Artery

The **ulnar artery** is the larger of the two terminal branches of the brachial artery. It arises in the apex of the antecubital fossa. In the forearm, it runs deep to the pronator teres and flexor digitorum superficialis, to the ulnar side, where it continues deep to the flexor carpi ulnaris. It passes through the Guyon canal to the palm, where it divides into two branches and contributes to the superficial and deep palmar arterial arches (▶ Fig. 11.6).

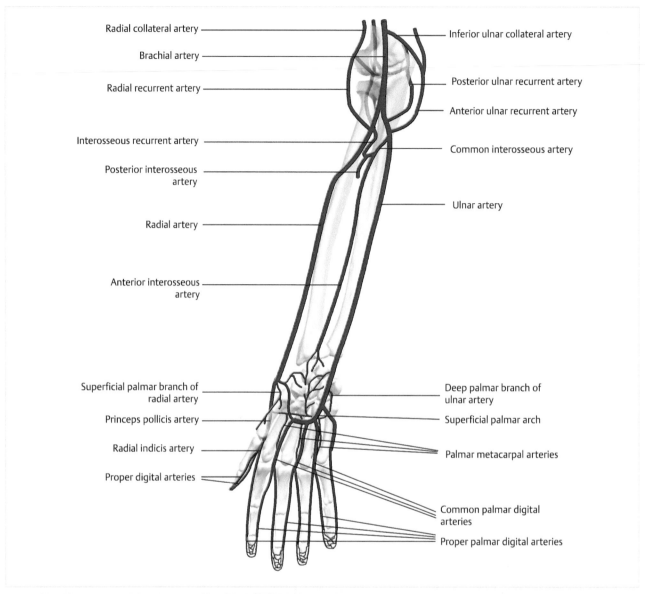

Radial collateral artery

Brachial artery

Radial recurrent artery

Interosseous recurrent artery

Posterior interosseous artery

Radial artery

Anterior interosseous artery

Superficial palmar branch of radial artery

Princeps pollicis artery

Radial indicis artery

Proper digital arteries

Inferior ulnar collateral artery

Posterior ulnar recurrent artery

Anterior ulnar recurrent artery

Common interosseous artery

Ulnar artery

Deep palmar branch of ulnar artery

Superficial palmar arch

Palmar metacarpal arteries

Common palmar digital arteries

Proper palmar digital arteries

Fig. 11.6 Schematic view of the arteries of forearm and hand.

The ulnar artery consistently supplies the skin of the medial forearm. There are four to nine perforators; 69% of these arteries are musculocutaneous and penetrate the flexor carpi ulnaris muscle. The mean superficial length is 27 ± 14 mm.[4] An ulnar pedicled or free flap or a perforator-based flap may be harvested from this territory.[15]

The ulnar nerve joins the artery at the distal end of the proximal third of the vessel and is located on its ulnar side. The artery is accompanied by two venae comitantes.

In the forearm, the ulnar artery gives rise to the ulnar recurrent, common interosseous, palmar carpal, and dorsal carpal arteries.

There are **two ulnar recurrent branches**, anterior and posterior. The anterior recurrent branch courses between the lateral edge of pronator teres and brachialis and supplies both muscles; it anastomoses anterior to the medial epicondyle with the inferior ulnar collateral artery. The posterior branch is larger than the anterior branch; it runs between the flexor digitorum superficialis and profundus and lies with the ulnar

nerve between the two heads of the origin of the flexor carpi ulnaris. It supplies adjacent muscles, the elbow joint, and the ulnar nerve, and forms the cubital articular network anastomosing with the superior and inferior ulnar collateral, interosseous recurrent, and middle collateral arteries.

The **common interosseous branch** is a short trunk about 1.2-cm long that arises from the posterior aspect of the ulnar artery, about 2.5 cm from its origin; it passes dorsally and distally between the flexor digitorum profundus and flexor pollicis longus. It branches into anterior and posterior interosseous arteries.

The **anterior interosseous branch** runs distally along the anterior surface of the interosseous membrane. It supplies the flexor digitorum profundus and the flexor pollicis longus. It divides into two branches at the proximal border of the pronator quadratus, the anterior and posterior terminal branches. It is accompanied by a vena comitans and medially by the anterior interosseous branch of the median nerve (▶Fig. 11.7).

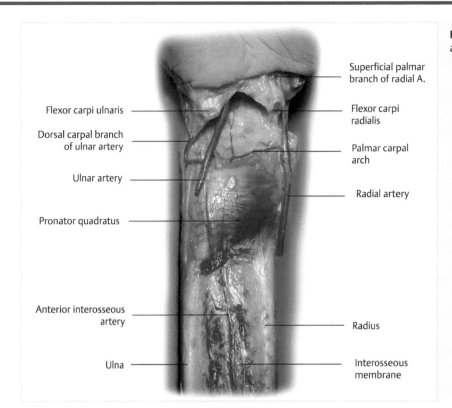

Fig. 11.7 Cadaver dissection of the anterior aspect of distal forearm.

Labels on figure:
- Flexor carpi ulnaris
- Dorsal carpal branch of ulnar artery
- Ulnar artery
- Pronator quadratus
- Anterior interosseous artery
- Ulna
- Superficial palmar branch of radial A.
- Flexor carpi radialis
- Palmar carpal arch
- Radial artery
- Radius
- Interosseous membrane

The skin territory for this anterior interosseous artery is over the distal dorsal forearm via its dorsal perforating branch. It has two to three perforators which emerge between the muscles of the first extensor compartment and the extensor digitorum communis tendons. The superficial length of the perforators is 21 ± 10 mm, with an average diameter of 0.5 ± 0.1 mm.

The **median artery** is a long thin vessel that arises from the anterior interosseous artery and runs distally between the flexor digitorum profundus and flexor pollicis longus to the median nerve and supplies it. In about 4 to 8% of cases,[3,7] the median artery is a large vessel that continues up to the hand, traversing the carpal ligament and participates in the formation of the superficial palmar arch. In 7 of 31 cases of a reported series, the median artery pierced the median nerve in the proximal third of the forearm.[7]

A median artery that passes completely through the median nerve in the forearm may produce pronator syndrome; and when bilateral, the median artery may produce symptoms of carpal tunnel syndrome.[16]

The **anterior terminal branch** passes between the pronator quadratus and the interosseous membrane and continues into the palmar carpal rete, where it anastomoses with the palmar carpal branches of the radial and ulnar arteries and the recurrent branch of the deep palmar arch.

The **posterior terminal branch** pierces the interosseous membrane and continues to the dorsum of the wrist, where it anastomoses to the dorsal carpal branch of the radial and ulnar arteries, in the dorsal carpal rete.

The **posterior interosseous branch** runs dorsally through the space formed by the interosseous membrane, oblique ligament, and ulna. It emerges between the abductor pollicis longus and supinator and continues distally between the deep and superficial extensors. An early branch is usually a recurrent interosseous artery that joins the arterial rete around the

elbow; most of the remaining branches are muscular, supplying the superficial flexor muscles close to their origin from the medial epicondyle of the humerus. Most of the blood supply of the deeper muscles in the dorsum of the forearm is from the radial and radial recurrent arteries rather than from the posterior interosseous. The posterior interosseous nerve accompanies this artery. Near the wrist, this artery may anastomose with the anterior interosseous artery which is the basis of the pedicled posterior interosseous artery flap.

There are approximately three to five communicating vessels between the anterior and posterior interosseous arteries, traversing the interosseous membrane.[4] The posterior interosseous artery can give origin to a cutaneous flap from the posterior aspect of the forearm, based on the distal anastomosis of this artery with the anterior interosseous.[17] The skin of the posterior forearm is supplied by about five perforators of the posterior interosseous artery.[4] The posterior interosseous flap can be used as cutaneous and osteocutaneous flap.[18,19]

The **palmar carpal branch** is a branch of the posterior interosseous artery. It courses across the carpal ligaments in the floor of the carpal canal, where it anastomoses with other carpal arteries to form a palmar carpal arch.

The dorsal carpal branch runs around the ulna to anastomose at the dorsal carpal arch with the dorsal carpal branch of the radial artery and posterior terminal branch of the anterior interosseous artery. The ulnar artery lies radial to the ulnar nerve as it crosses the wrist. At the palm, the ulnar artery lies deep to the hypothenar fascia and divides into two branches, superficial and deep.

The **superficial palmar arch** courses between the palmar aponeurosis and the flexor tendons, approximately at the level of the ulnar end of the proximal palmar crease and a few millimeters distal to the flexor retinaculum. Within the central compartment of the hand, the arch lies anterior to the branches of the median nerve and gives off three common palmar digital arteries to the adjacent sides of the four fingers (▶ Fig. 11.8a–d).

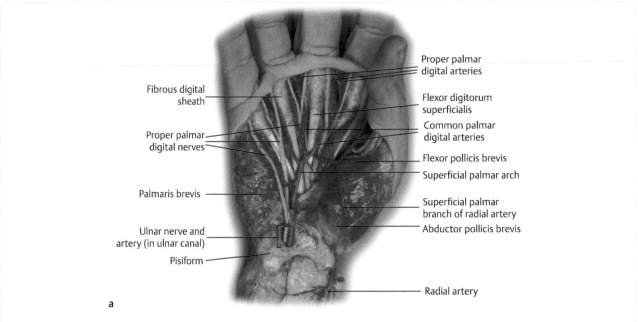

Proper palmar
digital arteries

Fibrous digital
sheath

Flexor digitorum
superficialis

Common palmar
digital arteries

Proper palmar
digital nerves

Flexor pollicis brevis

Superficial palmar arch

Palmaris brevis

Superficial palmar
branch of radial artery

Abductor pollicis brevis

Ulnar nerve and
artery (in ulnar canal)

Pisiform

Radial artery

a

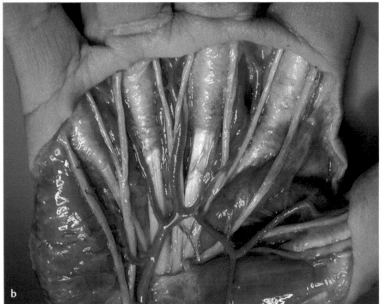

b

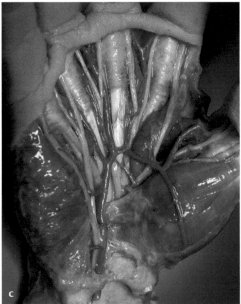

c

Fig. 11.8 (a) Cadaver dissection of superficial palmar arch and palmar arteries. (b) detailed view of the palm showing the superficial palmar arch and the palmar arteries. Note the palmar artery in the 3rd interspace going through a split in the common digital nerve. (c) The ulnar artery and ulnar nerve in the Guyon's canal. The ulnar artery contributing to the superficial palmar arch.

These start superficial to the nerves but then run deep, running dorsally to the nerves in the fingers. This arch may be completed with the superficial palmar branch of the radial artery (30%) or by union with the deep palmar arch through the princeps pollicis artery (42%).[3] It branches in the common digital branch and palmar proper digital branches. It is well known that the vascular anatomy of the palmer arches show great variability and thus have been classified into two groups (▶ Fig. 11.9). Group I, with the arch complete, was encountered in 78.5% of cases,[20] with five subdivisions:

- Type A: the classical arch formed by the superficial volar branch of the radial artery and the larger ulnar artery (34.5%).
- Type B: formed entirely by the ulnar artery (37%).
- Type C: ulnar artery and enlarged median artery (3.8%).

- Type D: radiomediulnar intercommunications (1.2%).
- Type E: well-formed arch initiated by the ulnar artery and completed by a large vessel derived from the deep arch (2%).

The volar interosseous artery was not noted to contribute to the arch formation, and no case of complete absence of the arch was found.

Group II is an incomplete arch, in which the contributing arteries do not anastomose or the ulnar artery does not reach the thumb and index finger. It was encountered in 21.5%, with patterns similar to those of group I, except for type E (▶ Fig. 11.9).

Perforator arteries of this arch supply the skin over the palm and the ulnar three fingers, the ulnar half of the index finger, and the skin over the dorsum of the fingers.[4] When the superficial palmar arch is insufficient to supply a digital space, this territory is taken by palmar metacarpal arteries from the deep palmar arch.

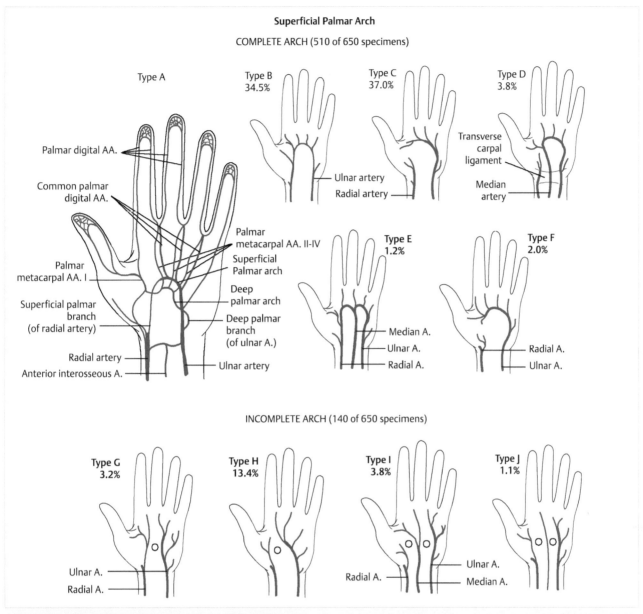

Fig. 11.9 Types of superficial volar arterial arch of the hand.

The **common digital arteries** arise from the convexity of the superficial palmar arch (usually being three in number), join the three corresponding metacarpal arteries, and give rise to a pair of palmar proper digital arteries.

The **palmar proper digital branches** continue distally, on the adjacent sides of the ulnar four digits. A palmar proper digital artery arises independently from this arch and supplies the ulnar side of the little finger.

The palmar proper digital arteries lie between the palmar and dorsal digital nerves. These arteries anastomose on the proximal side of each interphalangeal joint; they supply the flexor tendons and the integument. A dorsal digital branch supplies the dorsum of the digits at the middle of the proximal phalanx, and a second smaller branch supplies the distal phalanx.

The **deep branch of the ulnar artery** enters the hypothenar musculature between the abductor digiti minimi and flexor digiti

minimi brevis and supplies the hypothenar muscles. It anastomoses with the radial artery to form the deep palmar arch.

A **superficial ulnar artery** may be present in 0.7 to 9.4% of the population.[21] This superficial course occurs in almost every case in which the ulnar artery has a high origin. When this artery is present, the interosseous artery arises from the radial artery.[3]

11.5 Radial Artery

The **radial artery** is the continuation of the brachial artery into the forearm and is the smaller of the two branches of the brachial artery (▶Fig. 11.10). It begins in the midline of the antecubital fossa, lateral to the biceps tendon, and continues into the forearm until the styloid process of the radius. At the wrist, it turns dorsally to pass deep to the abductor pollicis and extensor pollicis brevis tendons, and it enters the palm between the two

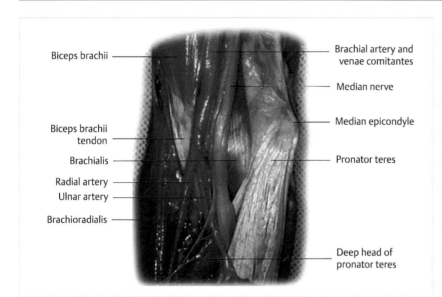

Biceps brachii

Biceps brachii tendon

Brachialis

Radial artery

Ulnar artery

Brachioradialis

Brachial artery and venae comitantes

Median nerve

Median epicondyle

Pronator teres

Deep head of pronator teres

Fig. 11.10 Cadaver dissection of structures in the right antecubital fossa.

heads of the first interosseous muscle. It extends across the palm to anastomose with the deep branch of the ulnar artery and form the deep palmar arch.[6]

In the forearm, the artery arches laterally and lies on the volar surface of the radius, accompanied by the superficial radial nerve, deep to the medial (ulnar) side of brachioradialis. It emerges from brachioradialis in the lower third of the forearm and continues superficially lateral to the flexor carpi radialis tendon. The branches of the radial artery in the forearm are the radial recurrent, muscular, superficial palmar, and palmar carpal.

Septocutaneous and musculocutaneous perforator arteries from the radial artery supply the lateral (radial) half of the forearm. The number of perforators of the radial artery ranges from 4 to 10, and average vessel diameter is 0.6 ± 0.2 mm, with a superficial length of 32 ± 25 mm.[4,22] The perforators arise from the radial artery throughout its course. In the proximal forearm, the perforators pass through the forearm musculature and are therefore musculocutaneous perforators, and in the distal forearm, the perforators are fasciocutaneous, passing directly to skin. Any of the perforators could be incorporated into a local or free skin flap.

The **radial recurrent branch** arises from the lateral (radial) side of the radial artery, just after its origin. It curves laterally and divides into three branches. The first branch travels proximally between the brachioradialis and brachialis, accompanied by the radial nerve, to anastomose with the radial collateral artery and supply the surrounding muscles and the elbow joint. The second branch passes laterally (radially) between the superficial and deep radial nerves to the brachioradialis and extensor carpi radialis longus and brevis, supplies these muscles, and anastomoses with the interosseous recurrent artery. The third branch descends with the superficial radial nerve, supplying it.[3]

The radial recurrent and interosseous recurrent arteries supply the lateral aspect of the elbow in an inverse relationship. For example, if one artery is larger, the other is correspondingly smaller in size and distribution.[4] The radial recurrent artery anastomoses with the posterior radial collateral artery and has

been used as the source vessels for the harvesting of the reversed lateral arm flap.[23]

Perforator flap techniques have recently focused attention on harvesting flaps based on a single perforator and maintaining an intact radial artery. There are two consistent perforator arteries, proximal and distal. The proximal perforator arises about 2 to 4 cm proximal to the radial styloid process. These septocutaneous perforators form a longitudinal chain-linked vascular plexus along the course of the artery that can be developed as an adipofascial pedicle for distal forearm flaps.[24]

The **muscular branches** supply the muscles on the lateral side of the forearm.

The **superficial palmar branch** arises from the distal end of the radial artery at the level of the radial styloid process. It enters the thenar muscle compartment and supplies the muscles. It may join the superficial branch of the ulnar artery and complete the superficial palmar arch in 32%.[3] It may end at the thenar musculature or continue to directly supply the radial digits.

The **palmar carpal branch** arises at the distal end of the pronator quadratus, courses across the radial carpal ligament, and anastomoses with the palmar carpal branch of the ulnar artery to form the **palmar carpal arch**. This rete is a local arterial arcade usually limited to arterial supply to the anterior carpal region. It is located deep in the carpal tunnel, with its venous counterpart, where it is subject to the same pressure as the median nerve in carpal tunnel syndrome.[25]

In the wrist, the radial artery turns dorsally after the styloid process of the radius and enters the palm by perforating the first dorsal interosseous muscle. It is crossed by the tendons of the abductor pollicis longus and extensor pollicis brevis. At the wrist, it gives rise to the dorsal carpal and first dorsal metacarpal arteries.

The **dorsal carpal branch** arises near where the radial artery is crossed by the extensor pollicis longus tendon. It runs to the ulnar side of the wrist in the groove between the distal and proximal carpal bones. It anastomoses with the dorsal carpal branch of the ulnar artery and the posterior terminal branch of the anterior interosseous artery, forming the **dorsal carpal arch**. This system is larger than the palmar carpal arch and lies distal to the extensor retinaculum.[25] Six patterns of vascular anatomy of the dorsal carpal arch have been described[20]:

- Type 1: formed by the dorsal carpal branch of the radial artery, carpal branches of the dorsal interosseous artery, and terminal branches of the volar interosseous (49.4%).
- Type 2: formed by dorsal carpal branches of the radial, ulnar, and interosseous arteries. This is the "classical" form (30.6%).
- Type 3: formed only by the dorsal carpal branch of the radial artery (8%).
- Type 4: formed by the dorsal carpal branches of the radial and ulnar arteries (5.3%).
- Type 5: formed by the dorsal carpal branches of ulnar artery and carpal branches of interosseous arteries (2.7%).
- Type 6: no arch (4%).

The dorsal carpal arch, together with the local segment of the radial artery, supplies metacarpal digital branches to the dorsum of the hand. These branches are supported by the perforating arteries, dorsal branches from the deep palmar arch, which may replace the branches from the dorsal carpal arch, which are usually quite small.[25]

The **dorsal metacarpal branches** are located with their corresponding dorsal interosseous muscles; each of these arteries receives a proximal perforating branch from the **palmar metacarpal arteries**. At the proximal end of the phalanges, they receive a distal perforating branch from the common digital and palmar metacarpal arteries and then divide into two dorsal digital branches. The dorsal surface of each interspace may receive as many as four perforating vessels from the volar arteries or just a single vessel. The size of the dorsal carpal vessel varies inversely with the number of the forating arteries. The dorsal metacarpal arteries are a consistent and reliable vascular source of dorsal metacarpal artery flaps. The first dorsal metacarpal artery was present in all hands, and the second dorsal metacarpal artery was present in 95%.[25] The fourth dorsal metacarpal artery is less consistent, so its presence should be verified using a handheld Doppler probe prior to dorsal metacarpal artery flap harvest.

The **dorsal digital branches** course distally on the dorsal aspect of the second to fifth digits. These are very thin branches and terminate about the midpoint of the middle phalanx.

The **first dorsal metacarpal branch** supplies the first dorsal interosseous and divides into two branches. The larger branch runs on the dorsal and then radial side of the index finger. The smaller branch courses over the dorsal aspect of the thumb.

In the palm, the radial artery passes between the origin of the oblique and transverse heads of the adductor pollicis. On the ulnar side of the palm, it joins the deep ulnar artery to complete the deep palmar arch.

The **deep palmar arch** lies about 1.5 cm proximal to the superficial arch. It lies deep to the palmar interosseous fascia, the ulnar bursa, and the flexor tendons of the digits. This arch describes a curve that roughly follows the bases of the metacarpal bones (▶ Fig. 11.11a–c). Its branches are the princeps pollicis, radialis indicis, palmar metacarpal, recurrent, proximal

perforating, and distal perforating arteries. The classical deep palmar arch is formed by the anastomoses of the terminal radial artery with the deep palmar branch of the ulnar artery, but many variations have been observed in the conformation of this arch (▶ Fig. 11.12). Two deep branches of the ulnar artery were encountered as contributors to this arch in 63.5% of specimens.[20] Anatomical variations have been classified in two groups: group I (arch is complete, observed in 97% of dissections)[20] and group II (incomplete deep palmar arch and the contributing arteries do not anastomose; 3%).

Group I is further subdivided into four types:

- Type A: formed by the radial artery and the superior ramus of the deep branch of the ulnar artery (34.5%).
- Type B: formed by the radial artery and inferior ramus of the deep branch of the ulnar artery (49%).
- Type C: formed by the ramus of the deep branch of the ulnar artery and the radial artery (13%).
- Type D: formed by the superior ramus of the deep branch of the ulnar artery and an enlarged superior perforating artery of the second intermetacarpal space (0.5%).

Group II is subdivided in two types:

- Type A: the inferior deep branch of the ulnar artery joins the perforating branch of the second intermetacarpal space (1.5%).
- Type B: the deep volar branch of the radial artery joins the perforating artery of the second intermetacarpal space, and the deep branch of the ulnar artery joins the perforating branch of the third intermetacarpal space (1.5%).

This arch supplies the palmar aspect of the thumb and index finger and the dorsal aspect of the hand. The dorsal metacarpal arteries supply the proximal two-thirds of the hand. The dorsal perforating branches of the deep palmar arch supply the distal third of the dorsal hand and proximal dorsal fingers. The dorsal cutaneous branches of the palmar digital arteries and the dorsal digital branches of the dorsal metacarpal arteries supply the dorsal aspect of the fingers.[26,27]

The **princeps pollicis** branch arises from the radial artery between the first dorsal interosseous and the adductor pollicis muscles. It divides at the metacarpophalangeal joint into two branches that become the palmar digital arteries of the thumb.

The **radialis indicis branch** arises from the deep arch in about 45% of cases, and 12% of these may arise from a common trunk with the princeps pollicis. It may arise from the superficial arch in 13% and receive contributions from both arches in 42%.[3] A longer branch extends distally between the lumbricals and long flexor tendon, along the radial aspect of the index finger. The shorter branch joins the common digital artery to supply the adjacent side of the second and third fingers.

The three **palmar metacarpal branches** arise from the convexity of the deep palmar arch and terminate by joining with the palmar common digital arteries to form the superficial arch. They vary considerably and may fail to join the corresponding palmar common digital artery; also, two volar metacarpal arteries may join the same palmar common digital artery. The metacarpal arteries usually extend only as far as the metacarpophalangeal joints, being primarily nutritive to the interosseous

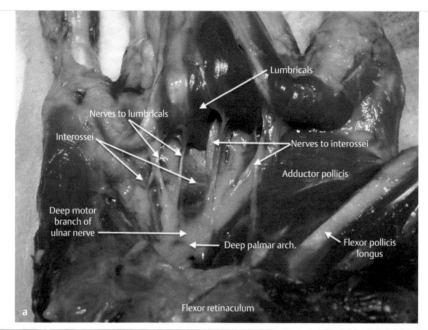

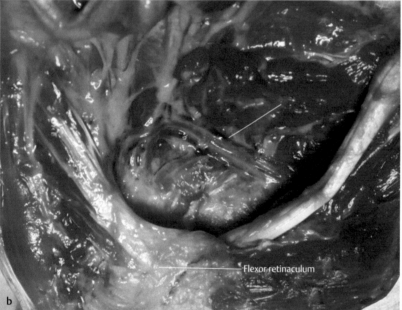

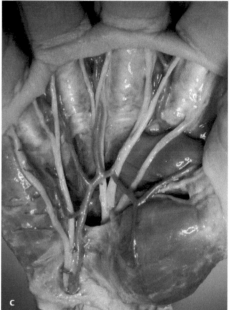

Fig. 11.11 (a–c) Relationship of the deep palmar arch to other structures in the palm.

muscles; second, third, and fourth lumbrical musclesl; metacarpal bones; and capsules of metacarpophalangeal joints. Volar metacarpal arteries were found to be the most variable vessels in the hand. In fact, few hands contained matching patterns. One consistent feature was the presence of the first and second volar metacarpal arteries in 95% of specimens.[20] The dorsal surface of each interspace may, therefore, receive as many as four perforators from the volar arteries, or merely a single vessel.

The carpal rete is formed by contributions of the anterior interosseous artery, posterior interosseous artery, and carpal rami of the radial and ulnar arteries. In 75 specimens, there were contributions from the dorsal carpal branch of radial artery in 93%, from the dorsal and volar interosseous in 83%, and from the dorsal carpal branch of ulnar artery in 39%.

There are two to three recurrent branches arising from the concavity of the deep palmar arch and passing to the wrist to anastomose with the palmar carpal arch and the branches of the anterior interosseous artery.[20]

As the palmar digital artery approaches the finger, it lies deep to the palmar fascia, between the flexor tendons, where

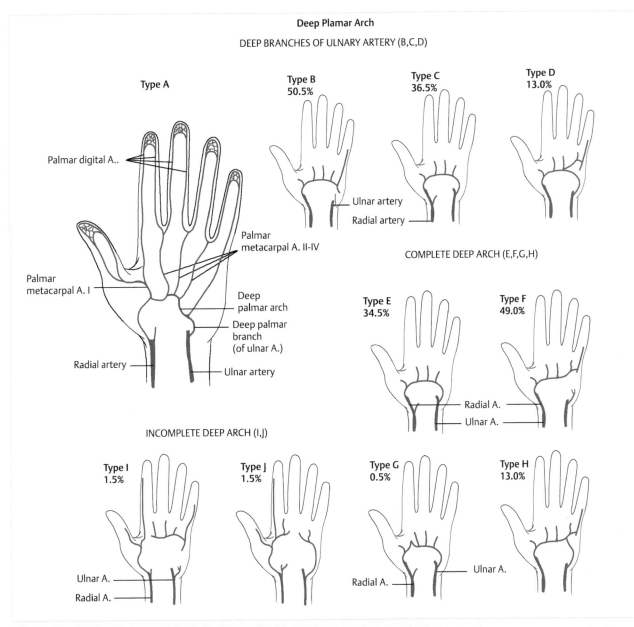

Fig. 11.12 Types of deep volar arterial arch of the hand.

it is protected from the pressure during gripping. When it emerges from behind the transverse fibers of the palmar aponeurosis, it lies in the loose connective tissue. Approximately at the level of the metacarpal heads, it is often joined by a palmar metacarpal artery and then divides into two branches, one to the adjoining sides of each finger, coming to lie dorsal to the nerves. Then it runs on between the fasciculi from the palmar aponeurosis to the fingers and anterior to the base of the phalanx (▶ Fig. 11.13). Then it runs dorsally to

lie between the palmar and dorsal digital cutaneous ligaments. Distally, the arteries give both palmar and dorsal retia, which is most marked around the joints, named by Edwards as the proximal and distal transverse digital arteries at the necks of the proximal and intermediate phalanx (▶ Fig. 11.14).[28] They run deep to the tendons and are closely related to the proximal part of the joint capsules. At the fingertips, there is a rich branching of the arteries, with multiple anastomosis-like arcades.

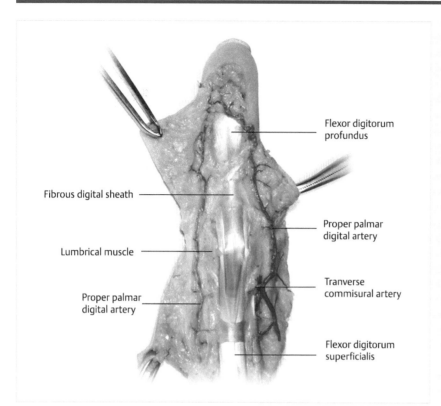

Fig. 11.13 Cadaver dissection of arteries of the fingers.

Flexor digitorum profundus

Fibrous digital sheath

Proper palmar digital artery

Lumbrical muscle

Tranverse commisural artery

Proper palmar digital artery

Flexor digitorum superficialis

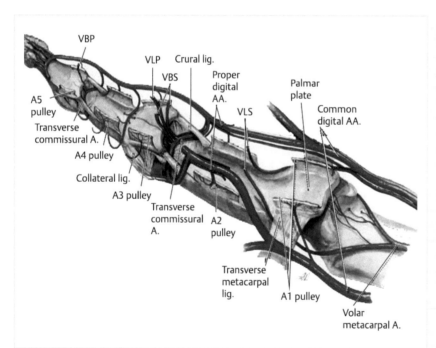

Fig. 11.14 The digital arteries with Edwards' arcades connecting the two digital arteries at the joint metacarpophalangeal and inter-carpal levels located proximal to the volar plates deep to the check rein ligaments. (The image is provided courtesy of Kleinert Institute, Louisville, KY.)

VBP

VLP   Crural lig.

VBS

Proper digital AA.

Palmar plate

A5 pulley

VLS

Common digital AA.

Transverse commissural A.

A4 pulley

Collateral lig.

A3 pulley

Transverse commissural A.

A2 pulley

Transverse metacarpal lig.

A1 pulley

Volar metacarpal A.

11.6 Veins of the Upper Extremity

The veins of the upper extremity are divided into two systems: superficial and deep. These two systems have several communications between them. The superficial system is located between the two layers of the superficial fascia. The deep system is formed by the venae comitantes which accompany each main artery. Both the superficial and deep systems have valves that help to carry the blood in a proximal direction to the heart. These valves are more numerous in the deep system than in the superficial.[29,30]

11.6.1 The Superficial Veins of the Upper Extremity

The superficial veins of the upper extremity are the digital, metacarpal, cephalic, basilic, and median (▶Fig. 11.15).

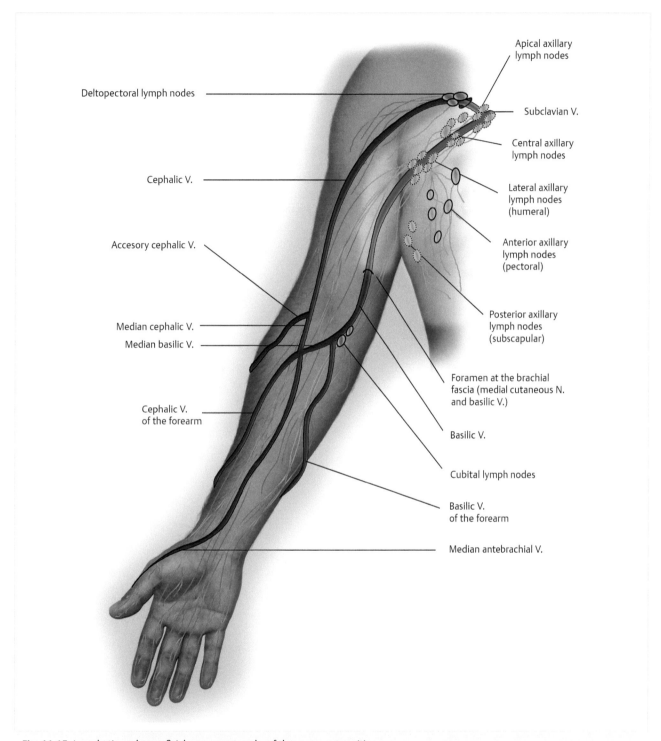

Fig. 11.15 Lymphatic and superficial venous networks of the upper extremities.

Superficial volar (▶Fig. 11.16a) and dorsal (▶Fig. 11.16b) veins of the pulp and the distal finger drain into cascading superficial veins (▶Fig. 11.17) on the palmar and dorsal aspect of the fingers. These veins have valves mostly at the junctions (▶Fig. 11.18).[29] They all tend to drain to the web vein (▶Fig. 11.19) and then on to the dorsal venous network.

The dorsal digital veins pass along the lateral aspect of the fingers and are joined to one another by oblique communicating branches. The veins from the adjacent sides of the fingers join to form three dorsal metacarpal veins, which end in a dorsal venous network at the level of the metacarpal bones. The radial part of the network is joined by the dorsal digital vein from the radial side of the index finger and by the dorsal digital veins of the thumb and is prolonged proximally as the cephalic vein. The ulnar part of the network receives the dorsal digital vein of the ulnar side of the little finger and continues proximally as the basilic vein. A communicating branch frequently connects the dorsal venous network with the cephalic vein about the middle of the forearm.[30]

The volar digital veins on each finger are connected to the dorsal digital veins by oblique intercapitular veins. They drain into a venous plexus which is situated over the thenar and hypothenar eminences and across the volar aspect of the wrist.

The cephalic vein arises in the radial part of the dorsal venous network and runs proximally on the radial aspect of the forearm, receiving tributaries from both surfaces. Below it reaches the elbow and gives off the median basilic vein, which receives a communicating branch from the deep veins of the forearm and passes across to join the basilic vein. The cephalic vein then ascends in the anterior elbow in the groove between

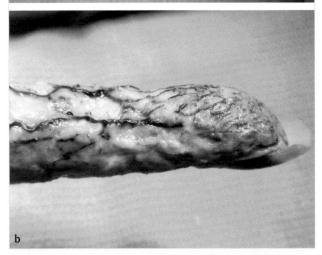

Fig. 11.16 (a, b) Superficial volar and dorsal veins of the pulp and fingertip.

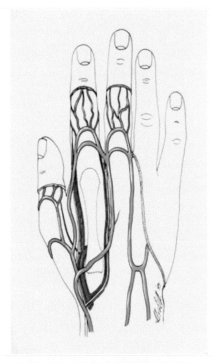

Fig. 11.17 Dorsal venous network of the finger. (The image is provided courtesy of Kleinert Institute, Louisville, KY.)

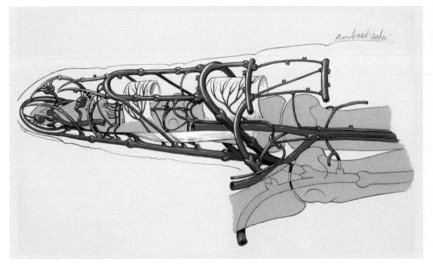

Fig. 11.18 Superficial and deep venous network of the finger. There are valves at vein junctions. (The image is provided courtesy of Kleinert Institute, Louisville, KY.)

the brachioradialis and the biceps brachii. It crosses superficial to the musculocutaneous nerve and ascends in the groove along the lateral border of the biceps brachii. In the upper third of the arm, it runs in the deltopectoral groove, where it is accompanied by the deltoid branch of the thoracoacromial artery. It pierces the coracoclavicular fascia and, crossing the axillary artery, ends in the axillary vein just below the clavicle. Sometimes it communicates with the external jugular vein by a branch which ascends in front of the clavicle.[30]

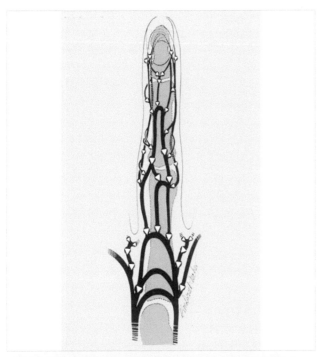

Fig. 11.19 Sequential venous drainage to the web veins. (The image is provided courtesy of Kleinert Institute, Louisville, KY.)

The accessory cephalic vein arises either from a small tributary plexus on the back of the forearm or from the ulnar side of the dorsal venous network and joins the cephalic vein distal to the elbow. In some cases, the accessory cephalic vein originates from the cephalic vein proximal to the wrist and rejoins it again more proximally. A large oblique branch frequently connects the basilic and cephalic veins on the dorsum of the forearm.[6]

The basilic vein arises in the ulnar part of the dorsal venous network. It runs up the posterior surface of the ulnar side of the forearm and inclines forward to the anterior surface distal to the elbow, where it is joined by the median ulnar vein. It then ascends obliquely in the groove between the biceps brachii and pronator teres and crosses the brachial artery, from which it is separated by the lacertus fibrosus; filaments of the medial antebrachial cutaneous nerve pass both in front of and behind this portion of the vein. It travels proximally along the medial border of the biceps brachii and perforates the deep fascia a little below the middle of the arm and, ascending on the medial side of the brachial artery to the lower border of the teres major, is continued onward as the axillary vein.

The median antebrachial vein drains the venous plexus on the volar surface of the hand. It ascends on the ulnar side of the front of the forearm and ends in the basilic vein or in the median ulnar vein; in a small proportion of cases, it divides into two branches, one of which joins the basilic, and the other branch joins the cephalic vein, distal to the elbow (▶Fig. 11.20).

11.7 The Deep Veins of the Upper Extremity

The **deep veins** follow the course of the arteries, forming their venae comitantes. They are generally arranged in pairs and are situated one on either side of the corresponding artery, connected at intervals by short transverse branches.

The superficial and deep palmar arterial arches are each accompanied by a pair of venae comitantes which constitute,

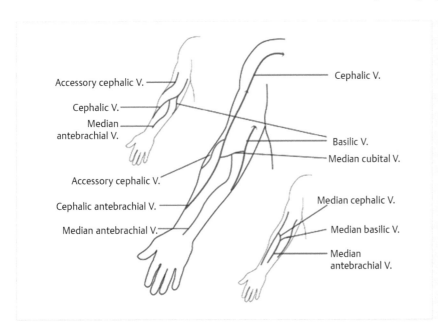

Fig. 11.20 Anatomical variations of the superficial venous system of the forearm.

Accessory cephalic V.

Cephalic V.

Median antebrachial V.

Accessory cephalic V.

Cephalic antebrachial V.

Median antebrachial V.

Cephalic V.

Basilic V.

Median cubital V.

Median cephalic V.

Median basilic V.

Median antebrachial V.

respectively, the **superficial** and **deep palmar venous arches** and receive the veins corresponding to the branches of the arterial arches; thus, the **common palmar digital veins**, formed by the union of the **proper palmar digital veins**, open into the superficial, and the **palmar metacarpal veins** into the deep, palmar venous arches. The **dorsal metacarpal veins** receive perforating branches from the palmar metacarpal veins and end in the radial veins and in the superficial veins on the dorsum of the wrist.

The **deep veins of the forearm** are the venae comitantes of the radial and ulnar veins and constitute, respectively, the proximal continuations of the deep and superficial palmar venous arches; they join in front of the elbow to form the brachial veins. The radial veins are smaller than the ulnar and receive the dorsal metacarpal veins. The ulnar veins receive tributaries from the deep palmar venous arches and communicate with the superficial veins at the wrist; near the elbow, they receive the volar and dorsal interosseous veins and send a large communicating branch, the profunda vein, to the median ulnar vein.

The **brachial veins** are situated on either side of the brachial artery, receiving tributaries corresponding with the branches given off from that vessel; near the lower margin of the subscapularis, they join the axillary vein; the medial one frequently joins the basilic vein.

These deep veins have numerous anastomoses, not only with each other but also with the superficial veins.[30]

The **axillary vein** begins at the lower border of the teres major as the continuation of the basilic vein, increases in size as it ascends, and ends at the outer border of the first rib as the subclavian vein. It runs medially to the axillary artery and completely overlaps the artery anteriorly when the arm is abducted. Near the lower border of the subscapularis, it receives the brachial veins (venae comitantes) and, close to its termination, superior to the pectoralis minor, the cephalic vein; its other tributaries correspond with the branches of the axillary artery. It lies on the medial side of the artery, which it partly overlaps; between the two vessels are the medial cord of the brachial plexus, the median, the ulnar, and the medial anterior thoracic nerves. It is provided with a pair of valves opposite the lower border of the subscapularis; valves are also found at the ends of the cephalic and subscapular veins.[30]

11.8 Lymphatic Vessels of the Upper Extremity

The lymphatic network of the upper limb consists essentially of superficial and deep components; they are separated anatomically and functionally by the superficial fascia. The two networks join in the axillary nodes (▶ Fig. 11.15).

The lymph collecting vessels are situated in the subcutaneous fat tissue, and their diameters remain similar throughout their course. They are often concentrated near the major draining veins, especially the cephalic and basilic. No lymph communications between the superficial and deep lymphatics have been observed.[31] Suami et al, in their work, found that without exception, all lymph vessels reach the lymph nodes in the axillary region. Most of the lymph vessels coursing along the anterior surface of the limb flowed into a large sentinel node. However, some on the posterior surface bypassed this node and flow into smaller sentinel glands.[31]

The deep network consists of deep collecting channels that run together with the neurovascular bundles. There are several nodes in their course and transverse anastomoses connect them.

In the hand, the deep collecting channels run at first with the digital and interosseous arteries. At the level of the palm, they form two networks. A superficial one accompanies the superficial palmar arch and branches in two main collecting channels, which run with the radial and ulnar arteries, respectively. These are joined at the wrist by the two trunks which originate from the deep palmar arch and follow the ulnar artery and termination of the radial artery as it curves around the first metacarpal. In the forearm, they follow the main vascular axes: radial, ulnar, anterior, and posterior interosseous. There are usually within each vascular sheath as two lymphatic trunks which anastomose freely and are interspersed with lymph nodes.[25]

The ulnar lymphatics drain into the superior ulnar node at the crease of the elbow. The radial lymphatics often run into a node at the level of the elbow crease but sometimes drain directly into a humeral node.

In the arm, two or three channels arise from the nodes at the elbow crease and follow the humeral and deep humeral vessels. At the lower third of the arm, they receive a few superficial lymphatics from the epitrochlear nodes via the foramen of the medial cutaneous nerve of the arm.

There are three to four deep lymphatic nodes at the elbow crease; the superior ulnar node drains the ulnar and posterior and anterior interosseous networks. Four to six more nodes lie in the course of the brachial channels.[25]

The **deep lymph nodes** are chiefly grouped in the axilla, although a few may be found in the forearm; in the course of the radial, ulnar, and interosseous vessels; and in the arm along the medial side of the brachial artery.[6,30]

The **axillary nodes** are of large size, vary from 20 to 30 in number, and may be arranged in the following groups[30]:

- A **lateral group** of four to six glands lies in the medial and posterior aspects of the axillary vein; the afferents of these glands drain the whole arm, with the exception of that portion whose vessels accompany the cephalic vein. The efferent vessels pass partly to the central and subclavicular groups of axillary glands and partly to the inferior deep cervical glands.
- An **anterior** or **pectoral group** consists of four or five glands along the lower border of the pectoralis minor, in relation with the lateral thoracic artery. Their afferents drain the skin and muscles of the anterior and lateral thoracic walls, and the central and lateral parts of the breast gland; their efferents pass partly to the central and partly to the subclavicular groups of axillary glands.
- A **posterior** or **subscapular group** of six or seven glands is placed along the lower margin of the posterior wall of the axilla in the course of the subscapular artery. The afferents of this group drain the skin and muscles of the lower part of the back of the neck and of the posterior thoracic wall; their efferents pass to the central group of axillary glands.
- A **central** or **intermediate group** of three or four large glands is imbedded in the adipose tissue near the base of the axilla. Its afferents are the efferent vessels of all the preceding groups of axillary glands; its efferents pass to the subclavicular group.
- A **medial** or **subclavicular group** of 6 to 12 glands is situated partly posterior to the upper portion of the

pectoralis minor and partly above the upper border of this muscle. Its only direct territorial afferents are those which accompany the cephalic vein and one which drains the upper peripheral part of the breast, but it receives the efferents of all the other axillary glands. The efferent vessels of the subclavicular group unite to form the subclavian trunk, which opens either directly into the junction of the internal jugular and subclavian veins or into the jugular lymphatic trunk; on the left side, it may end in the thoracic duct. A few efferents from the subclavicular glands usually pass to the inferior deep cervical glands.

References

1. Tank PW, Gest TR. Lippincott Williams & Wilkins Atlas of Anatomy. Philadelphia, PA: Wolters Kluwer Health/Lippincott Williams & Wilkins; 2008:432

2. Manchot C. The Cutaneous Arteries of the Human Body. New York, NY: Springer-Verlag; 1983:149

3. Tountas CP, Bergman RA. Anatomic Variations of the Upper Extremity. New York, NY: Churchill Livingstone; 1993:286

4. Thomas, BP, Geddes, CR, Tang, M, Morris, SF. Vascular Supply of the integument of the upper extremity. Chapter 15, In: Blondeel, PN. Perforator Flaps: Anatomy, Technique, and Clinical Applications. St. Louis, MO: Quality Medical Pub; 2006

5. Meltem A, Metin G, Zeynep A, Cenk M, Betul UG. The free deltoid flap: clinical applications to upper extremity, lower extremity, and maxillary defects. Microsurgery 2007;27(5):420–424

6. Gray H, Williams PL, Gray H. Gray's Anatomy. 37th ed. New York, NY: Churchill Livingstone; 1989:1598

7. McCormack LJ, Cauldwell EW, Anson BJ. Brachial and antebrachial arterial patterns; a study of 750 extremities. Surg Gynecol Obstet 1953;96(1):43–54

8. Masquelet AC, Rinaldi S, Mouchet A, Gilbert A. The posterior arm free flap. Plast Reconstr Surg 1985;76(6):908–913

9. Masquelet AC, Rinaldi S. Anatomical basis of the posterior brachial skin flap. Anat Clin 1985;7(3):155–160

10. Sauerbier M, Unglaub F. Perforator flaps in the upper extremity. Clin Plast Surg 2010;37(4):667–676, vii

11. Saint-Cyr M, Gupta A. Indications and selection of free flaps for soft tissue coverage of the upper extremity. Hand Clin 2007;23(1): 37–48

12. Kaplan EN, Pearl RM. An arterial medial arm flap--vascular anatomy and clinical applications. Ann Plast Surg 1980;4(3):205–215

13. Karamürsel S, Bağdatli D, Demir Z, Tüccar E, Celebioğlu S. Use of medial arm skin as a free flap. Plast Reconstr Surg 2005;115(7):2025–2031

14. Small JO, Millar R. The radial artery forearm flap: an anomaly of the radial artery. Br J Plast Surg 1985;38(4):501–503

15. Yu P, Chang EI, Selber JC, Hanasono MM. Perforator patterns of the ulnar artery perforator flap. Plast Reconstr Surg 2012;129(1): 213–220

16. Eid N, Ito Y, Shibata MA, Otsuki Y. Persistent median artery: cadaveric study and review of the literature. Clin Anat 2011;24(5):627–633

17. Zancolli EA, Angrigiani C. Posterior interosseous island forearm flap. J Hand Surg [Br] 1988;13(2):130–135

18. Akin S, Ozgenel Y, Ozcan M. Osteocutaneous posterior interosseous flap for reconstruction of the metacarpal bone and soft-tissue defects in the hand. Plast Reconstr Surg 2002;109(3):982–987

19. Angrigiani C, Grilli D, Dominikow D, Zancolli EA. Posterior interosseous reverse forearm flap: experience with 80 consecutive cases. Plast Reconstr Surg 1993;92(2):285–293

20. Coleman SS, Anson BJ. Arterial patterns in the hand based upon a study of 650 specimens. Surg Gynecol Obstet 1961;113:409–424

21. Dartnell J, Sekaran P, Ellis H. The superficial ulnar artery: incidence and calibre in 95 cadaveric specimens. Clin Anat 2007;20(8): 929–932

22. Ho AM, Chang J. Radial artery perforator flap. J Hand Surg Am 2010;35(2):308–311

23. Prantl L, Schreml S, Schwarze H, et al. A safe and simple technique using the distal pedicled reversed upper arm flap to cover large elbow defects. J Plast Reconstr Aesthet Surg 2008;61(5):546–551

24. Chang SM, Hou CL, Zhang F, Lineaweaver WC, Chen ZW, Gu YD. Distally based radial forearm flap with preservation of the radial artery: anatomic, experimental, and clinical studies. Microsurgery 2003;23(4):328–337

25. Tubiana R. The Hand. Philadelphia, PA: Saunders; 1981:1–5

26. Yang D, Morris SF. Reversed dorsal digital and metacarpal island flaps supplied by the dorsal cutaneous branches of the palmar digital artery. Ann Plast Surg 2001;46(4):444–449

27. Yang D, Morris SF. Vascular basis of dorsal digital and metacarpal skin flaps. J Hand Surg Am 2001;26(1):142–146

28. Edwards EA. Organization of the small arteries of the hand and digits. Am J Surg 1960;99:837–846

29. Nyström A; von Drasek-Ascher G; Fridén J; Lister GD, The palmar venous anatomy. Scandinavian journal of plastic and reconstructive surgery and hand surgery [Scand J Plast Reconstr Surg Hand Surg], ISSN: 0284-4311, 1990; Vol. 24 (2), pp. 113–9

30. Moore KL, Agur AMR, Dalley AF. Essential Clinical Anatomy. 2nd ed. Philadelphia, PA: Lippincott Williams & Wilkins; 2002:691

31. Suami H, Taylor GI, Pan WR. The lymphatic territories of the upper limb: anatomical study and clinical implications. Plast Reconstr Surg 2007;119(6):1813–1822

Section IV

Regional Anatomy and Function

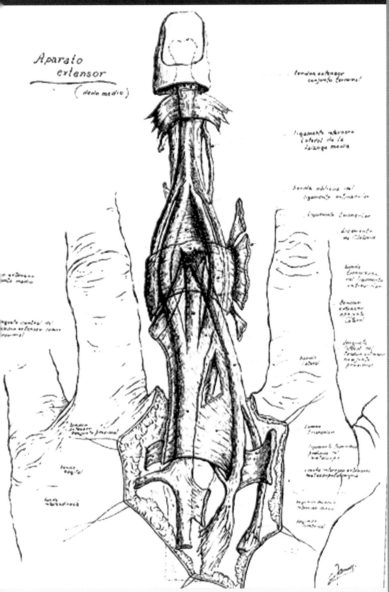

Aparato
extensor

(dedo medio)

Source: Drawing by Dr. Eduardo Alfredo Zancolli (Buenos Aires, Argentina).
Courtesy Zancolli family.

12 The Shoulder Joint

Mark Ross and Gregory I. Bain

12.1 Introduction

The miraculous functional capacity of the hand detailed elsewhere in this book is of less benefit without the ability to position the hand in space with a stable platform. It is the dual requirements of maximum range of motion and stability that make the shoulder joint so complex. In contrast to the hip, which primarily requires stability for locomotion with range of motion as a secondary consideration, the shoulder has little inherent bony stability. The demanding functional requirements of the shoulder are achieved through the interaction of the sternoclavicular joint, clavicle, acromioclavicular joint, scapulothoracic articulation, and, most important glenohumeral joint.

12.1.1 Clavicle and Sternoclavicular Joint

Due to their subcutaneous nature, there is a danger of underestimating the potential risk associated with surgical procedures on the clavicle and sternoclavicular joint. It is critical to have a complete understanding of the relational anatomy.

It should also be appreciated that even in the absence of catastrophic blood loss following injury to subclavian vessels, venous injury may cause air embolus leading to circulatory compromise or even death.[1] This is a particular consideration when surgery in this region is undertaken in an upright or semi-upright (beach chair) position and where spontaneous ventilation rather than positive pressure ventilation is utilized, with both of these technical aspects increasing the risk of air embolism.

The sternoclavicular joint is intimately related to the confluence of internal jugular and subclavian veins to form the brachiocephalic vein. This is readily appreciated in ▶Fig. 12.1, the joint capsule has been divided to allow the clavicle to be lifted superiorly. No tissue has been removed from between the posterior periosteum of the clavicle and the veins. The scant protection offered by the meager size of the subclavius muscle belly is evident.

The subclavian artery and axillary artery are divided into three parts by the scalenus anterior (▶Fig. 12.2) and pectoralis minor (▶Fig. 12.8), respectively.[2–4] The subclavian artery becomes the axillary artery at the lateral border of the first rib. The axillary artery then becomes the brachial artery at the lower border of the teres major. Iatrogenic injury to the artery from internal fixation of the clavicle would involve the subclavian artery at the sternoclavicular level, the first part of the axillary artery for midshaft fixation, and the second part of the axillary artery with coracoclavicular fixation.

The neurovascular bundle passes under the apex of the anterior curve of the **S**-shaped clavicle and traveled from superomedial to inferolateral (▶Fig. 12.1). Galley et al[5] assessed the relationship of the major vessels and the clavicle and noted considerable variability in the dimensions of the clavicle and the adjacent structures. As a consequence, the relative position of the vessels is best reported as a percentile of the entire length of the clavicle from the sternoclavicular joint. The mean length of the clavicle was 138 mm (range, 114–168). The subclavian vein lies under the junction of the medial and middle thirds of the clavicle at the 33rd percentile (range, 28–36) (▶Fig. 12.3), while the subclavian artery lies lateral to the vein but still medial to the midpoint of the clavicle, at the 42nd percentile (range, 37–46) (▶Fig. 12.4 and ▶Fig. 12.5). Therefore, from a surgical

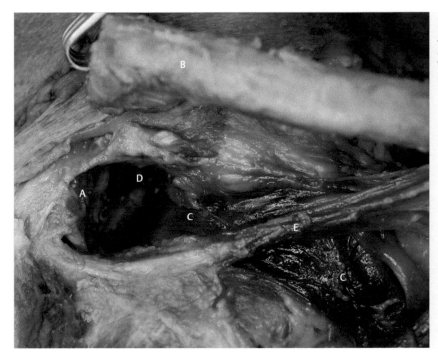

Fig. 12.1 Posterior sternoclavicular joint: *Sternoclavicular joint divided and clavicle retracted superiorly.* A: residual sternoclavicular disc; B: clavicle; C; subclavian vein; D: internal jugular vein; E: subclavius.

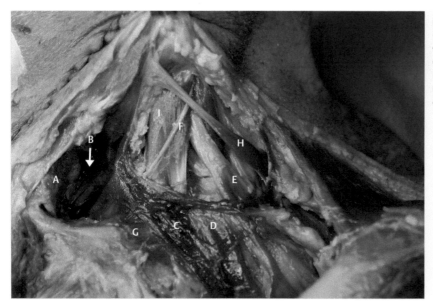

Fig. 12.2 Retroclavicular structures: *Anterior view, clavicle removed.* A: residual sternoclavicular disc; B: internal jugular vein; C: subclavian vein; D: subclavian artery; E: upper trunk of brachial plexus; F: phrenic nerve; G: first rib; H: omohyoid; I: scalenus anterior.

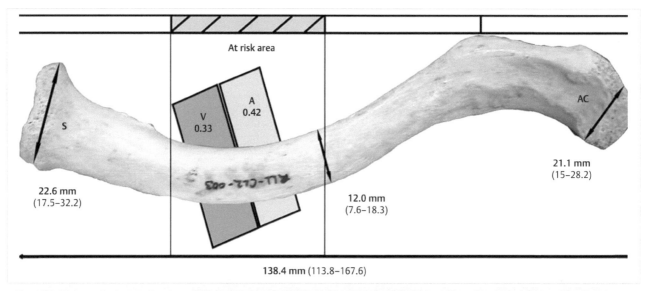

Fig. 12.3 Diagrammatic superior view of left clavicle length, width, and vessels: Median width and length measurements of the dry bone clavicles are shown. The position of the axillary vein (V) and artery (A) is represented as a ratio of clavicle length. AC, acromial end; S, Sternal end.

safety point of view, the surgeon needs to be aware that the vessels are at significant risk from the 28th to 46th percentile.[5] This represents 28 to 84 mm from the sternoclavicular joint. To make it easier to remember, at-risk zone is the second quarter, which is to say between the medial quarter and the midclavicle.[5]

The distance from the superior surface of clavicle to the superior aspect of the subclavian artery was 26 mm (range, 22–34). This was due to the thickness of the clavicle (15 mm; range, 11–16) and the subclavius muscle (11 mm; range, 7–15).

Sinha et al[6] utilized three-dimensional CT arteriograms to study the relation between the clavicle and vessels. At the medial end of the clavicle, they noted the vessels lying posterior to the clavicle. In some of the scans, the subclavian vein was in direct contact with the posterior periosteum. This is a critical point, as any violation of this significant vein that lies adjacent on the posterior clavicle could cause profuse venous bleeding, which is very difficult to control.

In the middle third, the three-dimensional relationship was more variable, with the artery and vein lying at a mean angle of 50° (range, 12–80°) and 70° (range, 38–100°), respectively, to the horizontal. This posteroinferior relationship is demonstrated in ▸ Fig. 12.6. Also seen in this figure is a branch from the subclavian vein passing superiorly, posterior to the clavicle, which may be tethered as a result of a clavicle fracture and cause tearing during surgical dissection, especially in subacute cases.

Sinha et al[6] also observed that at the lateral aspect of the clavicle, the vessels were inferior to the clavicle, with the artery and vein at mean distances of 64 mm (range, 47–97 mm) and 76 mm (range, 50–109 mm), respectively.

In summary, anatomic considerations would dictate the following precautions for safer clavicle surgery:
- Extreme upright positioning should be avoided and positive pressure ventilation employed.

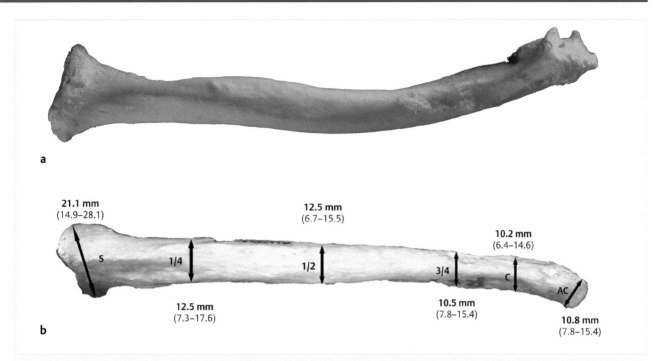

Fig. 12.4 (a,b) Diagrammatic anterior view of left clavicle thickness: Median thickness measurements of the dry bone clavicles are shown. AC, acromial end.; 1/4, one fourth of total length of clavicle from sternal end; 1/2, mid clavicle; 3/4, three fourths of total length of clavicle from sternal end; C, conoid ligament insertion; S, Sternal end .

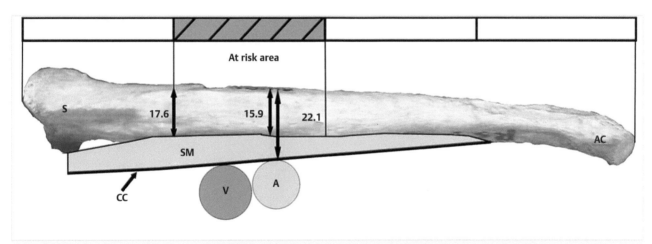

Fig. 12.5 Diagrammatic anterior view of left clavicle and vessels: Values are in millimeters. The minimum distance measured from the superior clavicle to the superior aspect of the axillary artery (A) was 22.1 mm. The thickest clavicle measured over the axillary artery was 15.9 mm. The thickest clavicle in the area of a clavicular plate was 17.6 mm. A, axillary artery; AC, acromial end; CC, costocoracoid membrane S, Sternal end; SM, subclavius muscle; V, axillary vein.

- Breaching the periosteum of the posterior clavicle in the second quarter must be avoided.
- Be mindful of the direction of drilling, specifically in relation to the foregoing three-dimensional relationships. In general terms, it is safest to direct medial screws from superior to inferior, to consider unicortical screws in the second quarter, and to direct lateral screws from anterior to posterior.

12.2 Acromioclavicular Joint

The clavicle serves as a stabilizing strut for the shoulder girdle via the scapula. The acromioclavicular joint is a synovial joint possessing an intra-articular fibrocartilaginous disc. The capsule of this synovial cavity may provide some degree of secondary stability; however, the main force transfer between the scapula and the clavicle occurs via the coracoclavicular ligaments.[4] The conoid ligament is more medial and posterior. It is an inverted cone with a smaller origin at the base of the coracoid and a larger insertion on the conoid tubercle on the posterior aspect of the lateral clavicle. The origin of the trapezoid ligament is more lateral on the coracoid and extends in a more horizontal fashion toward the trapezoid ridge on the clavicle (▶ Fig. 12.7). This complex ligamentous arrangement allows the clavicle to perform a suspensory function and

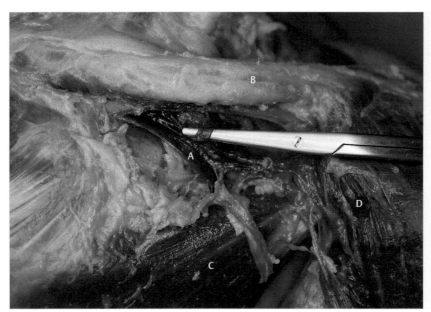

Fig. 12.6 Subclavian vein middle third of clavicle: *Anterior view, pectoralis major removed*. A: subclavian vein; B: clavicle; C: pectoralis minor; D: deltoid.

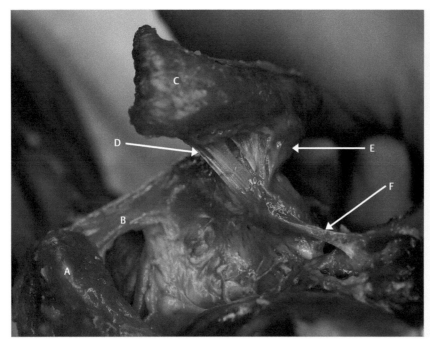

Fig. 12.7 Coraco clavicular ligaments: *Superior View, AC joint capsule divided and clavicle rotated anteriorly*. A: acromion; B: coracoacromial ligament; C: lateral clavicle; D: trapezoid ligament; E: conoid ligament; F: transverse scapular ligament across scapular notch.

prevents medial collapse of the scapula, throughout the range of scapulothoracic positioning.

As already described, the risk of damage to vascular structures is less in relation to the lateral clavicle than more medially. However, surgical procedures in the vicinity of the coracoclavicular ligaments (such as passage of grafts or sutures around the coracoid process for acromioclavicular joint reconstruction) require greater caution with regard to nerves. ▶ Fig. 12.8 demonstrates that the musculocutaneous nerve (a branch of the lateral cord of the brachial plexus) is closer to the coracoid than the axillary vessels. In this specimen, the nerve enters the coracobrachialis muscle 5 cm distal to the coracoid; however, this relationship is extremely variable and may be as little as 2 cm. In addition, care must be taken at the medial aspect of the base of the coracoid process due to the proximity of the suprascapular nerve (▶ Fig. 12.9).

12.3 Glenohumeral Joint

The principal focus of surgical anatomy in the shoulder region is the glenohumeral joint.

The most common surgical approach to the glenohumeral joint is the anterior deltopectoral approach. Identification and development of the plane between the medial border of the deltoid muscle and the lateral border of the pectoralis major muscle is usually defined by the presence of the cephalic vein within the deltopectoral interval (▶ Fig. 12.10). Depending on body habitus, there may be deposition of fat associated with the interval. As can be seen from this specimen, however, in the absence of significant adipose tissue, the interval may be hard to define, especially where the cephalic vein is deep, vestigial, or absent. The orientation of deltoid and pectoral muscle fibers

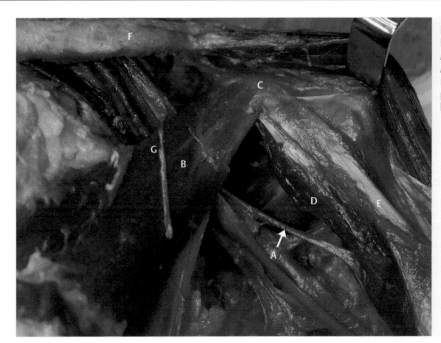

Fig. 12.8 Infraclavicular plexus and musculocutaneous nerve: *Anterior view, pectoralis major removed, anterior deltoid retracted laterally.* A: musculocutaneous nerve; B: pectoralis minor; C: tip of coracoid process; D: coracobrachialis; E: short head of biceps; F: clavicle; G: lateral pectoral nerve.

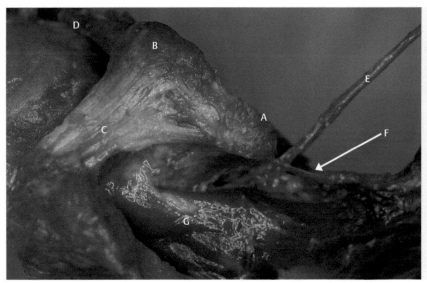

Fig. 12.9 Coracoacromial ligament and suprascapular nerve: *Superior view, clavicle removed.* A: base of coracoid process; B: tip of coracoid process; C: coracoacromial ligament; D: short head of biceps; E: suprascapular nerve; F: transverse scapular ligament; G: supraspinatus muscle belly.

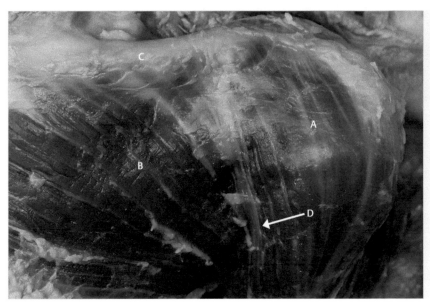

Fig. 12.10 Deltopectoral groove: *Anterior view.* A: anterior third deltoid; B: pectoralis major; C: clavicle; D: cephalic vein.

converges distally and the interval is easier to define proximally, closer to the clavicle. Palpating the underlying coracoid process may also assist in locating the interval.

It is easier to dissect between the cephalic vein and the pectoralis major muscle, as most of the tributaries of the vein run between the lateral aspect of the vein and the deltoid muscle. There is, however, one shortcoming in taking the vein laterally, and that is if the procedure is more extensive, requiring an extensile exposure such as in complex trauma or major shoulder arthroplasty. In such a circumstance, at the superior aspect of the exposure, once the deltoid and pectoralis muscles are separated, the cephalic vein will be crossing the deltopectoral interval from lateral to medial, and it will be at risk of injury and may limit proximal exposure. For that reason, if it is anticipated that more extensive exposure is required, then it may be preferable to spend a little more time ligating the tributaries on the lateral aspect of the vein and separating the vein from the deltoid and taking it with the pectoralis major.

Having defined and developed the deltopectoral interval, the principal anatomy of the anterior aspect of the shoulder as it relates to the deltopectoral approach may be defined by two critical bony landmarks. One of these landmarks is fixed and the other mobile, and both are of equal importance in developing appropriate surgical exposures in this region.

The fixed bony landmark is the coracoid process. It is encountered in the proximal aspect of the deltopectoral interval as soon as the two muscles are separated. The coracoid process has four key attachments, one from each

direction. From the medial aspect is the tendon of pectoralis minor (▶Fig. 12.8). Superiorly and more toward the root of the coracoid process are the conoid and trapezoid coracoclavicular ligaments (▶Fig. 12.7). Laterally is the coracoacromial ligament (▶Fig. 12.9), and inferiorly is the conjoint tendon of the short head of biceps and the coracobrachialis muscle (▶Fig. 12.8).

The mobile landmark which further facilitates identification of critical structures is the bicipital groove. The location of the groove depends on the rotation of the humerus; however, in general it is directly anterior when the humerus is in neutral rotation, as judged by the position of the forearm with the elbow flexed. The bicipital groove and related structures are in a deeper plane than the coracoid process, and their identification requires division of the clavipectoral fascia, particularly lateral to the coracoid and inferior to the coracoacromial ligament. The groove is occupied by the long head of biceps tendon, and this tendon may be traced superiorly to identify the rotator interval between the subscapularis and supraspinatus tendons and is one of the critical intervals for developing exposure to the glenohumeral joint. The medial aspect of the bicipital groove is formed by the lesser tuberosity, to which is attached the subscapularis tendon superiorly, with subscapularis muscular attachment to the humerus inferior to that (▶Fig. 12.11a). As the biceps tendon is traced more distally to the shallower portion of the bicipital groove, the tendon is covered by the pectoralis major tendon which inserts on the lateral lip of the bicipital groove. The pectoralis major tendon insertion is quite complex, with crossing over of

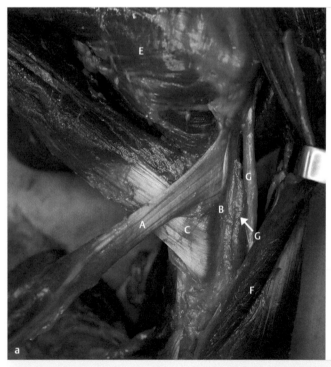
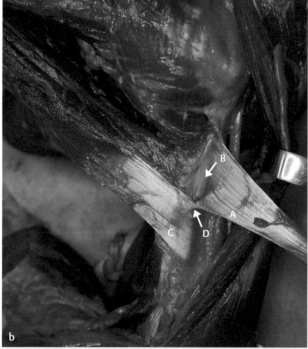

Fig. 12.11 (a) Bicipital groove, latissimus and teres major: *Anterior view, coracobrachialis and short head of biceps retracted laterally.* A: latissimus dorsi tendon; B: bicipital groove; C: teres major tendon; D: divided stump of insertion of pectoralis major; E: subscapularis; F: coracobrachialis; G: long head of biceps displaced laterally out of groove. (b) Latissimus and teres major tendons: *Anterior view, coracobrachialis and short head of biceps retracted laterally, latissimus dorsi reflected laterally.* A: undersurface of latissimus dorsi tendon; B: bursa on humeral shaft deep to latissimus tendon; C: teres major tendon; D: tenuous connection between latissimus and teres major tendons.

the fibers such that the costal fibers tend to insert more superiorly and the sternal and clavicular fibers to insert more inferiorly. At this level within the floor of the bicipital groove is the insertion of the flat ribbon like latissimus dorsi tendon, and closely related to the latissimus dorsi insertion and just inferior to the subscapularis muscle insertion is the insertion of the teres major tendon into the medial lip of the bicipital groove. Although closely related and sometimes harvested together as a dual tendon transfer, these tendons are almost completely separate (▶ Fig. 12.11b), and there is a well-defined bursa between the posterior aspect of the latissimus tendon and the medial aspect of the humeral shaft.

Most surgical approaches to the glenohumeral joint require some form of manipulation of the subscapularis tendon, whether through horizontal splitting of the muscle/tendon unit, tenotomy, or lesser tuberosity osteotomy. Exposure of the subscapularis is possible after division of the clavipectoral fascia. Mobilization of the subscapularis muscle and tendon requires dissection along the lateral border of the conjoint tendon. Loss of glenohumeral joint external rotation range of motion may be contributed by contracture around subscapularis in association with arthrosis or scar from previous surgery. Mobilization of subscapularis is advocated; however, experience in shoulder arthroplasty has suggested that aggressive mobilization may risk denervation.[7] The motor nerve supply to subscapularis is generally attributed to the upper and lower subscapular nerves, both branches of the posterior cord of the brachial plexus. This nerve supply is variable. ▶ Fig. 12.12 demonstrates the multiple and vulnerable nature of this nerve supply and even shows a branch from the axillary nerve to the subscapularis. Due to concerns regarding the nerve supply, dissection along the anterior aspect of the subscapularis muscle belly should be minimized, particularly medial to the conjoint tendon. Most releases are performed along the superior aspect of the subscapularis tendon and the posterior surface of the tendon, where it is intimately related to the anterior capsule of the glenohumeral joint, as well as the posterior aspect of the muscle belly, where the plane between the muscle and the subscapularis fossa of the anterior scapula may safely be developed well medial to the glenoid. Indeed, development of this plane is an important adjunct to intraoperative orientation of glenoid version in shoulder arthroplasty. The interval between anterior capsule and the

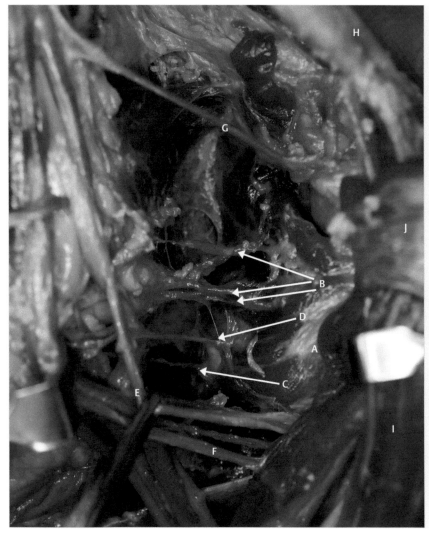

Fig. 12.12 Nerves to subscapularis: *Anterior view, pectoralis major removed , pectoralis minor/conjoint tendon and deltoid reflected laterally.* A: anterior surface of subscapularis muscle belly; B: branches of upper subscapular nerve; C: branch from axillary nerve to subscapularis ; D: lower subscapular nerve; E: axillary nerve (retracted); F: musculocutaneous nerve; G: suprascapular nerve; H: clavicle; I: deltoid; J: reflected pectoralis minor.

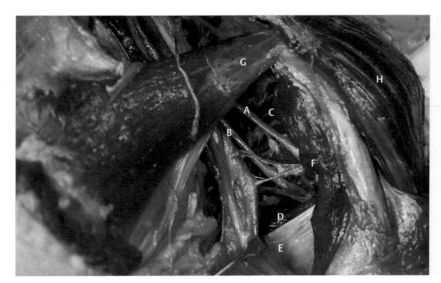

Fig. 12.13 Anterior quadrilateral space: *Anterior view, pec major removed, conjoint tendon retracted laterally.* A: musculocutaneous nerve; B: axillary nerve; C: subscapularis muscle belly; D: teres major; E: latissimus dorsi; F: coracobrachialis; G: pec minor; H: deltoid.

subscapularis tendon is more easily developed medially, where the two structures diverge at the level of the glenoid labrum.

When operating in the region of the glenoid neck and subscapularis, it is essential to appreciate the proximity of the axillary nerve. The axillary nerve is one of two terminal branches of the posterior cord of the brachial plexus. It passes from the axilla to the posterior aspect of the shoulder via the quadrilateral space. This space is defined by the subscapularis muscle superiorly, the teres major inferiorly, the long head of triceps medially, and the humeral shaft laterally (▶Fig. 12.13). The thickness of subscapularis separating the axillary nerve from the glenohumeral joint capsule is variable and decreases as the nerve runs posteriorly and closer to the glenoid. It may be directly related to the inferior capsule (▶Fig. 12.14). The axillary nerve is held to the shoulder capsule with loose areolar tissue in the zone between the 5 and 7 o'clock positions and is at risk in any arthroscopic or open procedure in this interval.[8] The nerve exits the quadrilateral space posteriorly, primarily to supply the deltoid muscle. The posterior boundaries of the quadrilateral space vary in one regard to the anterior boundaries: the superior margin is defined by teres minor instead of subscapularis (▶Fig. 12.15a).

The other terminal branch of the posterior cord is the radial nerve. It passes anterior to latissimus and teres major before reaching the posterior aspect of the shoulder by passing through a triangular space. The triangular space is bounded by the inferior aspect of teres major, the long head of triceps medially, and the shaft of the humerus laterally (▶Fig. 12.15b).

Once the axillary nerve enters the posterior aspect of the shoulder, it wraps around the proximal humerus, closely applied to the deep surface of the deltoid muscle (▶Fig. 12.16). It travels with the posterior circumflex humeral vessels. There is a constant vessel branching from the circumflex humeral vessels deep to the anterior third of deltoid (▶Fig. 12.17). The significance of this vessel is twofold. Most surgical procedures via a deltopectoral approach require definition and mobilization of the subdeltoid space. This

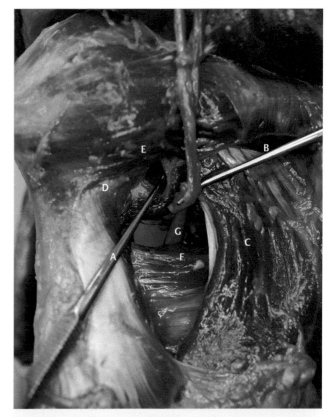

Fig. 12.14 Axillary nerve and inferior capsule: *Posterior view of quadrilateral space with deltoid reflected cephalad.* A: probe in postero-inferior capsular recess; B: probe on axillary nerve; C: long head of triceps; D: medial neck of humerus; E: teres minor; F: teres major; G: radial nerve.

vessel is a frequent cause of troublesome bleeding, which may be avoided if it is identified and controlled rather than incidentally disrupted during subdeltoid mobilization. Care should be taken, however, not to damage the axillary nerve when controlling this vessel, particularly when using

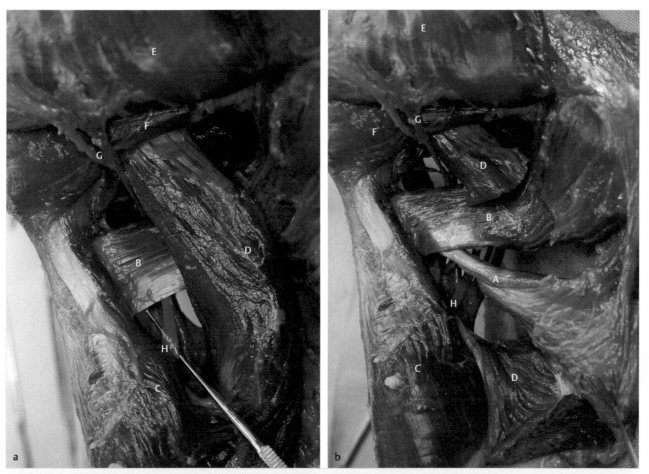

a

b

Fig. 12.15 (a) Posterior view of quadrilateral and triangular spaces, teres major, and latissimus dorsi: *Posterior view, deltoid retracted superiorly.* B: teres major; C: lateral head of triceps; D: long head of triceps; E: deltoid reflected superiorly; F: teres minor; G: axillary nerve; H: radial nerve. (**b**) Posterior view of quadrilateral and triangular spaces, teres major, and latissimus dorsi: *Posterior view, deltoid retracted superiorly, long head of triceps divided midsubstance.* A: latissimus dorsi tendon; B: teres major; C: lateral head of triceps; D: divided long head of triceps; E: deltoid reflected superior; F: teres minor; G: axillary nerve; H: radial nerve.

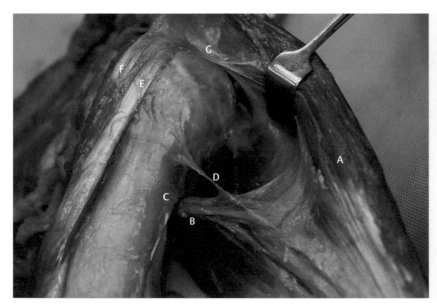

Fig. 12.16 Posterior axillary nerve and deltoid: *Lateral view, deltoid detached distally and hinged posteriorly* A: deltoid; B: axillary nerve and circumflex humeral vessels; C: meta-diaphyseal junction of humerus; D: humeral branch from posterior circumflex vessels; E: long head of biceps; F: conjoint tendon; G: coracoacromial ligament.

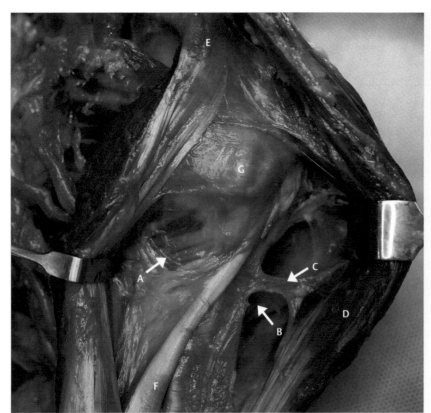

Fig. 12.17 Humeral branch from circumflex vessels: *Anterior view, deltoid retracted laterally, conjoint tendon retracted medially.* A: anterior circumflex humeral vessels; B: posterior circumflex humeral vessels; C: humeral branch of posterior circumflex humeral vessels; D: deltoid; E: tip of coracoid with attached conjoint tendon; F: long head of biceps; G: lesser tuberosity with attached subscapularis tendon.

electrocautery. In addition, this vessel can be used as a marker of the level of the axillary nerve on the deep surface of deltoid. The distance from the lateral margin of the acromion to the axillary nerve is variable but may be a little as 5 cm. ▶ Fig. 12.18 demonstrates the nerve lying approximately 6 cm distal to the acromion, where it is at risk in surgical approaches that split the deltoid. The axillary nerve is certainly at risk if dissection between the deltoid and the lateral humerus proceeds in the wrong plane. This is particularly the case in revision surgery, where there is frequently scarring in the subdeltoid space. The correct plane for subdeltoid dissection may be best identified between the coracoacromial ligament and the supraspinatus medially, with dissection sweeping laterally from the subacromial to subdeltoid space. This plane may also be developed inferiorly if there is difficulty identifying the plane between subscapularis and the conjoint tendon, again, in revision surgery.

Another frequent contributor to loss of external rotation is contracture within the rotator interval. The rotator interval lies between the superior margin of the subscapularis tendon and the anterior margin of the supraspinatus. These two tendons diverge medially to pass either side of the base of the coracoid. The long head of biceps passes through this interval to enter the glenohumeral joint on its way to inserting on the superior glenoid (▶ Fig. 12.19) and the interval is bridged by glenohumeral joint capsule. Thickenings in this capsule form the coracohumeral ligament, which passes between the humeral head laterally and the posterolateral surface of the coracoid process medially (▶ Fig. 12.20). Pathological contracture of the coracohumeral ligament is one of the most potent causes of loss of external rotation, and release of this structure is an extremely safe and effective contributor to restoration of that motion. In the patient with a retracted rotator cuff tear, it tethers the cuff,

and prevents reduction of the tendon. Releasing the coracohumeral ligament from the coracoid is an important aspect of mobilization of the cuff.

12.4 Glenoid, Labrum, and Capsule

Stability of the glenohumeral joint relies on a complex interplay between static and dynamic stabilizers. Congruence between the humeral head and the glenoid at a bony level is poor, with only a sixth of the surface area of the humeral head being covered by the bony glenoid. This coverage is increased by the glenoid labrum, to deepen the concavity of the glenoid.[9,10] The labrum also serves as an anchor for capsular attachment, contributing to both static restraint and dynamic stability through proprioceptive input.

Bain et al[11] performed a cadaveric study of 20 dry bone scapulae and 19 cadaveric shoulders, including histological examination. An external capsular circumferential ridge, 7 to 8 mm medial to the glenoid rim, marked the attachment of the capsule. A separate internal labral circumferential ridge 4 mm central to the glenoid rim marked the interface between the labrum and articular cartilage. A superoposterior facet was found consistently on the glenoid (▶ Fig. 12.21a, b). Two-thirds of the long head of biceps arose from the supraglenoid tubercle, 6.6 mm from the glenoid face, and the remainder from the labrum. The superior labrum was noted to be concave and loosely attached to the articular cartilage and glenoid rim. Clefts and foramens were common superiorly. In contrast, the anteroinferior labrum was convex, attached 4 mm central to the glenoid rim, and had a strong attachment to articular cartilage and bone. Sublabral clefts, recesses, and holes are common, but only in the superoanterior labrum. Lesions in other regions of the labrum are potentially pathological. It was postulated that the inferior

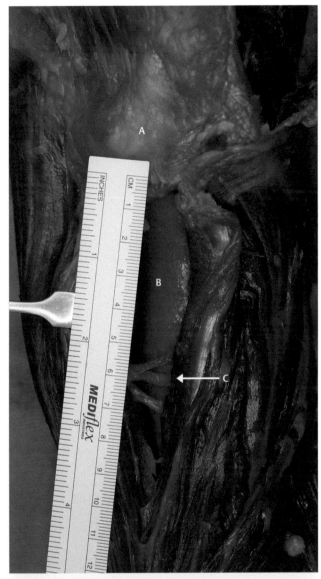

Fig. 12.18 Axillary nerve from acromion: *Superolateral view of shoulder, deltoid split in middle third.* A: lateral acromion; B: lateral humeral shaft; C: axillary nerve and circumflex humeral vessels.

labrum (5–10 o'clock positions) is rounded with a convex surface, designed to provide a bumper effect that increases the glenoid depth by up to 50%.[9,10] It has an adherent interface to the articular cartilage and has a rigid bony foundation, which prevents mobility of the labrum.

The authors proposed a new concept of labral mechanics (▶ Fig. 12.22).[11] The inferior labrum is a fixed organ of compression. In contrast, they noted that the superior labrum had a loose mobile interface with no bony foundation and attaches off the rim, away from the glenoid articular margin. It is concave in cross section and more meniscal in nature, and it follows the contour of the glenoid surface. The superior labrum is a mobile organ of tension. The long head of the biceps tendon is a dynamic structure that is anchored to the superior glenoid tubercle, but it can pull on the superior labrum and the attached glenohumeral ligaments and enhance stability throughout the range of motion[12]

▶ Fig. 12.23(a) shows the intimate relationship between the long head of biceps, labrum, and middle glenohumeral ligament. It also demonstrates the attachment of the biceps/superior labral complex to the superoposterior articular facet.[11] Although the long head of biceps is clearly an intracapsular structure, the long head of triceps tendon, inserting onto the infraglenoid tubercle, is clearly extracapsular, and is not visible until removal of the capsule, shown in ▶ Fig. 12.23(b).

Nonetheless, the long head of triceps insertion is important in exposure for shoulder arthroplasty, particularly when using a reverse or metal-backed platform implant that requires placement of inferior screws into the scapular neck. Clearance of capsule, labrum, and triceps tendon from the inferior aspect of the glenoid is essential to prevent implant impingement and subsequent risk of dislocation of reverse shoulder arthroplasty. In addition, clearance allows better appreciation of glenoid neck morphology, which may assist in decisions regarding glenosphere offset. Vertical glenoid neck morphology is more likely to be associated with inferior impingement leading to instability and notching. Finally, definition of the glenoid neck allows more accurate inferior screw placement.

The long head of triceps has an extensive lateral–medial insertion (▶ Fig. 12.24); thus, in spite of aggressive mobilization in this area, there is minimal risk of complete detachment.

Fig. 12.19 Rotator interval and LHB: *Anterosuperior view.* A: long head of biceps; B: supraspinatus; C: subscapularis; D: coracoid process; E: anterior acromion.

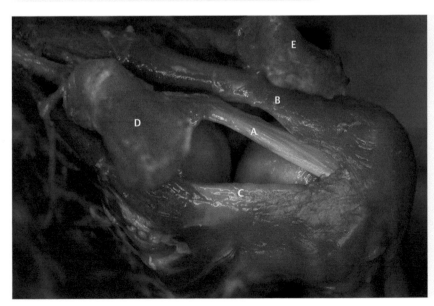

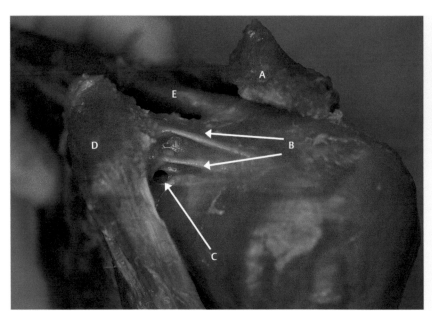

Fig. 12.20 Coracohumeral ligament: *Anterior view of rotator interval, clavicle and coracoacromial ligament removed.* A: anterior acromion; B: coracohumeral ligament; C: superior margin of subscapularis visible through small hole in capsular reflection; D: tip of coracoid process with attached conjoint tendon (short head of biceps and coracobrachialis; E: superior margin of supraspinatus tendon.

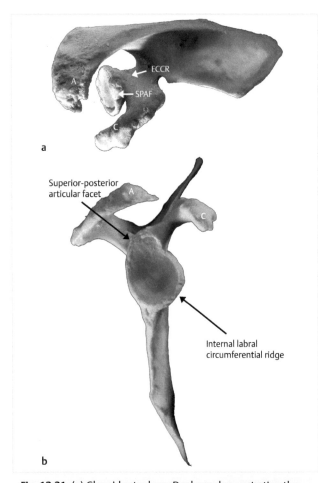

Fig. 12.21 (a) Glenoid osteology: Dry bone demonstrating the superior–posterior articular facet and internal labral circumferential ridge. (b) Glenoid osteology: A, acromion; C, coracoid; ECCR, external capsular circumferential ridge; SPAF, superior–posterior articular facet. Dry bone demonstrating the oblique superior–posterior articular facet which contains the superior labrum biceps complex. The external capsular circumferential ridge marks the capsular attachment.

12.5 Rotator Cuff

The rotator cuff contributes to dynamic stability of the glenohumeral joint and fine control of motion of the humeral head. It functions to centralize the humeral head in the glenoid and balances the superior displacement force of the deltoid. It is composed of the supraspinatus superiorly, infraspinatus posteriorly (with a minor contribution from teres minor), and subscapularis anteriorly. The rotator cuff functions within the subacromial space. This space is narrowed by the coracoacromial ligament (▶ Fig. 12.25 and ▶ Fig. 12.26). Mechanical impingement between the superior aspect of the cuff and the coracoacromial ligament is thought to contribute to rotator cuff degeneration, although it is clear that biological factors, including degenerative and vascular factors, play a significant role. The innervation of the subscapularis has been discussed previously. The supraspinatus and infraspinatus are innervated by the suprascapular nerve, the sole branch of the upper trunk of the brachial plexus. The relationship between the suprascapular nerve and the superior margin of subscapularis, the base of the coracoid, and the scapular notch has also been described (▶ Figs. 12.9 and 12.12). After passing through the suprascapular notch, the nerve innervates the supraspinatus and then passes lateral to the spine of the scapula through the spinoglenoid notch (▶ Fig. 12.27). It may be compressed in this location by cysts forming in relation to tears of the superoposterior labrum. Tethering of the cuff to the labrum and capsule may need to be released in order to mobilize retracted rotator cuff tears prior to repair. This tethering can be significant at the superoposterior aspect, where there is already a significant anatomic thickening of the connection between the supraspinatus tendon and the capsule (▶ Fig. 12.28). The suprascapular nerve is at risk of damage in this location if mobilization superior to the labrum is undertaken too medial to the glenoid.

The shoulder crane is a concept that has been developed to help understand the form and function of the shoulder (▶ Fig. 12.29).[13,14]

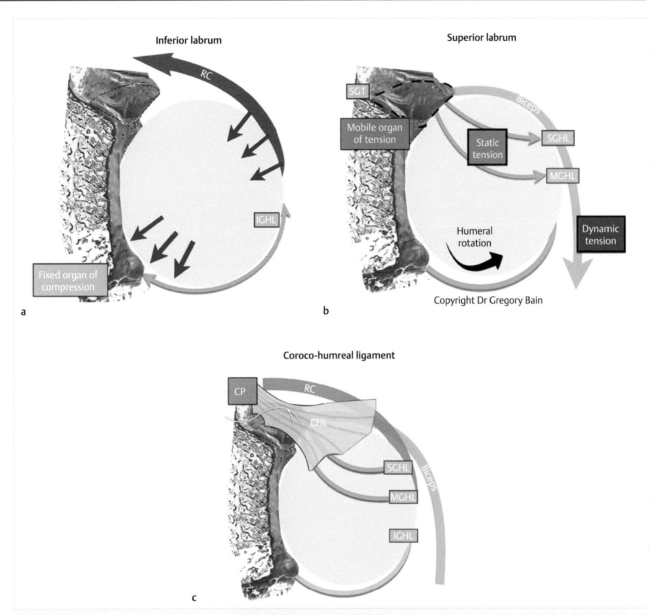

Fig. 12.22 Inferior and superior and labrum composite histology image of the glenoid labrum at 5 and 12 o'clock. (**a**) The inferior labrum is a fixed organ of compression. The convex bumper of the inferior labrum is mounted onto of the osseous glenoid. There is no defect between the glenoid, labrum and articular surface. (**b**) Superior labrum is a mobile organ of tension, attached off the glenoid face, with a synovial fined cleft between the labrum and the glenoid. It is a mobile organ of tension. The superior labrum is continuous with the static restraints (SGHL and MGHL), which become taut at the extremes of rotation. Biceps contraction pulls the mobile superior labrum onto the humeral head to increase containment and secondarily tightens the associated static restraints (SGHL and MGHL). The coracohumeral ligament (CHL) is closely associated with the biceps, SGHL and rotator cuff attachments to provide sensory feedback. (Copyright Dr Gregory Bain). (**c**) The CHL drapes the rotator cuff, biceps tendon, superior labrum, SGHL and MGHL. This sensory organ is perfectly positioned to receive the feedback on the tension in the rotator cuff and the ligament, the position of the humeral head and if it is subluxating. This servomechanism can fine tune rotator cuff function for function and elite performance. MGHL, middle glenohumeral ligament; SGHL, superior glenohumeral ligament. Reprinted from Journal of ISAKOS: Joint Disorders & Orthopaedic Sports Medicine, Vol 4, no. 2, Bain GI, Phadnis J, Itoi E, Di Giacomo G, Sugaya H, Sonnabend DH, McLean J, Shoulder crane: a concept of suspension, stability, control and motion, p. 68, Copyright 2019, with permission from BMJ Publishing Group Ltd.

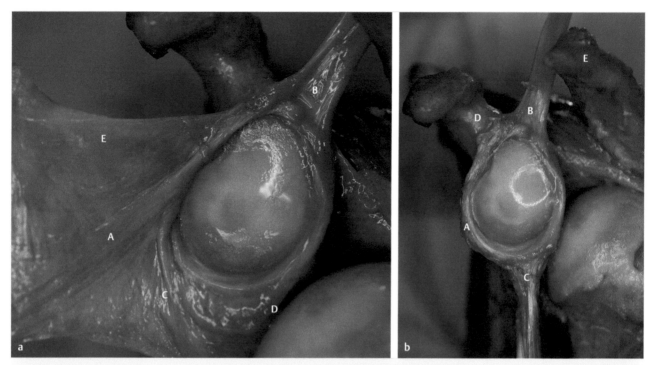

Fig. 12.23 (a) Glenoid, labrum, and attachments: *Antero inferior capsulolabral structures, capsule detached from humeral insertion and humeral head retracted posterior* A: middle glenohumeral ligament; B: long head of biceps; C: anterior band of inferior glenohumeral ligament; D: posterior band of inferior glenohumeral ligament; E: superior glenohumeral ligament. (b) Glenoid, labrum, and attachments (b): *Direct lateral view, humeral head displaced directly posterior* A: glenoid labrum; B: long head of biceps; C: long head of triceps; D: base of coracoid process; E: acromion.

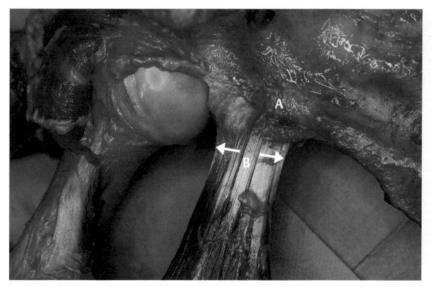

Fig. 12.24 Long head triceps: *Posterior view, deltoid and infraspinatus removed.* A: glenoid neck and infraglenoid tubercle; B: long head of triceps.

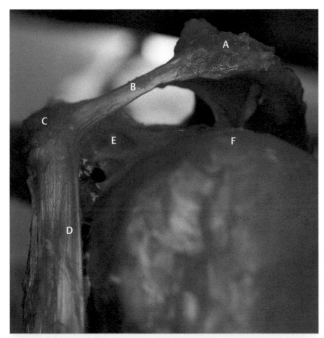

Fig. 12.25 Coracoacromial ligament: *Direct lateral view, deltoid removed, clavicle removed.* A: acromion; B: coracoacromial ligament; C: coracoid process; D: conjoint tendon; E: coracohumeral ligament; F: supraspinatus.

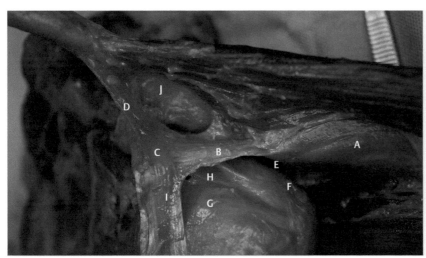

Fig. 12.26 Cuff and coracoacromial ligament: *Anterior view, deltoid detached distally and reflected laterally.* A: undersurface of reflected deltoid; B: coracoacromial ligament; C: coracoid process; D: coracoclavicular ligament (conoid); E: subacromial space; F: supraspinatus; G: subscapularis; H: coracohumeral ligament; I: conjoint tendon; J: undersurface lateral clavicle.

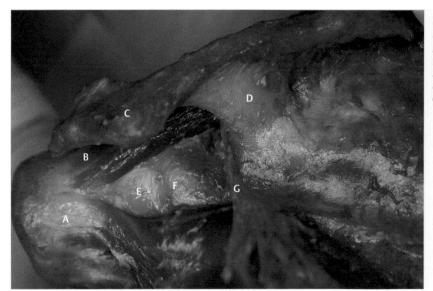

Fig. 12.27 Spinoglenoid notch and suprascapular nerve: *Posterior view, deltoid removed, infraspinatus reflected inferiorly.* A: infraspinatus tendon; B: supraspinatus; C: posterior acromion; D: scapular spine; E: posterior capsule; F: posterior labrum and glenoid; G: suprascapular nerve.

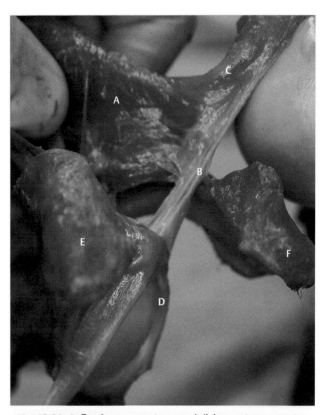

Fig. 12.28 Cuff tether to superior capsule/labrum: *Anterosuperior view, humeral head displaced posteriorly.* A: supraspinatus muscle belly; B: thickening in posterosuperior capsule; C: supraspinatus tendon merging with capsule; D: posterior labrum; E: coracoid process; F: anterior acromion.

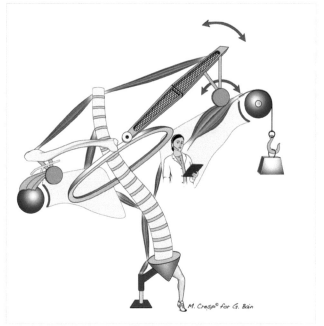

Fig. 12.29 The shoulder crane. The crane is constructed on top of the pelvic base and leg outriggers, which provide for stability and mobility. The articulated spinal tower and thoracic platform are stabilized by the core and periscapular muscles, respectively. The clavicular boom articulates with the anterior platform, at the sternoclavicular joint, and is elevated by the trapezius from the posterior tower. The scapula is suspended and swivels on the coracoclavicular ligaments, positioned by the powerful periscapular muscles, and traverses the 'scapular track'. These factors are all designed to enable the rotator cuff to mobilize the shoulder while it keeps the glenoid aligned and stabilized with the humeral head throughout motion and loading (Copyright Dr Gregory Bain). Reprinted from Journal of ISAKOS: Joint Disorders & Orthopaedic Sports Medicine, Vol 4, no. 2, Bain GI, Phadnis J, Itoi E, Di Giacomo G, Sugaya H, Sonnabend DH, McLean J, Shoulder crane: a concept of suspension, stability, control and motion, p. 64, Copyright 2019, with permission from BMJ Publishing Group Ltd.

References

1. Bain GI, Eng K, Zumstein M. Fatal air embolus during internal fixation of the clavicle: a case report. JBJS Case Connector 2013;3(1):e24

2. Daseler EH, Anson BJ. Surgical anatomy of the subclavian artery and its branches. Surg Gynecol Obstet 1959;108(2):149–174

3. Jobe CM, Coen MJ. Gross anatomy of the shoulder. In: Rockwood CA, Matsen FA III, Wirth MA, Lippitt SB, eds. The Shoulder. 3rd ed. Philadelphia, PA: Saunders; 2004:77–81

4. Last RJ. Lasts Anatomy: Regional and Applied. Edinburgh, Scotland: Churchill Livingstone; 1994

5. Galley IJ, Watts AC, Bain GI. The anatomic relationship of the axillary artery and vein to the clavicle: a cadaveric study. J Shoulder Elbow Surg 2009;18(5):e21–e25

6. Sinha A, Edwin J, Sreeharsha B, Bhalaik V, Brownson P. A radiological study to define safe zones for drilling during plating of clavicle fractures. J Bone Joint Surg Br 2011;93(9):1247–1252

7. Gerber C, Yian EH, Pfirrmann CAW, Zumstein MA, Werner CML. Subscapularis muscle function and structure after total shoulder replacement with lesser tuberosity osteotomy and repair. J Bone Joint Surg Am 2005;87(8):1739–1745

8. Uno A, Bain GI, Mehta JA. Arthroscopic relationship of the axillary nerve to the shoulder joint capsule: an anatomic study. J Shoulder Elbow Surg 1999;8(3):226–230

9. Howell SM, Galinat BJ. The glenoid-labral socket. A constrained articular surface. Clin Orthop Relat Res 1989;(243):122–125

10. Mileski RA, Snyder SJ. Superior labral lesions in the shoulder: pathoanatomy and surgical management. J Am Acad Orthop Surg 1998;6(2):121–131

11. Bain GI, Galley IJ, Singh C, Carter C, Eng K. Anatomic study of the superior glenoid labrum. Clin Anat 2013;26(3):367–376

12. Elser F, Braun S, Dewing CB, Giphart JE, Millett PJ. Anatomy, function, injuries, and treatment of the long head of the biceps brachii tendon. Arthroscopy 2011;27(4):581–592

13. Bain GI, Phadnis J, Sonnabend DH. The functional shoulder. In: Bain GJ, Itoi E, Di Giacomo G, Sugaya H (Eds.) Normal and Pathological Anatomy of the Shoulder. Springer-Verlag: Berlin Heidelberg, 2015.

14. Bain GI, Phadnis J, Itoi E, Di Giacomo G, Sugaya H, Sonnabend DH, McLean J. Shoulder crane: a concept of suspension, stability, control and motion. J ISAKOS: Joint Dis Orthop Sports Med. 2019 Mar 1;4(2):63–70.

13 The Anatomy of the Arm

John T. Capo and Ben Shamian

13.1 Humerus

The humerus is the largest bone in the upper limb. It articulates with the scapula (▶Fig. 13.1) at the glenohumeral joint proximally and the radius and the ulna distally at the elbow joint. The proximal end of the humerus consists of three parts: the articular head, lesser tuberosity, and greater tuberosity (▶Fig. 13.2). The hemispherical head articulates with the glenoid cavity of the scapula. The junction of the articular portion and the remaining head is called the anatomic neck, while the junction between the entire head fragment and the shaft, below the tuberosities, is called the surgical neck. The surgical neck is the most common site of fractures. The axillary nerve runs along the posterior aspect of the surgical neck.

The greater tuberosity is located lateral to the bicipital groove. It is the point of attachment of three rotator cuff muscles: the supraspinatus and infraspinatus (both innervated by suprascapular nerve) and the teres minor (innervated by axillary nerve). The lesser tuberosity, located medial

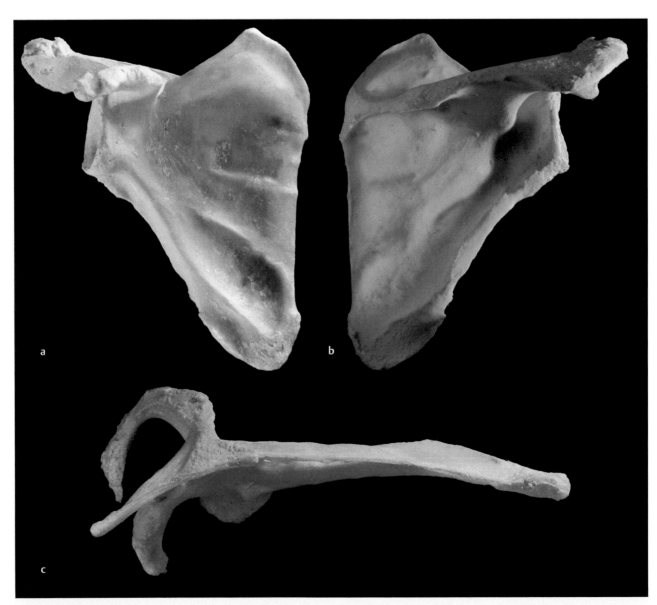

Fig. 13.1 **(a)** Anterior aspect of the right scapula. **(b)** Posterior aspect of the right scapula. **(c)** Medial aspect of the right scapula.

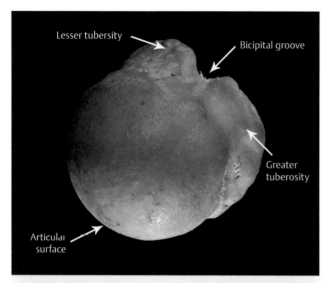

Fig. 13.2 End on view of the head of the humerus with markings showing the articular surface, greater and lesser tuberosities, and bicipital groove.

to the bicipital groove, is the site of subscapularis insertion (innervated by the upper and lower subscapular nerves). The shaft of the humerus (▶Fig. 13.3) is tubular and has two important prominent features: the deltoid tuberosity laterally for attachment of the deltoid muscle and the oblique radial groove (spiral groove) posteriorly, in which the radial nerve and deep brachial artery of the arm cross. The distal end of the humerus fans out into two columns and then supports the elbow articular surface. This joint includes the spooled trochlea (articulates with the ulna medially), the capitellum (articulate with the head of the radius laterally), and three fossae (radial fossa and coronoid fossa anteriorly, and olecranon fossa posteriorly). The following areas of the humerus are clinically important, as they are in direct contact with the indicated nerves:

- Surgical neck: axillary nerve
- Radial groove: radial nerve
- Medial epicondyle: ulnar nerve posterior to it
- Lateral epicondyle: radial nerve anterior to it

13.2 Cutaneous Innervations of the Arm

Posterior surface of the arm:
- Superior lateral cutaneous nerve of arm (branch of axillary nerve)
- Posterior cutaneous nerve of arm (branch of radial nerve)
- Inferior lateral cutaneous nerve of arm (branch of radial nerve)

Lateral surface of the arm:
- Superior lateral cutaneous nerve of arm (branch of axillary nerve)
- Inferior lateral cutaneous nerve of arm (branch of radial nerve)

Medial surface of the arm:
- Intercostobrachial nerve (lateral cutaneous branch of T2)
- Medial brachial cutaneous nerve of arm (from medial cord of brachial plexus)
- Medial antebrachial cutaneous nerve of arm (from medial cord of brachial plexus)

13.3 Muscles of the Arm

The *anterior compartment* contains three flexor muscles, all innervated by the musculocutaneous nerve (▶Fig. 13.4).

Biceps brachii: It consists of a short head and a long head, each with different sites of origin. The short head is attached to the coracoid process of the scapula, while the long head originates from the supraglenoid tubercle of scapula. Distally, the biceps muscle terminates into one tendon and a fascial extension. The true tendon attaches to the bicipital tuberosity on the radius, while the fascial bicipital aponeurosis fans onto the ulnar part of the antebrachial fascia and medial epicondyle. The blood supply of the biceps brachii is via the brachial artery.

Brachialis: This muscle originates on the anterior surface of humerus and inserts on to the coronoid process of ulna. The brachialis is the main flexor of the elbow. The brachial artery and radial recurrent artery are the blood supply to the brachialis muscle (▶Fig. 13.5).

Coracobrachialis: Originating from the coracoid process of scapula, it inserts on to the middle third of medial surface of humerus. This muscle has two important anatomical landmarks. The musculocutaneous nerve pierces it 5 to 6 cm from its origin (▶Fig. 13.6a). Its distal attachment indicates the location of the nutrient foramen of the humerus, where the main nutrient artery penetrates the bone, and the location where the ulnar nerve courses from anterior to posterior and penetrates the intermuscular septum. It is supplied by the brachial artery.

The *posterior compartment* contents include two muscles innervated by the radial nerve.

Triceps brachii: The long head originates from the infraglenoid tubercle of scapula, the lateral head (strongest) originates from the posterior surface of humerus, and the medial head originates from the lower half of the posterior surface of humerus inferior to the radial groove (▶Fig. 13.7). The three heads converge to form one tendon, which inserts onto the proximal end of the ulna at the olecranon process. Its blood supply is the profunda brachii artery of the arm.

Anconeus: This small triangular muscle originates on the lateral epicondyle of humerus and insert to lateral surface of the olecranon. It is supplied by the interosseous recurrent artery.

13.4 Nerves of the Arm

The arm contains four main nerves (median, ulnar, musculocutaneous, and radial), two of which (median and ulnar) supply no branches to the upper arm. The majority of the nerves and arteries in the arm are on the medial aspect of the anterior compartment (▶Fig. 13.6b).

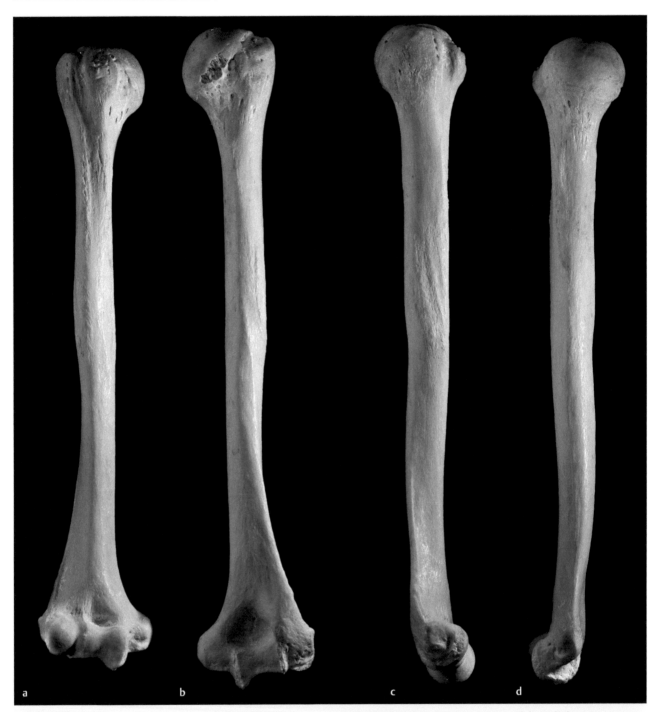

Fig. 13.3 (a) Anterior aspect of the right humerus. (b) Posterior aspect of the right humerus. (c) Lateral aspect of the right humerus. (d) Medial aspect of the right humerus.

13.5 Musculocutaneous Nerve (C5–C6)

The musculocutaneous nerve arises from the lateral cord of the brachial plexus. Proximally, it is located lateral to the median nerve (▶Fig. 13.6c). As it descends to the arm, it pierces the coracobrachialis approximately 5 to 8 cm distal to the coracoid.[1] The prevalence of cases of musculocutaneous nerve outside (not piercing) the coracobrachialis muscle is reported to be 0 to 8% in anatomical dissections.[2–4] In the proximal third of the arm, it is located between the biceps brachii and the coracobrachialis. It supplies motor innervation to the flexor muscles of the arm (coracobrachialis, biceps brachii, and brachialis). After supplying all three muscles of the anterior compartment of the arm, it terminates as the lateral cutaneous nerve (purely sensory nerve) of the forearm, which innervates the radial side of the forearm (▶Fig. 13.8).

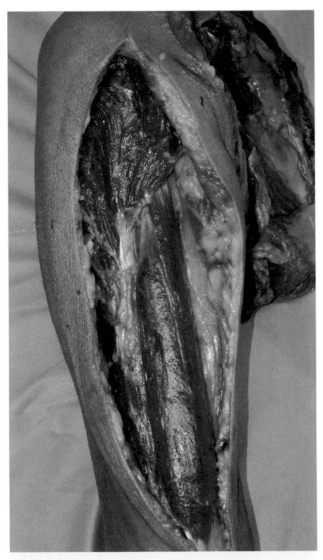

Fig. 13.4 Anterior compartment of the arm showing the biceps muscle superficial to the brachialis muscle. The deltoid muscle is also seen.

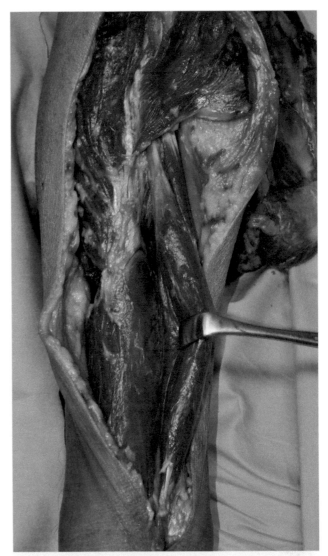

Fig. 13.5 The biceps brachialis muscle has been retracted medially, exposing the entire brachialis muscle.

Variation exists with regard to communication between the musculocutaneous nerve and the median nerve. In an anatomical[5] dissection of 56 upper limbs, communications were seen between the musculocutaneous and median nerves in 53.6% of the arms.

13.6 Median Nerve in the Arm (C6–T1)

The median nerve, from the medial and lateral cords of the brachial plexus, runs lateral to the brachial artery on top of the coracobrachialis muscle until it reaches the middle of the arm, where it crosses to the medial side as it encounters the brachialis muscle (▶ Fig. 13.9). It runs along the medial edge of the biceps brachii, with the brachial artery lying lateral to it. In the antecubital fossa, the median nerve lies deep to the bicipital aponeurosis; medial to the antecubital vein, the brachial artery, and the biceps tendon; and lateral to the common origin of the flexor and pronator muscles.[1] The median nerve has no branches in the arm, but it does supply articular branches to the elbow joint. The median nerve may become entrapped proximally at two locations in the arm, the ligament of Struthers and the lacertus fibrosis. The ligament of Struthers is an abnormal structure that is located 5 cm proximal to the medial epicondyle. It is a fibrous band originating from an aberrant supracondylar process on the medial aspect of the distal humerus that connects to the medial epicondyle.[1] The lacertus fibrosis is a normal fascial sleeve that extends from the biceps tendon to the medial epicondyle and covers the median nerve and brachial artery. The median nerve is lateral to the brachial artery in the upper part, anterior to it in the middle part, and medial to it in the lower arm. The median nerve supplies no muscular innervation in the upper arm.

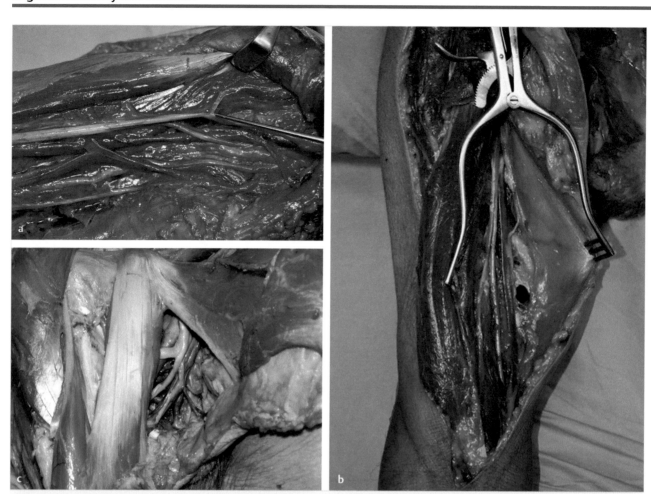

Fig. 13.6 (a) Medial aspect of the arm showing the musculocutaneus nerve. (b) Anteromedial aspect of the arm showing the nerves and arteries. (c) The musculocutaneous nerve arises from the lateral cord of the brachial plexus. Proximally, it is located lateral to the median nerve.

13.7 Ulnar Nerve in the Arm (C8–T1)

The ulnar nerve branches from the medial cord of the brachial plexus and runs medial to the brachial artery (▶Fig. 13.10). Proximally, it descends medial to the coracobrachialis and anterior to the long head of the triceps. In the middle of the arm, at the level of the distal attachment of the coracobrachialis to the humerus, together with the superior ulnar collateral artery, the nerve pierces the medial intermuscular septum to enter the posterior compartment of the brachium.[1] This point has been found to average 10 cm proximal to the medial epicondyle.[6] Distally, the ulnar nerve passes lateral and posterior to the medial epicondyle of the humerus and medial to the olecranon process in the cubital tunnel. In this area, the nerve is superficial, easily palpable, and vulnerable to injury. Like the median nerve, the ulnar nerve has no branches in the arm, but it also supplies articular branches to the elbow joint.

The ulnar nerve can become entrapped in two anatomic locations along its course in the arm: the medial intermuscular septum and the arcade of Struthers (▶Fig. 13.11). The arcade of Struthers is an area of transverse fascial fibers that connect the medial head of the triceps to the intermuscular septum approximately 8 to 10 cm proximal to the medial epicondyle.[7] The

thickness of these fibers is quite variable among patients. A true arcade is found in approximately 60 to 70% of the population.[8] The arcade of Struthers is much more common than the ligament of Struthers (median nerve entrapment), which is found in 1% of the population.[9]

13.8 Radial Nerve in the Arm (C5–T1)

The radial nerve, arising from the posterior cord of the brachial plexus, supplies all the muscles in the posterior compartment of the arm and forearm (▶Fig. 13.12). It enters the arm posterior to the brachial artery, medial to the humerus, and anterior to the long head of the triceps. It gives branches that innervate the long and the lateral head of triceps brachii before it crosses the humerus. The radial nerve then passes around the humeral shaft in the radial groove with the deep brachial artery of the arm in direct contact with the humeral shaft. After crossing the humerus, it pierces the lateral intermuscular septum approximately 10 to 12 cm from the lateral epicondyle[10–12] from posterior to anterior. This point is between the deltoid insertion and the brachioradialis origin. It then runs between the brachialis and brachioradialis to lie anterior to the lateral condyle of the humerus. One to 3 cm distal to the lateral epicondyle and deep to the brachioradialis, the radial nerve splits into the superficial

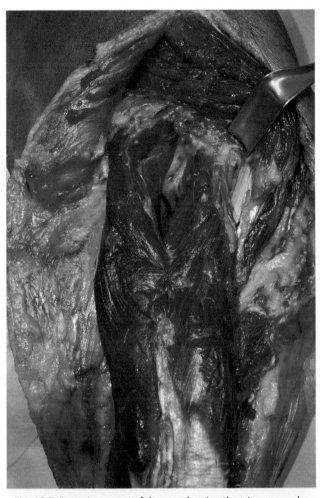

Fig. 13.7 Posterior aspect of the arm showing the triceps muscle.

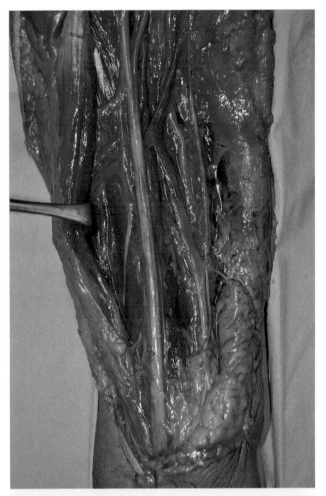

Fig. 13.8 The musculocutaneus nerve supplies motor innervation to the flexor muscles of the arm (coracobrachialis, biceps brachii, and brachialis). After supplying all three muscles of the anterior compartment of the arm, it terminates as the lateral antebrachial cutaneous nerve (LABCN), a purely sensory nerve of the forearm, which innervates the radial side of the forearm.

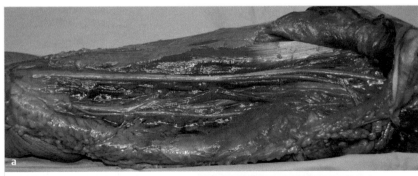

Fig. 13.9 (a) Anteromedial aspect of the arm showing the musculocutaneus nerve, the median nerve. (b) Detailed dissection of the anteromedial aspect of the arm showing the biceps muscle, the median nerve, the ulnar nerve and the medial brachial cutaneous nerve of arm and the medial antebrachial cutaneous nerve of the arm.

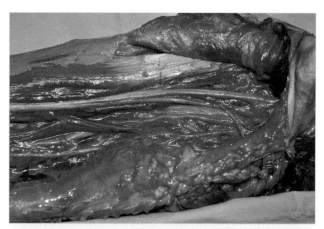

Fig. 13.10 Anteromedial dissection of the arm showing the close up of the musculocutaneus nerve, the median nerve, the radial nerve, the ulnar nerve and the brachial artery.

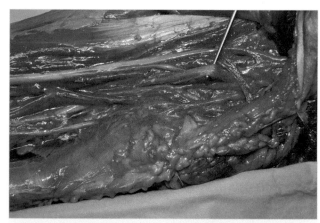

Fig. 13.12 The radial nerve in the proximal arm.

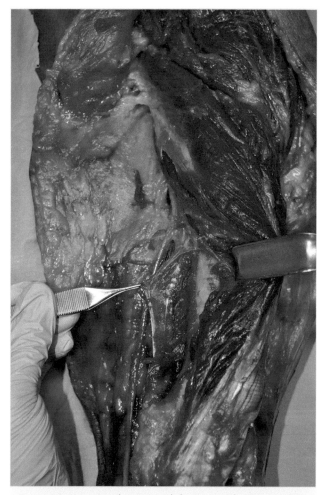

Fig. 13.11 Dissection showing medial intermuscular septum of the arm and the ulnar nerve.

radial nerve and the posterior interosseous nerve.[13,14] The deep branch (posterior interosseous nerves) of the radial nerve is

entirely a motor nerve. The superficial branch of the radial nerve is entirely a sensory nerve.

Among the major nerves in the upper extremity, radial nerve entrapment is the least common. Radial nerve palsy in the arm most commonly is caused by fractures of the humerus, especially in the middle third (Holstein–Lewis fracture). It can also be compressed by the lateral intermuscular septum. Although rare, an anomalous muscle, the accessory subscapularis–teres–latissimus, has been reported to cause compression of the radial nerve at this level.[15]

The axillary nerve branches off the posterior cord of the brachial plexus, runs along the anterior aspect of the subscapularis muscle, and goes into the quadrangular space the latissimus dorsi tendon (▶ Fig. 13.13). The nerve then courses under the inferior aspect of the glenohumeral joint capsule, around the humeral neck and into the posterior aspect of the deltoid muscle (▶ Fig. 13.14).

13.9 Arteries of the Arm

13.9.1 The Brachial Artery

The teres major marks the end of the axillary artery and beginning of the brachial artery. During its course through the arm, the brachial artery lies anterior to the triceps brachii and brachialis muscles, and is overlapped by the biceps brachii and coracobrachialis muscles. Proximally, the artery lies medial to the humerus. As it descends, accompanying the median nerve, the artery is located in an anterior position relative to the humerus. It terminates in the cubital fossa under the bicipital aponeurosis, dividing into the two major arteries of the forearm at the level of the neck of the radius, the radial and ulnar arteries. Major branches in the arm are the deep artery of the arm (profunda brachii artery), the superior ulnar collateral artery, the inferior ulnar collateral artery, and the nutrient humeral artery. The profunda brachii artery travels with the radial nerve and is the largest branch of the brachial artery. The superior ulnar collateral artery, arising from the brachial artery, accompanies the ulnar nerve, piercing the medial intermuscular septum, to end proximally posterior to the medial

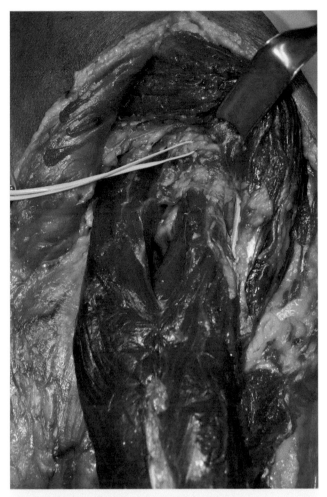

Fig. 13.13 The axillary nerve in the proximal arm.

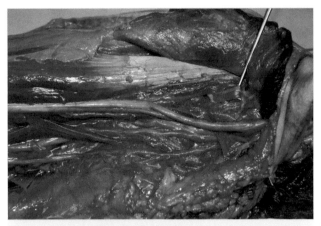

Fig. 13.14 The relationship of the axillary nerve in the proximal arm to the other neurovascular structures.

epicondyle of the humerus. The ulnar artery gives rise to both the anterior ulnar recurrent artery, which joins the inferior ulnar collateral anterior to the medial epicondyle of the humerus, and the posterior ulnar recurrent artery, which joins the superior ulnar collateral artery posterior to the medial humeral epicondyle.[16] The radial artery gives off the radial recurrent artery, which joins with the radial recurrent branch of the deep artery of the arm anterior to the lateral epicondyle.

13.10 Superficial Veins of the Arm

The veins of the arm are divided into superficial and deep. The two systems anastomose frequently with each other. The superficial veins are located immediately beneath the skin. The deep veins accompany the arteries. The two main superficial veins are the basilic and the cephalic veins. The basilic vein, visible through the skin, runs on the medial aspect of the arm. It ascends in the groove between the biceps brachii and pronator teres. It perforates the deep fascia and runs on the medial side of the brachial artery. It finally drains into the axillary vein. The cephalic vein ascends on the lateral side of the arm in front

of the elbow in the groove between the brachioradialis and the biceps brachii. It continues up in the deltopectoral groove piercing the clavipectoral fascia to drain into axillary vein.

13.11 Summary

The anterior (flexor) compartment contents include the following:

- The *flexor muscles*: coracobrachialis, biceps brachii, and brachialis
- The *brachial artery* and *branches*
- The *median nerve*
- The *ulnar nerve (proximally)*
- The *musculocutaneous nerve*
- The *basilic vein*

The posterior (extensor) compartment contents include the following:

- The *extensor muscles*: triceps
- The *radial nerve* and *branches*
- The *profunda brachii artery*
- The *ulnar nerve (distally)*

13.12 Surgical Approaches

Various approaches to the humerus have been described: the anterior approach, the anterolateral approach, the posterior approach, and the lateral approach. The radial nerve is at greatest risk during exposure of the humeral shaft in the posterior and lateral approaches.

13.13 Anterior Approach to the Humerus

For the anterior approach, an incision is made longitudinally from the tip of the coracoid process distally in line with the deltopectoral groove and continued along the lateral aspect of the biceps muscle and tendon, stopping 3 cm proximal to the anterior elbow flexion crease. The deep dissection

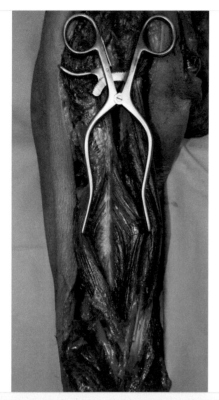

Fig. 13.15 The brachialis split in the anterior approach to the humerus.

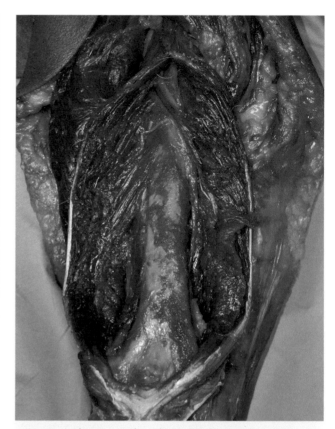

Fig. 13.16 The triceps split in the posterior approach to the humerus.

involves splitting of the brachialis muscle in its central portion (▶Fig. 13.15). This is an internervous plane, as the medial side of the brachialis is innervated by the musculocutaneous nerve and the later aspect is innervated by the radial nerve. Through this approach, the humerus can be exposed from the humeral head to the humeral shaft distally to the coronoid fossa. The uses of the anterior approach include the following[17]:

- Anterior plating of fractures of the humerus
- Osteotomy of the humerus
- Biopsy and resection of bone tumors
- Treatment of osteomyelitis

13.14 Anterolateral Approach to the Humerus

The anterior lateral approach begins with a curved longitudinal incision over the lateral border of the biceps, starting about 10 cm proximal to the flexion crease of the elbow and extending to the lateral epicondyle. The deep interval is between the brachialis and the brachioradialis. The radial nerve travels in this interval and needs to be protected as it courses from posterior to anterior. This approach exposes the distal fourth of the humerus distally down to the lateral epicondyle.[18] Through this interval the radial nerve can be traced from the midhumerus to the proximal forearm. Care must be taken distally not to injure the lateral antebrachial cutaneous nerve as it exits between the biceps and brachialis muscles.

The radial nerve is likewise at risk from distal extension and must be identified between the brachialis and brachioradialis at the lateral epicondyle.[18]

13.15 Posterior Approaches to the Humerus

An incision is made in the midline of the posterior aspect of the arm, from 8 cm below the acromion to the olecranon fossa. These approaches provide excellent access to the lower three-fourths of the posterior aspect of the humerus. The posterior approach is complicated by the vulnerability of the radial nerve, which spirals around the back of the bone. The deep interval involves management of the triceps and can be accomplished in several ways.

Triceps split: The deep dissection involves separating the two superficial heads of the triceps brachii muscle, the long and lateral heads. The spiral groove contains the radial nerve; thus, the radial nerve actually separates the origins of the lateral and medial heads of the triceps (▶Fig. 13.16). The critical aspect of this approach is identification of the radial nerve as it exits the spiral groove approximately 14 cm proximal to the lateral epicondyle and pierces the intermuscular septum 10 cm from the articular surface.[18] The nerve can be reliably identified at a point two fingerbreadths proximal to the beginning of the triceps tendon, described as the "point of confluence."[19] The humeral shaft can be exposed proximal to the nerve up to the

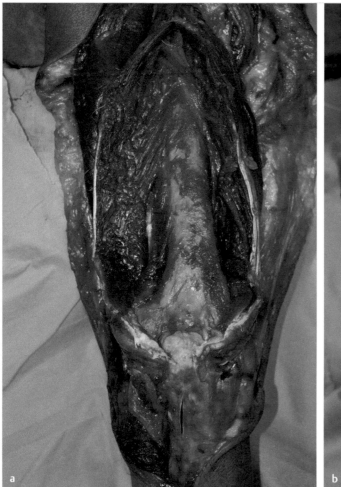
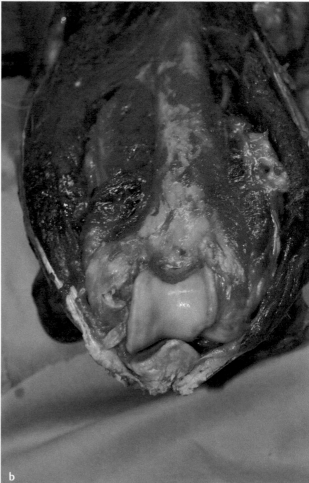

Fig. 13.17 (a,b) Extended triceps split exposure of the distal humerus.

proximal third and distal to the nerve to the olecranon fossa. The exposure can be extended distally by splitting the triceps tendon along the olecranon.[20] Through this extension, the medial and lateral columns and the proximal aspect of the articular surface can be exposed (▶Fig. 13.17).

Paratricipital approach: The medial and lateral aspects of the triceps can be elevated from either side, and the humeral shaft and the distal aspect of the humeral columns can be exposed. The ulnar nerve must be identified on the medial column and traced proximally to the intermuscular septum and distally to the cubital tunnel (▶Fig. 13.18). The medial humeral shaft and medial humeral column are easily exposed through this exposure (▶Fig. 13.19). The lateral exposure is along the laterals aspect of the triceps muscle and will encounter the radial nerve approximately 12 cm proximal to the lateral epicondyle. The triceps muscle can be retracted medially and laterally to expose the humeral shaft (▶Fig. 13.20). This exposure is ideal for distal third humeral shaft and extra-articular supracondylar fractures. Simple intra-articular fractures of the distal humerus can be addressed using this approach. The joint surface can be visualized by hyperflexion of the elbow and retraction of the triceps with elbow extension.

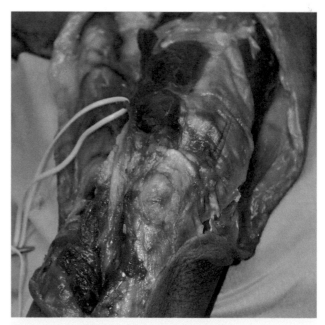

Fig. 13.18 Exposing the ulnar nerve in the medial exposure.

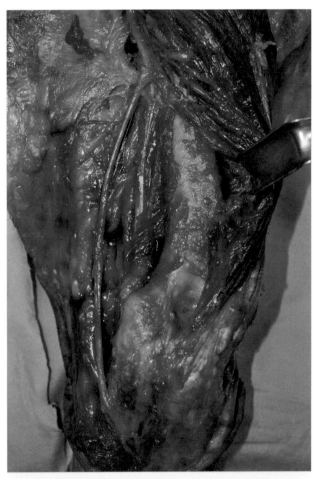

Fig. 13.19 Extended medial exposure of the distal humerus.

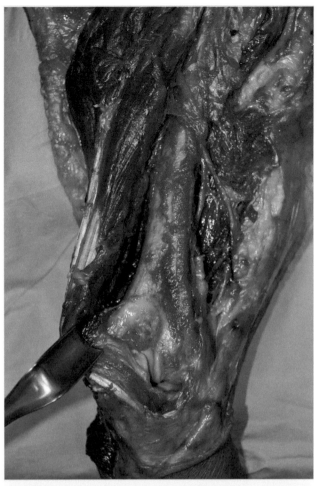

Fig. 13.20 The lateral head of the triceps is reflected from the lateral to medial side to expose the lateral column of the distal humerus.

13.16 Extended Posterolateral Approach

This recently described approach gives an extensile approach of nearly the entire humeral shaft. The superficial dissection begins with identifying the posterior antebrachial cutaneous on the superficial aspect of the lateral triceps and tracing it down to the radial nerve proper. The lateral head of the triceps is reflected from lateral to medial, exposing the humeral shaft from the neck of the humerus to distal aspect of the lateral column (▶ Fig. 13.21). Approximately 94% of the humeral diaphysis can be exposed with this approach.[21] The radial nerve can be identified throughout its entirety from the medial humerus to the radial tunnel. It is an excellent approach to plate the humeral diaphysis while exploring the radial nerve. Fixation of the humerus can be accomplished from the humeral neck, to the lateral column distally to the posterior aspect of the capitellum. The profunda brachii artery runs with the radial nerve in the spiral groove and must also be protected.

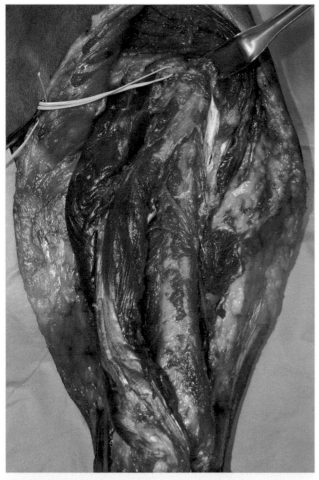

Fig. 13.21 The lateral head of the triceps is reflected from the lateral to medial side to expose the lateral column of the distal humerus.

References

1. Mazurek MT, Shin AY. Upper extremity peripheral nerve anatomy: current concepts and applications. Clin Orthop Relat Res 2001;(383):7–20

2. Remerand F, Laulan J, Couvret C, et al. Is the musculocutaneous nerve really in the coracobrachialis muscle when performing an axillary block? An ultrasound study. Anesth Analg 2010;110(6):1729–1734

3. Krishnamurthy A, Nayak SR, Venkatraya Prabhu L, et al. The branching pattern and communications of the musculocutaneous nerve. J Hand Surg Eur Vol 2007;32(5):560–562

4. Macchi V, Tiengo C, Porzionato A, et al. Musculocutaneous nerve: histotopographic study and clinical implications. Clin Anat 2007;20(4):400–406

5. Guerri-Guttenberg RA, Ingolotti M. Classifying musculocutaneous nerve variations. Clin Anat 2009;22(6):671–683

6. Contreras MG, Warner MA, Charboneau WJ, Cahill DR. Anatomy of the ulnar nerve at the elbow: potential relationship of acute ulnar neuropathy to gender differences. Clin Anat 1998;11(6):372–378

7. Gabel GT, Amadio PC. Reoperation for failed decompression of the ulnar nerve in the region of the elbow. J Bone Joint Surg Am 1990;72(2):213–219

8. De Jesus R, Dellon AL. Historic origin of the "arcade of Struthers." J Hand Surg Am 2003;28(3):528–531

9. Terry RJ. A study of the supracondyloid process in the living. Am J Phys Anthropol 1921. https://doi.org/10.1002/ajpa.1330040203

10. Uhl RL, Larosa JM, Sibeni T, Martino LJ. Posterior approaches to the humerus: when should you worry about the radial nerve? J Orthop Trauma 1996;10(5):338–340

11. Robson AJ, See MS, Ellis H. Applied anatomy of the superficial branch of the radial nerve. Clin Anat 2008;21(1):38–45

12. Guse TR, Ostrum RF. The surgical anatomy of the radial nerve around the humerus. Clin Orthop Relat Res 1995;(320):149–153

13. Abrams RA, Ziets RJ, Lieber RL, Botte MJ. Anatomy of the radial nerve motor branches in the forearm. J Hand Surg Am 1997;22(2):232–237

14. Low CK, Chew JTH, Mitra AK. A surgical approach to the posterior interosseous branch of the radial nerve through the brachioradialis—a cadaveric study. Singapore Med J 1994;35(4):394–396

15. Kameda Y. An anomalous muscle (accessory subscapularis-teres-latissimus muscle) in the axilla penetrating the brachial plexus in man. Acta Anat (Basel) 1976;96(4):513–533

16. Yamaguchi K, Sweet FA, Bindra R, Morrey BF, Gelberman RH. The extraosseous and intraosseous arterial anatomy of the adult elbow. J Bone Joint Surg Am 1997;79(11):1653–1662

17. Hoppenfeld S, deBoer P. Surgical Exposures in Orthopaedics: The Anatomic Approach. Lippincott Williams & Wilkins; 2003

18. Zlotolow DA, Catalano LW III, Barron OA, Glickel SZ. Surgical exposures of the humerus. J Am Acad Orthop Surg 2006;14(13):754–765

19. Seigerman DA, Choung EW, Yoon RS, et al. Identification of the radial nerve during the posterior approach to the humerus: a cadaveric study. J Orthop Trauma 2012;26(4):226–228

20. McKee MD, Wilson TL, Winston L, Schemitsch EH, Richards RR. Functional outcome following surgical treatment of intra-articular distal humeral fractures through a posterior approach. J Bone Joint Surg Am 2000;82-A(12):1701–1707

21. Gerwin M, Hotchkiss RN, Weiland AJ. Alternative operative exposures of the posterior aspect of the humeral diaphysis with reference to the radial nerve. J Bone Joint Surg Am 1996;78(11):1690–1695

14 The Elbow Joint

Hill Hastings II

14.1 The Confluent Layered Anatomy of the Elbow

The student of elbow anatomy will quickly realize that it is difficult to see all portions of the joint without taking down or dividing many of the more superficial structures. The many vessels and nerves that traverse the joint, particularly medially and anteriorly, have branches to the proximal musculature that prevent deep dissection without division of some of the branches that innervate the proximal musculature. The tendons that appear separate in the middle and distal forearm are inseparable proximally, since many of them converge and take origin close to the flexion/extension axis of the elbow. In addition, there is no easily identifiable plane between superficial and deep structures of the most proximal medial and lateral elbow tendon origins. Tendon fibers underlap or overlap each other to allow for each to arise close to the elbow flexion/extension axis. Also, the tendon fibers of the flexor pronator and extensor supinator origins arise not only from bone but also from the deeper medial and lateral ligament structures.

The following dissections will cover the superficial and deep anatomy of the elbow. To do so, the more superficial layers have been removed to allow for visualization of the deeper ligamentous anatomy.

Nerve and vascular anatomy is covered in chapters 9 and 11, so it will only be mentioned here when particularly relevant to the elbow structures.

14.2 Articular Anatomy

The elbow joint contains three different portions or articular components, all within the same capsular synovial cavity.

Ulnohumeral joint: The trochlea is shaped like a grooved spool positioned between the medial epicondyle and the lateral epicondyle (▶ Fig. 14.1a). The trochlea, which articulates with the coronoid and olecranon of the proximal ulna (trochlear notch), provides a stable surface for flexion and extension of the elbow. The medial part of the trochlear groove is wider and deeper anteriorly and medially than on its shorter lateral surface. It is separated from the capitellum by a small ridge of bone.

Radiocapitellar joint: The capitellum articulates with the radial head to form the second portion of the elbow joint (radiocapitellar articulation) that allows for rotation of the radial head and for flexion and extension (▶ Fig. 14.1b).

Proximal radioulnar joint: Third, the circumferential surface of the radial head articulates with the sigmoid notch of proximal ulna to comprise the proximal radioulnar joint. The radial head is stabilized to the ulna at the "sigmoid notch" (▶ Fig. 14.2a,b) by the strong or stout annular ligament that encircles the radial head by arising from ulna anteriorly and attaching to ulna posteriorly. The annular ligament exists as part of the "lateral collateral ligament complex" and contains also the fibers of origin of

the supinator as well as the extensors in the forearm. The radial fossa subtends an arc of 66° of the radial head, or 18% of the radial head circumference. And 215° of the radial head consists of articular surface that articulates through full pronation to full supination.[1]

The radial head is slightly oblong in shape and is concentrically located in the sigmoid notch in neutral rotation. It shifts anteriorly with pronation and posteriorly with supination.

14.3 Effect of Elbow Joint Morphology on Elbow Alignment

The morphology of the trochlea and capitellum provides for valgus elbow alignment with elbow extension and varus alignment in flexion. In the coronal plane, the medial trochlea extends more distal than the lateral trochlea and capitellum (▶ Fig. 14.1b). In elbow extension, this places the elbow in a valgus carrying angle, which facilitates holding or carrying objects away from the body (▶ Fig. 14.1b). When the elbow flexes, the anterior part of the capitellum, which projects more anteriorly than does the trochlea, swings the forearm into slight varus, which facilitates placing the hand close to the head or mouth (▶ Fig. 14.1a).

14.4 Structures That Provide for Varus/Valgus Stability

Valgus stability depends on the intact ulnar collateral ligament medially and the buttressing effect of the radial head laterally (▶ Fig. 14.1b). In the opposite direction, stability against varus stress requires an intact medial coronoid and lateral collateral ligament complex (▶ Fig. 14.1b).

14.5 Structures That Resist Posterolateral Elbow Dislocation

When the intact surfaces of the trochlea and trochlear notch of ulna are compressed together by muscle forces of brachialis and triceps, the joint is remarkably stable. The coronoid process and radial head both function as an anterior buttress constraint against posterior dislocation (▶ Fig. 14.1a,c). The lateral collateral ligament complex (▶ Fig. 14.11a) prevents opening of the lateral and posterolateral elbow joint. When disrupted, the ulnohumeral joint opens laterally (ulnohumeral supination). As this occurs, the radial head falls posterior to the capitellum and loses its buttressing support with the capitellum (▶ Fig. 14.1c).

Because of the projections of the radial head and coronoid process, an adequate fossa is required for both to allow for full elbow flexion. The normal elbow has an abundant anterior coronoid recess and capitellar (radial) recess to facilitate flexion (▶ Fig. 14.1b). An abundant triangular olecranon fossa is

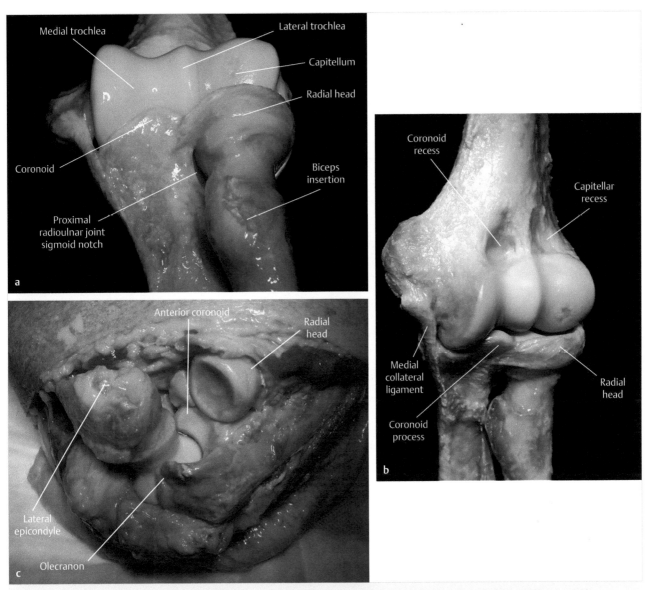

Fig. 14.1 (a) Coronoid process, medial trochlea, lateral trochlea, capitellum, proximal radioulnar joint sigmoid notch, and biceps tendon. (b) Coronoid recess, ulnar collateral ligament, capitellar recess, coronoid process, and radial head. (c) Anterior coronoid and radial head.

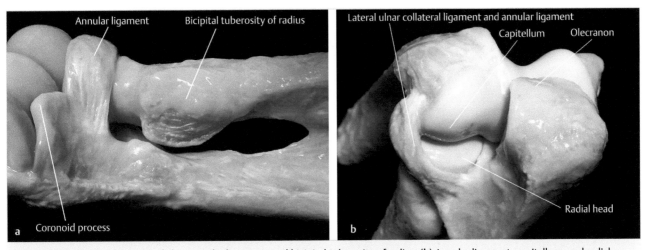

Fig. 14.2 (a) Coronoid process of ulna, annular ligament, and bicipital tuberosity of radius. (b) Annular ligament, capitellum, and radial head.

required to provide or allow for full elbow extension without abutment of the olecranon against the posterior humerus (▶ Fig. 14.3a,b). The coronoid fossa anteriorly and olecranon fossa posteriorly are separated by a thin lamina of bone that at times may have a perforation known as the supratrochlear foramen.

Posteriorly, the triceps tendon inserts onto the olecranon process, not on the tip of the process, but in a small subtle transverse sulcus approximately 5 to 10 mm anterior to the posterior-most proximal ulna (▶ Fig. 14.3a). In the normal elbow, the anterior capsule in front of the elbow and the posterior capsule (▶ Fig. 14.3b) are normally quite soft, compliant, and thin.

▶ Fig. 14.3c–e shows the end-on anatomy of the distal humerus, the olecranon, and the proximal ulna and the radial head.

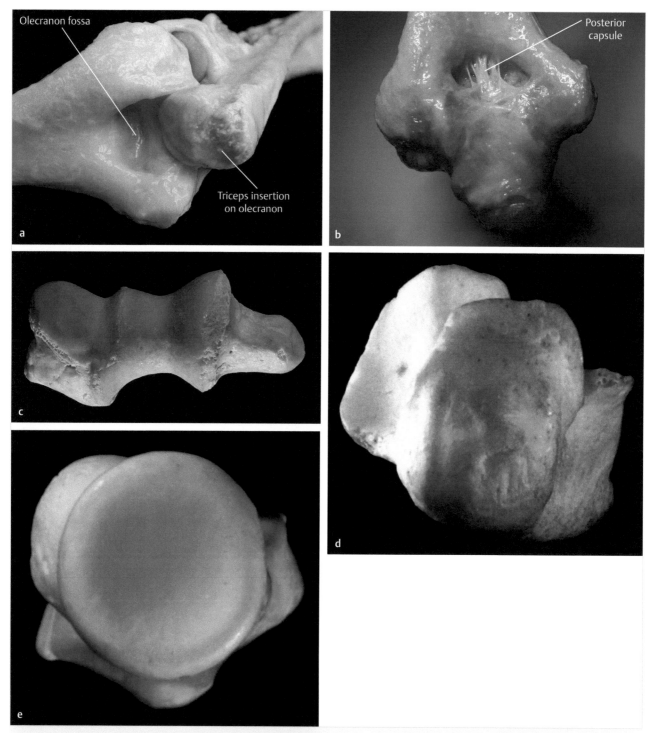

Fig. 14.3 (a) Olecranon fossa and attachment of triceps tendon. (b) Posterior capsule. (c) End-on view of distal humerus. (d) End-on view of olecranon and proximal ulna. (e) End-on view of radial head.

14.5.1 Posteromedial Anatomy

Proximal to the elbow, the intermuscular septum (▶Fig. 14.4a) separates the posterior compartment with triceps from the anterior compartment, which contains the brachialis and biceps muscles. The ulnar nerve lies posterior to the intermuscular septum (▶Fig. 14.4b) and is covered by a fascial layer that extends from the medial triceps to the intermuscular septum. Around 3 to 10 cm proximal to the medial epicondyle, a 2- to 5-cm thickening, termed the arcade of Struthers (▶Fig. 14.4c), may exist which can potentially compress the ulnar nerve. When present, it derives from a thickening fascia of the distal part of the arm, by superficial muscle fibers of the medial head of the triceps muscle arising from the medial intermuscular septum, and by attachments of the internal brachial ligament.[2]

As the ulnar nerve approaches the elbow, it gains segmental vascular supply from the inferior ulnar collateral vessels (▶Fig. 14.4b). Just distal to the medial epicondyle, the ulnar nerve passes beneath the ligament of Osborne, a ligamentous structure between olecranon and medial epicondyle, and the fascial aponeurosis between the humeral and ulnar heads of the flexor carpi ulnaris (▶Fig. 14.4b). In elbow extension (as shown in the figure), the ligament is lax, but with elbow flexion it tightens, as does the posterior band of the ulnar collateral ligament just deep to the ulnar nerve. In flexion, the tightening of these two structures compresses the ulnar nerve. At the level of the ligament of Osborne, the ulnar nerve delivers innervation to the proximal ulnar head of the flexor carpi ulnaris and then more distally to the more anterior humeral head of the flexor carpi ulnaris (▶Fig. 14.4c). In this figure, the fascia and the ulnar head of the flexor carpi ulnaris have been reflected to expose the ulnar nerve along its course from the medial epicondyle distally. The nerve at the level of the released ligament of Osborne in this specimen has been compressed and there is precompressive neuromatous enlargement of the nerve just proximally. The first most relevant branch to the deeper humeral head of the flexor carpi ulnaris enters muscle 5- to 7-cm distal to the medial epicondyle. The posterior band of the ulnar collateral ligament serves as the floor of the cubital tunnel deep to the ulnar nerve. The anterior band of the ulnar collateral ligament lays one fingerbreadth anterior to the ulnar nerve under the flexor pronator origin. Access to the anterior band of the ulnar collateral

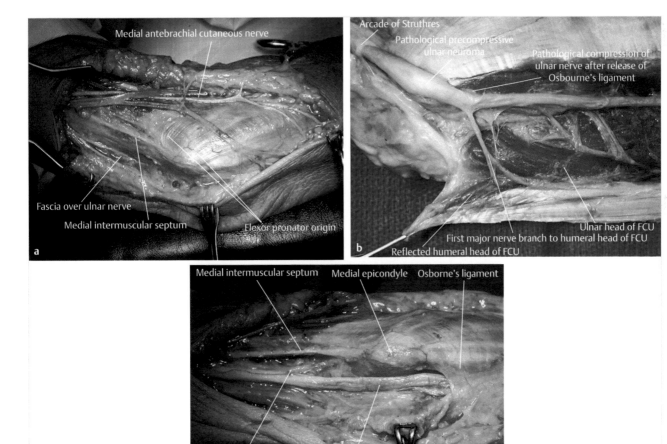

Fig. 14.4 (a) Intermuscular septum, fascial covering ulnar nerve, and flexor pronator origin. (b) Ligament of Osborne, medial epicondyle, inferior ulnar collateral vessels to ulnar nerve, ulnar nerve (fascia removed), and intermuscular septum. (c) Arcade of Struthers, pathologic precompressive ulnar neuroma, pathologic compression of ulnar nerve seen after release of ligament of Osborne, reflected humeral head of flexor carpi ulnaris, first major nerve branch to humeral head of head of flexor carpi ulnaris, and ulnar head of flexor carpi ulnaris.

ligament and to the medial coronoid is most easily obtained leaving the ulnar nerve in situ rather than by transposing it anteriorly, where the branches, as shown here, would be in the way of deeper dissection.

14.5.2 Medial Anatomy

Superficial Medial Anatomy

Five major muscle tendon groups (flexor pronator origin) arise from the medial aspect of the elbow (▶ Fig. 14.4a). While the individual tendons are separately identifiable at the distal forearm and wrist, their tendon fibers arise together and are not easily distinguishable or identifiable in the surgical setting because of their confluent origin.

The flexor pronator muscles consist of the flexor carpi radialis, pronator teres, palmaris longus, flexor digitorum superficialis, and flexor carpi ulnaris (▶ Figs. 14.4a and 14.5a). The flexor carpi radialis and the humeral head of the pronator teres arise from the medial epicondyle and distal intermuscular septum. The pronator teres also has a deep or ulnar head that takes origin off of the medial border of the coronoid process. Most anteriorly lies the flexor carpi radialis, followed by the pronator teres. Most tendinopathies of medial tennis elbow involve the origin of these two muscles. More posteriorly and superficially lies the palmaris longus origin and deep to that the flexor digitorum superficialis origin followed by the humeral origin of the flexor carpi ulnaris. The flexor digitorum superficialis muscles arise as an arch more posteriorly and deeply from the proximal anteromedial ulna, interosseous membrane, and deep forearm fascia and anteriorly from the radius (▶ Fig. 14.5b). The flexor

carpi ulnaris has a humeral head of origin off of the medial epicondyle and ulnar head off of the proximal ulna. The median nerve passes between the deep and superficial heads of the pronator teres and more distally deep to the arch formed by the heads of origin of the flexor digitorum superficialis. It is susceptible to compression at both sites (▶ Fig. 14.5c).

14.6 Deep Medial Anatomy

The ulnar collateral ligament consists of three structures[3–6] (▶ Fig. 14.6a,b). The posterior band of the ulnar collateral ligament contributes very little to elbow stability and only when the elbow is flexed. It can become shortened and thickened after elbow trauma and at times therefore limit elbow flexion. More anteriorly lies the prime medial stabilizer of the elbow, the anterior band of the ulnar collateral ligament (▶ Fig. 14.6a,b). This arises from the medial epicondyle deep to the flexor pronator origin and inserts on the supinator crest of proximal ulna. Between these two structures lies a relatively unimportant transverse band (▶ Fig. 14.6a,b). ▶ Fig. 14.6b shows all three portions of the ulnar collateral ligament complex, with the overlying flexor pronator origins having been dissected away. (Note the relatively taut anterior band of the ulnar collateral ligament and the lax posterior band of the ulnar collateral ligament of this specimen in elbow extension.) The anterior band of the ulnar collateral ligament consists of two bundles with various fibers within those bundles being taut throughout the arc of motion from extension to flexion. The flexor pronator origin, as seen elevated in ▶ Fig. 14.6a, more distally is separate from the supinator crest and anterior band of ulnar collateral ligament insertion, but

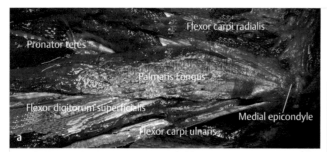

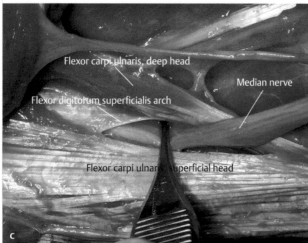

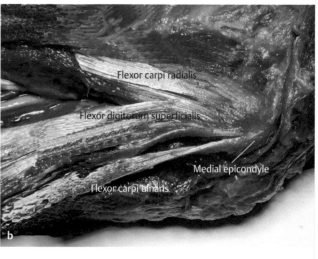

Fig. 14.5 (a and b) Pronator teres, flexor digitorum superficialis, palmaris longus, flexor carpi ulnaris, and flexor carpi radialis. Palmaris longus and pronator teres removed in (b). (c) Flexor digitorum superficialis arch, deep head of flexor carpi ulnaris, median nerve, and superficial head of flexor carpi ulnaris.

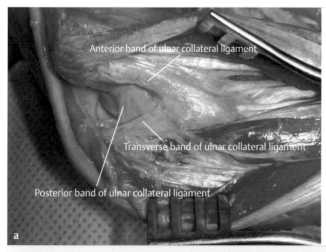

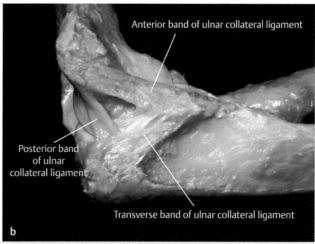

Fig. 14.6 **(a)** Posterior band of ulnar collateral ligament, anterior band of ulnar collateral ligament, and transverse band of ulnar collateral ligament. **(b)** Posterior band of ulnar collateral ligament, anterior band of ulnar collateral ligament, and transverse band of ulnar collateral ligament.

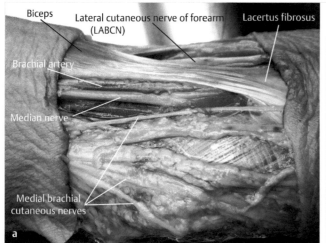

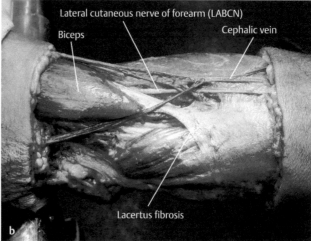

Fig. 14.7 **(a)** Median nerve, brachial artery, biceps, lateral cutaneous nerve of forearm (also called lateral antebrachial cutaneous nerve (LABCN)), lacertus fibrosis, and medial brachial cutaneous nerves. **(b)** Biceps, lateral cutaneous nerve of forearm, cephalic vein, and lacertus fibrosis.

its fibers more proximally take origin from the proximal part of the ligament as well as from the medial epicondyle. Complete dislocation of the elbow disrupts the anterior band of the ulnar collateral ligament but often spares the more elastic myotendinous origin of the flexor pronator. Because of the attachments between the proximal aspect of the ulnar collateral ligament and the overlying flexor pronator musculature myotendinous structures, the intact flexor pronator origin can support and facilitate healing of the underlying collateral ligament.

14.6.1 Anterior Anatomy

Branches of the medial brachial cutaneous nerve (Chapter 9) pass across the anteromedial elbow, with the most common relevant branches usually lying one fingerbreadth distal to the medial epicondyle (▶Fig. 14.7a). The short head of the biceps provides a consistent fascial extension into the fascia of the flexor pronator, termed the lacertus fibrosus (▶Fig. 14.7a,b),[7] one potential site for compression of the median nerve. (Note in this specimen the location of the

median nerve and, just lateral to the median nerve, the brachial artery.) Lateral to the biceps tendon, the lateral cutaneous nerve of the forearm emanates (▶Fig. 14.7b), a branch of the musculocutaneous nerve (Chapter 9). Irritation of this nerve represents the most common complication of biceps tendon rupture and repair.

Just anterior and medial to the flexor pronator origin lies the anteromedial elbow joint, including the coronoid process (▶Fig. 14.8a) and brachialis muscle. The brachialis muscle and its insertional footprint lie distal to the anterior tip of the coronoid process. In this figure, the flexor pronator origin has been removed to show the deeper anatomy. The brachialis muscle has two heads, with a larger superficial head arising off the proximal humerus proximal to a smaller deep head. The larger superficial head is thought to have a mechanical advantage over the deeper head due to its more proximal origin and more distal insertion. It provides the major strength of elbow flexion. The smaller oblique deep head has a more anterior insertion on the coronoid, which may facilitate initiation of elbow flexion from an extended position.[8]

14.7 Distal Biceps Tendon

Distal to the proximal neck of radius and beneath the supinator lies the bicipital tuberosity, which swings into close approximation to the ulna in pronation (▶ Fig. 14.2a). In almost half of cases (48%), the distal biceps tendon has two distinct parts, with the fibers from the short head of biceps inserting at the anteroinferior (distal) margin and the long head in the posterosuperior (proximal) portion.[9,10]

Anterior to the flexor pronator origin lies the brachialis muscle (▶ Fig. 14.8b), on top of which passes the median nerve, which then gives off muscular branches to the different components of the flexor pronator origin. The nerve has a deeper smaller branch (anterior interosseous nerve) and a larger continuation of the median nerve. Both pass between the humeral and ulnar heads of the pronator teres (▶ Fig. 14.5c). Note in ▶ Fig. 14.8b the tension of the deeper humeral origin of the flexor carpi ulnaris on the median nerve and the more distal flexor digitorum superficialis origin, which also can compress the median nerve.

If one splits away the anterior half of the flexor pronator origin, the medial elbow can be visualized with the anteromedial tip of the coronoid and the overlying brachialis muscle that inserts distal to the coronoid (▶ Fig. 14.10).

14.7.1 Lateral Anatomy

Proximal to the elbow, the brachioradialis and extensor carpi radialis longus take origin off of the humerus (▶ Fig. 14.9a–c). The extensor carpi radialis longus takes origin from the lateral supracondylar ridge of humerus, the lateral intermuscular septum, and, most distally, a few fibers from the anterior lateral epicondyle. It is distinguishable from the proximal extensor carpi radialis brevis by its muscular appearance, in distinction from the tendinous appearance of the extensor carpi radialis brevis. This allows both the brachioradialis muscle and the extensor carpi radialis longus to contribute to elbow flexion. Almost all of the remaining extensor supinator muscle tendon origins arise from the region of the lateral epicondyle. As in the flexor pronator group, tendons that are separately identifiable distally converge toward their point of origin, with tendon fibers difficult to distinguish from one another (▶ Fig. 14.9c). In almost all elbows, the brachioradialis and extensor carpi radialis longus have a muscular type of appearance at the level of the

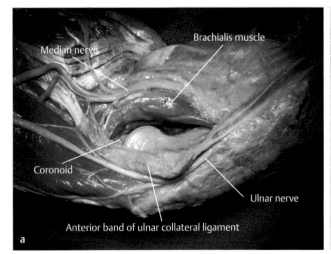
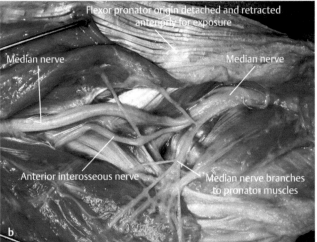
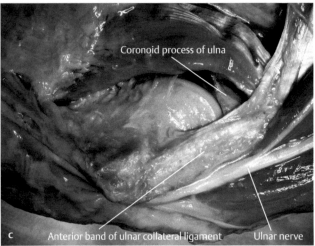

Fig. 14.8 (a) Coronoid process of ulna, anterior band of ulnar collateral ligament, ulnar nerve, median nerve, and brachialis muscle. (b) Continuation of median nerve, anterior interosseous nerve, median nerve, and median nerve branches to flexor pronator muscles. (c) Coronoid process of ulna, ulnar nerve, and anterior band of ulnar collateral ligament.

elbow. More posteriorly, the tendinous origins of the extensor carpi radialis brevis, extensor digitorum communis, and extensor digiti quinti appear tendinous in nature (▶Fig. 14.9a). Posterior to this and once again in muscular appearance lie the extensor carpi ulnaris and, then, the anconeus. Since the tendon origins take place at or near the axis of the elbow, the converging fibers of the extensors underlap and overlap to take origin at or near the same axis. The fibers of the extensor carpi radialis brevis lie deep to the extensor digitorum communis (▶Fig. 14.9c). In ▶Fig. 14.9c, the extensor digitorum communis and extensor digiti quinti have been excised to show the more proximal extensor carpi radialis brevis tendon origin and supinator muscle below. Tennis elbow lesions, therefore, while at times visible arthroscopically from the deep articular side, are not evident or visible immediately from the lateral side, since the primary involvement (extensor carpi radialis brevis) lies deep to the more superficial fibers of the extensor digitorum communis.

The posterolateral elbow is covered by the triangular anconeus muscle, which takes tendinous origin off of the posterolateral surface of the lateral epicondyle and inserts into the proximal lateral ulna (▶Fig. 14.10a,b). The anterior part of the muscle is tendinous for two-thirds of its length.[11,12] Three arterial pedicles supply the anconeus (▶Fig. 14.10b,c): the recurrent branch of the posterior interosseous artery, the medial collateral artery, and the posterior branch of the radial collateral artery. Based on the medial collateral artery, it can be used as a pedicle flap for adjacent coverage of the elbow.[11]

By taking down the tendinous and muscular origin of the anconeus off the humerus, the lateral elbow is easily visualized along with the lateral collateral annular complex[13] (▶Fig. 14.11a).

14.8 Lateral Collateral Ligament Complex

The lateral stabilizers of the elbow consist of a complex of tendon and ligamentous fibers that are intimately related and interwoven with each other. This includes the obliquely oriented supinator muscle, the transversely oriented annular ligament (▶Fig. 14.11a,b), the lateral collateral ligament, and the extensor myotendinous origins. If one looks closely at the

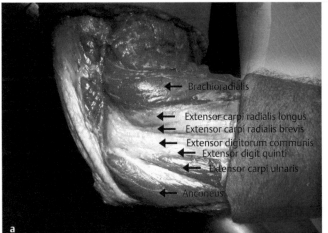
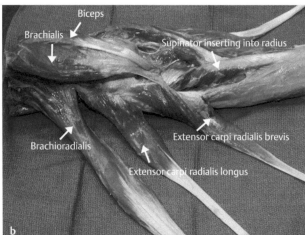
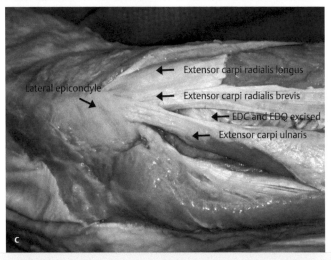

Fig. 14.9 Coronoid process of ulna, annular ligament, and bicipital tuberosity of radius. (a) Brachioradialis, extensor carpi radialis longus, extensor carpi radialis brevis, extensor digitorum communis, extensor digiti quinti, extensor carpi ulnaris, and anconeus. (b) Brachialis, biceps, brachioradialis, extensor carpi radialis longus, and extensor carpi radialis brevis. (c) Lateral epicondyle, extensor carpi radialis longus, extensor carpi radialis brevis, extensor digitorum communis and extensor digiti quinti excised, extensor carpi ulnaris, and anconeus.

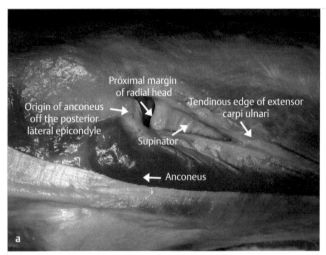
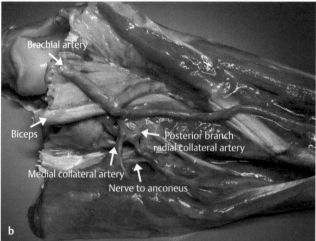
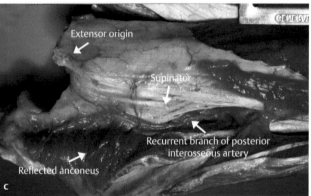

Fig. 14.10 (a) Origin of anconeus off of posterior lateral epicondyle, anconeus, proximal margin of radial head, supinator, and tendinous edge of extensor carpi ulnaris. (b) Brachial artery, medial collateral artery, nerve to anconeus, and posterior branch of radial collateral artery. (c) Extensor origin, supinator, reflected anconeus, and recurrent branch of posterior interosseous artery.

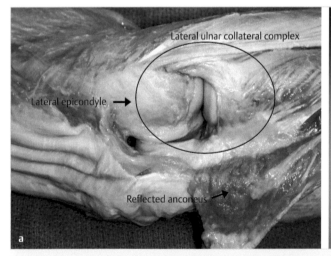
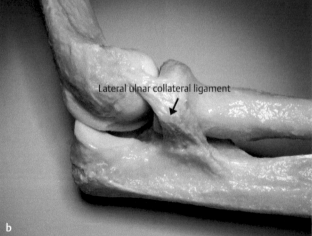

Fig. 14.11 (a) Lateral collateral ligament complex: interdigitation of fibers of lateral collateral ligament, annular ligament, supinator, and common extensor origin; lateral epicondyle; and reflected anconeus. (b) Lateral collateral ligament with annular ligament (other components of lateral collateral ligament complex have been excised).

annular ligament, which stabilizes the radial head, one will see transverse fibers of the annular ligament interwoven with oblique fibers of origin of the supinator as well as oblique fibers from the lateral collateral ligament that course through and along with the annular ligament attach to the proximal ulna. The annular ligament has a single or a unipennate attachment to the proximal ulna 55% of the time and a bipennate attachment with a band attaching slightly more distally along the supinator crest 45% of the time[13] (▶Fig. 14.11b). Anatomically speaking, therefore, it is more accurate to describe the stabilizing structures of the lateral elbow as a "lateral collateral ligament complex."[13] A "lateral ulnar collateral ligament" has been described,[14] which represents the distal coursing fibers of the lateral collateral annular complex. It is not responsible for lateral elbow stability. Instead, it is the proximal fibers of the lateral collateral deep to the extensor supinator origin that play a primarily role in stabilizing the posterolateral elbow. The lateral collateral ligament and annular ligament are the primary stabilizers that maintain stability and reduction of the radial head and capitellum when the elbow is loaded in supination.[13,15–18] The secondary stabilizers are the extensor muscles with their fascial bands and intermuscular septae.[13]

The extensor carpi ulnaris has a fascial bend on its undersurface that arises off of the inferior lateral epicondyle and inserts into the ulna around 5 cm distal to the radial head. Its oblique course provides additional rotational support to the lateral elbow.

14.8.1 Posterior Anatomy

The posterior elbow is covered by the triceps tendon that is the only extensor of the elbow (▶Fig. 14.12). This tripennate muscle has three origins: the long head arises from the scapular infraglenoid tubercle and joins distally with the lateral head that arises from the proximal posterior humerus. Together, they blend into one tendon; the medial head arises from the lower posterior humerus and often has a separate insertion deep or anterior to the combined tendon of the long and lateral heads of triceps.[19] In 47% of cases, the medial head inserts into the combined tendon fibers of the long and lateral heads, with its contribution representing the deeper tendon fibers. In 53% of cases, it has a distinguishable separate deep insertion.[20] Rupture or avulsion of the triceps tendon can involve the entire distal tendon, just the combined tendinous insertion of long and lateral heads, or just the deep medial head insertion. Rupture of the deep medial head will give weakness to elbow extension from a fully flexed position.

Deep to the triceps and superficial to the posterior capsule is a collection of fat, termed the posterior fat pad. It is usually not evident on a lateral X-ray of the elbow. When seen, it represents distention of the elbow capsule due to a joint effusion or, in the case of trauma, hemarthrosis.

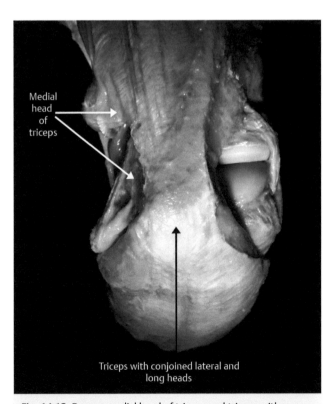

Medial head of triceps

Triceps with conjoined lateral and long heads

Fig. 14.12 Deeper medial head of triceps and triceps with conjoined lateral and long heads.

References

1. Weiss APC, Hastings H II. The anatomy of the proximal radioulnar joint. J Shoulder Elbow Surg 1992;1(4):193–199
2. Siqueira MG, Martins RS. The controversial arcade of Struthers. Surg Neurol 2005;64(Suppl 1):17–20
3. Miyake J, Moritomo H, Masatomi T, et al. In vivo and 3-dimensional functional anatomy of the anterior bundle of the medial collateral ligament of the elbow. J Shoulder Elbow Surg 2012; 21(8): 1006–1012
4. Farrow LD, Mahoney AJ, Stefancin JJ, Taljanovic MS, Sheppard JE, Schickendantz MS. Quantitative analysis of the medial ulnar collateral ligament ulnar footprint and its relationship to the ulnar sublime tubercle. Am J Sports Med 2011;39(9):1936–1941
5. Dugas JR, Ostrander RV, Cain EL, Kingsley D, Andrews JR. Anatomy of the anterior bundle of the ulnar collateral ligament. J Shoulder Elbow Surg 2007;16(5):657–660
6. Armstrong AD, Ferreira LM, Dunning CE, Johnson JA, King GJW. The medial collateral ligament of the elbow is not isometric: an in vitro biomechanical study. Am J Sports Med 2004;32(1):85–90
7. Athwal GS, Steinmann SP, Rispoli DM. The distal biceps tendon: footprint and relevant clinical anatomy. J Hand Surg Am 2007;32(8):1225–1229
8. Leonello DT, Galley IJ, Bain GI, Carter CD. Brachialis muscle anatomy. A study in cadavers. J Bone Joint Surg Am 2007;89(6): 1293–1297
9. Cho C-H, Song K-S, Choi I-J, et al. Insertional anatomy and clinical relevance of the distal biceps tendon. Knee Surg Sports Traumatol Arthrosc 2011;19(11):1930–1935
10. Mazzocca AD, Cohen M, Berkson E, et al. The anatomy of the bicipital tuberosity and distal biceps tendon. J Shoulder Elbow Surg 2007;16(1):122–127
11. Schmidt CC, Kohut GN, Greenberg JA, Kann SE, Idler RS, Kiefhaber TR. The anconeus muscle flap: its anatomy and clinical application. J Hand Surg Am 1999;24(2):359–369
12. Coriolano MGWS, Lins OG, Amorim MJAAL, Amorim AA Jr. Anatomy and functional architecture of the anconeus muscle. Int J Morphol 2009;27(4):1009–1012
13. Cohen MS, Hastings H II. Rotatory instability of the elbow. The anatomy and role of the lateral stabilizers. J Bone Joint Surg Am 1997;79(2):225–233
14. O'Driscoll SW, Horii E, Morrey BF, Carmichael SW. Anatomy of the ulnar part of the lateral collateral ligament of the elbow. Clin Anat 1992;5:296–303

15. Kim P-T, Isogai S, Murakami G, et al. The lateral collateral ligament complex and related muscles act as a dynamic stabilizer as well as a static supporting structure at the elbow joint: an anatomical and experimental study. Okajimas Folia Anat Jpn 2002;79(2–3):55–61

16. Seki A, Olsen BS, Jensen SL, Eygendaal D, Søjbjerg JO. Functional anatomy of the lateral collateral ligament complex of the elbow: configuration of Y and its role. J Shoulder Elbow Surg 2002;11(1):53–59

17. Olsen BS, Vaesel MT, Søjbjerg JO, Helmig P, Sneppen O. Lateral collateral ligament of the elbow joint: anatomy and kinematics. J Shoulder Elbow Surg 1996;5(2 Pt 1):103–112

18. Imatani J, Ogura T, Morito Y, Hashizume H, Inoue H. Anatomic and histologic studies of lateral collateral ligament complex of the elbow joint. J Shoulder Elbow Surg 1999;8(6):625–627

19. Madsen M, Marx RG, Millett PJ, Rodeo SA, Sperling JW, Warren RF. Surgical anatomy of the triceps brachii tendon: anatomical study and clinical correlation. Am J Sports Med 2006;34(11): 1839–1843

20. Athwal GS, McGill RJ, Rispoli DM. Isolated avulsion of the medial head of the triceps tendon: an anatomic study and arthroscopic repair in 2 cases. Arthroscopy 2009;25(9):983–988

15 The Forearm Fascia and Retinacula

Alexis Laungani, Alain Carlier, Nirusha Lachman, and Michel Saint-Cyr

15.1 General Considerations for Fascia

At the turn of the century, the term *fascia* was used in the general sense to describe all connective tissue sheaths and envelopes of the body.[1-3] The term *fascia* is derived from the Latin for a band or bandage.[4] Anatomically, it was considered a soft tissue layer that had to be dissected away in order to expose the underlying structures.[3,5,6] Since the actual function of this enveloping fascia was not clearly understood, early descriptions in anatomical studies were often confusing.[7] However, as proper understanding of anatomical structure, function, and relations continues to guide surgical technique, the last decade has seen a resurgence of interest in the fascial systems of the body.[3,8,9] While its exact role is still misunderstood, many authors agree that the fascia within the extremities plays an active role in achieving and providing tendon stability during movement.[7-12]

The description proposed by the Fascia Research Society defines the fascia as "*the soft tissue component of the connective tissue system that permeates the human body forming a whole body continuous three dimensional matrix of structural support.*"[11] Based on this definition, we explore the concept of the fascias of the human body as organized in "fascial systems" as a representation of the external equivalent of the bony skeleton.

Fascial systems provide critical and unique anatomical support for the underlying musculature and vary in density and thickness based on their location and distribution. The reader should be aware of the ambiguous terminology when referring to fascia. In the literature, the term *fascia* has been used to describe a wide range of connective tissue, which is confusing.[13] This might be explained by the diversity of disciplines involved in the field of "fascia research." We will refer in this chapter to the terminology proposed by Langevin and Huijing,[3] who avoid using the term *fascia*, preferring a description of the structure as mentioned in ▶ Table 15.1.

Different classifications of the fascias can be found in the textbooks, some of them referring to the relationship with the skin (superficial and deep) and some referring to the biomechanical and histological properties ("loose" or areolar and dense connective tissues).[3] Nevertheless, it is common to

Table 15.1 Recommended use of terms regarding fascial structures

Designation	Description of the tissue
Dense connective tissue	Connective tissue containing closely packed, irregularly arranged (that is, aligned in many directions) collagen fibers.
Non dense (areolar) connective tissue	Connective tissue containing sparse, irregularly arranged collagen fibers.
Superficial fascia	Enveloping layer directly beneath the skin, containing dense and areolar connective tissue and fat.
Deep fascia	Continuous sheet of mostly dense, irregularly arranged connective tissue that limits the changes in shape of underlying tissues. Deep fasciae may be continuous with epimysium and intermuscular septa and may also contain layers of areolar connective tissue.
Intermuscular septa	A thin layer of closely packed bundles of collagen fibers, possibly with several preferential directions predominating, arranged in various layers. The septa separate different, usually antagonistic, muscle groups (for example, flexors and extensors) but may not limit force transmission.
Interosseal membrane	Two bones in a limb segment can be connected by a thin collagen membrane with a structure similar to the intermuscular septa.
Periost	Surrounding each bone and attached to it is a bilayered collagen membrane similar in structure to the epimysium.
Neurovascular tract	The extramuscular collagen fiber reinforcement of blood and lymph vessels and nerves. This complex structure can be quite stiff. The diameter and, presumably, the stiffness of neurovascular tracts decrease along limbs from proximal to distal parts. Their stiffness is related to the angle or angles of the joints that they cross.
Epimysium	A multilayered, irregularly arranged collagen fiber sheet that envelopes muscles and that may contain layers of both dense and areolar connective tissue.
Intra- and Extramuscular aponeurosis	A multilayered structure with densely laid down bundles of collagen with major preferential directions. The epimysium also covers the aponeuroses but is not attached to them. Muscle fibers are attached to intramuscular aponeuroses by their myotendinous junctions.
Perimysium	A dense, multilayered, irregularly arranged collagen fiber sheet that envelopes muscle fascicles. Adjacent fascicles share a wall of the tube (like the cells of a honeycomb).
Endomysium	Fine network of irregularly arranged collagen fibers that form a tube enveloping and connecting each muscle fiber. Adjacent muscle fibers share a wall of the tube (like the cells o f a honeycomb).

Source: Used with permission from Langevin and Huijing.[3]

describe the fascial systems of the body as organized into three distinct layers:

- The *superficial fascia* is located under the skin, contains a variable amount of fat, and is sometimes also called "panniculus adiposus."[7] This fatty layer is thicker in upper extremities, on the posterior aspect of the body, and in females.[8]
- The *deep fascia* forms an intricate network separating muscles, nerves, and vessels and acts as a component-binding structure.[8] Some authors therefore describe a "muscular fascia" that enables the gliding of muscles against each other and also against other structures.[5,11]
- The *epimysium* is the outermost layer of the muscle and sometimes provides attachments to muscle insertions. The most common example is the "lacertus fibrosus" aponeurosis, which extends from the biceps tendon and then merges with the antebrachial fascia.[5,8]

Based on this description of the generic structure of the fascial system, it is easier to understand the specificities of each region of the body. The fascial system of the forearm is described in this chapter.

15.2 The Fascial System of the Forearm

Three compartments (the anterior compartment, the posterior compartment, and the mobile wad) are defined by nonextensible intermuscular and intramuscular fascial sheaths that compose the antebrachial fascia, or "fascia antebrachii"[5,8,11] (▶ Fig. 15.1). This nonextensibility of the fascia has a clinical relevance, since it is the reason acute compartment syndromes may occur.[14,15] The deep fascias are reinforced around the joints, in the form of *retinacula* that can be considered as pulleys preventing the bowstringing of the tendons.[8]

15.2.1 Retinacula System

As mentioned previously in the general considerations, there is a whole variety of terms used to describe all types of connective tissues. While some authors consider the terms *flexor*

retinaculum, carpal transverse ligament, volar, or *anterior annular ligament* as being interchangeable,[16,17] others consider the use of the term *flexor retinaculum* to be incorrect, believing that it does not correspond to any properly defined anatomical structure.[16] In this chapter, however, the term *flexor retinaculum* will be used to describe the fascial band on the volar aspect of the wrist.

The Flexor Retinaculum

The flexor retinaculum is composed of two layers, superficial or deep, depending on its relation to the ulnar nerve and vessels.[17,18]

The *superficial layer* is referred to as the "palmar carpal ligament" and comprises the thickened antebrachial fascia proximally and the palmar fascia distally.

The *deep layer* is composed of three distinct adjacent segments:

- The **proximal** segment that represents continuity with the deep fascia of the forearm.
- The **central** segment, properly called "transverse carpal ligament" (▶ Fig. 15.2), which has attachments to the pisiform and the hamate on the ulnar side and to the scaphoid and the trapezium on the radial side of the wrist. This central segment is often referred to as "flexor retinaculum" in anatomy textbooks.[16,19] It converts the anterior concavity of the carpus into the carpal tunnel, through which the tendons of the flexor digitorum profundus, flexor digitorum superficialis, and median nerve pass.[17]
- The distal segment is an aponeurosis lying between the thenar and hypothenar muscles.

The flexor retinaculum merges distally with the palmar aponeurosis (▶ Fig. 15.3). Its proximal boundaries are difficult to define due a proximal thinning as well as a merging with the antebrachial fascia. Moreover, the course of the palmaris longus tendon below the antebrachial fascia and then above its distal third may compromise the visualization of the transition between the antebrachial fascia and the flexor retinaculum.[20] Therefore, Won et al[21] described the flexor retinaculum as consisting of proximal and distal parts that actually

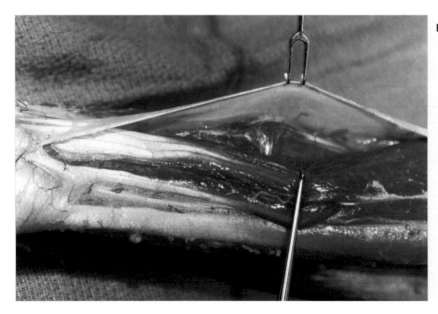

Fig. 15.1 Aspect of the fascia of the forearm.

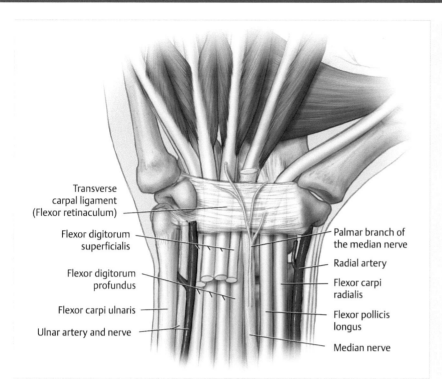

Fig. 15.2 The transverse carpal ligament.

Transverse carpal ligament (Flexor retinaculum)

Flexor digitorum superficialis

Flexor digitorum profundus

Flexor carpi ulnaris

Ulnar artery and nerve

Palmar branch of the median nerve

Radial artery

Flexor carpi radialis

Flexor pollicis longus

Median nerve

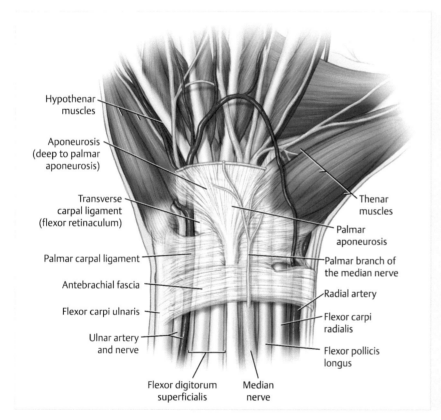

Fig. 15.3 Palmar view of the wrist, showing the relation between palmar aponeurosis and flexor retinaculum.

Hypothenar muscles

Aponeurosis (deep to palmar aponeurosis)

Transverse carpal ligament (flexor retinaculum)

Palmar carpal ligament

Antebrachial fascia

Flexor carpi ulnaris

Ulnar artery and nerve

Flexor digitorum superficialis

Median nerve

Thenar muscles

Palmar aponeurosis

Palmar branch of the median nerve

Radial artery

Flexor carpi radialis

Flexor pollicis longus

correspond to the central and distal segments described by Cobb et al.[17] The flexor retinaculum is vascularized through a deep network from the superficial palmar arch, a superficial network formed by branches of the ulnar artery.[22] The flexor retinaculum, by its position, defines a carpal tunnel underneath. This carpal tunnel leads the way to the flexor tendons of the fingers and to the median nerve.

There are two common sites of potential compression of the median nerve at the wrist: proximally at the proximal edge of the transverse carpal ligament and distally at the level of the hook of the hamate, where the canal is narrowest.[17]

The flexor retinaculum has a dorsal equivalent: the *extensor retinaculum* (▶ Fig. 15.4).

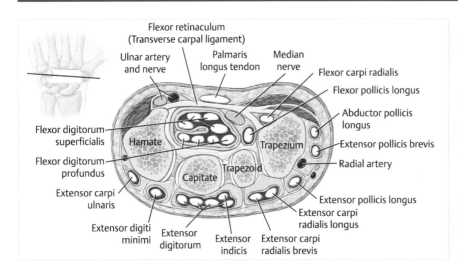

Fig. 15.4 Transverse view of the wrist at the level of the retinacula.

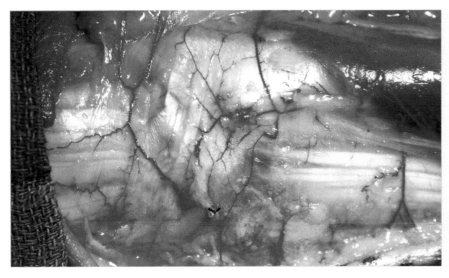

Fig. 15.5 The extensor retinaculum and its vascularization.

The Extensor Retinaculum

The extensor retinaculum is a reinforcement of the antebrachial fascia[1,12,23,24] (▶ Fig. 15.5) that prevents bowstringing of the extensor tendons across the wrist joint.[2,12,24] It is made of a superficial and a deep layer, referred to as supratendinous retinaculum and infratendinous retinaculum. The supratendinous part of the extensor retinaculum lies just under the skin and gets thicker from proximal to distal. Its fibers are transversely oriented in the proximal part, while they are more oblique distally.[23] On the ulnar side, the supratendinous part of the extensor retinaculum does not attach to the ulna itself but has three distinct insertions: the antebrachial fascia proximally, the triquetrum and pisiform bones centrally, and the fascia of abductor digiti minimi and fifth metacarpal bone distally. On the radial side, the supratendinous part of the extensor retinaculum also presents with three insertions: a proximal continuity with the antebrachial fascia, a central insertion on the radius, and distally a merge with the fascia overlying the thenar muscles.[23]

From the supratendinous part of the flexor retinaculum arise vertical sheaths which connect to the radial periosteum, creating six delimited compartments[1,2,12,23,25] well described in the literature with five osteofibrous and one fibrous canal (▶ Fig. 15.6):

- First compartment: extensor pollicis brevis and abductor pollicis longus.
- Second compartment: wider, the two radial wrist extensors.
- Third compartment: narrow, with only extensor pollicis longus.
- Fourth compartment: extensor indicis proprius and extensor digitorum.
- Fifth compartment: only fibrous, with extensor digiti minimi.
- Sixth compartment: the extensor carpi ulnaris is contained within a duplication of the infratendinous retinaculum, a fibrous tunnel that extends from the base of the ulnar styloid to the triquetrum.[23]

The deep infratendinous layer is a thinner and narrower part that extends from the radiocarpal joint to the carpometacarpal joint. It has a common insertion on the triquetrum and receives extensions from the three ulnar compartments delimited by the supratendinous layer.[2,23]

The extensor retinaculum possesses an identical histological three-layer architecture as the flexor pulleys of the digital sheaths.[24] It has therefore been proposed by Lister[26] to be used in reconstructive procedures of those pulleys.

15.2.2 Lacertus Fibrosus

The distal part of the muscular part of fascia brachii presents a reinforcement that is attached to the biceps aponeurosis and

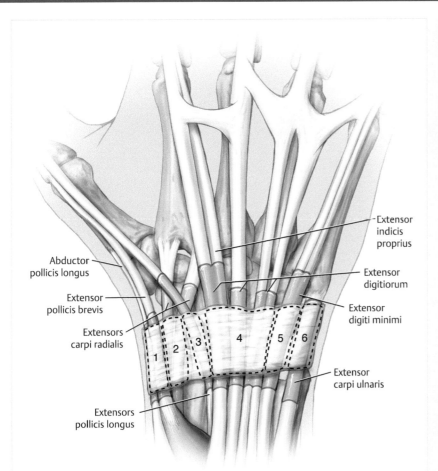

Fig. 15.6 The six compartments delimited by the extensor retinaculum.

Extensor indicis proprius

Extensor digitiorum

Extensor digiti minimi

Abductor pollicis longus

Extensor pollicis brevis

Extensors carpi radialis

Extensor carpi ulnaris

Extensors pollicis longus

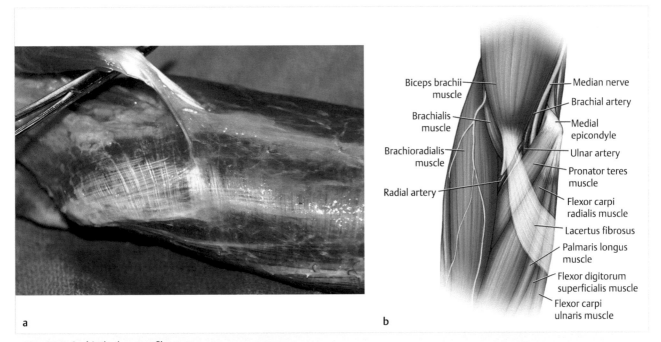

Biceps brachii muscle

Brachialis muscle

Brachioradialis muscle

Radial artery

Median nerve

Brachial artery

Medial epicondyle

Ulnar artery

Pronator teres muscle

Flexor carpi radialis muscle

Lacertus fibrosus

Palmaris longus muscle

Flexor digitorum superficialis muscle

Flexor carpi ulnaris muscle

a

b

Fig. 15.7 (a, b) The lacertus fibrosus.

tendon (▶Fig. 15.7a). This complex structure, called the "lacertus fibrosus," is a fascia that extends from the musculotendinous junction connecting the arm and forearm fascias[11,27] (▶Fig. 15.7b).

When the biceps muscle contracts, this structure tightens, thus maintaining the tendon against the bone and avoiding the bowstringing of the tendon. The powerful biceps tendon is then surrounded by two hard structures, the bone and the fascia, which leads to the best functional efficiency.[27,28]

The lacertus fibrosus appears as a crisscross ligament at the elbow crease, in which one can distinguish several directions in the collagen bundles[11]:

- The main group in oblique direction, downward and medially
- The second group parallel to the median line of the forearm

Due to its position in the elbow crease, the lacertus fibrosus may be the origin of neurovascular compressions. Indeed, compressions of the brachial artery by the lacertus fibrosus have been reported in two cases,[27,29] whereas the compression of median nerve is more common.[27,30,31] Interestingly, it was historically known as preventing injuries while performing bloodlettings on the cubital vein and was thus called "Grace a Dieu" (Thanks to God) aponeurosis.

15.3 Conclusion

The fascial system of the forearm should be seen as a component of the fascial system complex of the forearm with distinctive properties, playing a unique role in its achievement of movement. Besides the biomechanical and protective properties, the proprioceptive properties of the fascia, well known to physical therapists, are now also a topic of great interest to reconstructive surgeons. The resurgence of interest in and increasing research on fascial structure will promote better understanding of its anatomical properties and the range of motion of the forearm complex.

References

1. Testut L, ed. Traite d'anatomie humaine. Paris: Doin; 1889
2. Doyle JR, Botte MJ. Surgical Anatomy of the Hand and Upper Extremity. Philadelphia, PA: Lippincott Williams & Wilkins; 2003
3. Langevin HM, Huijing PA. Communicating about fascia: history, pitfalls, and recommendations. Int J Ther Massage Bodywork 2009;2(4):3–8
4. Hyrtl J, ed. Onomatologica: Geschichte und Kritik der Anatomischen Sprache der Gegenwart. Vienna: Wilhelm Braumller; 1880
5. van der Wal J. The architecture of the connective tissue in the musculoskeletal system—an often overlooked functional parameter as to proprioception in the locomotor apparatus. Int J Ther Massage Bodywork 2009;2(4):9–23
6. Stecco C, Duparc F. Fasciae anatomy. Surg Radiol Anat 2011;33(10):833–834
7. Singer E, ed. Fasciae of the Human Body and Their Relations to the Organs They Envelop. Baltimore, MD: The Williams & Wilkins Company; 1935
8. Stecco C, Macchi V, Porzionato A, Duparc F, De Caro R. The fascia: the forgotten structure. Ital J Anat Embryol 2011;116(3): 127–138
9. Benjamin M. The fascia of the limbs and back—a review. J Anat 2009;214(1):1–18
10. Findley T, Chaudhry H, Stecco A, Roman M. Fascia research—a narrative review. J Bodyw Mov Ther 2012;16(1):67–75
11. Stecco A, Macchi V, Stecco C, et al. Anatomical study of myofascial continuity in the anterior region of the upper limb. J Bodyw Mov Ther 2009;13(1):53–62
12. Palmer AK, Skahen JR, Werner FW, Glisson RR. The extensor retinaculum of the wrist: an anatomical and biomechanical study. J Hand Surg [Br] 1985;10(1):11–16
13. Schleip R, Jäger H, Klingler W. What is 'fascia'? A review of different nomenclatures. J Bodyw Mov Ther 2012;16(4):496–502
14. Duckworth AD, Mitchell SE, Molyneux SG, White TO, Court-Brown CM, McQueen MM. Acute compartment syndrome of the forearm. J Bone Joint Surg Am 2012;94(10):e63
15. Botte MJ, Gelberman RH. Acute compartment syndrome of the forearm. Hand Clin 1998;14(3):391–403
16. Stecco C, Macchi V, Lancerotto L, Tiengo C, Porzionato A, De Caro R. Comparison of transverse carpal ligament and flexor retinaculum terminology for the wrist. J Hand Surg Am 2010;35(5): 746–753
17. Cobb TK, Dalley BK, Posteraro RH, Lewis RC. Anatomy of the flexor retinaculum. J Hand Surg Am 1993;18(1):91–99
18. Denman EE. The volar carpal ligament. Hand 1979;11(1): 22–27
19. Nigro RO. Anatomy of the flexor retinaculum of the wrist and the flexor carpi radialis tunnel. Hand Clin 2001;17(1):61–64, vi
20. Stecco C, Lancerotto L, Porzionato A, et al. The palmaris longus muscle and its relations with the antebrachial fascia and the palmar aponeurosis. Clin Anat 2009;22(2):221–229
21. Won HS, Han SH, Oh CS, Chung IH, Suh JS, Lim SY. Morphological study of the proximal boundary of the flexor retinaculum and of its constituent parts. J Hand Surg Eur Vol 2012;37(1):35–41
22. Zbrodowski A, Gajisin S. The blood supply of the flexor retinaculum. J Hand Surg [Br] 1988;13(1):35–39
23. Taleisnik J, Gelberman RH, Miller BW, Szabo RM. The extensor retinaculum of the wrist. J Hand Surg Am 1984;9(4):495–501
24. Klein DM, Katzman BM, Mesa JA, Lipton JF, Caligiuri DA. Histology of the extensor retinaculum of the wrist and the ankle. J Hand Surg Am 1999;24(4):799–802
25. Hanz KR, Saint-Cyr M, Semmler MJ, Rohrich RJ. Extensor tendon injuries: acute management and secondary reconstruction. Plast Reconstr Surg 2008;121(3):109e–120e
26. Lister GD. Reconstruction of pulleys employing extensor retinaculum. J Hand Surg Am 1979;4(5):461–464
27. Bassett FH III, Spinner RJ, Schroeter TA. Brachial artery compression by the lacertus fibrosus. Clin Orthop Relat Res 1994;(307):110–116
28. Eames MH, Bain GI, Fogg QA, van Riet RP. Distal biceps tendon anatomy: a cadaveric study. J Bone Joint Surg Am 2007;89(5):1044–1049
29. Biemans RG. Brachial artery entrapment syndrome. Intermittent arterial compression as a result of muscular hypertrophy. J Cardiovasc Surg (Torino) 1977;18(4):367–371
30. Swiggett R, Ruby LK. Median nerve compression neuropathy by the lacertus fibrosus: report of three cases. J Hand Surg Am 1986;11(5):700–703
31. Laha RK, Lunsford D, Dujovny M. Lacertus fibrosus compression of the median nerve. Case report. J Neurosurg 1978;48(5): 838–841

16 Anatomy of the Forearm

Luke P. Robinson and Russell A. Shatford

16.1 Osteology

The exact knowledge of the bones is the foundation of all anatomy.
J. B. Winslow (1669-1760).

The forearm skeleton consists of the radius and ulna (▶Figs. 16.1, 16.2). The two bones articulate proximally at the proximal radial ulnar joint (PRUJ) and distally at the distal radial ulnar joint (DRUJ). Stability is conferred by the bony anatomy, the annular ligament, the interosseous membrane (IOM), the triangular fibrocartilage complex, and, to a certain extent, the elbow collateral ligaments, which reduce sheer forces across the IOM. The design allows constant tension between the radius and ulna, creating stability throughout pronosupination. Bony anatomic alignment of the PRUJ and DRUJ is critical for stability, as demonstrated by the contribution of anatomic reduction to the stability of Galeazzi and Monteggia fractures.

The radius is curved in both coronal and sagittal planes. The apex lateral (radial) bow is approximately 10° and the apex dorsal bow is approximately 4°, although the curve is accentuated by the larger metaphyses and narrowed central diaphysis. Malunion that alters the normal curvature of the radius can result in limitations of pronosupination or instability at the DRUJ.[1] Furthermore, rotational malunions can occur, leading to positional instability, where the DRUJ will be stable in some positions during pronosupination but lax in others. These rotational malunions can be difficult to appreciate given the limited radiographic landmarks.

The bicipital tuberosity anatomy facilitates supination of the forearm. There is a cam effect at the bicipital tuberosity, with an apex medial configuration. This cam provides greater mechanical advantage to the biceps insertion than a straight radius would provide. The apex medial curvature of the proximal radius is most evident in the anteroposterior view at approximately full supination. The biceps tendon inserts on the posteromedial aspect of the bicipital tuberosity. Although a single bicipital tuberosity is present the vast majority of the time (88%), the tuberosity can be absent (6%) or bifid (6%).[2] The bicipital tuberosity begins approximately one diameter of the radial head from the articular surface (articular head diameter average 22 mm and distance to start of bicipital tuberosity averages 23 mm), and it is approximately one radial head diameter long (21 mm).[3]

The center of the bicipital tuberosity is anterior to 180° from the radial styloid, sometimes even markedly so. Because of the posteromedial insertion, the biceps tendon insertion is not as anterior as the center of the bicipital tuberosity. In bifed tuberosities, the two ridges may not be of equal size, and the actual biceps attachment may be smaller. This apparent major anterior tuberosity could lead to confusion during biceps tendon reinsertion or to difficulty in judging rotation in radial shaft fractures, malunions, or nonunions. Comparison with the contralateral side, if uninjured, can be useful.

The difficulty in using the bicipital tuberosity for assessing rotational reduction is that the bicipital tuberosity is bulbous, making radiographic determination of the exact point of maximal prominence difficult to distinguish. Maximum prominence of the radial styloid also can be somewhat difficult to assess radiographically, but the dorsal and volar lip of the sigmoid notch usually provide clear radiographic landmarks. Further complicating intraoperative assessment of proximal and distal radial rotation, most image intensifiers used in the operating room have a field view too small to simultaneously visualize both the radial styloid and bicipital tuberosity in an adult forearm.

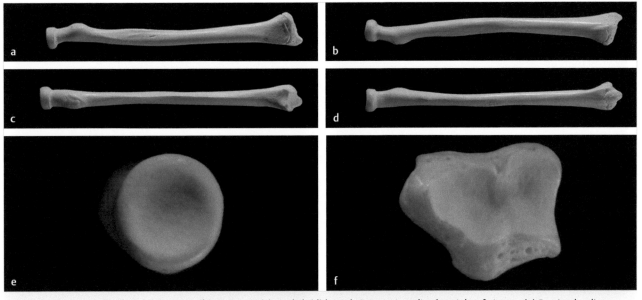

Fig. 16.1 Six views of radius. **(a)** Anterior, **(b)** posterior, **(c)** medial, **(d)** lateral. Orientation: distal to right of picture. **(e)** Proximal radius. Orientation: lateral to right of picture, anterior at top. **(f)** Distal radius, viewed distally. Orientation: lateral to left of picture, anterior at top. (All images have been oriented as right upper limbs, regardless of whether the limb was right or left. Left upper limb images have been reversed to make all specimens appears as right upper limbs. Furthermore, an attempt has been made to rotate all photographs such that the orientation remains consistent. Backgrounds have been simplified, or replaced, in some images to reduce distractions).

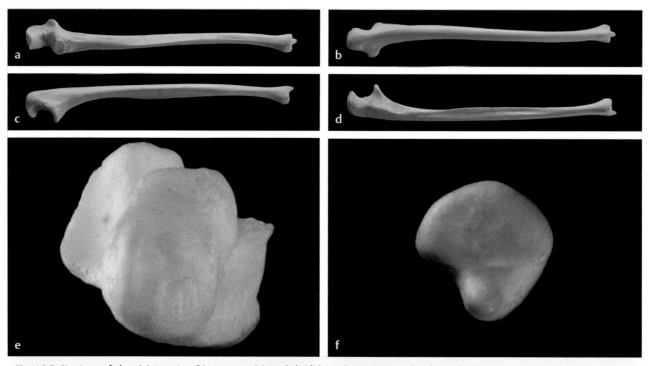

Fig. 16.2 Six views of ulna. (**a**) Anterior, (**b**) posterior, (**c**) medial, (**d**) lateral. Orientation: distal to right of picture. (**e**) Proximal ulna. Orientation: lateral to right of picture, anterior at top. (**f**) Distal ulna, viewed distally. Orientation: lateral to left of picture, anterior at top.

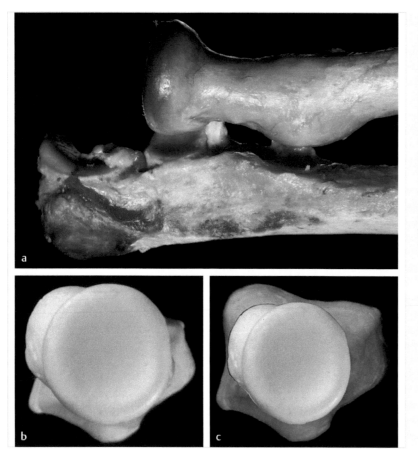

Fig. 16.3 (**a**) Lateral view of elbow showing the proximal radial ulnar joint—slightly splayed for visualization. The bicipital tuberosity, the insertion of the biceps tendon, can be seen. Orientation: distal at right of picture, anterior at top. (**b**) Photograph showing relationship of bicipital tuberosity and radial styloid. The radial head is large in comparison with the distal radius secondary to parallax, and obscures some of the distal radius. Orientation: viewed from proximal. Distal radial styloid laterally at right of picture, volar at top of picture. (**c**) Radial head and bicipital tuberosity digitally superimposed on distal radius composite image showing actual relative size and relationship of bicipital tuberosity and radial styloid. Orientation: viewed from proximal, radial styloid laterally at right of picture, volar at top of picture.

The radial head articulates with the ulna at the PRUJ and with the humerus at the radiocapitellar joint (▶ Fig. 16.3). The full circumference of the radial head does not engage the ulna at the PRUJ. The extra-articular portion of the radial head correlates with a 110° arc between the radial styloid and Lister's tubercle. This *safe zone* for hardware placement is covered with

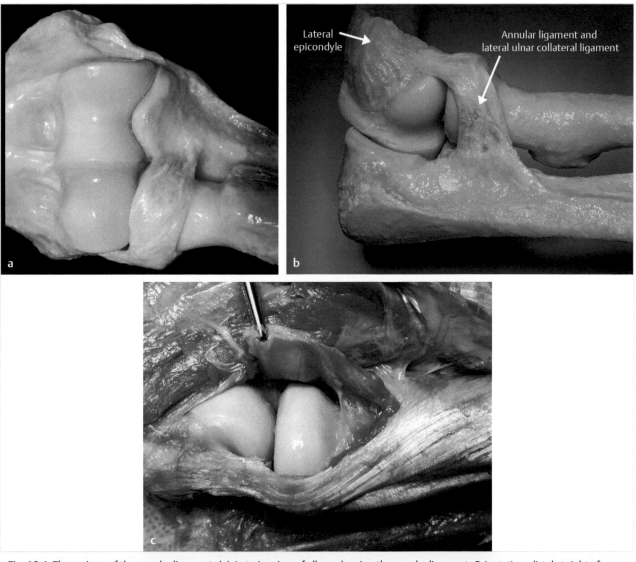

Fig. 16.4 Three views of the annular ligament. (**a**) Anterior view of elbow showing the annular ligament. Orientation: distal at right of picture, medial at top. (**b**) Lateral view of elbow showing the annular ligament. Orientation: distal at right of picture, anterior forearm at top. (**c**) Lateral view of elbow with the annular ligament opened showing deep surface. Orientation: distal at right of picture, anterior forearm at top.

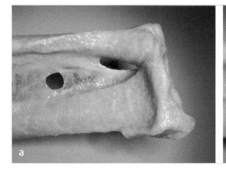 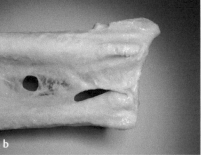

Fig. 16.5 View of distal forearm and interosseous membrane. (**a**) View of volar distal radius and medial ulna. Orientation: distal at right of picture, ulnar at top. (**b**) View of dorsal distal radius and lateral ulna. Orientation: distal at right of picture, radial at top.

thinner cartilage that "articulates" with the annular ligament. Prominent hardware, even in the *safe zone*, can hinder pronosupination (▶Fig. 16.4).[4,5]

The ulna has a sigmoid curve in the coronal plane starting at the proximal ulna with an apex lateral (radial) bow of varying severity (11–23°) and terminating with an apex medial bow distally. In the sagittal plane, there is an apex posterior bow that averages 4.5° (1–14°) at the proximal ulna.[6] Unlike the more volar radial styloid, the ulnar styloid process is a posterior structure (Figs. 16.5, 16.6).

Pronosupination is approximately 160° following a nearly circular arc. The axis of rotation of the forearm approximates a

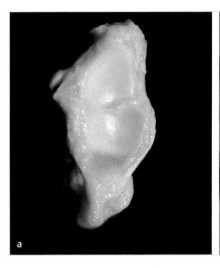
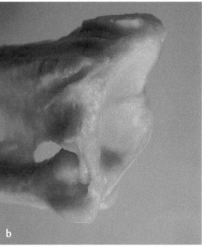

Fig. 16.6 Distal forearm. (**a**) End-on view of distal forearm showing scaphoid facet (*top*), lunate facet (*middle*), and triangular fibrocartilage complex (*bottom*). Lister's tubercle, and path of extensor pollicis longus can be seen on the dorsal radius (*left*). Orientation: dorsal at left of picture, radial at top. (**b**) Dorsal distal view of distal radius, again showing scaphoid facet (*top*), lunate facet (*middle*), and triangular fibrocartilage complex (*bottom*). Lister's tubercle, and oblique path of extensor pollicis longus (EPL) can be seen, along with grooves for extensor carpi radialis longus (ECRL) and extensor carpi radialis brevis (ERCB) in the floor of the second compartment radial to Lister's tubercle. The floor of the fourth compartment lies ulnar to Lister's tubercle. Orientation: distal at right of picture, radial at top.

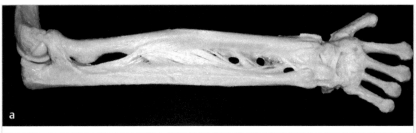
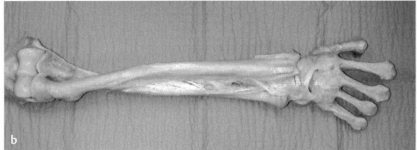
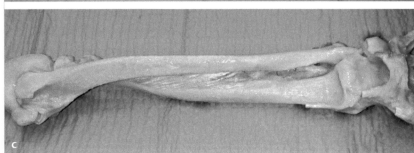

Fig. 16.7 The interosseous membrane, distal at right of picture. (**a**) Forearm in neutral rotation, viewed from lateral with respect to the humerus/ulna, with radial at top. Orientation: lateral view of the ulna and posterior view of the radius. (**b**) Forearm in pronation viewed from anterior with respect to the humerus/ulna. Orientation: anterior view of the ulna and posterior view of the radius. (**c**) Forearm in pronation viewed from posterior with respect to the humerus/ulna. Orientation: posterior view of the ulna with anterior view of the radius.

line from the center of the radial head to the fovea of the ulnar head. At the DRUJ, differences between the radius of curvature of the ulnar head and the sigmoid notch lead to a less constrained joint than the PRUJ. The ulnar head has a radius of approximately 1 cm, and the sigmoid notch of the radius has a radius of approximately 1.5 cm. This incongruity between the ulnar head and the sigmoid notch allows the radius to translate relative to the ulna.

The IOM helps maintain the relationship between the radius and the ulna. There is a knifelike bony prominence along the ulnar shaft, from which the main ligamentous band of the IOM arises. This crista is along the axis of forearm rotation, allowing the three distal bundles of the IOM (central band, accessory band, and distal oblique bundle) to remain nearly isometric during pronosupination, an anatomic feature that has consequences for IOM reconstruction (▶Fig. 16.7).[7] The proximal portion of the IOM is not isometric, furling and unfurling during pronosupination. Trauma to the membranous portion may result in scarring and potential limitation of pronosupination.[8]

16.2 Myology

16.2.1 Volar

Two muscles insert on the proximal volar forearm. The brachialis inserts just distal to the coronoid process of the ulna. The proximal margin of the insertion is about 11 mm from the coronoid tip and extends 2 cm onto the proximal ulna.[9] The biceps inserts on the posteromedial aspect of the bicipital tuberosity of the radius, with the biceps insertion approximately 7 mm wide. The biceps muscle rotates 90° to insert, with the tendinous contribution from the long head inserting distal and the short head contribution inserting proximal on the bicipital tuberosity. The short head also gives rise to the lacertus fibrosus.[3]

The remainder of the volar forearm can be conceptualized in layers, either three or four, depending on how the structures are categorized. Any conceptualization of a three-dimensional structure in two dimensions is an oversimplification. For instance, the pronator teres is both a superficial muscle (with a partial superficial origin) and a deep muscle with an insertion onto the radial shaft. However, considering the muscles in layers can aid conceptualization.

When dividing the volar forearm into four layers, the superficial layer can be considered as (from lateral to medial) pronator teres, flexor carpi radialis (FCR), palmaris longus (when present), and flexor carpi ulnaris (FCU). These four muscles arise from the common flexor origin at the medial epicondyle. The pronator teres and the FCU also have deep heads that originate from the proximal ulna. The pronator teres inserts on the midshaft radius, while the other muscles insert distal to the forearm (▶ Fig. 16.8).

The pronator teres is bounded by the antecubital fossa laterally (with the pronator teres forming the medial border of the antecubital fossa), the FCR medially, and the flexor digitorum superficialis (FDS) deep (▶ Fig. 16.9). The median nerve travels between the superficial and deep heads of the pronator teres, and the ulnar artery passes deep to pronator teres. The FCR, in the proximal forearm, lies medial to the pronator teres, lateral to the palmaris longus or FCU, and superficial to the FDS. In the distal forearm, the FCR is bounded radially by the radial artery and ulnarly by the palmaris longus, with the median nerve lying deep between the FCR and palmaris longus.

The palmaris longus, when present, lies in the proximal forearm between the FCR and FCU. In the proximal forearm, the palmaris longus lies superficial to the FDS. Distally, the palmaris longus lies superficial to the carpal tunnel contents, lying just superomedial to the median nerve, and superficial to the FDS (▶ Fig. 16.10, ▶ Fig. 16.11, and ▶ Fig. 16.12). In the absence of

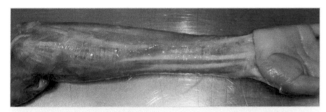

Fig. 16.8 Volar forearm with skin removed but fascia intact. Distally, at the wrist, visible through the fascia, are the tendons of the (from *top* to *bottom*) flexor carpi ulnaris (FCU), palmaris longus, flexor carpi radialis (FCR), and abductor pollicis longus (APL). At the junction of middle and distal forearm, a segment of tendon of the flexor digitorum superficialis (FDS) can be seen deep to the fascia between the FCU and palmaris longus. Orientation: distal at right of picture, ulnar at top.

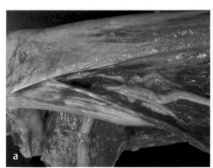

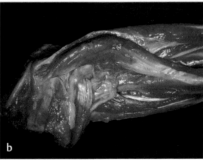

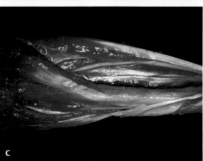

Fig. 16.9 Pronator teres. (**a**) Medial view of proximal forearm showing proximal pronator teres and median nerve. The triangular tendon is the origin of the pronator teres. The vermiform structure passing beneath the tendon is the median nerve, passing through the substance of the pronator teres. Orientation: distal at right of picture, posterior forearm at top. (**b**) Medial view of proximal forearm showing pronator teres origin and insertion. Orientation: distal at right of picture, posterior medial forearm at top. (**c**) Anterior view of forearm, showing insertion of pronator teres on midshaft radius. Orientation: distal at right of picture, medial at top.

the palmaris longus, the median nerve has been misidentified as the palmaris longus and harvested as a tendon graft.[10] Not only is palmaris longus variably present, but the position of the muscle belly can vary as well.[11]

The FCU is the most ulnar muscle of the superficial layer and is bounded laterally by either the palmaris longus or the FCR. The FCU lies superficial and medial to the FDS and flexor digitorum profundus (FDP). The FCU arises from both the common flexor origin and the proximal ulna. At the elbow, the ulnar nerve passes deep to the FCU, between the two heads. In the proximal forearm, the ulnar nerve is joined by the ulnar artery. This neurovascular bundle continues deep to the FCU with the ulnar nerve lying ulnar and dorsal to the artery at the wrist. Unlike most other tendons at the wrist, the FCU is an extrasynovial tendon; while spared from stenosing tenosynovitis, the FCU is susceptible to calcific tendonitis and tendinosis commonly seen in other extrasynovial tendons (▶Fig. 16.13).[12]

The second layer of the volar forearm is the FDS. The FDS originates from a broad, obliquely oriented fibrous arcade that includes the common flexor origin, the coronoid process, and the proximal radius. Superficial to the FDS lie the four muscles of the superficial layer. The FDP and flexor pollicis longus (FPL) lie deep to the FDS. The median nerve is found between the second (FDS) and the third layers (FDP and FPL) of the volar forearm.[13]

The third layer of the volar forearm can be considered as the FDP and the FPL. The FDP has a broad origin. The FDP originates just distal to the brachialis insertion, on both the IOM and the anterior ulna, including the medial coronoid. The FDP origin extends distally to the pronator quadratus crest on the distal ulna. The FPL has a broad origin, including the medial border of the radius, along the anterior oblique line just distal to the radial head. The FPL origin extends distally along the smooth anterior surface of the radius to just proximal to the pronator quadratus.[13] An accessory origin of the FPL, Gantzer's muscle, can also be found arising from the medial epicondyle (and sometimes coronoid) in approximately half of limbs. Gantzer's muscle remains innervated by

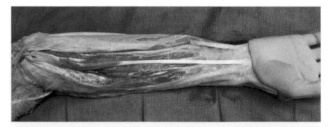

Fig. 16.11 Volar forearm with palmaris dissected. Orientation: distal at right of picture, posterior elbow and ulnar wrist at top.

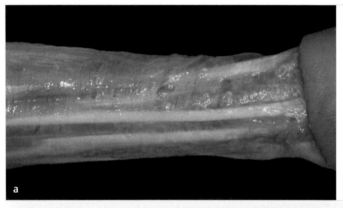
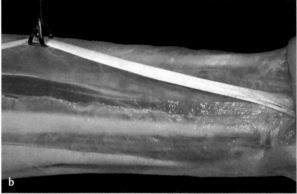

Fig. 16.10 Anterior forearm showing palmaris longus. (a) Palmaris longus within fascia. (b) With fascia released and the palmaris longus retracted ulnarly. Through the fascia, the flexor carpi ulnaris tendon can be seen (top). Deep to the path of the palmaris longus lies the FDS muscle. Radially, next to the palmaris longus path lie the tendon of the flexor carpi radialis, the radial artery, brachioradialis, and extensor carpi radialis longus proximally and the abductor pollicis longus and extensor pollicis brevis distally (bottom). Orientation: distal at right of picture, ulnar at top.

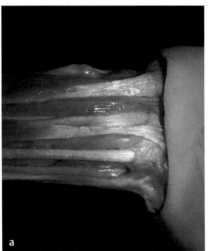
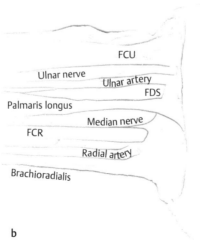

Fig. 16.12 (a, b) Volar wrist. Orientation: distal at right of picture, ulnar at top.

FCU
Ulnar nerve
Ulnar artery
FDS
Palmaris longus
Median nerve
FCR
Radial artery
Brachioradialis

the anterior interosseous nerve (AIN) and always lies posterior to the median nerve and AIN.[14]

The fourth layer is the pronator quadratus. The pronator quadratus arises from the pronator ridge of the ulna and inserts on the radius. Superficially, the pronator quadratus is bounded by the FDP and FPL (▶ Fig. 16.14). The third and fourth layers are sometimes descriptively grouped together, but this conceptualization limits appreciation of Parona's space. Between the pronator quadratus and the overlying tendons of the FDP lies this potential space that can allow communication of infected spaces and bursae within the hand, as well as become an abscess.

The common flexor tendon represents the origin of several volar flexors. The common flexor origin can be divided into an anterior and a posterior tendon. The anterior common tendon consists of a robust convergence of the pronator teres, FCR, palmaris longus, and FDS tendons and runs parallel to the anterior bundle of the medial ulnar collateral ligament. The intermuscular fascia between the FDS and FCU also coalesces to form a thinner posterior common tendon located at the inferior end of the medial epicondyle and medial joint capsule.[15]

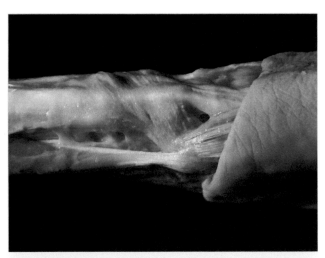

Fig. 16.13 Ulnar view of wrist showing flexor carpi ulnaris (FCU) insertion. At bottom of picture, the FCU can be seen inserting on the pisiform. Orientation: distal at right of picture, dorsal at top.

16.2.2 Dorsal

Just as the biceps and brachialis insert just distal to the elbow on the volar forearm, the triceps brachii terminates on the olecranon on the proximal dorsal forearm, providing elbow extension (▶ Fig. 16.15). While the vast majority of the triceps muscle is proximal to the forearm, the triceps can have prominent slips at the medial head insertion, which have been suggested as a potential source of ulnar nerve irritation.[16,17]

Excluding the triceps insertion, the dorsal forearm extensor muscles can be conceptualized as superficial and deep groups. The superficial layer can be further subdivided into the three muscles in the lateral group and the three muscles in the superficial long extensor group.

The lateral group includes the brachioradialis, extensor carpi radialis longus (ECRL), and the extensor carpi radialis brevis (ECRB). The brachioradialis arises from the lateral epicondylar ridge of the humerus, starting at approximately the junction of the middle and distal thirds of the humerus, and inserts on the radial styloid. The ECRL arises from the lateral epicondylar ridge of the humerus more distally and inserts on the dorsal base of the second metacarpal. The ECRB arises from the common extensor origin at the lateral epicondyle and inserts on the dorsal base of the third metacarpal.

The brachioradialis forms the lateral border of the antecubital fossa. The brachioradialis is bounded posteriorly by the ECRL. In the proximal forearm, the brachioradialis overlies the supinator. In the proximal and middle forearm, the pronator teres passes deep to the brachioradialis. In the mid-forearm, the brachioradialis overlies the insertion of the pronator teres. In the distal forearm, the brachioradialis passes radial to the FPL and pronator quadratus to insert on the radial styloid. The abductor pollicis longus (APL) and extensor pollicis brevis (EPB) pass obliquely and superficial to the brachioradialis (and also pass superficial to ECRL and ECRB). The radial artery and dorsal sensory branch of the radial nerve (DSBRN) course just deep to the brachioradialis proximally. The DSBRN pierces the antebrachial fascia to become superficial between the brachioradialis and ECRL, at approximately the junction of middle and distal thirds of the forearm. However, even in the mid-forearm, the DSBRN lies

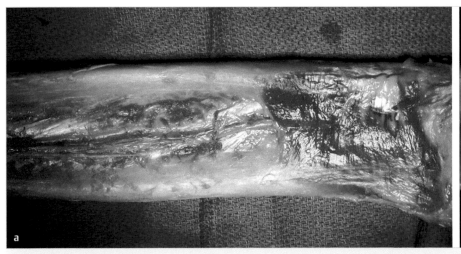
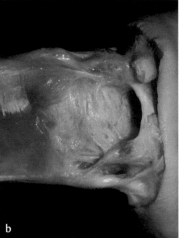

Fig. 16.14 (a, b) Volar view of forearm/wrist showing pronator quadratus. All overlying muscles have been removed, exposing the pronator quadratus, interosseous membrane, and anterior interosseous artery (injected). Orientation: distal at right of pictures, ulnar at top.

barely deep to the brachioradialis. The radial artery continues distally with the brachioradialis, becoming medial to the brachioradialis tendon in the distal forearm (▶Fig. 16.16). The ECRL originates between the brachioradialis and the ECRB on the distal humerus. The ECRB arises from the common extensor tendon at the lateral epicondyle. Both muscles continue distally just superficial to the radius. In the distal forearm, the APL and EPB cross superficial to the ECRL and ECRB. The ECRL and ECRB then continue through the second dorsal compartment of the wrist to insert on the bases of the second and third metacarpals, respectively (▶Fig. 16.17, ▶Fig. 16.18, ▶Fig. 16.19, and ▶Fig. 16.20).

The remaining muscles in the superficial group, the superficial long extensors, arise from the lateral epicondyle and include the extensor digitorum communis (EDC), the extensor digit minimi (EDM), also called the extensor digiti quinti, and the extensor carpi ulnaris (ECU). The EDC and EDM, along with the ECRB, arise from a common extensor origin on the superior aspect of the lateral epicondyle. The ECU arises from the posteroinferior lateral epicondyle.[18]

The EDC lies medial to the ECRB and lateral to the EDM. In the proximal forearm, the EDC lies superficial to the supinator. More distally, the EDC passes superficial to the APL, the extensor pollicis longus (EPL), the EPB, and the extensor indicis proprius (EIP), also known as the extensor indices. The EDM lies between the EDC and the ECU. Similar to the EDC, the EDM passes superficial to the supinator, then to the APL, the EPL, and the EIP. The ECU lies medial to the EDM and overlies the supinator, APL, EPL, and EIP. The origin of the EPB is not as ulnar as the other muscles of the deep layer (▶Fig. 16.21, ▶Fig. 16.22, ▶Fig. 16.23, ▶Fig. 16.24, ▶Fig. 16.25, ▶Fig. 16.26, and ▶Fig. 16.27).

The deep layer, from proximal to distal, lying directly on bone and/or IOM, includes the anconeus (although the anconeus is

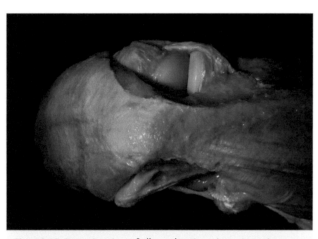

Fig. 16.15 Posterior view of elbow showing triceps insertion. Orientation: distal at right of picture, lateral at top.

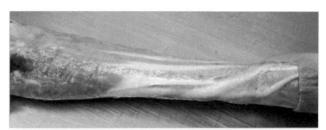

Fig. 16.17 Radial view of forearm with skin removed but fascia intact, showing brachioradialis (*center*). Anterior to the brachioradialis are the flexor carpi radialis and palmaris longus tendons (*top*). Posterior to the brachioradialis are the radial wrist extensors, with the extensor carpi radialis longus (ECRL) seen through the fascia. In the distal forearm, the abductor pollicis longus and extensor pollicis brevis can be seen crossing the extensor carpi radialis brevis (ECRB), ECRL and the brachioradialis. At the wrist, the extensor pollicis longus (EPL) can be seen crossing the radial wrist extensors to continue distally to the thumb. Orientation: distal at right of picture, anterior at top.

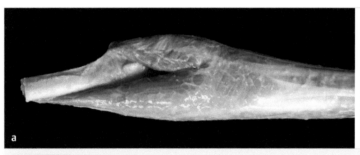

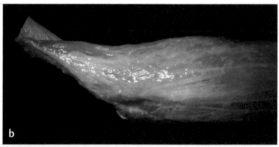

Fig. 16.16 (a) Antecubital fossa with proximal soft tissues removed, leaving the muscles bounding the antecubital fossa, the pronator teres (*top*), and brachioradialis (*bottom*). Distally, the tendons of the flexor carpi radialis (*top*), brachioradialis (*middle*), and extensor carpi radialis brevis longus (*bottom*) can be seen along with the muscle belly of the ECRB. Orientation: distal at right of picture, medial at top. (b) Lateral elbow, with brachial muscles excised, showing origin from the distal humerus of the brachioradialis (most proximally) extensor carpi radialis longus, and muscles arising from the common extensor origin at the lateral epicondyle. Orientation: distal at right of picture, anterior at top.

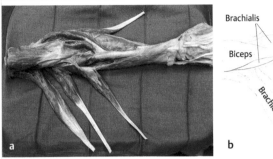
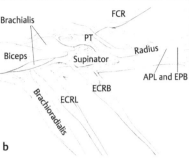

Fig. 16.18 (a, b) Anterior view of forearm showing brachioradialis, extensor carpi radialis longus (ECRL), and extensor carpi radialis brevis (ECRB) muscle origin, biceps and brachialis insertions, and supinator and pronator teres, with its insertion on the radius. The insertions of the brachioradialis, ECRL, ECRB, and flexor carpi radialis have been divided. The median nerve has been removed, leaving its empty path through the substance of the pronator teres. Orientation: distal at right of picture, medial elbow at top.

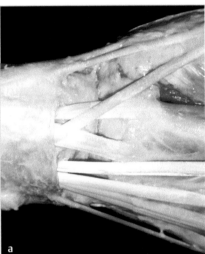
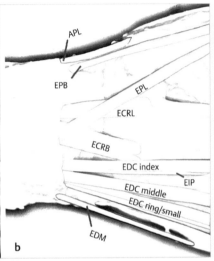

Fig. 16.19 (a, b) Dorsal view of wrist showing insertion of extensor carpi radialis longus and extensor carpi radialis brevis into the bases of the second and third metacarpals, respectively. Extensor indicis proprius (EIP) can be seen just on the ulnar edge and deep to extensor digitorum communis (EDC) to index. Orientation: distal at right of picture, radial at top.

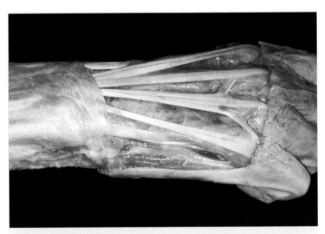

Fig. 16.20 Dorsal ulnar view of wrist showing insertion of extensor carpi ulnaris (ECU) on base of fifth metacarpal. From *bottom* to *top*, the tendons are the ECU, extensor digit minimi, extensor digitorum communis (EDC) to ring/small, EDC to middle, extensor indicis proprius, and EDC to index, with a segment of the extensor carpi radialis brevis visible at the radial side of the wrist (*top*). Orientation: distal at right of picture, radial at top.

also superficial since it has no overlying muscles), the supinator, the APL, the EPL, the EPB, and the EIP. The APL, EPL, EPB, and EIP all have oblique origins, from the ulna, IOM, and medial radius, with the muscles angling from ulnar proximal to radial distal. The APL is larger than the other deep extensor muscles that insert distal to the wrist. The EIP is classically considered the most distal muscle to be innervated or reinnervated and is used to monitor posterior interosseous nerve recovery, although the EPB is innervated at approximately the same level as the EIP. Patients who have undergone index extensor tendon transfer to replace EPL function after tendon rupture may retain some independence of both the reconstructed thumb and donor index finger, suggesting that independent index extension may not always require a functional EIP.[20]

The first dorsal compartment contains the tendons of the APL (which often has multiple slips—up to 14 have been reported) and the EPB (which is dorsal and often much smaller, although variable in size). The APL and EPB usually lie together within the first compartment. However, the EPB may lie within its own subcompartment with a septum between the two tendons, a variant found in 20% of limbs in one cadaver study (▶ Fig. 16.28 and ▶ Fig. 16.29).[21]

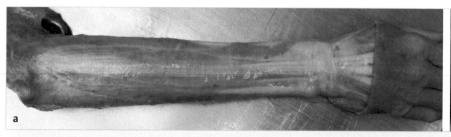
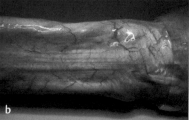

Fig. 16.21 Dorsal forearm with the skin removed overlying the extensor digitorum communis (EDC) and extensor digit minimi (EDM). From *bottom* to *top*, in the forearm, the extensor carpi ulnaris, EDM (seen best at the wrist), extensor digitorum communis, and extensor pollicis brevis/abductor pollicis longus can be seen through the fascia. (**a**) Dorsal forearm. Orientation: distal at right of picture, radial at top. (**b**) Dorsal distal forearm. Orientation: distal at right of picture, radial at top.

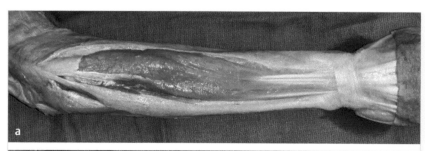
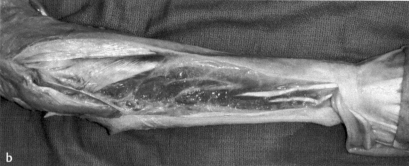

Fig. 16.22 (**a**) Dorsal forearm with the fascia removed, showing the extensor digitorum communis and extensor digit minimi (EDM). Orientation: distal at right of picture, radial at top. (**b**) Dorsal forearm with the fascia removed and the ED and EDM reflected distally, exposing the deep muscle layer. At the wrist, the longer tendon is the extensor pollicis longus (*top*) and the shorter tendon is the extensor indicis proprius (*bottom*). Orientation: distal at right of picture, radial at top.

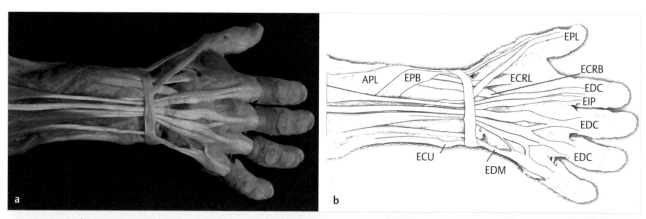

Fig. 16.23 (**a, b**) Extensor pollicis longus can be seen in the distal forearm, just radial to the extensor digitorum communis (EDC) index. A well-defined separate EDC to small is not always present, especially in the presence of a sturdy junctura from the ring.[15] Orientation: distal at right of picture, radial at top.

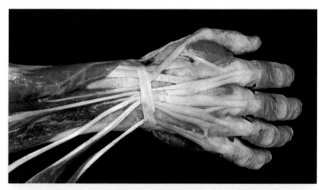

Fig. 16.24 Proximal extensor digitorum communis (EDC) index retracted ulnarly, exposing the proximal extensor pollicis longus. EDC middle retracted ulnarly, exposing the extensor indices proprius (EIP). Abductor pollicis longus (APL) and extensor pollicis brevis (EPB) cross obliquely superficial to the extensor carpi radialis brevis (ECRB), the extensor carpi radialis longus (ECRL) and the brachioradialis (BR). Orientation: distal at right of picture, radial at top.

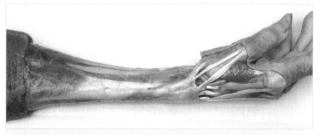

Fig. 16.25 Abductor pollicis longus (APL) and extensor pollicis brevis (EPB) insertions on thumb. Proximally, the muscle belly of the brachioradialis can be seen, continuing distally as a tendon. Dorsal to the brachioradialis lies the extensor carpi radialis longus (ECRL; *bottom*); ulnarly, the flexor carpi radialis. Distally, distal to the APL and EPB, the extensor pollicis longus can be seen crossing the extensor carpi radialis longus and extensor carpi radialis brevis and extending distally onto the thumb, ulnar to the EPB. Orientation: distal at right of picture, anterior at top.

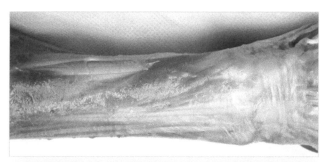

Fig. 16.26 Abductor pollicis longus and extensor pollicis brevis seen deep to fascia, crossing superficial to extensor carpi radialis longus, extensor carpi radialis brevis, and brachioradialis. Orientation: distal at right of picture, radial at top.

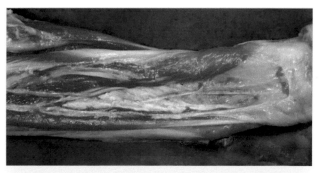

Fig. 16.27 Deep layer of dorsal forearm with extensor pollicis longus and extensor indices proprius removed. Orientation: distal at right of picture, radial at top.

The second dorsal compartment contains the tendons of the ECRL and ECRB. The dorsal radius, between the first and second compartments, can be harvested as a vascularized bone graft based on a pedicle from the radial artery, using the 1,2 inter-compartmental supraretinacular artery.[22,23] The third dorsal compartment contains the EPL tendon. The fourth dorsal compartment contains the tendons of the EDC along with the tendon of the EIP (which is oblique and deep to the tendons of the EDC). The fifth dorsal compartment contains the EDM (usually a split tendon distally) (▶Fig. 16.30, ▶Fig. 16.31, and ▶Fig. 16.32). The sixth compartment, which lies in a groove in the ulna, does not rotate with the radius and contains the ECU (▶Fig. 16.33).

A summary of the extensor tendon and their insertions is shown (▶Fig. 16.34 and ▶Fig. 16.35). Anatomic cross-sections showing the muscular relationships at the elbow, midproximal third, junction of proximal and middle thirds, mid-forearm, junction of middle and distal thirds, mid-distal third, and wrist, are shown (▶Fig. 16.36, ▶Fig. 16.37, ▶Fig. 16.38, ▶Fig. 16.39, ▶Fig. 16.40, ▶Fig. 16.41, and ▶Fig. 16.42). The seven cross-sections are courtesy of the National Library of Medicine Visible Human Project™. Of note, in these images, the forearm is not positioned in "anatomic position" (with the shoulder in neutral and the forearm fully supinated). Instead, the shoulder is internally rotated and the forearm rotation is near neutral instead of supinated. In addition, the elbow is flexed mildly, creating oblique sections through the forearm, rather than true transverse sections, with the obliquity more apparent at the wrist, where the cross-section is just proximal to the articular surface of the radius, nearly parallel with the articular surface, but cuts obliquely through the ulnar neck.

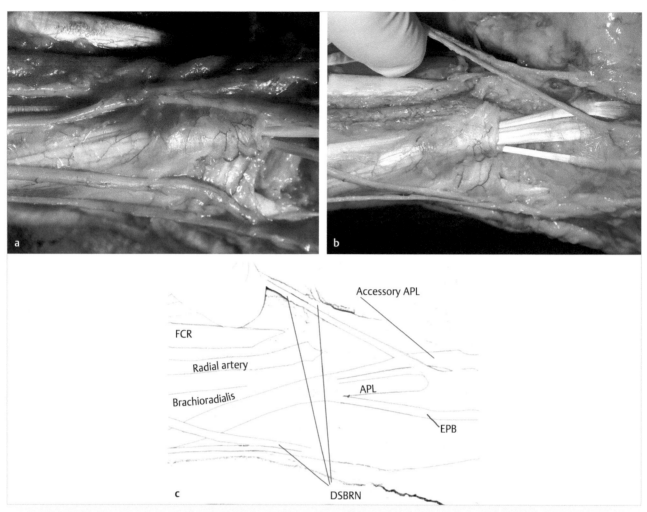

Fig. 16.28 **(a)** Radial wrist view showing first dorsal compartment with overlying radial sensory branches. Orientation: distal at right of picture, anterior at top. **(b, c)** Radial wrist view showing first dorsal compartment with multiple abductor pollicis longus slips, with insertion into base of first metacarpal and volar tendon inserting onto thenar musculature. The volar branches of the dorsal sensory branch of the radial nerve (DSBRN) are retracted volarly. Orientation: distal at right of picture, anterior at top.

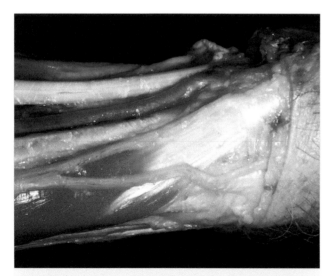

Fig. 16.29 Radial wrist view showing first dorsal compartment muscles with overlying fascia removed. Radial artery lies between brachioradialis, which is just under the abductor pollicis longus, and the flexor carpi radialis tendon (*top*). Orientation: distal at right of picture, anterior at top.

16.3 Arteries

The forearm arterial supply is primarily from the radial and ulnar arteries, both of which branch from the brachial artery. Although there can be a high bifurcation of the brachial artery, the common level of bifurcation is usually in the antecubital fossa. Just distal to the bifurcation, the ulnar artery gives rise to the common interosseous artery, which bifurcates into the anterior and posterior interosseous arteries. There are four recurrent arteries that arise just distal to the elbow and turn proximally, with the ulnar artery, or its branches, responsible for three of the four. There are two ulnar recurrent arteries, anterior and posterior, a single radial recurrent, and the interosseous recurrent. The ulnar recurrent branches form arterial loops around the elbow by joining branches of the brachial artery. The posterior ulnar recurrent joins the superior ulnar collateral artery, and the anterior ulnar recurrent joins the inferior ulnar collateral artery. The interosseous recurrent and radial recurrent form loops with branches of the profunda brachii; the interosseous recurrent anastomoses with the radial collateral branch and the radial recurrent with the anterior branch of the profunda brachii.

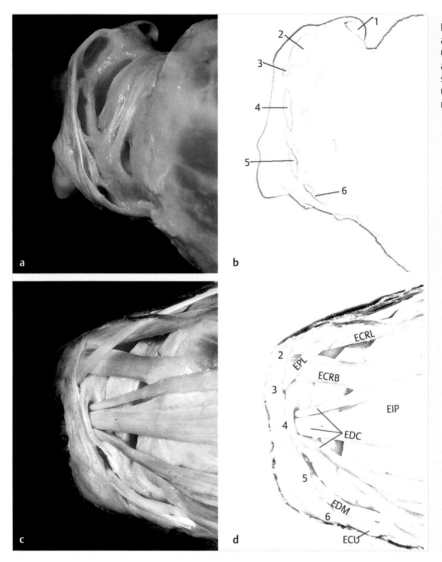

Fig. 16.30 (a, b) View dorsal compartments as seen from distally, with tendons removed. Orientation: distal at right of picture, radial at top. (c, d) Dorsal distal view of wrist showing dorsal compartments 2 through 6, with their contents. Orientation: distal at right of picture, radial at top.

The radial artery in the proximal forearm lies just deep to the brachioradialis, medial to the ECRL. The radial artery lies superficial to the pronator teres and FDS. Distally, the artery lies deep to the fascia, medial to the brachioradialis tendon, lateral to the FCR, and superficial to the FPL (▶ Fig. 16.43 and ▶ Fig. 16.44).

Coursing distally from the elbow, the ulnar artery passes deep to the pronator teres and joins the ulnar nerve in the proximal forearm, deep to the FCU, in the ulnar groove between the FDS and FDP (▶ Fig. 16.45). The ulnar artery is just radial and superficial to the ulnar nerve at the wrist. Both the radial artery and the ulnar artery have perforators that perfuse the overlying skin, passing between the muscles to the skin. These perforators can be used as the basis for pedicled flaps. For instance, between 2 to 5 cm proximal to the pisiform, the ulnar artery gives off a perforator that passes posterior to the FCU, along with the dorsal sensory branch of the ulnar nerve. This perforator is the basis for the Becker dorsal ulnar artery flap.[24]

The anterior interosseous artery arises from the ulnar artery via the common interosseous artery just distal to the elbow at the level of the bicipital tuberosity. The anterior interosseous artery then courses anterior to the IOM (as its name implies) between the FDP and the FPL. The anterior interosseous artery accompanies the anterior interosseous nerve, and both enter the wrist via the ligament of Testut. (This ligament may be more properly referred to as the synovial fold of Testut, since the ligament of Testut is not a true ligamentous structure.[25])

The posterior interosseous artery arises from the common interosseous artery (although the posterior interosseous artery can occasionally arise directly from the ulnar artery)[26] and perforates the IOM to gain access to the posterior forearm where it courses longitudinally between the radius and ulna. The artery lies between the superficial and deep layers. Approximately 2 cm proximal to the DRUJ, there is commonly an anastomosis with the anterior interosseous artery, and this anastomosis provides perfusion to the reversed posterior interosseous artery flap. In this flap, fascia and skin perfusion is based on perforators lying in the septum between the EDM, and the ECU (▶ Fig. 16.46).[27]

16.4 Veins

The venous plexus of the forearm is highly variable, with most of the veins without established names. The basilic, cephalic,

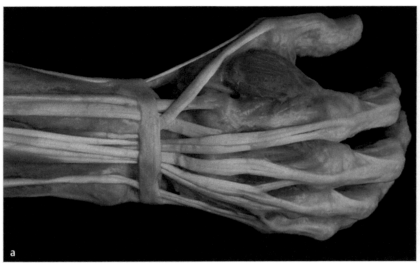

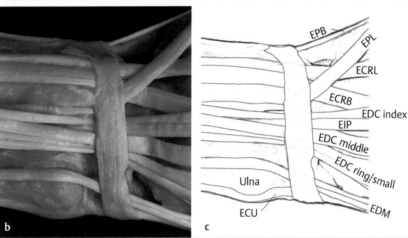

Fig. 16.31 (a) Dorsal view of extensor tendons passing under intact segment of retinaculum. Orientation: distal at right of picture, radial at top. (**b, c**) Detail view of dorsal wrist. Orientation: distal at right of picture, radial at top.

antecubital, and medial antebrachial veins are the exceptions. The cephalic vein is formed at the radial wrist and continues proximally in the forearm to the lateral elbow, then continues proximally to the deltopectoral groove, and finally drains into the axillary vein. The basilic vein classically forms at the ulnar wrist, then continues proximally to the medial elbow, finally joining the brachial vein to form the axillary vein. The medial antebrachial vein accompanies the medial antebrachial cutaneous nerve of the forearm, lying longitudinal in the anteromedial forearm. The deep veins of the forearm are smaller than the superficial veins and accompany arteries as venae comitans (▶ Fig. 16.47).

16.5 Nerves

16.5.1 Cutaneous Nerves of the Forearm

Three nerves contribute the majority of the forearm cutaneous sensation: the medial antebrachial cutaneous nerve, the lateral antebrachial cutaneous nerve, and the posterior antebrachial cutaneous nerve.

The medial antebrachial cutaneous nerve and the ulnar nerve are the terminal branches of the medial cord, which gives off the medial antebrachial cutaneous nerve and then continues

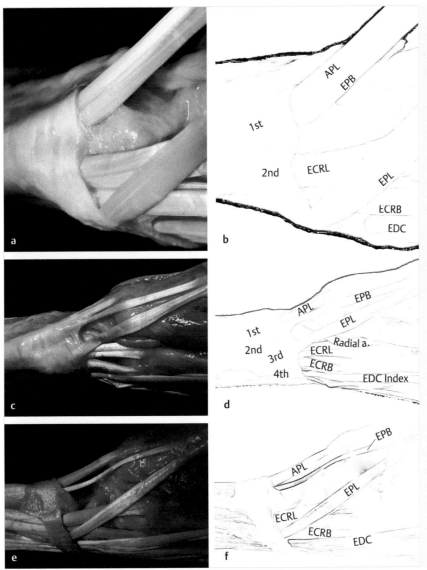

Fig. 16.32 (**a, b**) Radial view of wrist showing first and second compartments. Here, the abductor pollicis brevis and abductor pollicis longus (APL) are of relatively equal size. Orientation: distal to right of picture, anterior at top of picture. (**c, d**) Radial view of wrist. Here the extensor pollicis brevis (EPB) is smaller than the APL, with multiple slips of the APL. Orientation: distal at right of picture, anterior at top. (**e, f**) The proximal tendons have been exposed, leaving a segment of retinaculum left intact overlying the compartments. Here the APL is much larger than the EPB. Orientation: distal at right of picture, radial at top.

distally as the ulnar nerve. The medial antebrachial cutaneous nerve initially accompanies the ulnar nerve and medial brachial cutaneous nerve and then becomes superficial, accompanying the medial antebrachial vein to innervate the anteromedial forearm.

The lateral antebrachial cutaneous nerve is the terminal branch of the musculocutaneous nerve that, after innervating the anterior brachial muscles, becomes the lateral antebrachial cutaneous nerve. The lateral antebrachial cutaneous nerve becomes superficial, just lateral to the biceps tendon in the antecubital fossa, then courses longitudinally along the forearm, providing sensation to the lateral anterior forearm.

The radial nerve gives off the posterior antebrachial cutaneous nerve, which provides sensation to the posterior elbow and forearm. The radial nerve also divides into superficial and deep branches. While the DSBRN primarily provides sensation

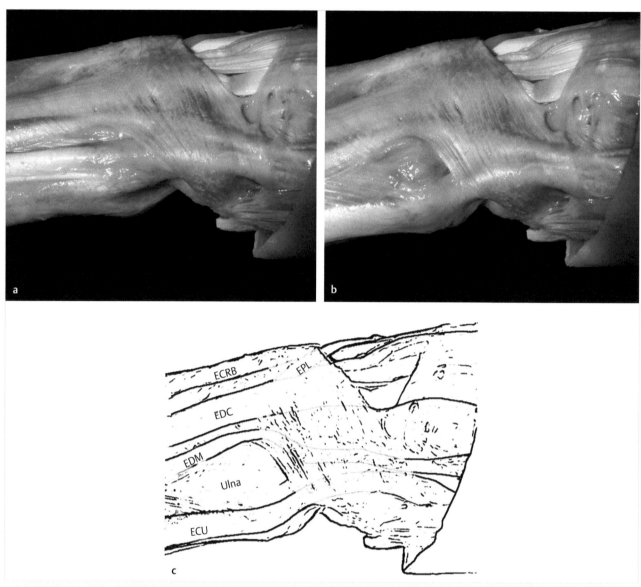

Fig. 16.33 The extensor digit minimi (EDM) retains its relationship with the radius in the extensor retinaculum, while the extensor carpi ulnaris (ECU), restrained to the ulna by the ulnar bony anatomy and the ECU subsheath, maintains its orientation with respect to the ulna, leading to splaying of the EDM and ECU during pronation. (a) Ulnar wrist viewed in supination. Orientation: distal at right of picture, dorsal radius at top. (b, c) Picture shown with forearm in pronation—the view is the same with respect to the radius in both pictures but not with respect to the ulna, which is in a different rotation in the two pictures. Orientation: distal at right of picture, dorsal radius at top.

to the dorsal radial hand, the innervation includes a variable amount of the radial distal forearm. The DSBRN travels deep to the brachioradialis muscle, until approximately the junction of the middle and distal thirds of the forearm, where the DSBRN pierces the fascia becoming subcutaneous between the brachioradialis and the ECRL tendons. The DSBRN then arborizes,

giving two branches to the dorsal thumb, as well as branches to the dorsal radial hand. Occasionally, the DSBRN may provide sensation to the ulnar dorsal hand as well (▶ Fig. 16.48).[28]

The division between brachial and antebrachial cutaneous branches is not a well-defined line between brachium and forearm, so the brachial innervation may be variable, extending into the proximal forearm. Similarly, innervation of the proximal hand may encroach on the distal forearm with the radial, ulnar, and median nerves extending their innervation proximally into the forearm into the antebrachial cutaneous nerve territory. The lateral antebrachial cutaneous nerve can also extend into the proximal thenar eminence (▸Fig. 16.49). Neuroanatomy can be further variable, with nerves sometimes reconnecting to

other nerves, similar to the motor contribution of the median to the ulnar nerve in the Martin-Gruber connection.[29]

Both the anterior and posterior interosseous nerves have sensory fibers, but neither nerve provides cutaneous innervation. The anterior interosseous terminal branch passes into the wrist in the ligament of Testut to innervate the scapholunate area. The posterior interosseous nerve passes into the wrist in the floor of the fourth compartment on the lateral side, deep to the EDC and EIP. The posterior interosseous nerve innervates the dorsal wrist capsule and the triangular fibrocartilage complex, which also has innervation from the ulnar nerve and dorsal cutaneous branch of the ulnar nerve.[30]

16.5.2 Deep Nerves of the Forearm
Radial Nerve and Posterior Interosseous Nerve

The radial nerve provides motor innervation to the posterior forearm, via the radial nerve proper; the nerve to triceps (which gives off a branch that innervates the anconeus); and the posterior interosseous nerve. Although classically considered a posterior structure, the radial nerve is anterior in the antecubital fossa, making the radial nerve vulnerable to anterior penetrating trauma. The radial nerve proper gives off muscular branches to the brachioradialis and the ECRL, with both of these muscles arising proximal to the elbow. The ECRB is variably innervated with its muscular branch arising near to the radial nerve bifurcation. The ECRB is usually innervated by the radial nerve proper, sometimes by the deep branch of the radial nerve, and occasionally even by a motor branch from the DSBRN.

The deep branch (posterior interosseous nerve) passes deep to the proximal fibrous edge of the supinator (arcade of

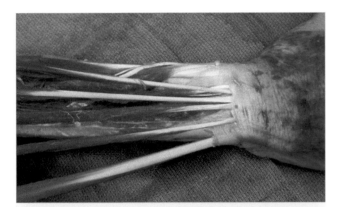

Fig. 16.34 Dorsal view of distal forearm. From top to bottom, distally, the abductor pollicis longus and extensor pollicis brevis can be seen crossing the extensor carpi radialis longus and extensor carpi radialis brevis (ECRB). At the wrist, the extensor pollicis longus can be seen ulnar to the ECRB, adjacent to the extensor digitorum communis (EDC) index. Between the EDC index and EDC middle, the tendon of the EIP can be seen. Only three definitive individual tendons are seen for the EDC, with the ulnar tendon presumably providing the ring extensor and the EDC contribution to the small finger extensor mechanism. Ulnar to the fourth compartment lies the EDM and, finally, ulnarly, the large tendon of the extensor carpi ulnaris (bottom). Orientation: distal at right of picture, radial at top.

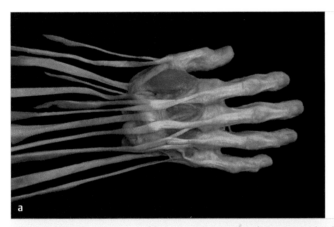
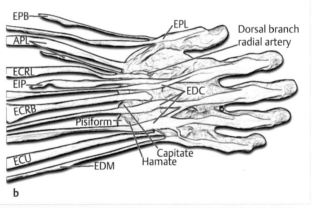

Fig. 16.35 (a, b) Summary of forearm extensor muscle insertions (excluding brachioradialis, which inserts on the distal radius at the radial styloid). The proximal tendons are no longer constrained by their origins and their dorsal compartments and are no longer in their anatomic order proximally, having been laid out from their distal insertions. Orientation: distal to right of picture, radial at top.

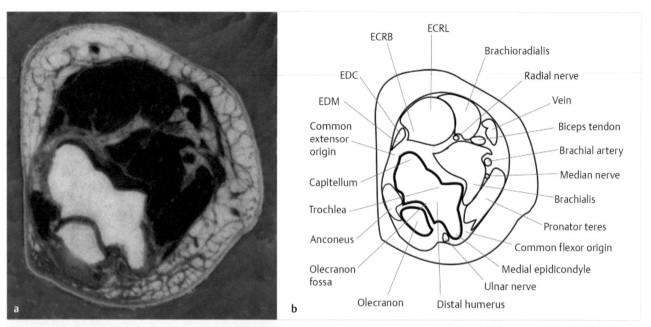

Fig. 16.36 (**a, b**) Cross-section through elbow, showing anatomic relationships of muscles. Here the brachial artery has not yet bifurcated. The biceps musculotendinous junction is proximal, leaving only tendon remaining. The ulnar nerve lies behind the medial epicondyle. (Nerves, especially the radial nerve in these sections, are difficult to distinguish from surrounding fat.) Orientation of all seven cross-sections: posteromedial at bottom of picture. (A cross-section courtesy of the National Library of Medicine Visible Human Project.)

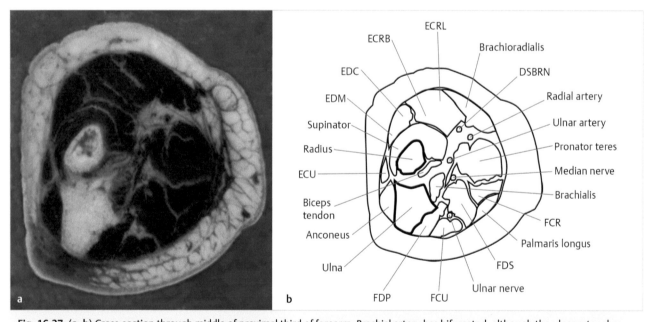

Fig. 16.37 (**a, b**) Cross-section through middle of proximal third of forearm. Brachial artery has bifurcated, although the ulnar artery has not yet joined the ulnar nerve. The ulnar artery is passing deep to pronator, while the median nerve passes through pronator. The radial nerve has divided into the DSBRN and the deep branch, with the deep branch not identified on these cross-sections. (A cross-section courtesy of the National Library of Medicine Visible Human Project.)

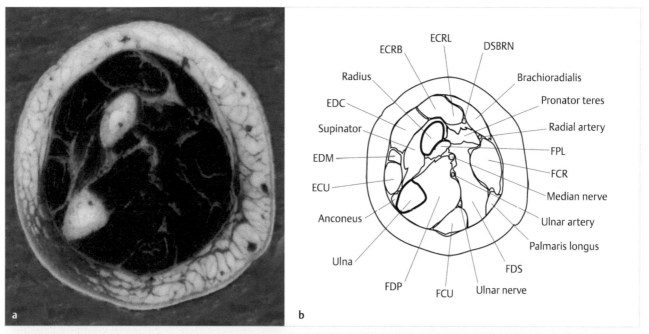

Fig. 16.38 (a, b) Cross-section at junction of proximal and middle thirds of forearm. (A cross-section courtesy of the National Library of Medicine Visible Human Project.)

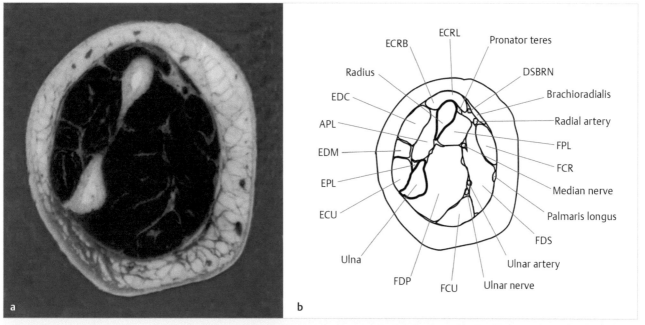

Fig. 16.39 (a, b) Cross-section through midforearm. (A cross-section courtesy of the National Library of Medicine Visible Human Project.)

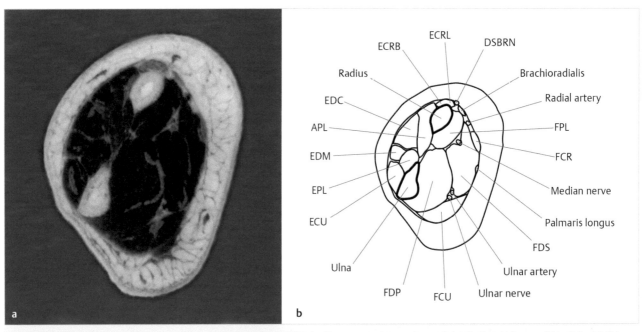

Fig. 16.40 (a, b) Cross-section at junction of middle and distal thirds. (A cross-section courtesy of the National Library of Medicine Visible Human Project.)

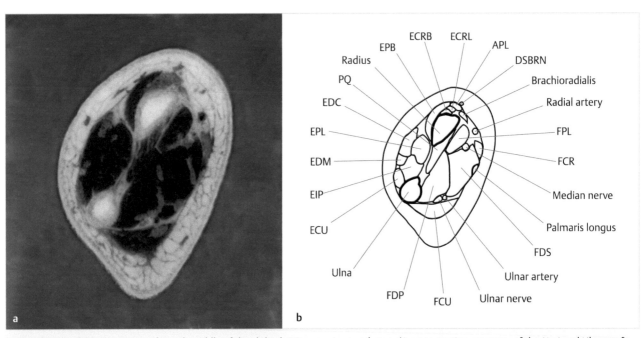

Fig. 16.41 (a, b) Cross-section through middle of distal third. PQ, pronator quadratus. (A cross-section courtesy of the National Library of Medicine Visible Human Project.)

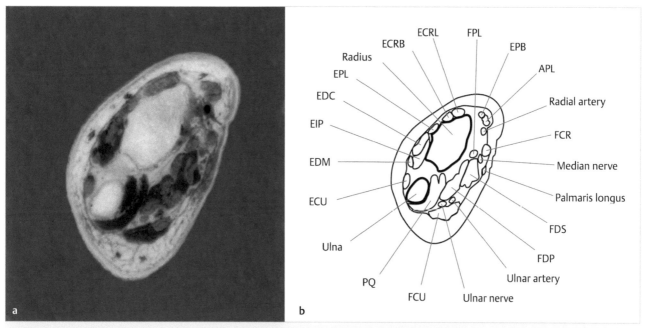

Fig. 16.42 **(a, b)** Cross-section through wrist. (A cross-section courtesy of the National Library of Medicine Visible Human Project.)

Frohse) (▶ Fig. 16.50). The posterior interosseous nerve gives off branches to the supinator, EDC, EDM, and ECU, in descending order. The posterior interosseous nerve then continues distally between the superficial and deep muscles of the dorsal forearm, providing branches to the APL, the EPL, the EPB, and the EIP. Occasionally, motor fibers may continue into the hand, innervating the radial dorsal interossei (first, second, and third) as the Froment–Rauber nerve.[31]

Median Nerve and Anterior Interosseous Nerve

The median nerve enters the volar forearm with the brachial artery, passing through the pronator teres at a variable depth, then deep to the FDS to lie between the FDS (second layer) and FDP (third layer) (▶ Fig. 16.51). The median nerve or its branch, the anterior interosseous nerve, provide motor innervation to the majority of the anterior forearm muscles (all muscles with the exception of the ulnar FDP and the FCU). The median nerve innervates the pronator teres, the FCR, the palmaris longus, and the FDS. The median nerve also gives off the palmar cutaneous sensory branch in the distal forearm, approximately 2 to 7 cm proximal to the distal wrist crease.[32] The remainder of the median nerve continues into the hand. A persistent median artery can sometimes be observed, which can be associated with abnormalities of the median nerve, including a bifurcated median nerve, or the artery can even perforate the nerve.[33] The anterior interosseous nerve arises from the median nerve

approximately 5 to 8 cm distal to the lateral epicondyle and provides motor innervation to the FDP to the index and variably middle, the FPL, and the pronator quadratus.[34]

Ulnar Nerve

The ulnar nerve enters the forearm posterior to the medial epicondyle, deep to Osborne's ligament passing between the two heads of the FCU to continue distally. The ulnar artery passes deep to the pronator teres, between the FDS and the FDP, to join the ulnar nerve (▶ Fig. 16.52, ▶ Fig. 16.53, and ▶ Fig. 16.54). The ulnar nerve gives off multiple branches in the forearm. The first branch can be an articular branch to the elbow joint within the cubital tunnel; although this branch is present infrequently, found in 13% in one study.[35] The ulnar nerve then provides innervation to the two heads of the FCU, with a mean of 3.4 branches to the FCU.[36] The ulnar nerve subsequently innervates the FDP to the ring and small fingers (and variably middle finger). In the proximal forearm, approximately 5 to 11 cm distal from the medial epicondyle, the ulnar nerve provides the nerve of Henle in approximately half of limbs, with the nerve of Henle continuing adjacent to the ulnar nerve and artery and supplying variable cutaneous innervation as well as consistent sympathetic innervation to the ulnar artery.[37,38]

In the distal forearm, the ulnar nerve gives off the dorsal sensory branch at approximately 1.5 to 8.7 cm proximal to the distal ulnar articular surface. The dorsal sensory branch passes between the ulna and the FCU (superficial to the ulna and deep to the FCU), becoming subcutaneous 0 to 3.4 cm proximal to the

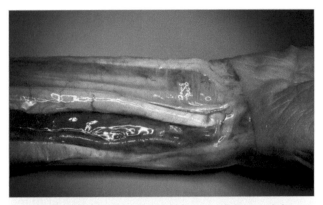

Fig. 16.43 View of volar radial distal forearm, showing radial artery lying between brachioradialis tendon (*bottom*), and flexor carpi radialis tendon. Flexor carpi ulnaris (FCU) tendon can be seen through fascia at the top of picture, with FDS lying radial to FCU. Orientation: distal at right of picture, antero-ulnar at top.

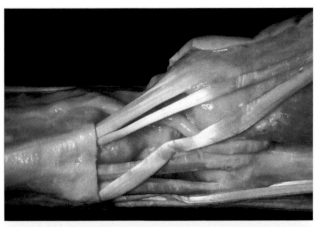

Fig. 16.44 Radial view of wrist showing distal course of radial artery, and dorsal branch of radial artery. Orientation: distal at right of picture, anterior at top.

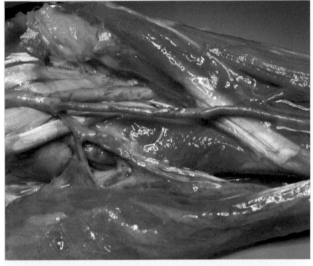

Fig. 16.45 View of proximal anterior right forearm with brachial artery dividing. The radial artery can be seen passing superficial to the tendon of pronator teres, while the ulnar artery passes deep to pronator teres. Orientation: distal at right of picture, medial at top.

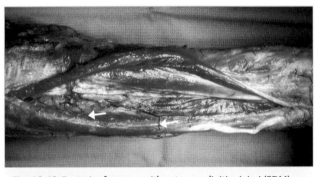

Fig. 16.46 Posterior forearm, with extensor digiti minimi (EDM) mobilized radially. Posterior interosseous artery has been injected, showing perforators in septum between EDM and extensor carpi ulnaris (*arrow*). Orientation: distal at right of picture, radial at top.

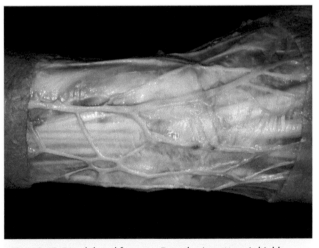

Fig. 16.47 Distal dorsal forearm. Dorsal vein pattern is highly variable. Orientation: distal at right of picture, radial at top.

distal ulnar articular surface. In pronation, all the longitudinal branches of the ulnar dorsal sensory nerve pass into the hand volar to the midline of the ulna, not crossing the ECU tendon dorsally until 0 to 2.8 cm distal to the distal ulnar articulation. There is a transverse branch to the DRUJ, which, while usually distal to the joint, can also cross proximal to the ulnar styloid tip.[39] Pronation does appear to increase the distance between the longitudinal branches of the ulnar sensory nerve and the distal ulna (▶Fig. 16.55).[40] The remainder of the ulnar nerve continues into the hand.[41]

The Martin-Gruber communication is between the median (or anterior interosseous) and the ulnar nerve. Generally,

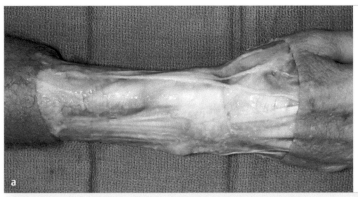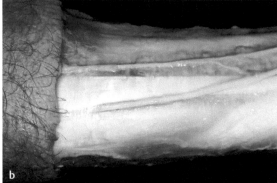

Fig. 16.48 Dorsal sensory branch of radial nerve piercing the forearm fascia between the brachioradialis and extensor carpi radialis longus (ECRL), becoming superficial at approximately the junction of middle and distal thirds of the forearm. (a) Distal forearm. Orientation: distal at right of picture, anteroradial at top. (b) Detail view of DSBRN piercing the fascia between the brachioradialis (*top*) and ECRL (*bottom*) to become superficial. Abductor pollicis longus can be seen crossing superficially distally. Orientation: distal at right, anterior at top of picture.

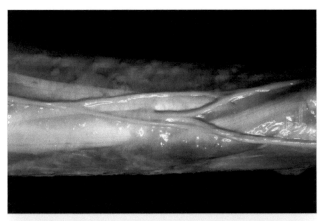

Fig. 16.49 An example of nonstandard neuroanatomy: Distal half of forearm viewed from radially, with the dorsal sensory branch becoming superficial between the brachioradialis (*above* the nerve) and ECRL (*below*), just proximal to the superficially crossing abductor pollicis longus and extensor pollicis brevis. The radial nerve is receiving contributions from the lateral antebrachial cutaneous nerve. Orientation: distal at right of picture, anterior at top.

the axons arise from the median nerve in the proximal forearm and join the ulnar nerve. Usually, the median nerve provides motor axons that would normally already be part of the ulnar nerve, most commonly axons to the first dorsal interosseous. Less commonly, the median nerve passes axons to the ulnar nerve that innervate the hypothenar musculature.[42]

16.6 Lymphatics

Forearm lymphatics have little notoriety and are seldom identified on anatomic drawings or dissections. This limited emphasis is in part because the lymphatics are not well seen on dissection, being collapsed in the normal forearm, with the little lymphatic fluid within them clear and virtually colorless. Even with peripheral edema, lymphatics are difficult to see and dissect. There are no standard named lymphatics in the forearm, although there are lymphatics in the skin, as well as larger lymphatic vessels accompanying major superficial veins—the cephalic, basilic, and antecubital veins—and deep lymphatics accompanying major arteries, including the radial, ulnar, anterior interosseous, and posterior interosseous arteries. The most distal lymph nodes in the upper limb, the epitrochlear nodes or cubital nodes, lie just proximal to the forearm in the distal medial brachium. Even these epitrochlear nodes are usually not readily apparent on dissection, unless enlarged by inflammation or hypertrophy.

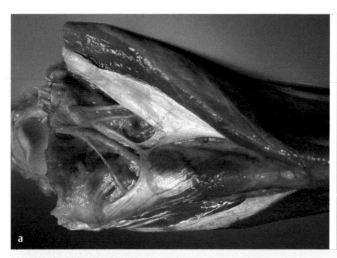 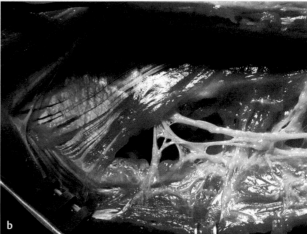

Fig. 16.50 (a) Deep branch of radial nerve passing deep to the arcade of Frohse, on the proximal edge of the supinator. Orientation: distal at right of picture, medial at top of picture. (b) Deep branch of radial nerve exiting deep to supinator and arborizing. Orientation: distal at right of picture, anterior at top.

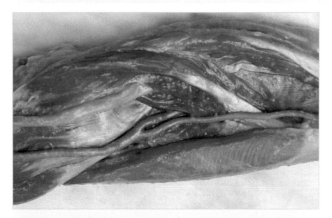

Fig. 16.51 Median nerve entering the pronator teres. Brachial artery has been mobilized laterally. Once again the ulnar artery can be seen diving deep to the pronator teres, while the median nerve passes through the pronator teres. Orientation: distal at right of picture, medial at top.

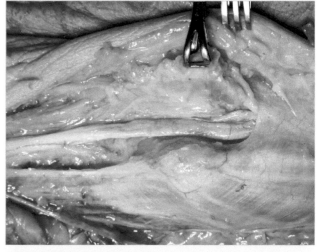

Fig. 16.53 View of posterior elbow showing ulnar nerve entering forearm between heads of flexor carpi ulnaris. Osborne's ligament has been removed. The medial epicondyle is just anterior to the ulnar nerve (*bottom*), while the olecranon is just lateral (*top*). Orientation: distal at right of picture, posterior at top.

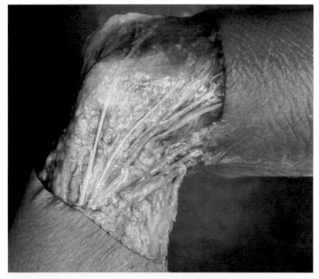

Fig. 16.52 Branches of the medial brachial cutaneous nerve lie superficial to the cubital tunnel and can be injured during medial approaches to the elbow. Orientation: distal at right of picture, posterior forearm at top.

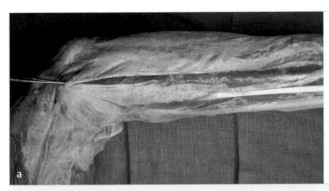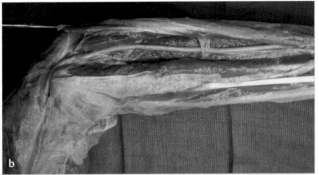

Fig. 16.54 View of medial elbow, showing ulnar nerve course in forearm. (a) Muscles in place. (b) Muscles retracted, showing nerve. Orientation: distal at right of picture, posterior forearm at top of picture.

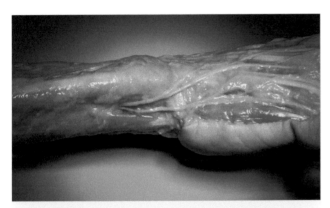

Fig. 16.55 Dorsal sensory branch of the ulnar nerve. The longitudinal branches of the nerve lie volar to the midpoint of the head of the distal ulna. Orientation: distal at right of picture, dorsal at top.

References

1. Rupasinghe A, Poon P. Radius morphology and its effect on rotation with contoured and noncontoured plating of the proximal radius. J Shoulder Elbow Surg. 2012;21:568–573
2. Mazzocca AD, Cohen M, Berkson E, Nicholson G, Carofino BC, Arciero R, Romeo AA. The anatomy of the bicipital tuberosity and distal biceps tendon. J Shoulder Elbow Surg. 2007 Jan-Feb;16(1):122–7
3. Athwal GS, Steinmann SP, Rispoli DM. The distal biceps tendon: footprint and relevant clinical anatomy. J Hand Surg Am. 2007 Oct;32(8):1225–9
4. Caputo AE, Mazzocca AD, Santoro VM. The nonarticulating portion of the radial head: anatomic and clinical correlations for internal fixation. J Hand Surg 1998;23:1082–1090
5. Smith GR, Hotchkiss RN. Radial Head and neck fractures: anatomic guidelines for proper placement of internal fixation. J Shoulder Elbow Surg 1996;5:113–117
6. Grechenig W, Clement H, Pichler W, Tesch NP, Windisch G. The influence of lateral and anterior angulation of the proximal ulna on the treatment of a Monteggia fracture: an anatomical cadaver study. J Bone Joint Surg Br. 2007 Jun;89(6):836–8
7. Moritomo H, Noda K, Goto A, Murase T, Yoshikawa H, Sugamoto K. Interosseous membrane of the forearm: length change of ligaments during forearm rotation. J Hand Surg Am. 2009 Apr;34(4):685–91
8. Nakamura T, Yabe Y, Horiuchi Y, Seki T, Yamazaki N. Normal kinematics of the interosseous membrane during forearm pronation-supination-a three-dimensional MRI study. Hand Surg. 2000 Jul;5(1):1–10
9. Cage DJ, Abrams RA, Callahan JJ, Botte MJ. Soft Tissue Attachments of the Ulnar Coronoid Process: An Anatomic Study with Radiographic Correlation. Clin Orthop Relat Res. 1995 Nov; 320:154–158
10. Vastamäki M. Median nerve as free tendon graft. The J Hand Surg Br. 1987 Jun;12(2):187–8
11. Tountas CP, Bergman RA. Anatomic Variations of the Upper Extremity. June, 1993, Churchill Livingstone
12. Shin AY, Deitch MA, Sachar K, Boyer MI. Ulnar sided wrist pain. Diagnosis and treatment. J Bone Joint Surg. 2004: 86A:1560–1574
13. Grant J, Method of Anatomy. 1938 William Wood and Company. Baltimore
14. al-Qattan MM. Gantzer's muscle. An anatomical study of the accessory head of the flexor pollicis longus muscle. J Hand Surg Br. 1996 Apr;21(2):269–70
15. Otoshi K, Kikuchi S, Shishido H, Konno S. The proximal origins of the flexor-pronator muscles and their role in the dynamic stabilization of the elbow joint: an anatomical study. Surg Radiol Anat. 2014 Apr;36(3):289–94
16. Matsuura S, Kojima T, Kinoshita Y. Cubital tunnel syndrome caused by abnormal insertion of triceps brachii muscle. J Hand Surg Br. 1994 Feb;19(1):38–9
17. O'Hara JJ, Stone JH. Ulnar nerve compression at the elbow caused by a prominent medial head of the triceps and an anconeus epitrochlearis muscle. J Hand Surg Br. 1996 Feb;21(1):133–5
18. Zoner CS, Buck FM, Cardoso FN, Gheno R, Trudell DJ, Randall TD, Resnick D. Detailed MRI-anatomic study of the lateral epicondyle of the elbow and its tendinous and ligamentous attachments in cadavers. AJR Am J Roentgenol. 2010 Sep;195(3):629–36
19. von Schroeder HP, Botte MJ. Anatomy of the extensor tendons of the fingers: variations and multiplicity. J Hand Surg Am. 1995 Jan; 20(1):27–34
20. Meads BM, Bogoch ER. Transfer of either index finger extensor tendon to the extensor pollicis longus tendon. Can J Plast Surg. 2004 Spring;12(1):31–4
21. Thwin SS, Fazlin Z, Than M. Multiple variations of the tendons of the anatomical snuffbox. Singapore Med J. 2014;55(1):37–40
22. Zaidemberg C, Siebert JW, Angrigiani C. A new vascularized bone graft for scaphoid nonunion. J Hand Surg Am. 1991;16:474–478
23. Shin AY, Bishop AT, Berger RA. Vascularized pedicled bone grafts for disorders of the carpus. Tech Hand Upper Extrem Surg 1998; 2:94–109
24. Becker C, Gilbert A. The ulnar flap – Description and applications. European Journal of Plastic Surgery. May 1988, Volume 11, Issue 2:79–82

25. Berger RA, Kauer JMG, Landsmeer JMF. Radioscapholunate ligament: A gross anatomic and histologic study of fetal and adult wrists. J Hand Surg Am. 1991 Mar;16(2):350–5

26. CV Penteado, AC Masquelet, JP Chevrel. The anatomic basis of the fascio-cutaneous flap of the posterior interosseous artery. Surgical and Radiologic Anatomy. 1986, Volume 8, Issue 4:209–215)

27. Angrigiani C, Grilli D, Dominikow D, Zancolli EA. Posterior interosseous reverse forearm flap: experience with 80 consecutive cases. Plast Reconstr Surg. 1993 Aug;92(2):285–93

28. Kuruvilla A, Laaksonen S, Falck B. Anomalous superficial radial nerve: a patient with probable autosomal dominant inheritance of the anomaly. Muscle Nerve. 2002 Nov;26(5):716–9

29. Bas H, Kleinert JM. Anatomic variations in sensory innervation of the hand and digits. J Hand Surg Am. 1999;24(6):1171–1184

30. Gupta R, Nelson SD, Baker J, Jones NF, Meals RA. The innervation of the triangular fibrocartilage complex: nitric acid maceration rediscovered. Plast Reconstr Surg. 2001 Jan;107(1):135–9

31. Guo BY, Ayyar DR, Grossman JAI. Posterior interosseus palsy with an incidental Froment–Rauber nerve presenting as a pseudoclaw hand. Hand (N Y). Sep 2011;6(3):344–347

32. Dowdy PA, Richards RS, McFarlane RM. The palmar cutaneous branch of the median nerve and the palmaris longus tendon: a cadaveric study. J Hand Surg Am. 1994 Mar;19(2):199–202

33. Singla RK, Kaur N, Dhiraj GS: Prevalence of the persistent median artery. J Clin Diagn Res 2012 Nov;6(9):1454–7

34. Spinner M: The median nerve. In Injuries to the Major Branches of Peripheral Nerves of the Forearm, Philadelphia, WB Saunders, 1972:76–111

35. Watchmaker GP, Lee G, Mackinnon SE. Intraneural topography of the ulnar nerve in the cubital tunnel facilitates anterior transposition. J Hand Surg Am. 1994 Nov;19(6):915–22

36. Tubbs RS, Custis JW, Salter EG, Blount JP, Oakes WJ, Wellons JC 3rd. J Quantitation of and landmarks for the muscular branches of the ulnar nerve to the forearm for application in peripheral nerve neurotization procedures. Neurosurg. 2006 May;104(5):800–3

37. McCabe SJ, Kleinert JM. The nerve of Henle. J Hand Surg Am. 1990 Sep;15(5):784–8

38. Balogh B, Valencak J, Vesely M, Flammer M, Gruber H, Piza-Katzer H. The nerve of Henle: an anatomic and immunohistochemical study. J Hand Surg Am. 1999 Sep;24(5):1103–8

39. Root CG, London DA, Strauss NL, Calfee RP. Anatomic Relationships and Branching Patterns of the Dorsal Cutaneous Branch of the Ulnar Nerve. J Hand Surg Am. Jun 2013;38(6):1131–1136

40. Puna R, Poon P The anatomy of the dorsal cutaneous branch of the ulnar nerve. J Hand Surg Eur 2010 Sep;35(7):583–5

41. Spinner M: The ulnar nerve. In Injuries to the Major Branches of Peripheral Nerves of the Forearm, Philadelphia, WB Saunders, 1972:113–132

42. Kazakos KJ, Xarchas KC, Dimitrakopoulou A, Verettas DA: Anastomosis between the median and ulnar nerves in the forearm. An anatomic study and literature review. Acta Orthop Belg. 2005 Feb;71(1):29–35

17 The Interosseous Membrane

David J. Slutsky

17.1 Interosseous Membrane Anatomy

In an anatomical study of 30 forearm specimens, Noda et al identified that the interosseous membrane (IOM) included five ligaments: the central band (CB), the accessory band (AB), the distal oblique bundle (DOB), the proximal oblique cord, and the dorsal oblique accessory cord (▶ Fig. 17.1a–c).[1] They further subdivided the IOM into proximal, middle, and distal portions. The middle ligamentous complex consists of the CB and the AB. The CB is the broadest and thickest of these ligaments. The CB originates from the interosseous crest of the radius, then courses distally and ulnarly to insert into the interosseous border of the ulna. The mean width was 9.7 ± 3 mm (range, 4.4–16 mm) and the mean thickness 1.3 ± 0.2 mm (range, 1–1.6 mm). The AB consists of several ligaments either proximal or distal to the CB that were often less than 1 mm in thickness and varied in location and number (▶ Fig. 17.2).

The DOB is an inconstant ligament that is present within the distal membranous portion. It originates from the distal sixth of the ulnar shaft, at the proximal border of the pronator quadratus muscle, blending into the capsule of the distal radioulnar joint (DRUJ) and inserting into the inferior rim of the sigmoid notch and dorsal and palmar radioulnar ligaments (▶ Fig. 17.3a,b). The mean width was 4.4 ± 1.1 mm (range, 2–6 mm) and the mean thickness 1.5± 0.5 mm (range, 0.5–2.6 mm). The DOB appeared to form an isometric collateral ligament with the triangular fibrocartilage complex (TFCC) to stabilize the forearm during rotation, because the ulnar insertions of these ligaments coincide with the axis of rotation.[2]

The proximal oblique cord (ligament of Weitbrecht) was seen in the proximal membranous portion. It originates from the anterolateral aspect of the coronoid process of the ulna and inserts just distal to the radial tuberosity (▶ Fig. 17.4a,b). The mean width was 3.7 ± 1.6 mm (range, 1.5–8 mm) and the mean thickness 1.1 ± 0.5 mm (range, 0.4–2 mm). A less constant dorsal oblique accessory cord was seen on the posterior aspect of the forearm, originating from the distal two-thirds of the ulnar shaft and inserting into the interosseous crest of the radius (▶ Fig. 17.5a,b). The mean width was 3.2 ±1 mm (range, 1.9–5 mm) and the mean thickness 0.9 ± 0.2 mm (range, 0.5–1 mm).

17.2 Kinematics

In a companion computed tomography (CT) study of nine forearms in seven volunteers, Moritomo et al found that the distal three ligaments, the CB, AB, and DOB, had little change in

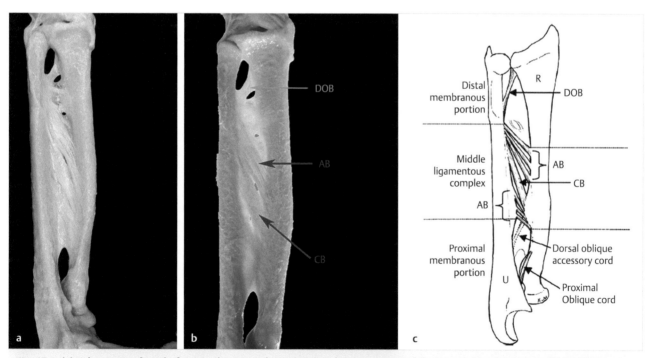

Fig. 17.1 (a) Volar aspect of a right forearm dissection demonstrating the components of the interosseous membrane. (b) Backlight specimen highlighting the distal oblique bundle (DOB), the thin accessory band (AB), and the thick central band (CB). (c) Schematic diagram. (Reproduced with permission from Noda et al.[1])

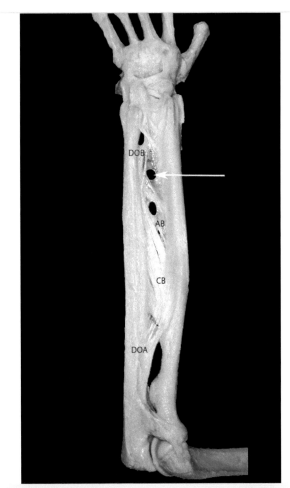

Fig. 17.2 Dorsal aspect of a left forearm dissection with labeling of the IOM components. The interosseous artery penetrates through a hole in the distal membrane (*arrow*). AB, accessory band; CB, central band; DOA, dorsal oblique accessory cord; DOB, distal oblique bundle.

length during forearm rotation and were isometric stabilizers of the forearm and coincided with the axis of rotation of the forearm.[2] The DOB (if present) was thought to aid in stabilizing the DRUJ. Conversely, the two proximal ligaments, the proximal oblique cord and dorsal oblique accessory cord, changed substantially in length, with their attachments being off the axis of rotation, potentially acting as a restraint to excessive forearm pronation.

Similarly, Nakamura et al[3] studied the in vivo dynamic shape changes of IOM during forearm rotation using three-dimensional magnetic resonance imaging (3D-MRI). They noticed wavy deformities in the membranous IOM (CB) in pronation, maximal supination, and neutral, whereas the tendinous part demonstrated *minimal* dynamic changes during rotation. There was some deformity of dorsal oblique cord at maximum pronation. They concluded that the tendinous part of the IOM is taut during rotation in order to provide stability between the radius and ulna, while the more deformable membranous part allows for smooth rotation, since it lies at a distance from the axis of forearm rotation.

17.3 Biochemistry and Biomechanics

McGinley et al performed a histological and biochemical analysis of the IOM from 21 forearm specimens.[4] The histologic organization of the IOM showed a dense connective tissue with an abundance of collagen arranged in parallel surrounded by an elastin sheath. This was composed of 84.1 ± 7.8% collagen. The relative amount of collagen increased from the distal to the proximal bundles. This group also performed a shear analysis of the CB and accessory bundles.[5] The average ultimate force was 1,101 ± 191 N, the ultimate strength was 13.98 ± 4.85 MPa, and elastic modulus was 135.29 ± 41.57 MPa. IOM sectioning led to increased bending of the radius and ulna during axial loading.[6] The CB has been shown to be the stiffest stabilizing structure of the forearm. Pfaeffle et al reported the CB of the IOM to have an average stiffness of 13.1 N/mm per millimeter width of the band.[7] The average CB width was 4.3 mm, which equated to 56.3 N/mm for the entire CB. Werner et al found the stiffness to range from 45 to 54 N/mm at different forearm positions in six specimens.[8]

The IOM functions as a longitudinal stabilizer of the forearm. It is also a dorsal–volar stabilizer of the DRUJ. Watanabe et al tested eight cadaver forearms both quantitatively and clinically in neutral and 60° of pronation or supination.[9] They found that the distal IOM (which variably contains a DOB) constrained volar and dorsal laxity of the radius at the DRUJ in all forearm rotation positions. Dorsal dislocation of the radius relative to the ulna strongly suggested a rupture of the distal IOM rupture. Disengagement of the radius from the DRUJ indicated injury to the distal and middle IOM. Kitamura et al tested 10 cadaver arms.[10] The DOB was present in four specimens consisting of an obvious thick fiber bundle, but there was considerable variation. The group with a DOB demonstrated a significantly greater DRUJ stability in the neutral position than the group without a DOB. In pronated and supinated forearm positions, no significant difference in DRUJ stability was obtained between the groups with and without a DOB. They surmised that after a TFCC injury or ulnar head resection, patients with a DOB might not experience signs or symptoms of DRUJ instability, pain, or dysfunction compared with patients who lack a DOB.

In a recent study, Yi et al[11] tested the ultimate load to failure in 10 potted cadaver forearms. They found that the CB ruptured in six specimens at a maximum load of 1,021.50 ± 250.13 N, with a stiffness of 138.24 ± 24.29 N/m and displacement of 9.77 ± 1.77 mm. A fracture at the fixed end of the ulna occurred in the other four specimens when the maximum load was 744.40 ± 109.85 N, with a stiffness of 151.17 ± 30.68 N/m and displacement of 6.51 ± 0.51 mm.

Rupture of the IOM has important clinical consequences. This is evident with an Essex-Lopresti fracture where there is a fracture of the radial head and disruption of the IOM. Shepard et al[12] performed a sectioning study on the IOM in 20 fresh frozen forearms which were instrumented with custom-designed load cells. Simultaneous measurements of load cell forces, radial head displacement relative to the capitellum, and local tension within the CB of the IOM were made as the wrist was loaded to 134 N, with the forearm at 90° of elbow flexion

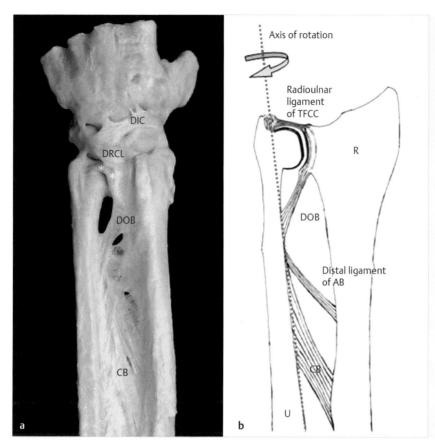

Fig. 17.3 (a) Dorsal aspect of a left forearm dissection showing the intimate relationship between the distal oblique bundle (DOB) blending with the dorsal radioulnar ligament and triangular fibrocartilage (*). CB, central band; DIC, dorsal intercarpal ligament; DRCL, dorsal radiocarpal ligament. (b) Schematic diagram demonstrating the axis of rotation which passes through the ulnar head. (Reproduced with permission from Moritomo et al.[2])

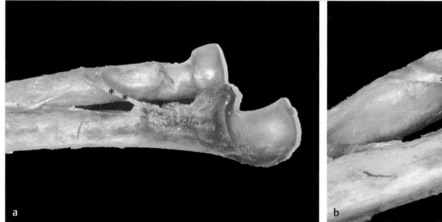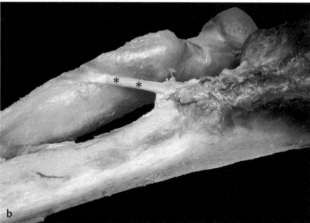

Fig. 17.4 (a) Proximal oblique cord (*) from the volar aspect of the elbow. (b) Proximal oblique cord (*) from the ulnar aspect of the elbow.

and in neutral pronation supination. For a valgus elbow alignment where the radial head was in contact with the capitellum, the mean force carried by the distal ulna was 7.1% of the applied wrist force and the mean force transferred from the radius to ulna through the IOM was 4.4%. For a varus elbow alignment with a mean gap of 2 mm between the radial head and the capitellum, the load was transferred to the IOM with a mean distal ulna force of 28% and a mean IOM force of 51%. The mean applied wrist force that was necessary to close the varus gap was 89 N. Sectioning of the proximal and distal thirds of the IOM had no significant effect upon the mean distal ulnar

force or mean IOM force. The mean applied wrist force that was necessary to close the varus gap decreased significantly after both partial IOM section (71 N) and total IOM section (25 N). The IOM became loaded only when the radius displaced proximally relative to the ulna, closing the gap between the radius and the capitellum. As the radius displaced proximally, the wrist became increasingly ulnar positive, which in turn led to direct loading of the distal ulna. They concluded that this shift of force to the distal ulna could present clinically as ulnar-sided wrist pain or as ulnar impaction after an IOM injury.

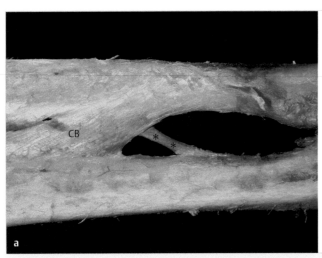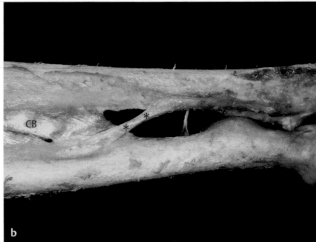

Fig. 17.5 (a) Dorsal oblique accessory cord (*) from the volar aspect of the proximal forearm. (b) Dorsal oblique accessory cord (*) from the dorsal aspect of the proximal forearm. CB, central band.

References

1. Noda K, Goto A, Murase T, Sugamoto K, Yoshikawa H, Moritomo H. Interosseous membrane of the forearm: an anatomical study of ligament attachment locations. J Hand Surg Am 2009;34(3): 415–422

2. Moritomo H, Noda K, Goto A, Murase T, Yoshikawa H, Sugamoto K. Interosseous membrane of the forearm: length change of ligaments during forearm rotation. J Hand Surg Am 2009;34(4):685–691

3. Nakamura T, Yabe Y, Horiuchi Y, Seki T, Yamazaki N. Normal kinematics of the interosseous membrane during forearm pronation-supination—a three-dimensional MRI study. Hand Surg 2000;5(1):1–10

4. McGinley JC, Heller JE, Fertala A, Gaughan JP, Kozin SH. Biochemical composition and histologic structure of the forearm interosseous membrane. J Hand Surg Am 2003;28(3):503–510

5. McGinley JC, D'addessi L, Sadeghipour K, Kozin SH. Mechanics of the antebrachial interosseous membrane: response to shearing forces. J Hand Surg Am 2001;26(4):733–741

6. Kaufmann RA, Kozin SH, Barnes A, Kalluri P. Changes in strain distribution along the radius and ulna with loading and interosseous membrane section. J Hand Surg Am 2002;27(1): 93–97

7. Pfaeffle HJ, Tomaino MM, Grewal R, et al. Tensile properties of the interosseous membrane of the human forearm. J Orthop Res 1996;14(5):842–845

8. Werner FW, Taormina JL, Sutton LG, Harley BJ. Structural properties of 6 forearm ligaments. J Hand Surg Am 2011;36(12): 1981–1987

9. Watanabe H, Berger RA, Berglund LJ, Zobitz ME, An KN. Contribution of the interosseous membrane to distal radioulnar joint constraint. J Hand Surg Am 2005;30(6):1164–1171

10. Kitamura T, Moritomo H, Arimitsu S, et al. The biomechanical effect of the distal interosseous membrane on distal radioulnar joint stability: a preliminary anatomic study. J Hand Surg Am 2011;36(10):1626–1630

11. Yi XH, Pan J, Guo XS. Anatomical and biomechanical study on the interosseous membrane of the cadaveric forearm. Chin J Traumatol 2011;14(3):147–150

12. Shepard MF, Markolf KL, Dunbar AM. The effects of partial and total interosseous membrane transection on load sharing in the cadaver forearm. J Orthop Res 2001;19(4):587–592

18 The Carpal Tunnel

Steven McCabe, Brett McClelland, and Amit Gupta

18.1 Introduction

The carpal tunnel is an important anatomical passageway that conveys the median nerve and nine flexor tendons (flexor digitorum superficialis [FDS] and flexor digitorum profundus [FDP] to the index, middle, ring, and little fingers, as well as the flexor pollicis longus [FPL] tendon to the thumb) from the forearm to the hand. A thorough knowledge of the anatomy of the carpal tunnel and that of the surrounding structures provides a critical base to all practitioners managing common upper extremity problems.

18.2 Anatomy

A thin layer of fascia, called the antebrachial fascia, covers the whole forearm (▶ Fig. 18.1). The fascia thickens as it approaches the palmar aspect of the wrist.

The carpal tunnel does form a distinct tunnel located on the flexor surface of the wrist. The carpal bones and intercarpal

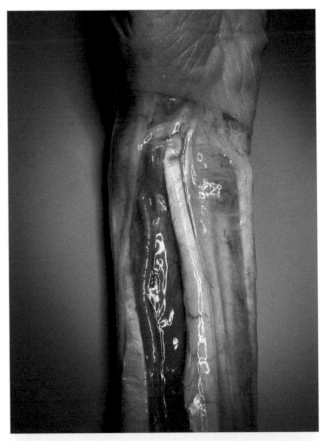

Fig. 18.1 The antebrachial fascia of the forearm thickens as it approaches the palmar part of the wrist proximal to the carpal tunnel.

ligaments that create a gentle arch concave toward the palm form the dorsal surface of the tunnel, commonly referred to as the floor. The positioning of the carpal bones also forms the walls of the tunnel. The volar surface, or roof, is formed by a strong transversely oriented fibrous layer known as the flexor retinaculum (▶ Fig. 18.2 a,b). The mean width of the tunnel is 24 mm at its proximal end (▶ Fig. 18.3), 20 mm at the narrowest region, and 25 mm at its distal border.[1] The depth of the tunnel also varies, being around 12 mm at the proximal end, 10 mm at the narrowest, and 13 mm at the distal end. At the proximal end, the depth of the carpal tunnel is 8 mm on the radial side, 12 mm in the center, and 10 mm on the ulnar side (▶ Fig. 18.4). The narrowest area of the tunnel is found 2.1 mm distal to the proximal pole of the capitate.[2]

Motion of the wrist changes the diameter and alters the pressures in the carpal tunnel (▶ Fig. 18.5a–c). In flexion of the wrist, the cross section of the carpal tunnel decreases as the flexor retinaculum comes closer to the carpal bones.[3] Gelberman et al[4] measured carpal tunnel pressures in normal subjects and patients with carpal tunnel syndrome. In control subjects, the pressure was 2.5 mm Hg that rose to 31 mm Hg with wrist flexion and 30 mm Hg in wrist extension. In contrast, in patients with carpal tunnel syndrome, the mean carpal tunnel pressure was 32 mm Hg that rose to 94 mm Hg with the wrist in 90° flexion and 110 mm Hg with the wrist in extension.

In many anatomical writings, the terms *transverse carpal ligament* (TCL), *palmar carpal ligament* (PCL), and *flexor retinaculum* are used interchangeably.[1,5] Schmidt and Lanz[3] make an anatomic distinction between the PCL and the flexor retinaculum. According to them, the superficial reinforcing bands of the forearm fascia form the PCL (▶ Fig. 18.6). This ligament extends from the insertion onto the tendon of flexor carpi ulnaris (FCU) to the ulnar border of palmaris longus. The PCL adheres very tightly to the flexor retinaculum radial to the palmaris longus (▶ Fig. 18.7a–d).

In a detailed study of the anatomy of the flexor retinaculum, Cobb et al[1] divide the covering of the palmar wrist into anatomical parts. The thin fascia covering the whole forearm is the *antebrachial fascia*. Distal to that, the *flexor retinaculum* has three components. The most proximal portion of the flexor retinaculum (called *palmar carpal ligament* [PCL] by Schmidt and Lanz[3]) is a thickening of the antebrachial fascia. This superficial sheet covers the ulnar artery and nerve and courses deep to the FCU. The flexor carpi radialis (FCR) tendon pierces the flexor retinaculum to enter its fibro-osseous tunnel. The middle part of the flexor retinaculum is distal and deeper to the PCL and is termed the transverse carpal ligament (TCL). It is attached to pisiform, hamate, the tubercle of the trapezium, and the tubercle of the scaphoid. The very distal portion of the flexor retinaculum is an *aponeurosis* between the thenar and hypothenar muscles.

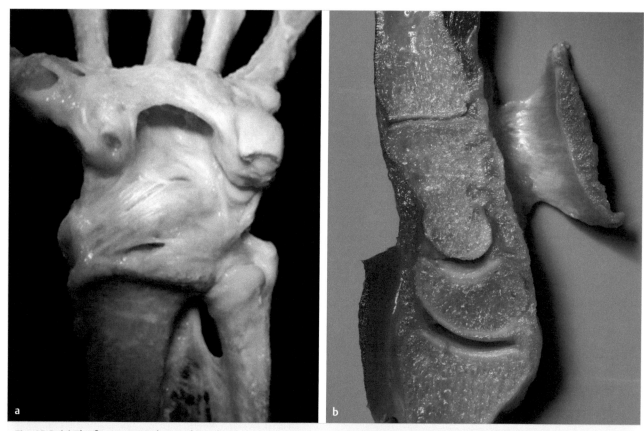

Fig. 18.2 (a) The flexor retinaculum and its relationship to the carpus and the palmar wrist ligaments. (b) The major thick part of the flexor retinaculum is situated opposite the capitate. The space between the carpus and the flexor retinaculum and the volume of the carpal tunnel is maximum in neutral position of the wrist.

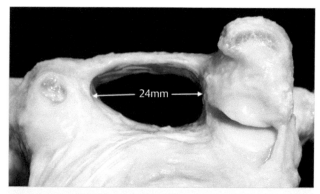

Fig. 18.3 Width of the carpal tunnel.

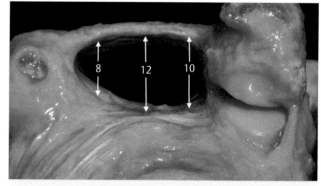

Fig. 18.4 Dimensions of the carpal tunnel.

The descriptions in the current literature are very confusing. After many dissections, a thorough study of the literature, and discussions with renowned anatomists and hand surgeons, we present our schema.

The antebrachial fascia covers the whole forearm with a thin lining. There is distinct condensation of this fascia in the palmar portion of the distal forearm that extends to envelop the ulnar neurovascular bundle and the FCU (▶ Fig. 18.7a–d). The palmaris longus is superficial to this portion of the fascial condensation. Schmidt and Lanz[3] have termed this fascial segment PCL.

Anatomically, it is a part of the antebrachial fascia (▶ Fig.18.6a,b, ▶ Fig. 18.7a–d).

This portion can cause compression of the median nerve, and prominent hand surgery teachers like Dr. Carroll and Dr. Kleinert advocated always dividing this ligament during carpal tunnel release.

The thick covering of the carpal tunnel is the flexor retinaculum (▶ Fig. 18.2a,b). It is a thick sheet that is attached to the ridge of the trapezium and ridge of the scaphoid on the radial side and to the pisiform and hamate on the ulnar side.

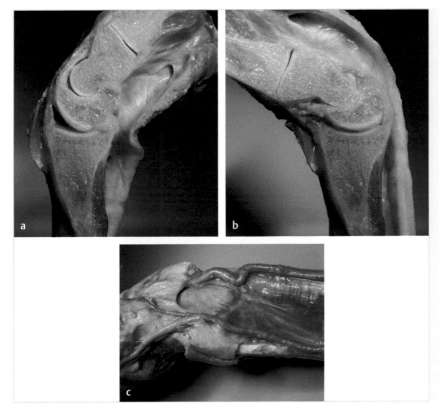

Fig. 18.5 (a) Flexion of the wrist shows the transverse carpal ligament and the dimensions of the carpal tunnel narrowing especially in the proximal part. (b) Extension of the wrist also narrows the dimensions of the carpal tunnel. (c) Hyperextension of the wrist flattens the dimensions of the carpal tunnel.

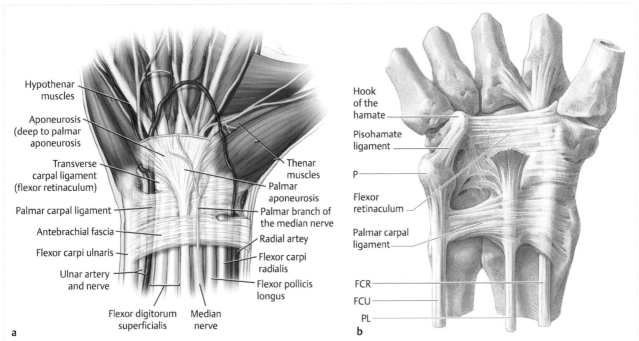

Fig. 18.6 (a,b) Superficial antebrachial fascia. Thickened deep palmar carpal ligament (Copyright Mayo Clinic). The flexor retinaculum and the distal muscle aponeurosis. P: Pisiform; PL: tendon of the palmaris longus; FCU: tendon of the flexor carpi ulnaris; FCR: tendon of the flexor carpi radialis. (From Schmidt H-M, Lanz U. Surgical Anatomy of the Hand. Thieme, 2004)

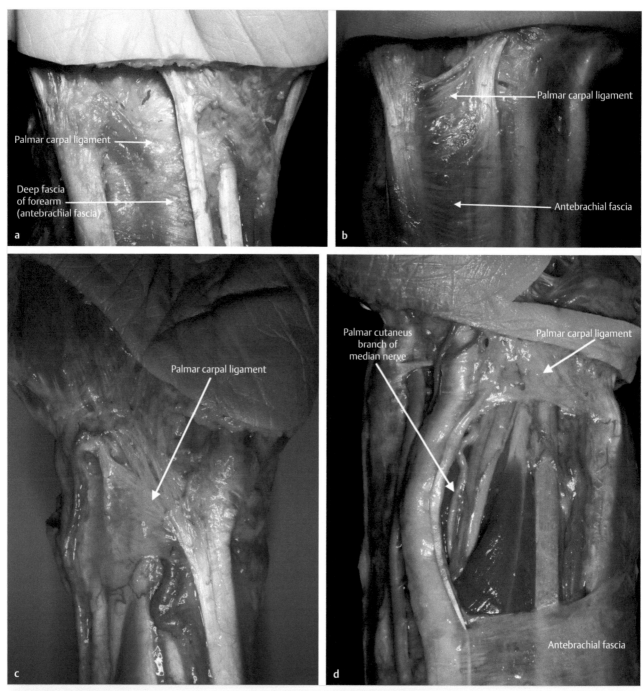

Fig. 18.7 (a–d) The antebrachial fascia and palmar carpal ligament.

The Terminology for Hand Surgery, by the IFSSH (2001), recognizes only flexor retinaculum as a terminology, and there is no mention of TCL. Therefore, the term *transverse carpal ligament* (TCL) is confusing and should not be used. Additionally, we feel that it is artificial to divide the flexor retinaculum into different anatomical components and that it serves no useful function. Thus, we believe that the antebrachial fascia and the palmar carpal ligament cover the forearm.

The Palmar carpal ligament (PCL) is a distinct component of the antebrachial fascia. The distal part and the true covering

of the carpal tunnel is the flexor retinaculum. There is an area in the distal part of the flexor retinaculum that consists of criss-crossing of muscle aponeurosis of the thenar and hypothenar muscles (▶ Fig. 18.9a,b). However, this segment is just the very distal part of the flexor retinaculum from which these muscles are taking origin. This happens in many areas of the body, and these areas do not deserve unique terminologies.

The flexor retinaculum is supplied by branches from the superficial branch of the radial artery and from the ulnar artery directly[3] (▶ Fig. 18.10).

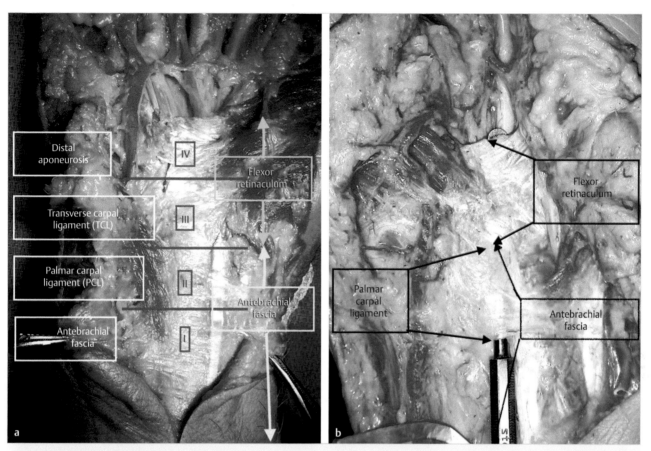

Fig. 18.8 (a) The antebrachial fascia and the three parts of the flexor retinaculum: the palmar carpal ligament, the transverse carpal ligament, and the distal thenar and hypothenar muscle aponeurosis (according to Cobb et.al[1]. PCL is defined by Scmidt and Lanz[3].). (b) Our schema includes the antebrachial fascia, the palmar carpal ligament (PCL) and the Flexor Retinaculum.

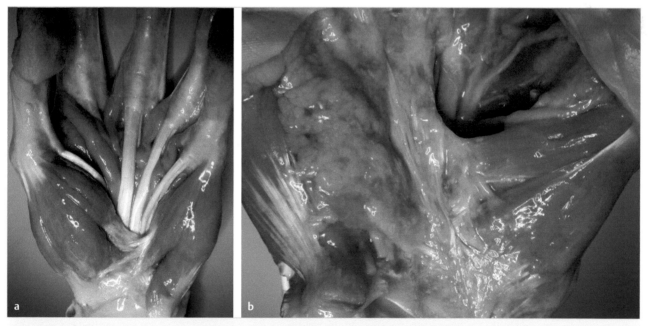

Fig. 18.9 (a, b) The distal muscle aponeurosis. The thenar motor branch of the median nerve is in its usual position.

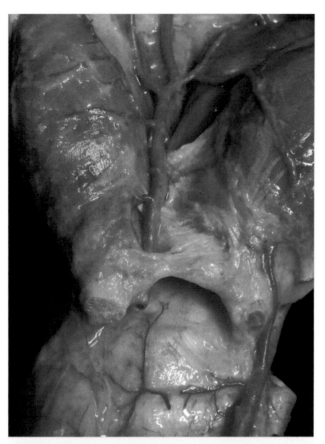

Fig. 18.10 Vascular supply of the flexor retinaculum with branches from the superficial branch of the radial artery and branches from the ulnar artery directly.

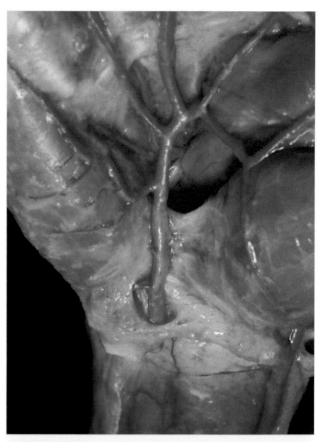

Fig. 18.11 The superficial palmar arch is on the average 12.5 mm away from the distal border of the flexor retinaculum.

At the distal margin of the flexor retinaculum, there is a fat pad[6] that separates the retinaculum from the median nerve and marks an anatomical landmark of the end of the flexor retinaculum and outlines the distal completion of carpal tunnel release. The end of the flexor retinaculum is within 2 mm of the fat pad.

The superficial palmar arch that is formed by the ulnar artery and the superficial branch of the radial artery lies about 12.5 mm from the distal margin of the flexor retinaculum[6–8] (▶ Fig. 18.11). The motor branch of the median nerve is 6.75 mm away.

18.3 Borders

The floor of the tunnel is formed by the capsule covering the central portions of both proximal and distal carpal rows, predominantly the scaphoid, lunate, and capitate (▶ Fig. 18.2). The walls are formed on the radial side by the scaphoid tubercle and trapezium and on the ulnar side by the pisiform and the hook of the hamate. The roof is formed by the flexor retinaculum (▶ Fig. 18.2, ▶ Fig. 18.8). This structure attaches ulnarly to the pisiform and hamate and radially to the scaphoid tuberosity and the medial aspect of the ridge of the trapezium. The ligament is 24 to 36 mm in length.[9]

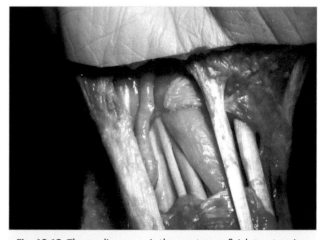

Fig. 18.12 The median nerve is the most superficial structure in the carpal tunnel.

18.4 Contents

The carpal tunnel contains the eight long finger flexor tendons, the long flexor to the thumb, and the median nerve. The median

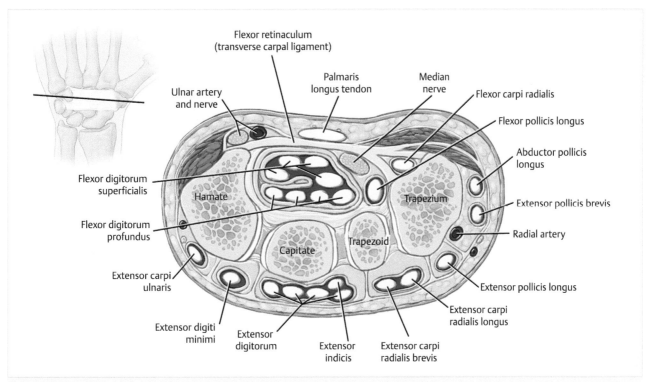

Fig. 18.13 Diagram of the transverse section through the carpal tunnel showing the contents of the carpal tunnel as well as Guyon's canal. (Copyright Mayo Clinic).

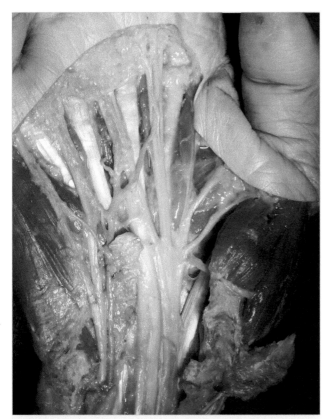

Fig. 18.14 The flexor pollicis longus is the most radial structure in the carpal tunnel.

nerve is the most superficial of the structures (▶ Fig. 18.12), and sits immediately below the palmaris longus tendon before entering the carpal tunnel.[10] The arrangement of the long flexors has some variation, but in general the deepest layer is formed by the index, middle, and ring FDP tendons, with the FDS and little finger FDP arranged above (▶ Fig. 18.13). The FPL tendon sits radial to the FDS tendons (▶ Fig. 18.14) The FPL is the most radial structure in the carpal tunnel. The FCR tendon is contained in a separate tunnel and does not usually enter the carpal tunnel. The motor fibers of the median nerve are located in the radiopalmar portion of the nerve in 60%, in a central location in 22%, and between the two locations in 18%[11] (▶ Fig. 18.15).

The variations in the position of thenar motor branch has been well documented by several investigators.[12,13] The classic article is by Lanz,[14] in which he points out the incidence of thenar branch variations in 100 cadaver to be extraligamentous in 46% (▶ Fig. 18.16a), subligamentous in 31%, and transligamentous in 23%, along with uncommon variations (▶ Fig. 18.16b). There are also unusual variations of the thenar branch of the median nerve that has been documented (▶ Fig. 18.16c).

18.5 Surgical Anatomy

As has been demonstrated in an elegant anatomical study,[15] there are a lot of variations in Kaplan's cardinal line (KCL). This line does not predict the deeper structures. The authors suggested drawing the KCL from the apex of the interdigital

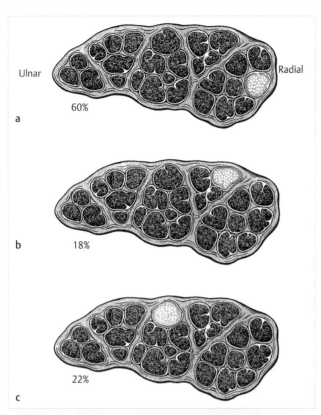

Fig. 18.15 (a–c) The position of the motor fibers in the median nerve inside the carpal tunnel. (Schmidt H-M, Lanz U. Surgical Anatomy of the Hand. Thieme, 2004)

space between the thumb and index finger to the hook of hamate (▶ Fig. 18.17). The motor branch of the median nerve is located proximal and ulnar to the landmark.

The median nerve can shift in the radial or ulnar direction as it passes through the tunnel, and with movement and positioning of the wrist.[16] The ulnar artery also moves with wrist deviation and can extend up to 7 mm radial to the hook of the hamate with ulnar deviation. The average distance from the TCL proximal margin to the origin of the thenar motor branch of the median nerve is 31.3 mm. The origin is usually on the anterolateral aspect of the nerve, but several variations have been described. The average distance from the distal edge of the TCL to the superficial palmer arch is 9.2 mm.[17] The volume of the carpal tunnel is roughly 5 mL but varies with the size of the hand.[18]

There have been many anatomical variations described of the carpal tunnel contents and pathways. Some of the more common anomalies are described in ▶ Table 18.1.[19]

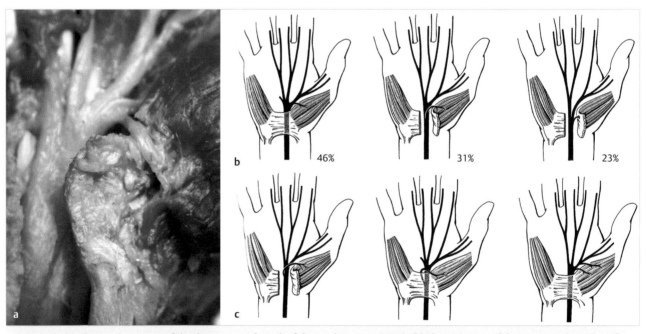

Fig. 18.16 (a) The usual anatomy of the thenar motor branch of the median nerve (46%). (b) The variations of thenar motor branches of the median nerve: extraligamentous in 46%, subligamentous in 31%, and transligamentous in 23%. (c) Unusual variations in the anatomy of the thenar moor branch of the median nerve. (b and c. Schmidt H-M, Lanz U. Surgical Anatomy of the Hand. Thieme, 2004)

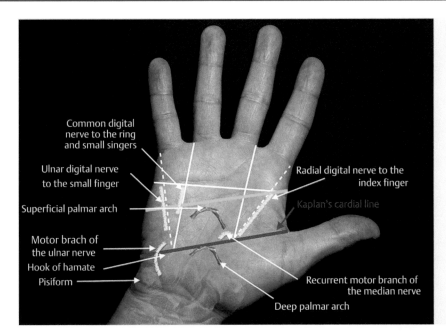

Fig. 18.17 Kaplan's cardinal line and surface markings of the palm.

Common digital nerve to the ring and small singers

Ulnar digital nerve to the small finger

Superficial palmar arch

Motor brach of the ulnar nerve

Hook of hamate

Pisiform

Radial digital nerve to the index finger

Kaplan's cardial line

Recurrent motor branch of the median nerve

Deep palmar arch

Table 18.1 Anatomical anomalies within and around the carpal tunnel

Nerve anomalies

High bifurcation of median nerve

Aberrant origin of motor branch of median nerve (▶ Fig. 18.16b and c).

Transligamentous palmer cutaneous branch of median nerve

Anomalous course of ulnar nerve

Ulnar-to-median nerve connection (Berrettini communication) (Fig. 18.18)

Tendon anomalies

Conjoint FPL and FDP II (Linburg–Comstock syndrome)

Vascular anomalies

Persistent median artery

Superficial ulnar artery

Muscle anomalies

Palmaris longus

Index lumbrical

Flexor digitorum superficialis indices

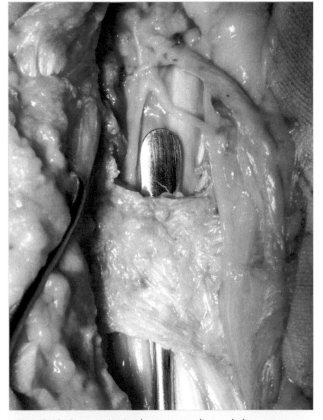

Fig. 18.18 Communication between median and ulnar nerve. (Berrettini Communication)

References

1. Cobb TK, Dalley BK, Posteraro RH, Lewis RC. Anatomy of the flexor retinaculum. J Hand Surg Am 1993;18(1):91–99

2. Morimoto KW, Budoff JE, Haddad J, Gabel GT. Cross-sectional area of the carpal anal proximal and distal to the wrist flexion crease. J Hand Surg Am 2005;30A:487–492

3. Schmidt H-M, Lanz U. Surgical Anatomy of the Hand. Stuttgart, Germany: Thieme; 2004

4. Gelberman RH, Hergenroeder PT, Hargens AR, Lundborg GN, Akeson WH. The carpal tunnel syndrome. A study of carpal canal pressures. J Bone Joint Surg Am 1981;63(3):380–383

5. Godfrey J, Rayan GM. Anatomy of the volar retinacular elements of the hand: a unified nomenclature. J Hand Surg Am 2018;43(3):260–270

6. Madhav TJ, To P, Stern PJ. The palmar fat pad is a reliable intraoperative landmark during carpal tunnel release. J Hand Surg Am 2009;34(7):1204–1209

7. Omokawa S, Tanaka Y, Ryu J, Suzuki J, Kish VL. Anatomy of the ulnar artery as it relates to the transverse carpal ligament. J Hand Surg Am 2002;27(1):101–104

8. Cobb TK, Knudson GA, Cooney WP. The use of topographical landmarks to improve the outcome of Agee endoscopic carpal tunnel release. Arthroscopy 1995;11(2):165–172

9. Johnson RK, Shrewsbury MM. Anatomical course of the thenar branch of the median nerve—usually in a separate tunnel through the transverse carpal ligament. J Bone Joint Surg Am 1970;52(2):269–273

10. Rotman MB, Donovan JP. Practical anatomy of the carpal tunnel. Hand Clin 2002;18(2):219–230

11. Mackinnon SE, Dellon AL. Anatomic investigations of nerves at the wrist: I. Orientation of the motor fascicle of the median nerve in the carpal tunnel. Ann Plast Surg 1988;21(1):32–35

12. Tountas CP, Bihrle DM, MacDonald CJ, Bergman RA. Variations of the median nerve in the carpal canal. J Hand Surg Am 1987; 12(5 Pt 1):708–712

13. Kozin SH. The anatomy of the recurrent branch of the median nerve. J Hand Surg Am 1998;23(5):852–858

14. Lanz U. Anatomical variations of the median nerve in the carpal tunnel. J Hand Surg Am 1977;2(1):44–53

15. Vella JC, Hartigan BJ, Stern PJ. Kaplan's cardinal line. J Hand Surg Am 2006;31(6):912–918

16. Schmidt H-M, Lanz U. Anatomy of the median nerve in the carpal tunnel. In: Richard H, Gelberman MD, eds. Operative Nerve Repair and Reconstruction. Vol II. Philadelphia, PA: JB Lippincott; 1991:889–897

17. Hong JT, Lee SW, Han SH, et al. Anatomy of neurovascular structures around the carpal tunnel during dynamic wrist motion for endoscopic carpal tunnel release. Neurosurgery 2006;58 (1, Suppl):ONS127–ONS133

18. Richman JA, Gelberman RH, Rydevik BL, Gylys-Morin VM, Hajek PC, Sartoris DJ. Carpal tunnel volume determination by magnetic resonance imaging three-dimensional reconstruction. J Hand Surg Am 1987;12(5 Pt 1):712–717

19. Mitchell R, Chesney A, Seal S, McKnight L, Thoma A. Anatomical variations of the carpal tunnel structures. Can J Plast Surg 2009;17(3):e3–e

19 The Hypothenar Area: Anatomy of the Ulnar Carpal Tunnel

Keichi Murata

19.1 Anatomy of the Ulnar Carpal Tunnel

The ulnar carpal tunnel[1] is composed of three distinct parts from a proximal to distal direction: Guyon's canal, the pisohamate tunnel, and the opponens tunnel (▶Fig. 19.1). The ulnar nerve passes through these tunnels, accompanying the ulnar artery.

19.1.1 Guyon's Canal (▶Fig. 19.2, ▶Fig. 19.3, ▶Fig. 19.4, ▶Fig. 19.5)

The anatomic space adjacent to the hypothenar eminence was described by Jean Casimir Félix Guyon, a French surgeon and urologist, as "loge de Guyon" in 1861.[2] As the term *loge* indicates, this space is a hiatus starting at the distal edge of the palmar

carpal ligament proximally and ending at the proximal fibrous arch of the hypothenar fascia distally. However, textbooks sometimes defined it to include the more proximal area where the palmar carpal ligament (PCL) exists. This area is also on the risk of nerve compression. The floor of the tunnel is the flexor digitorum profundus proximally, the flexor retinaculum (FR) distally (▶Fig. 19.4b). The radial boundary of the tunnel is the underlying flexor retinaculum (FR). The pisiform and the flexor carpi ulnaris form the ulnar boundary of the tunnel. The roof of the tunnel is composed of PCL, the palmaris brevis, and hypothenar fat and fibrous tissue. Within this tunnel, the ulnar nerve is accompanied by the ulnar artery radially (▶Fig. 19.2, ▶Fig. 19.3, ▶Fig 19.4) and divides into its deep motor branch and two superficial sensory branches. The superficial branch of the ulnar artery and the arterial branches to the palmaris brevis and the overlying skin pass through the fat tissue at the hiatus. In some hands, the motor branch to the abductor digiti minimi (ADM) is bifurcated

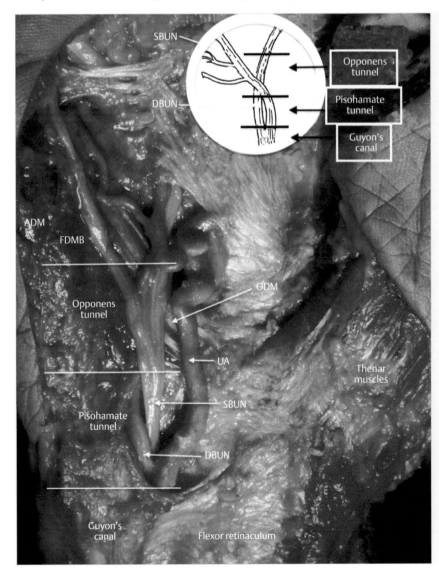

Fig. 19.1 Anatomic location of the ulnar carpal tunnel. (Right hand). ADM: Abductor digiti minimi; FDMB: Flexor digiti minimi brevis; ODM: Opponens digiti minimi; UA: ulnar artery; SBUN: Superficial branch of ulnar nerve; DBUN: Deep branch of ulnar nerve.

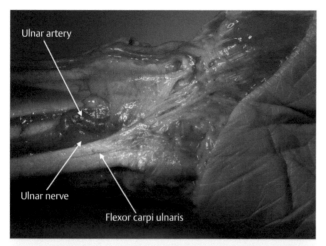

Fig. 19.2 Volar aspect of the distal forearm with the flexor carpi ulnaris (FCU) on the ulnar border of the ulnar artery and the ulnar nerve at entrance to the Guyon's canal.

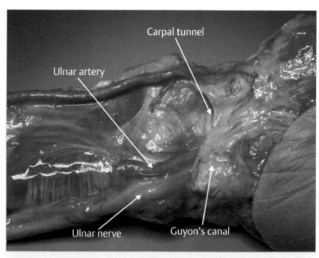

Fig. 19.3 Deeper dissection with structures of the carpal tunnel and FCU removed sahowing the entrance to Guyon's canal.

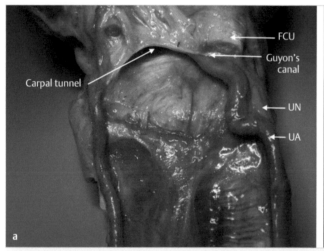

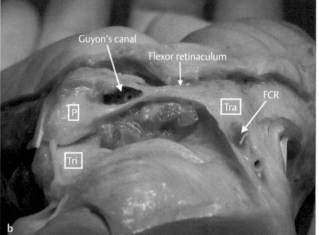

Fig. 19.4 (a) Different perspective at the entrance to Guyon's canal showing the relationship of the tortuous ulnar artery on the radial side of the ulnar nerve. (b) End on perspective showing the relationship of Guyon's canal to the carpal tunnel. The flexor retinaculum forms the roof of the carpal tunnel and the floor of Guyon's canal. FCR: flexor carpi radialis; P: pisiform; Tra: trapezium; Tri: triquetrum

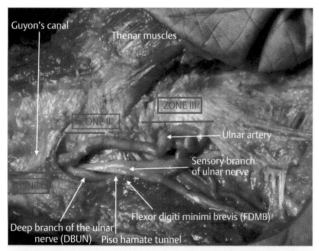

Fig. 19.5 The ulnar nerve divides into the deep branch (DBUN) and the superficial branch (SBUN). The DBUN enters the pisohamate tunnel.

from the main trunk of the ulnar nerve within this tunnel. Guyon's canal continues distally to the pisohamate tunnel, through which the deep branch of the ulnar nerve (DBUN) passes (▶Fig 19.2, ▶Fig. 19.3, ▶Fig. 19.4, ▶Fig. 19.5).[1,3–5]

19.1.2 The Pisohamate Tunnel (▶Fig. 19.6)

The pisohamate tunnel[6] is the middle segment of the ulnar carpal tunnel (▶Fig. 19.6, ▶Fig. 19.7, ▶Fig. 19.8, ▶Fig. 19.9) continuing from Guyon's canal proximally and the opponens tunnel distally. The entrance of the tunnel is formed by the fascial arcade or intermuscular space, consisting of the bony attachment of the hypothenar muscles. Ganglions and other masses in this tunnel can compress the DBUN and cause pure motor ulnar palsy (▶Fig. 19.7). The floor of the tunnel is formed by the pisohamate and pisometacarpal ligament and joint capsule between these bones (▶Fig. 19.9 and ▶Fig. 19.10). The hook of the hamate and the pisiform form the radial and ulnar boundary of the tunnel, respectively.[1,3–5]

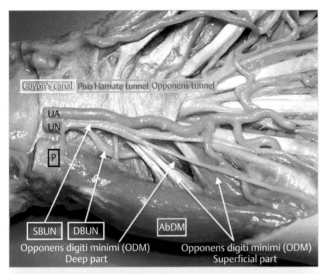

Fig. 19.6 The three parts of the ulnar carpal tunnel: 1. Guyon's canal; 2. the pisohamate tunnel; 3. the opponens tunnel. ADM: Abductor digiti minimi; DBUN: Deep branch of ulnar nerve; SBUN: Superficial branch of ulnar nerve; UA: Ulnar artery; UN: Ulnar nerve.

The structural patterns of the entrance (arcade) of the pisohamate tunnel can be classified into three types (►Fig. 19.11).[7] In type 1, it consists of the intermuscular space between the ADM and the flexor digiti minimi brevis (FDMB). In this type, the fascial continuity between the ADM and the FDMB forms the arched structure (fascial arch) across the hiatus and the DBUN passes under this fascial arch. This type is the most common. In type 2, it consists of the fascial arch between the two origins of the FDMB, the pisiform and the hook of the hamate. In type 3, it consists of the intermuscular space between the ADM and the opponens digiti minimi (ODM). There is no fibrous arcade at the entrance. In this type, the FDMB may be absent. The DBUN passes through this tunnel and then turns radially around the hook of the hamate. In some cases, an artery accompanies the DBUN in this tunnel.

19.1.3 The Opponens Tunnel (►Fig. 19.6)

The opponens tunnel is the third segment of the ulnar carpal tunnel continuing from the pisohamate tunnel distally. The ODM originates from the hook of the hamate, pisohamate ligament, and distal margin of the FR. This muscle splits into two

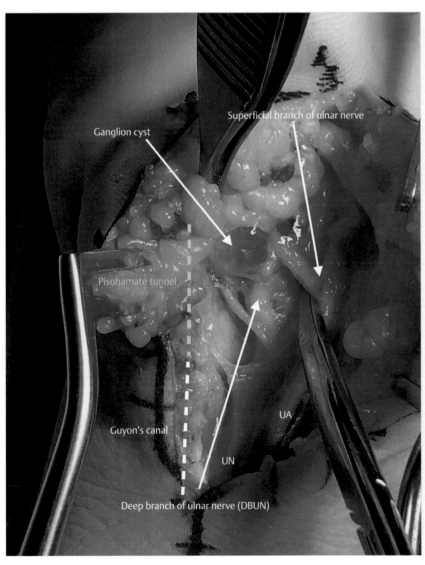

Fig. 19.7 Ganglion cyst compressing the deep branch of the ulnar nerve in the pisohamate tunnel, causing motor ulnar palsy without sensory symptoms.

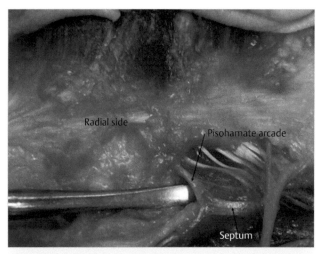

Fig. 19.8 The elevator shows the entrance to the pisohamate tunnel.

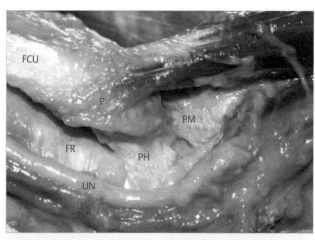

Fig. 19.9 The floor of the Guyon's canal and the pisohamate tunnel. ADM: abductor digiti minimi; FCU: flexor carpi ulnaris; P: Pisiform; FR: flexor retinaculum; PH: pisohamate ligament; PM: pisometacarpal ligament; UA: ulnar artery; UN: ulnar nerve.

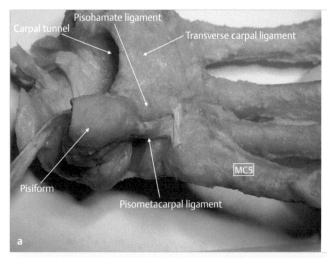

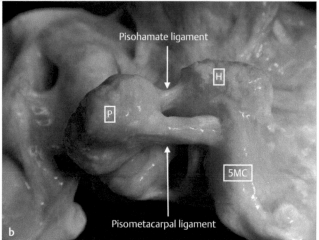

Fig. 19.10 (a, b) Pisohamate and pisometacarpal ligaments that form the floor of the pisohamate tunnel. (P: Pisiform; MC5: 5th metacarpal; 5MC: 5th metacarpal.)

fibromuscular lamellae (superficial and deep), which form a slitlike tunnel. The DBUN passes between the superficial and the deep layers of the ODM and continues radially and dorsally, branching several motor branches to the ODM.[1,3–5]

19.1.4 Anatomical Zones of the Ulnar Carpal Tunnel

The ulnar carpal tunnel has been divided in three zones based on the topography of the nerve and its relationship to the surrounding structures (▶ Fig. 19.12).[8] Zone I consists of the portion of the tunnel proximal to the bifurcation of the DBUN and superficial branches of the ulnar nerve (SBUN). Zone II encompasses the DBUN and surrounding structures. Zone III includes the SBUN and adjacent distal and lateral tissues.

Zone I

Zone I extends approximately 3 cm from the proximal edge of the palmar carpal ligament (PCL) to the bifurcation of the ulnar nerve into the DBUN and the SBUN. The ulnar nerve,

along with the ulnar artery, passes deep to the PCL to enter the ulnar carpal tunnel. The artery is located slightly superficial and radial to the nerve at this level. In Zone I, the ulnar nerve carries both motor and sensory fibers; the palmar–radial fibers contain the fascicles to become the SBUN, whereas the dorsal–ulnar fibers contain the fascicles to become the DBUN. Therefore, a lesion in Zone I will have a high likelihood of producing both motor and sensory deficits.

Zone II

Zone II encompasses the portion of the ulnar carpal tunnel distal to the bifurcation of the ulnar nerve, in the region where the DBUN passes. Zone II is consistent with combination of the pisohamate and the opponens tunnels. The DBUN in Zone II is purely motor; therefore, lesions in this zone produce only motor deficits.

Zone III

Zone III originates just distal to the bifurcation of the ulnar nerve. This zone encompasses the SBUN. This zone is located

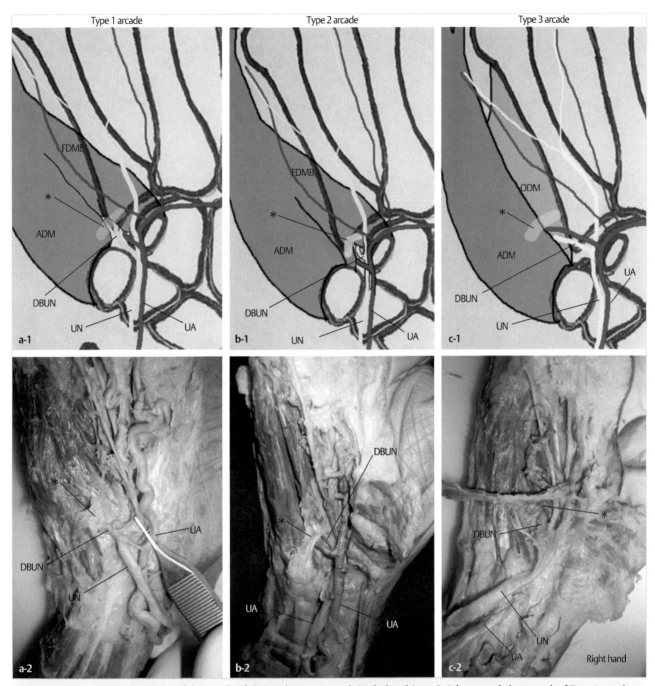

Fig. 19.11 The structural patterns of the arcade of the pisohamate tunnel. (Right hands) a-1,2: Scheme and photograph of Type 1 arcade, respectively. b-1,2: Scheme and photograph of Type 2 arcade, respectively. c-1,2: Scheme and photograph of Type 3 arcade, respectively. *Arcade, ADM: Abductor digiti minimi, FDMB: Flexor digiti minimi brevis, ODM: Opponens digiti minimi, DBUN: Deep branch of the ulnar nerve, UN: Ulnar nerve, UA: Ulnar artery.

in superficial layer between the hypothenar fascia dorsally and subcutaneous tissue palmarly. As the SBUN continues distally, it gives off small branches that innervate the palmaris brevis. The SBUN in Zone III contains mostly sensory fibers, along with motor fibers to the hypothenar muscles. Lesions in this zone will produce primarily sensory deficits, with possible motor weakness of the hypothenar muscles.

19.2 Muscle Anatomy

19.2.1 Palmaris Brevis

The palmaris brevis is a thin and small quadrangular muscle located between the hypothenar fascia and the skin at the ulnar side of the palm. The muscle fibers of this muscle are perpendicular to the axis of the upper extremity.[4,9,10]

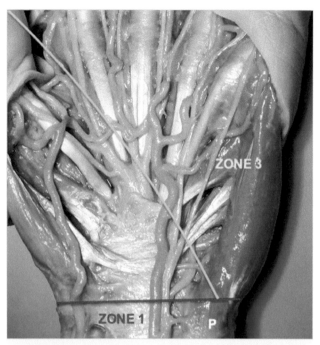

Fig. 19.12 Scheme of the three zones of the ulnar carpal tunnel.

Origin: The muscle arises from the FR and the medial border of the central part of the palmar aponeurosis.[4,9,10]

Insertion: The muscle fibers insert into the dermis on the ulnar border of the hand.

Function: It provides wrinkling of the skin on the ulnar side of the palm of the hand and deepens the hollow of the palm by accentuating the hypothenar eminence.[9,10]

Innervation: The nerve supply arises from the SBUN.[4,9,10]

Blood supply: The branch from the superficial palmar arch (SPA) gives blood supply to this muscle.[4,9,10]

Variations: The muscle varies greatly in size. This muscle may be absent or doubled. It sometimes inserts into the FDMB or the pisiform.[9,10] The palmaris brevis profundus muscle has been found to arise transversely from the FR and the palmar aponeurosis to the pisiform and may be located within Guyon's canal; therefore, it may cause ulnar nerve compression.[11]

19.2.2 Abductor Digiti Minimi

The ADM is the most ulnar of the three hypothenar muscles and lies on the ulnar border of the palm. It is a flat fusiform muscle.[4,9,10]

Origin: (▶ Fig 19.13 a–d) The muscle arises from the pisiform, the flexor carpi ulnaris tendon, and the pisohamate ligament.[4,9,10]

Insertion: The muscle insertion has two variations (▶ Fig. 19.13 b, c).[7,12,13] In a few hands, it has only one slip inserting onto the ulnar side of the base of the proximal phalanx of the small finger. In more hands, insertion of the muscle has two slips. In addition to the insertion to the proximal phalanx, the other slip continues distally and dorsally to join the aponeurosis of the extensor tendon of the small finger.

Function: The muscle adducts the small finger (proximal phalanx) from the ring finger (thus spreading the fourth web

space when the digits are extended). In the hand, its insertion connects to the extensor mechanism and provides flexion of the proximal phalanx and extension of the distal two phalanges.[9,10]

Innervation: The nerve supply arises from the DBUN. The branching patterns of the motor branch to the ADM vary as are described in the section of the nerve anatomy.[7,9,10]

Blood supply: The artery accompanying the deep branch of the ulnar nerve (AADBUN) or its branch, the ulnar artery, the SPA, and palmar digital artery of the small finger give blood supply to this muscle.[7,9,10]

Variations: The muscle may be absent or united with the FDMB. It occasionally has two or three muscle bellies.[7,9,10] Several types of the aberrant muscle have been reported.[7,9,14–19] The accessory ADM, which originates from the FR, the antebrachial fascia, or the tendon of the flexor carpi ulnaris or palmaris longus, is fused with the ADM distally (▶ Fig. 19.14a).[9] The pisiuncinatus, a small muscle occurring in 2 to 5% of hands, extends between the pisiform and the hook of the hamate.[9] This muscle may pass between the ulnar nerve and artery. The pisiannularis extends from the pisiform to the FR (▶ Fig. 19.14b).[9] Another small aberrant muscle originated from the pisiform and inserted onto the volar aspect of the head of small finger metacarpal dorsally to the ADM (▶ Fig. 19.14c).[7] These aberrant ADM may cause symptoms of compression neuropathy of the ulnar nerve.[14–16,18]

19.2.3 Flexor Digiti Minimi Brevis

The FDMB lies deep and adjacent to the ADM, along the radial border of the ADM and coursing in the same direction. It is a flat fusiform muscle. The muscle may have two bellies. It often fuses with the ADM; it has common insertions with the ADM. It may also fuses with the ODM at the place of origin. Its fusion with the ADM and with ODM can be combined.[4,9,10]

Origin: The muscle originates from the hook of the hamate, the adjacent ulnar portion of the FR, and/or the radial portion of the pisiform.[7,9,10] The FDMB occasionally is fused with ODM at the place of origin.[7] Two origins of the FDMB onto the pisiform and the hook of the hamate occasionally form the fascial arcade for the DBUN.[7]

Insertion: When the FDMB is fused distally with the ADM, it has common insertions with the ADM.[7] In the hand where the FDMB exists independently it inserts onto the volar aspect of the head of the fifth metacarpal.[4,7,9,10]

Function: The muscle flexes the proximal phalanx of the small finger. When the FDMB has common insertion with the ADM, it assists in extension of the two distal phalanges of the small finger.[9,10]

Innervation: The muscle is innervated by a branch from the SBUN or the DBUN. The nerve to the ADM and the FDMB may arise together as a single branch.[7,9,10]

Blood supply: The AADBUN or its branch, the ulnar artery, the SPA, and palmar digital artery of the small finger give blood supply to this muscle.[7,9,10]

Variations: The FDMB may be absent or fused with the ADM or the ODM.[7,9,10] The muscle may have an accessory slip from the forearm fascia and/or the metacarpal to the small finger.[9,10] The muscle may be replaced by a tendinous band that arises

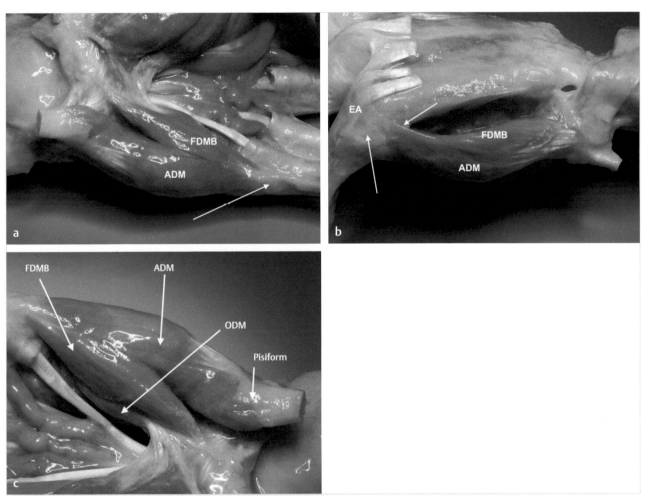

Fig. 19.13 (**a, b**) Two forms of the ADM insertion viewed from the ulnar side of the left hand. (**a**) ADM inserts only to the the proximal phalanx, (**b**) ADM inserts to both the proximal phalanx and dorsal slip to the aponeurosis of the extensor tendon. (**c**) Insertion of ADM and FDMB is integrated into the proximal phalanx. Viewed from voloulnar aspect of the left hand. ADM: abductor digiti minimi, FDMB: flexor digiti miniimi breis, ODM: opponens digiti minimi, EA: extensor aponeurosis.

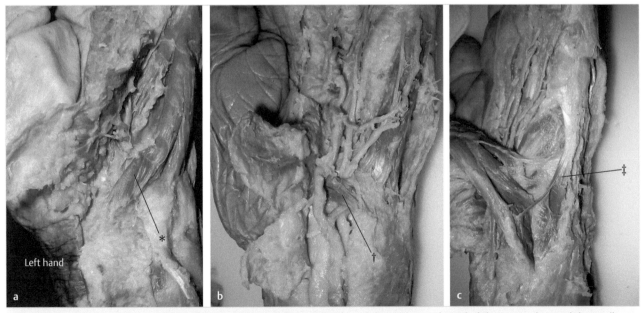

Fig. 19.14 Variation of aberrant abductor digiti minimi (AbDM). (Left hands) a: *The accessory AbDM, b: †The pisiannularis, c: ‡The small aberrant muscle originated from the pisiform and inserted onto the volar aspect of the head of small finger metacarpal dorsally to the AbDM.

from the flexor carpi ulnaris and inserts onto the base of the fifth proximal phalanx and the hook of the hamate.[9] The tensor capsularis articulationis metacarpophalangei digiti minimi is a small muscle that arises from the pisohamate ligament and inserts into the palmar surface of the metacarpophalangeal joint of the small finger.[9] The ulnaris externus brevis rarely exists, arising about 6.5 cm proximal to the distal end of the ulna. It inserts onto the fourth and fifth metacarpals.[9]

19.2.4 Opponens Digiti Minimi

The ODM lies deep to the ADM and the FDMB. It is triangular, broad at its base and tapering to the apex distally. It has two layers of the superficial and deep origins. The space between these layers is the opponens tunnel, through which the DBUN passes.[1,4,7]

Origin: The superficial and deep layers of the ODM originate from the distal part of the hook of the hamate and the part of the ulnar flexor compartment wall that is adjacent to the hook of the hamate, respectively.[1,4,7]

Insertion: The superficial and deep layer insert into the distal and proximal ulnar side of the fifth metacarpal shaft, respectively.[1,4,7]

Function: The ODM permits opposition of the small finger to the thumb. This is a combination movement of abduction, flexion, and lateral rotation of the metacarpal of the small finger.[9,10]

Innervation: The muscle is innervated by a branch from the DBUN before the nerve passes through the muscle.[7,9,10]

Blood supply: The AADBUN or its branch, the distal deep palmar branch of the ulnar artery (DDPBUA) or its branch, the SPA, and the deep palmar arch (DPA) give blood supply to this muscle.[9,10]

Variations: The width of deep layer's insertion to the fifth metacarpal varies greatly. It may be so thin that it looks like membrane.[7]

19.3 Nerve Anatomy

19.3.1 The Arborization of the Ulnar Nerve at the Hypothenar Area

The arborization of the ulnar nerve at the hypothenar area varies,[7,20] and can be classified into five types according to their morphologic characteristics (▶ Fig. 19.15).[7] In type 1, the ulnar

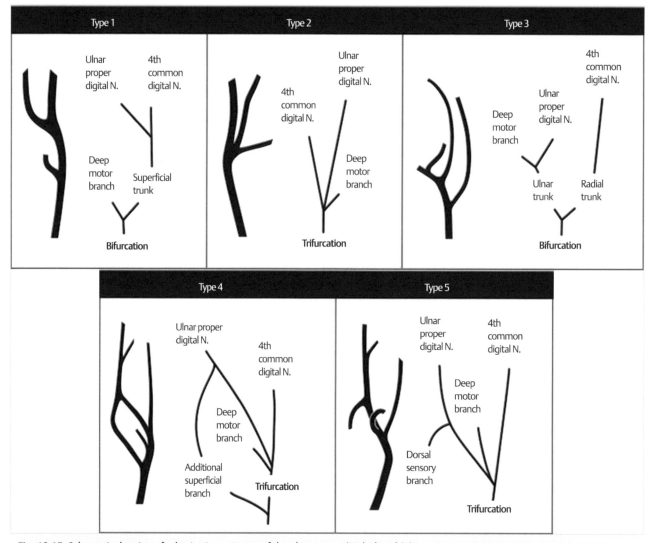

Fig. 19.15 Schematic drawing of arborization patterns of the ulnar nerve. (Right hands) (From Murata K, Tamai M, Gupta A. Anatomic study of variations of hypothenar muscles and arborization patterns of the ulnar nerve in the hand. J Hand Surg 2004;29A:500–509.)

nerve bifurcates into the DBUN and a superficial trunk just distal to the distal edge of the pisiform (►Fig. 19.16a). The superficial trunk bifurcates distally into two sensory branches: the fourth common digital nerve and the ulnar proper digital nerve of the small finger. This type is the most common. In type 2, the ulnar nerve trifurcates into the ring finger common digital nerve, the ulnar proper digital nerve of the small finger, and the DBUN just distal to the distal edge of the pisiform (►Fig. 19.16b). In type 3, the ulnar nerve bifurcates into radial and ulnar trunks just distal to the distal edge of the pisiform (►Fig. 19.16c). The radial trunk continues to the ring finger common digital nerve and the ulnar trunk bifurcates distally into the ulnar proper digital nerve of the small finger and the DBUN. In type 4, an additional superficial branch originates from the main trunk of the ulnar nerve in Guyon's canal and communicates with the ulnar proper digital nerve of small finger distally (►Fig. 19.16d). The main trunk trifurcates into the ring finger common digital nerve, the ulnar proper digital nerve of small finger, and the DBUN just distal to the distal

edge of the pisiform. In type 5, the dorsal sensory branch of the ulnar nerve connects with the ulnar proper digital nerve of the small finger (►Fig. 19.16e). The main trunk trifurcates into the ring finger common digital nerve, the ulnar proper digital nerve of the small finger, and the DBUN just distal to the distal edge of the pisiform.

19.3.2 The Branching Patterns of the Motor Branch to the ADM

The branching patterns of the motor branch to the ADM are classified into four types (►Fig. 19.17).[7] In type 1, a motor branch to the ADM originates from the DBUN within the pisohamate tunnel. In type 2, a main motor branch to the ADM originates from the DBUN within Guyon's canal and an additional motor branch to the ADM originates from the DBUN within the pisohamate tunnel. In type 3, the ulnar nerve

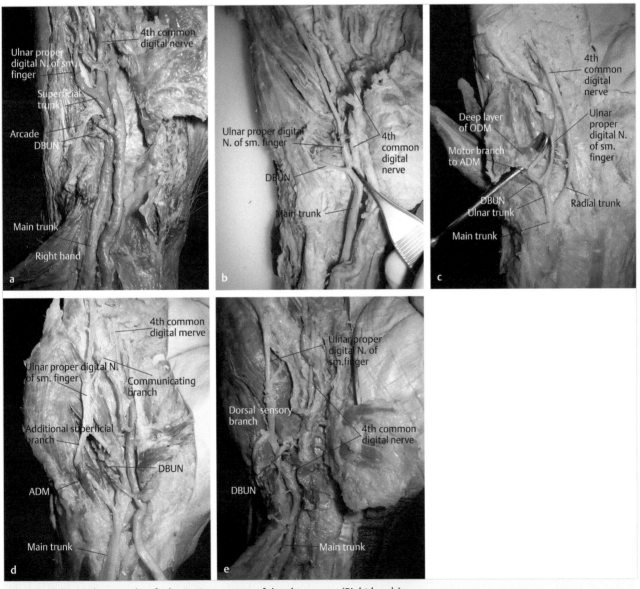

Fig. 19.16 (a–e) Photographs of arborization patterns of the ulnar nerve. (Right hands)

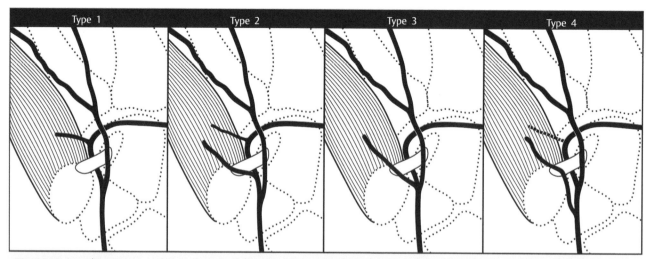

Fig. 19.17 Branching patterns of motor branch of abductor digiti minimi (ADM). (Right hands) (From Murata K, Tamai M, Gupta A. Anatomic study of variations of hypothenar muscles and arborization patterns of the ulnar nerve in the hand. J Hand Surg 2004;29A: 500–509. With permission.)

trifurcates into a superficial trunk, the DBUN, and a motor branch to the ADM in Guyon's canal. In type 4, a main motor branch to the ADM originates from the main trunk of the ulnar nerve within Guyon's canal. In hands classified as type 4, an additional motor branch to the ADM may originate from the DBUN within the pisohamate tunnel.

19.3.3 The Deep Branch of the Ulnar Nerve

The DBUN supplies one to several branches to the hypothenar muscles.[7,20] Many muscles receive cross-innervation from multiple motor branches, and many motor branches innervate multiple muscles. There is no correlation between the number of the hypothenar muscles and the number of hypothenar nerve branches. After the DBUN passes through the opponens tunnel, it runs deep to the extrinsic flexor tendons but palmar to the interossei. The DBUN innervates each of the seven interossei, the third and fourth lumbricals, the adductor pollicis, and the flexor pollicis brevis.[7] The terminal branch of the DBUN provides sensory afferent nerves to the ulnocarpal, intercarpal, and carpometacarpal joints.[1,5,7]

19.3.4 The Superficial Branch of the Ulnar Nerve

After deviation of the ulnar nerve into the DBUN and the SBUN, the SBUN lies superficial to the hypothenar fascia.[1,5,7] The SBUN provides several small twigs to innervate the skin on the ulnar side of the hand.[1,5] The motor branches to the palmaris brevis may branch off at this point.[5,20] The nerve continues distally and radially and divides into the proper digital nerve to the ulnar side of the small finger and the common palmar digital nerve to the fourth web space.[1,5,7] In the palm, the SBUN lies dorsal to the SPA and palmar to the flexor tendons.[1,5,7]

19.3.5 Other Communicating Branches

There may be a communicating branch between the two sensory branches to the fingers and/or between the dorsal sensory branch of the ulnar nerve and the ulnar proper digital nerve of the small finger (▶ Fig. 19.16e).[5,7] The SBUN and/or these communicating branches may pass through the muscle belly of the ADM.[7] In many hands, there may be a superficial communication branch between the median and ulnar nerves (▶ Fig. 19.16d).[5,7,21–23]

19.4 Vascular Anatomy

19.4.1 Anatomic Variations of the Ulnar Artery and Its Branches

The ulnar artery continues distally to the SPA, which starts after the ulnar artery branches off the deep branches of the ulnar artery.[1,24] Complex anatomical variations of the ulnar artery and its branches in the hypothenar area have been described.[24–28] Four arborization patterns of the ulnar artery in Guyon's canal and the hypothenar area are identified: 1UA, 2UA, 3UA, and 4UA (▶ Fig. 19.18).[28] In type 1UA, the AADBUN passes through the fascial arch of the hypothenar muscles and forms a DPA. No other branches enter the midpalmar space distally (▶ Fig. 19.19a). Feeding arteries of the ADM, the ODM, and/ or the FDMB originate from the AADBUN in this type. This type is most common. In type 2UA, the AADBUN continues to the feeding artery of the ADM and does not form a DPA (▶ Fig. 19.19b). In addition, a DDPBUA branches off distally and enter the retrotendinous midpalmar space between the flexor tendon sheath of the small finger and the FDMB. This arterial structure forms a DPA. In most hands of this type, the feeding artery of the FDMB originates from the SPA and occasionally from the ulnar palmar digital artery

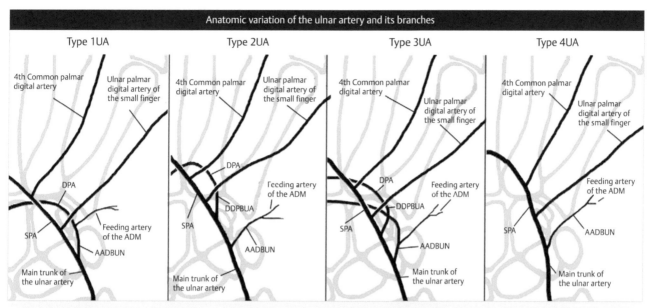

Fig. 19.18 Schematic drawing of anatomic variation of the ulnar artery and its branches. (Left hands)

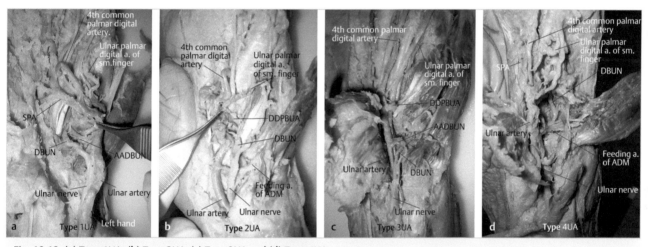

Fig. 19.19 (a) Type 1UA; (b) Type 2UA; (c) Type 3UA and (d) Type 4UA.

of the small finger. The feeding arteries of the ODM originate from the DPA in type 2UA. In type 3UA, both the AADBUN and the DDPBUA form DPAs (▶Fig. 19.19c). The feeding artery of the ADM originates from the AADBUN in type 3UA, and the feeding artery of the FDMB originates from the AADBUN or the SPA. The feeding arteries of the ODM originate from the DDPBUA in type 3UA. In type 4UA, the AADBUN continues to the feeding artery of the ADM. No

DDPBUA exists in this type and therefore neither does a DPA (▶Fig. 19.19d). The feeding artery to the FDMB and ODM originates from the SPA.

In addition, a dorsal perforating artery of the ulnar artery occasionally exists (▶Fig. 19.20). This branch originates from the AADBUN at the level of the distal edge of the pisiform, passing dorsally through the soft tissue of the triquetral–hamate joint and merging with the dorsal carpal arterial arch.[28]

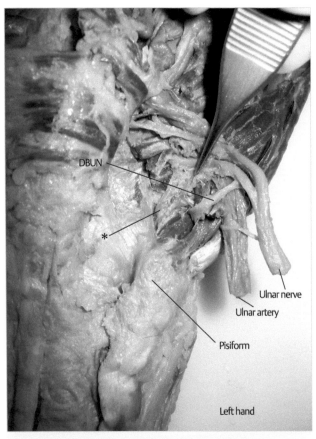

Fig. 19.20 The cut ulnar artery and ulnar nerve lifted up to expose*. *Dorsal perforating artery of the ulnar artery

References

1. Peripheral nerves. In: Chase RA, eds. Atlas of Hand Surgery. Vol 2. Philadelphia, PA: WB Saunders; 1984:102–1102.

2. Guyon F. Note sur une disposition anatomique proper a la face anterieure de la region du poignet et non encore decrite par le decteur. Bull Soc Anat Paris 1861;6:181–186

3. Botte MJ, Gelberman RH. Ulnar nerve compression at the wrist. In: Szabo RM, ed. Nerve Compression Syndromes, Diagnosis and Treatment. Thorofare, NJ: Slack Inc.; 1989:121–136

4. Williams PL, ed. Gray's Anatomy. 38th ed. New York, NY: Churchill Livingstone; 1995:737–900

5. Botte MJ. Nerve anatomy. In: Doyle JR, Botte MJ, eds. Surgical Anatomy of the Hand & Upper Extremity. Philadelphia, PA: Lippincott Williams & Wilkins; 2003:185–236

6. Uriburu IJ, Morchio FJ, Marin JC. Compression syndrome of the deep motor branch of the ulnar nerve. (Piso-Hamate Hiatus syndrome). J Bone Joint Surg Am 1976;58(1):145–147

7. Murata K, Tamai M, Gupta A. Anatomic study of variations of hypothenar muscles and arborization patterns of the ulnar nerve in the hand. J Hand Surg Am 2004;29(3):500–509

8. Gross MS, Gelberman RH. The anatomy of the distal ulnar tunnel. Clin Orthop Relat Res 1985;(196):238–247

9. Tountas CP, Bergman RA, eds. Anatomic Variations of the Upper Extremity. New York, NY: Churchill Livingstone; 1993:53–186

10. Botte MJ. Muscle anatomy. In: Doyle JR, Botte MJ, eds. Surgical Anatomy of the Hand & Upper Extremity. Philadelphia, PA: Lippincott Williams & Wilkins; 2003:92–184

11. Tonkin MA, Lister GD. The palmaris brevis profundus. An anomalous muscle associated with ulnar nerve compression at the wrist. J Hand Surg Am 1985;10(6 Pt 1):862–864

12. Kanaya K, Wada T, Isogai S, Murakami G, Ishii S. Variation in insertion of the abductor digiti minimi: an anatomic study. J Hand Surg Am 2002;27(2):325–328

13. von Schroeder HP, Botte MJ. The dorsal aponeurosis, intrinsic, hypothenar, and thenar musculature of the hand. Clin Orthop Relat Res 2001;(383):97–107

14. Fahrer M, Millroy PJ. Ulnar compression neuropathy due to an anomalous abductor digiti minimi-clinical and anatomic study. J Hand Surg Am 1981;6(3):266–268

15. James MR, Rowley DI, Norris SH. Ulnar nerve compression by an accessory abductor digiti minimi muscle presenting following injury. Injury 1987;18(1):66–67

16. Luethke R, Dellon AL. Accessory abductor digiti minimi muscle originating proximal to the wrist causing symptomatic ulnar nerve compression. Ann Plast Surg 1992;28(3):307–308

17. Sañudo JR, Mirapeix RM, Ferreira B. A rare anomaly of abductor digiti minimi. J Anat 1993;182(Pt 3):439–442

18. Netscher D, Cohen V. Ulnar nerve compression at the wrist secondary to anomalous muscles: a patient with a variant of abductor digiti minimi. Ann Plast Surg 1997;39(6):647–651

19. Curry B, Kuz J. A new variation of abductor digiti minimi accessorius. J Hand Surg Am 2000;25(3):585–587

20. Lindsey JT, Watumull D. Anatomic study of the ulnar nerve and related vascular anatomy at Guyon's canal: a practical classification system. J Hand Surg Am 1996;21(4):626–633

21. Bonnel F, Vila RM. Anatomical study of the ulnar nerve in the hand. J Hand Surg [Br] 1985;10(2):165–168

22. Meals RA, Shaner M. Variations in digital sensory patterns: a study of the ulnar nerve-median nerve palmar communicating branch. J Hand Surg Am 1983;8(4):411–414

23. Ferrari GP, Gilbert A. The superficial anastomosis on the palm of the hand between the ulnar and median nerves. J Hand Surg [Br] 1991;16(5):511–514

24. Coleman SS, Anson BJ. Arterial patterns in the hand based upon a study of 650 specimens. Surg Gynecol Obstet 1961; 113:409–424

25. Gelberman RH, Panagis JS, Taleisnik J, Baumgaertner M. The arterial anatomy of the human carpus. Part I: The extraosseous vascularity. J Hand Surg Am 1983;8(4):367–375

26. König PS, Hage JJ, Bloem JJ, Prosé LP. Variations of the ulnar nerve and ulnar artery in Guyon's canal: a cadaveric study. J Hand Surg Am 1994;19(4):617–622

27. Gellman H, Botte MJ, Shankwiler J, Gelberman RH. Arterial patterns of the deep and superficial palmar arches. Clin Orthop Relat Res 2001;(383):41–46

28. Murata K, Tamai M, Gupta A. Anatomic study of arborization patterns of the ulnar artery in Guyon's canal. J Hand Surg Am 2006;31(2):258–263

20 Anatomy of the Wrist Joint

Nathan Polley and Amit Gupta

20.1 Bones of the Wrist

The wrist is generally described as a joint with motion between the eight individual carpal bones and between the proximal and distal rows. These eight carpal bones can be divided into two rows, the proximal and distal carpal rows. The proximal row consists of the scaphoid, lunate, triquetrum, and pisiform. The distal row is comprised of the trapezium, trapezoid, capitate, and hamate. (▶Fig. 20.1, ▶Fig. 20.2, ▶Fig. 20.3).[1]

20.1.1 Extensor Retinaculum

The extensor retinaculum forms the dorsal strap of the wrist, helping anchor the extensors of the wrist and fingers in separate compartments. Unlike descriptions in anatomical texts with diagrams, the extensor retinaculum is a three-dimensional structure (▶Fig. 20.4a). The first compartment contains the extensor pollicis brevis (EPB), the abductor pollicis longus (APL), and frequently multiple tendons of accessory APL. This compartment may be subdivided into two, with the EPB running in its own compartment.

The second compartment contains the extensor carpi radialis longus and the extensor carpi radialis brevis. The third compartment contains the extensor pollicis longus tendon. The fourth compartment contains the extensor digitorum communis (EDC) and the extensor indicis tendons. A more superficial fifth compartment contains the extensor digiti minimi tendon. (▶Fig. 20.4b).

The sixth compartment is very special. It divides into two layers to enclose the extensor carpi ulnaris tendon. The deep layer of the compartment is intimately related to the triangular fibrocartilage (TFC) and forms the peripheral layer of the TFC. Whereas the other five compartments are fixed to the radius, the sixth compartment moves with the ulna in pronation and supination, staying relatively fixed by the subsheath to the ulna.

20.1.2 Flexor Retinaculum

The carpus is curved on the palmar surface. The space between the scaphoid and trapezium on the radial side and the hook of the hamate and pisiform on the ulnar side is the area of the carpal tunnel and is bounded on the palmar aspect by the flexor retinaculum (▶Fig. 20.5a). The flexor retinaculum consists of three fibrous bands that extend between the trapezium and the

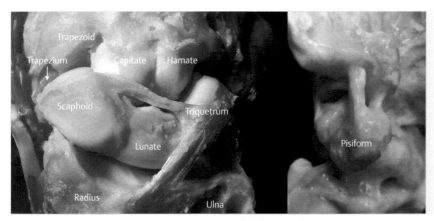

Fig. 20.1 Dorsal and palmar view of the bones of the right wrist.

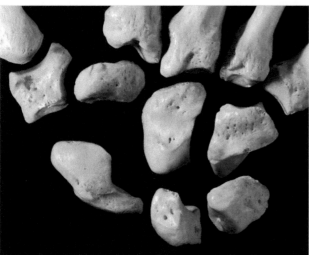

Fig. 20.2 Bones of the right wrist. Dorsal View.

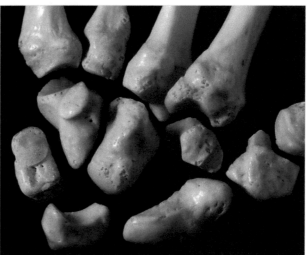

Fig. 20.3 Bones of the right wrist. Volar View.

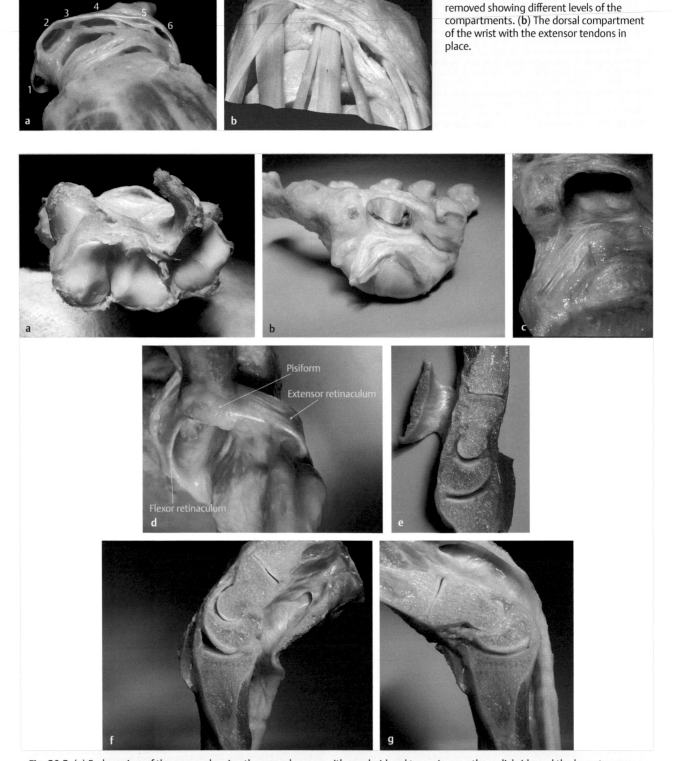

Fig. 20.4 (a) The dorsal compartments of the extensor retinaculum with the tendons removed showing different levels of the compartments. (b) The dorsal compartment of the wrist with the extensor tendons in place.

Fig. 20.5 (a) End-on view of the carpus showing the curved carpus with scaphoid and trapezium on the radial side and the hamate especially the hook on the ulnar side. (b) The flexor retinaculum and the curved carpus. (c) The relationship between the volar ligaments of the carpus and the flexor retinaculum. (d) The extensor and flexor retinaculum encircle the wrist like a watch strap and meet at their insertion into the pisiform. (e–g) The space between the carpus and the flexor retinaculum is maximum in the neutral position of the wrist (e); the space and thus the volume decreases in flexion (f) and extension (g) of the wrist.

hamate, the trapezium and the pisiform, and the scaphoid and the hamate (▶Fig. 20.5b,c).

The pisiform forms a key structure. The extensor and flexor retinaculum encircle the wrist like a watch strap and meet at their insertion into the pisiform (▶Fig. 20.5d).

In the neutral position, the carpal tunnel volume and the space between the flexor retinaculum and the carpus are at their maximum. These parameters decrease in flexion and extension especially in hyperextension (▶Fig. 20.5e,f,g).

20.1.3 Ligaments of the Wrist

There are countless articles, academic texts, and cadaveric and anatomic studies attempting to define the complex anatomy, function, and orientation of the ligaments of the wrist.

Verbal communication from Taleisnik to Berger was discussed in an article by Berger in 2001, stating that "anatomy does not change, only our descriptions of anatomy change."[2] Taleisnik defined the wrist ligaments as extrinsic and intrinsic, which are based on anatomic location.[3] Extrinsic ligaments originate proximal to the carpal bones and course distally to insert onto the carpal bones (▶Fig. 20.6), while intrinsic ligaments are found solely within the boundaries of the carpal bones (▶Fig. 20.7).[1] Berger and Landsmeer consider the majority of the wrist ligaments to be intracapsular ligaments, which essentially means they are confined between the synovium and fibrous layer of the joint capsule.[4]

20.2 Extrinsic Ligaments

The volar extrinsic ligaments consist of the radioscaphocapitate (RSC), long radiolunate (LRL), radioscapholunate (RSL), short radiolunate (SRL) and the ulnocarpal ligaments (UCL). The ulnocarpal ligaments will be discussed in Chapter 24. The dorsal radiocarpal ligament makes up the dorsal extrinsic system. In regard to origin and insertion, we will refer to origin as proximal and insertion as distal. The volar extrinsic ligaments are difficult to see when viewed from a volar approach. The volar wrist appears as a homogenous layer (▶Fig. 20.8). In situ, these ligaments can be identified through a dorsally inserted arthroscope (▶Fig. 20.9) or dorsal capsulotomy with hyperflexion (▶Fig. 20.10).

20.3 Radioscaphocapitate Ligament

The radioscaphocapitate (RSC) ligament (▶Fig. 20.11, ▶Fig. 20.12) has also been termed the radioscaphoid, radiocapitate, arcuate, and deltoid ligament.[5] The name radioscaphocapitate is largely recognized and used in most literature, thereby adequately describing the ligamentous attachments to the respective carpal bones. The RSC ligament originates from the radial

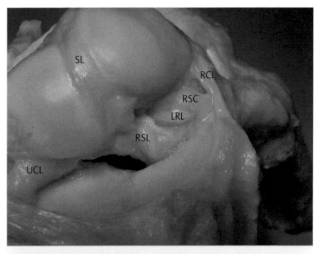

Fig. 20.7 The intrinsic ligaments of the wrist (scapholunate ligament) and the extrinsic volar radiocarpal ligaments from the dorsal wrist with the wrist hyper flexed. SL: Scapholunate ligament, RCL: Radial Collateral Ligament, RSC: Radioscaphocapitate Ligament, LRL: Long Radiolunate Ligament, RSL: Radioscapholunate ligament, UCL: Ulnar carpal Ligaments.

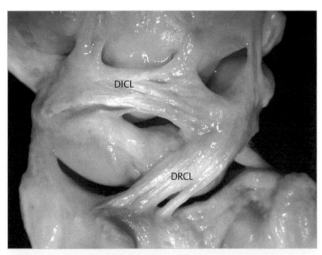

Fig. 20.6 Dorsal extrinsic ligaments of the right wrist. DICL: Dorsal Intercarpal Ligament, DRCL: Dorsal Radiocarpal Ligament.

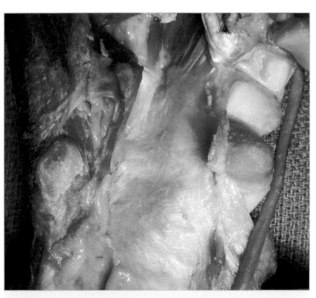

Fig. 20.8 The volar carpal ligaments appear as a homogeneous layer when viewed from the volar aspect.

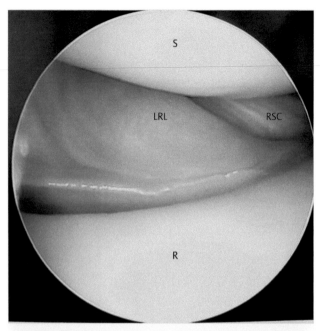

Fig. 20.9 The volar carpal ligaments seen through an arthroscope.

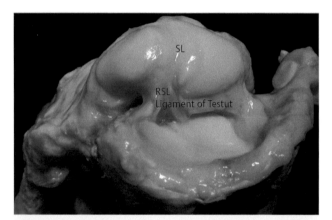

Fig. 20.10 The volar carpal ligaments can also be seen from the dorsal side after hyper flexing the right wrist. SL: Scapholunate Ligament, RSL: Radioscapholunate Ligament.

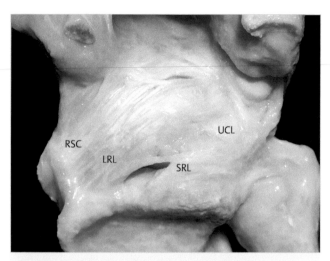

Fig. 20.11 Volar extrinsic ligaments showing the radioscaphocapitate ligament, the long radiolunate and the ulnocarpal ligaments (left wrist). LRL: Long Radiolunate Ligament, RSC: Radioscaphocapitate Ligament, SRL: short radiolunate ligament, UCL: Ulnar carpal Ligaments.

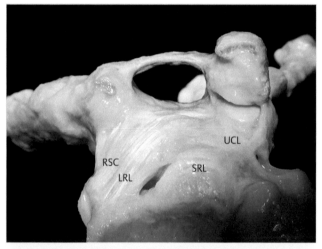

Fig. 20.12 The relationship of the carpal tunnel to the volar extrinsic ligaments (left wrist). LRL: Long Radiolunate Ligament, RSC: Radioscaphocapitate Ligament, SRL: short radiolunate ligament, UCL: Ulnar carpal Ligaments.

styloid of the distal radius with the radial most fibers inserting onto the waist of the scaphoid. Although debated, this portion is referred to as the collateral component of the lateral wrist: radial collateral ligament (RCL) (▶Fig. 20.13). The remaining fibers are oriented obliquely and ulnarly toward the capitate. Radially, these fibers will coalesce with the scaphocapitate ligament[6] and some fibers will largely interdigitate with fibers of the ulnocapitate ligament and meet at the base of the capitate (▶Fig. 20.13, ▶Fig. 20.14).

This coalescence of the RSC with the ulnocapitate ligament, gives the classic arch or inverted **V** shape and has been historically termed the "arcuate" or "deltoid" ligament. Controversy exists over whether there is direct attachment of the RSC to the capitate (▶Fig. 20.15). A small percentage of fibers attach to the waist of the capitate, but whether these are directly from the RSC itself, are coalescences from the scaphocapitate ligament and RSC, or are merely synovial reflections from the RSC is debated. These anatomical variations may be purely academic, and it is unknown whether these contribute to any significant

biomechanical stability, as this attachment, being at the proximal nonarticular neck of the capitate, is thought to act only as a "sling" for support of the capitate.[1,5] This insertion completes what Berger and Landsmeer described as three major components of the RSC ligament: radial collateral, radioscaphoid, and radiocapitate.[4] The ligament runs on the waist of the scaphoid and acts as a fulcrum for flexion of the scaphoid (▶Fig. 20.16, ▶Fig. 20.17, ▶Fig. 20.18, ▶Fig. 20.19).

20.4 Long Radiolunate Ligament

The long radiolunate ligament (LRL) is immediately ulnar to the RSC ligament (▶Fig. 20.9, ▶Fig. 20.13, ▶Fig. 20.14, ▶Fig. 20.15), courses over the proximal pole of the scaphoid anteriorly, and attaches to the volar horn on the radial half of the lunate. This ligament was once thought to be a continuous ligament that coursed ulnarly to insert with the lunotriquetral

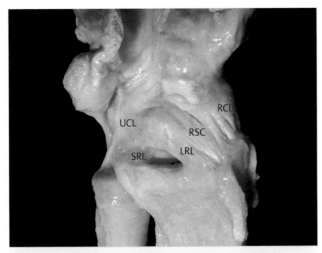

Fig. 20.13 The radioscaphocapitate (RSC) ligament, the long radiolunate ligament (LRL) and the collateral ligament of the right wrist. RCL: radial collateral ligament, SRL: short radiolunate ligament, UCL: ulnocarpal ligaments.

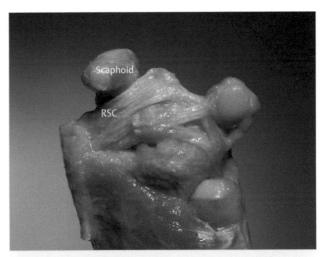

Fig. 20.16 The RSC (Radioscaphocapitate) ligament runs on the waist of the scaphoid and acts as a fulcrum for flexion of the scaphoid (left wrist).

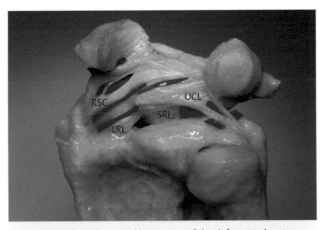

Fig. 20.14 The volar carpal ligaments of the left wrist showing the details of the radioscaphocapitate ligament. LRL: long radiolunate ligament, RSC: radioscaphocapitate ligament, SRL: short radiolunate ligament, UCL: Ulnar carpal Ligaments.

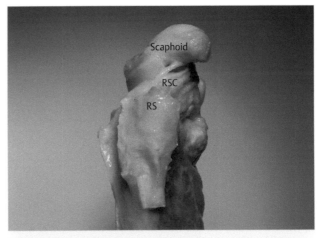

Fig. 20.17 Lateral view of the wrist showing the RSC running on the waist of the scaphoid. RS: radial styloid, RSC: radioscaphocapitate ligament.

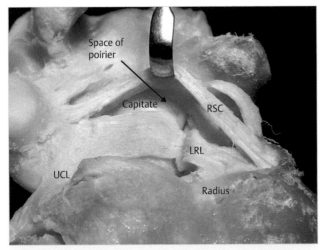

Fig. 20.15 The "deltoid" or "arcuate" RSC ligament. The RSC has very few attachments to the capitate. The space of Poirier is between the RSC and the long radiolunate ligament (right wrist). RSC: radioscaphocapitate ligament, LRL: long radiolunate Ligament, UCL: ulnocarpal ligaments.

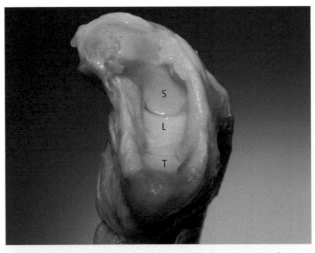

Fig. 20.18 View of the midcarpal joint with the capitate and hamate taken out. The scaphoid (S), lunate (L) and triquetrum (T) are seen. The dorsal and palmar wrist ligaments form a cradle for the midcarpal joint. The RSC runs in the waist of the scaphoid. Dorsal to the RSC is the palmar scaphotriquetral ligament.

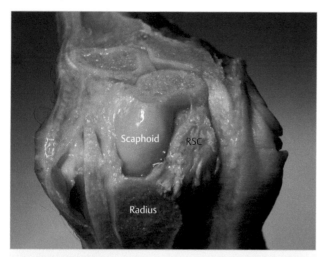

Fig. 20.19 The RSC is running on the waist of the scaphoid. RSC: radioscaphocapitate ligament.

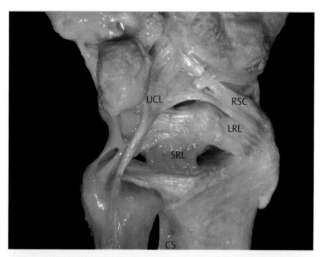

Fig. 20.20 The long radiolunate ligament and the RSC ligament. The short radiolunate ligament and the ulnocarpal ligaments are seen (right wrist). RSC: radioscaphocapitate ligament, LRL: long radiolunate ligament, SRL: short radiolunat ligament, UCL: ulnocarpal ligaments.

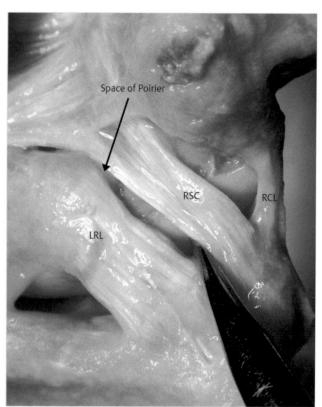

Fig. 20.21 The radial collateral ligament, the radioscaphocapitate ligament and the long radiolunate ligament. The instrument is in the space of Poirier. (Right wrist). RCL: radial collateral ligament, RSC: radioscaphocapitate ligament, LRL: long radiolunate ligament.

interosseous (LTI) ligament, hence the prior name radiotrique-tral ligament.[1] In fact, the terminal insertion ends by giving slight augmentation to the scapholunate interosseous (SLI) ligament, with the remainder being a thin layer of fibrous joint capsule over the palmar surface of the lunate.[4] The LRL is separated from the RSC by a deep longitudinal division called the interligamentous sulcus, which is not readily seen from a volar viewpoint but is clearly demarcated through a dorsal approach or arthroscopy. With traumatic separation, the space of Poirier is created, a weak area where perilunate dislocations can occur (▶Fig. 20.20, ▶Fig. 20.21).[5,7]

20.5 Radioscapholunate Ligament

The radioscapholunate ligament (RSL) or ligament of Testut (▶Fig. 20.22, ▶Fig. 20.23, ▶Fig. 20.24) is located just ulnar to the LRL, between the LRL and short radiolunate ligament, and originates from the volar rim of the radius and is oriented perpendicular to the LRL and the SRL.[5,8] The RSL has been debated extensively in the literature over its role in function, anatomy, and contributions to stability of the wrist, specifically of the proximal carpal row.[9] The RSL attaches upon the volar joint capsule and courses between the LRL and SRL and eventually interdigitates with the SLI ligament. Histologically, the collagen fibers are not as densely oriented as the extrinsic ligaments like the LRL and the RSC. Therefore, some argue that it is not a true ligament. The collagenous and synovial fibers run perpendicular to the joint capsule and house a rich neurovascular network. Histological sectioning of the fetal wrist has shown that the RSL contains terminal extensions of the anterior interosseous artery and nerve, and the proximal carpal branch of the radial artery.[4] Landsmeer chose not to define this structure as a ligament based on sectioning of fetal wrists, where he described the RSL as a "vascular pedicle" to supply the SLI ligament.[9,10] Several years following this publication, Berger et al confirmed this finding with cadaveric dissection, showing that the RSL attaches onto the proximal margin of the SLI ligament as well as the scaphoid and lunate, although no vasculature was found to supply either the scaphoid or lunate.[8,9,11] Fifty cadaveric wrists dissected by Berger et al consistently found terminal contributions from the anterior interosseous nerve within the RSL. Prior literature has pointed to a possible role of pain perception specifically within the scapholunate complex.[12,13] A recent in vivo study helped confirm this hypothesis by use of nerve conduction recordings prior to and after sectioning of SLI ligaments in patients undergoing wrist arthrodesis.[14]

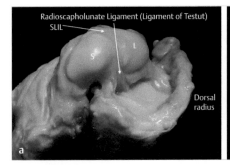

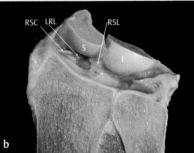

Fig. 20.22 (a) The Radioscapholunate (RSL) ligament (Ligament of Testut) from the inside of the wrist joint. (b) The RSL and the volar carpal ligaments from the radiocarpal joint.

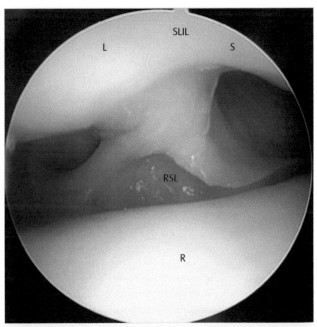

Fig. 20.23 Arthroscopic view of the RSL ligament.

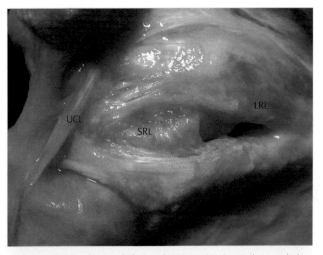

Fig. 20.25 The short radiolunate ligament (SRL). LRL: long radiolunate ligament, UCL: ulnocarpal ligaments.

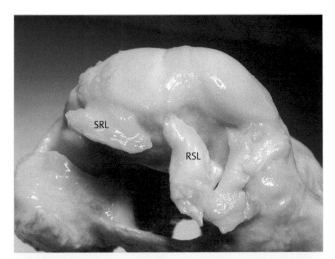

Fig. 20.24 The RSL ligament and the short radiolunate ligament.

20.6 Short Radiolunate Ligament

The short radiolunate ligament (SRL) spans the palmar radiolunate joint interspace originating from the volar lip of the radius and inserting onto the junction of the nonarticular and articular surface of the proximal lunate (▶Fig. 20.24, ▶Fig. 20.25, ▶Fig. 20.26). The SRL shares fibers with the

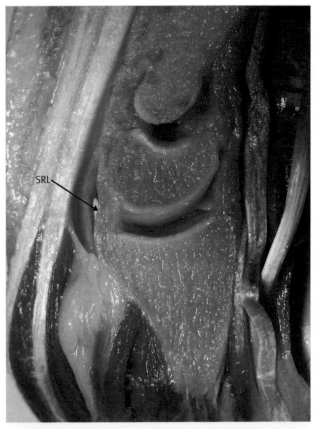

Fig. 20.26 Sagittal longitudinal section of the wrist showing the short radiolunate ligament (SRL).

adjacent LRL and lunotriquetral ligaments at its insertion onto the lunate as well as fibers of the ulnolunate ligament and TFC complex that insert onto the ulnar side of the volar lunate. The SRL has been described as a flat ligamentous sheet contiguous with the volar capsule, but histologic studies have shown it to be a thick, robust ligament.[4] The SRL is thought to be the primary restraint of the lunate maintaining close proximity to the radius in traumatic lunate–perilunate dislocations described by Mayfield et al.[15]

20.7 Dorsal Radiocarpal Ligament

There is a paucity of publications regarding the dorsal ligaments of the wrist when compared with the volar ligaments, as the latter are larger and deemed more anatomically significant. The dorsal radiocarpal ligament (DRC) originates from the dorsal rim of the distal radius, with the origin between the ulnar aspect of Lister's tubercle, and the dorsal lip of the sigmoid notch. The DRC then traverses the radiocarpal joint in an oblique and ulnar direction to insert on the dorsal aspect of the lunate and triquetrum. The origin and insertion are highly variable and were classified into subtypes based on anatomical dissections of 50 cadaveric wrists.[16] Some authors suggest this

ligament as having two components: a superficial radiotriquetral and a deep radiolunotriquetral band.[1]

Mizuseki and Ikuta[16] classified the DRC into four types:
- Type I: Fibers arise from the fourth compartment and the dorsoulnar border of the radius and insert into the dorsal tubercle of the triquetrum (44%) (▶ Fig. 20.27).
- Type II: In addition to type I structure, thin deltoid fibers cover the proximal part of the scaphoid, converging on the triquetrum (30%) (▶ Fig. 20.28).
- Type III: Like type II, with thickened proximal part that covers the proximal scaphoid (14%) (▶ Fig. 20.29).
- Type IV: Two groups of fibers run from the dorsoulnar border of the radius toward the triquetrum (12%) (▶ Fig. 20.30).

Although the anatomy was reported as variable in regard to the attachments, all subtypes had origins along the distal radius and insertions upon the triquetrum with frequent attachment to the lunate and LTI ligament.[16,17] Functional and biomechanical studies have also been reported and have linked associations between certain pathologic states and the DRC ligament,

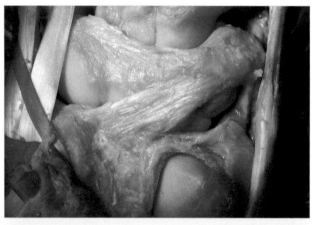

Fig. 20.27 The Dorsal Radiocarpal Ligament. Type I DRCL (right wrist).

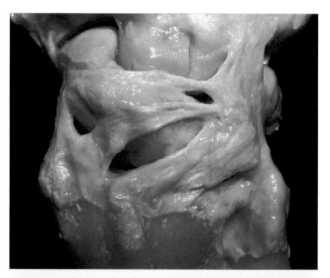

Fig. 20.29 The Dorsal Radiocarpal Ligament. Type III DRCL (right wrist).

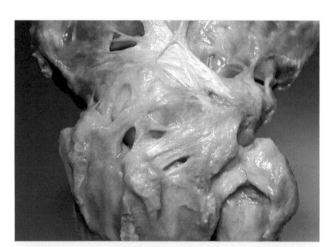

Fig. 20.28 The Dorsal Radiocarpal Ligament. Type II DRCL (right wrist).

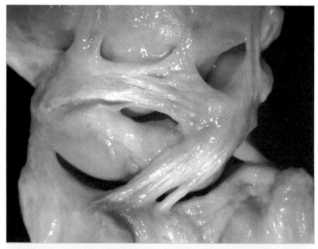

Fig. 20.30 The Dorsal Radiocarpal Ligament. Type IV DRCL (right wrist).

along with the dorsal intercarpal (DIC) ligament. Ulnar translation of the carpus in rheumatoid arthritis is seen as a result of attenuation of the DRC ligament.[16,18] The study of Mizuseki and Ikuta reminds the surgeon that when entering the dorsal capsule care should be taken to approximate this ligament if sectioned, to prevent ulnar translation.[16] Recent biomechanical and kinematic studies have demonstrated that static volar intercalated segment instability (VISI) requires disruption of both the DRC and the DIC ligaments.[17,19,20]

20.8 Intrinsic Ligaments

Within the proximal carpal row, the intrinsic ligaments consist of the DIC ligament, SLI ligament, LTI ligament, and scaphotriquetral (ST) ligament. Ligaments that connect the proximal and distal rows (midcarpal ligaments) include the scaphotrapeziotrapezoidal (STT) ligament, scaphocapitate ligament, triquetrohamate ligament, and triquetrocapitate ligament (TC). Distal row ligaments are comprised of the trapeziotrapezoid ligament, capitotrapezoid ligament, and capitohamate ligament.

20.9 Dorsal Intercarpal Ligament

Taleisnik[3] considers the DIC as an intrinsic ligament. The anatomy of the DIC ligament osseous attachments, especially the insertion, is variable, based on several cadaveric studies. The DIC ligament is generally described as having two bands, proximal and distal, both of which originate from the dorsal tubercle of the triquetrum.[2,17] The proximal band, as reported by Viegas et al, was the thicker of the two bands and found consistent insertion upon the distal lunate, the scaphoid, and the proximal lip of the trapezium, based on 90 cadaveric wrists. It also had insertions onto the SLI and LTI ligaments (▶Fig. 20.30, ▶Fig. 20.31).

As discussed earlier, these latter insertions, in concert with the DRC ligament, are postulated to contribute to carpal stability, both in VISI and dorsal intercalated segment instability

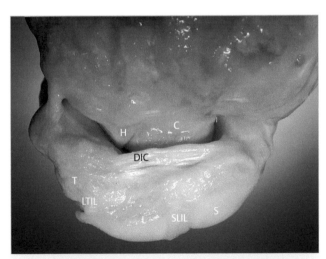

Fig. 20.31 The dorsal left wrist with the proximal and distal carpal rows. The SLIL (scapholunate interosseous ligament) and the LTIL (lunotriquetral interosseous ligament) and part of the Dorsal Intercarpal Ligament are seen (left wrist). S: scaphoid, L: lunate, T: triquetrum, C: capitate, H: hamate.

(DISI) deformities.[17,19,21] As a result, many authors recommend surgical repair of these dorsal structures when there is evidence of scapholunate dissociation.[22,23] The distal, thinner band inserts upon either the trapezoid or capitate, or both.[21] The variability in anatomy seems to be the rule rather than the exception (▶Fig. 20.27, ▶Fig. 20.28, ▶Fig. 20.29, ▶Fig. 20.30). Similar to the DRC, classification systems have also been implemented to account for the anatomical variations found in the DIC.[21,24]

The DRC and DIC are closely related in regard to biomechanical stability and work as a unit to maintain carpal stability, especially in the stabilization of the scaphoid. Depending on the position of the wrist, the angle between the DRC and DIC changes. The DRC and DIC relationship construct has been described as the "lateral V configuration," with the DRC and DIC forming the proximal and distal limbs of the "V," respectively.[25] The angle of this "V" decreases and increases with wrist extension and flexion, respectively. This unique construct provides a linkage system from the radius to the scaphoid and is postulated to offer indirect scaphoid stability without sacrificing scaphoid mobility.[2,21,26]

20.10 Scapholunate Interosseous Ligament

The SLI ligament is found between the ulnar aspect of the scaphoid and the radial aspect of the lunate, and aids in maintaining intimate association between these carpal bones. With sectioning of 37 wrists, Berger[27] described this ligament as having three anatomic regions: dorsal, volar, and proximal. The ligament is arranged in a C-shape that is open on the distal end (▶Fig. 20.32).[28] The dorsal and volar portions are considered true ligaments and have transverse- and oblique-oriented collagen fascicles, respectively. The dorsal ligament was found to be the stronger and thicker portion with fibrous attachments to the DRC and DIC ligaments. The proximal portion was found to be composed of mainly fibrocartilage with a relatively small percentage of collagen and was considered to have little bearing on mechanical strength.[27] This fibrocartilaginous area provides attachment for the RSL, which is hypothesized to serve as a neurovascular conduit for the SLI ligament.[8,11,27]

The SLI ligament's contribution to SL stability has been widely reported in the literature. An isolated tear of the SLI ligament is unlikely to cause static diastasis, but progressive and abnormal biomechanics within the proximal carpal row can lead to pathologic stress to secondary stabilizers. If left untreated, progression from dynamic to static SL instability will likely ensue.[19,29,30] Although there is discord within the literature over which ligament(s) provide primary stabilization of the SL interval, no doubt the SLI is clinically important.

20.11 Lunotriquetral Interosseous Ligament

The lunotriquetral interosseous (LTI) ligament (▶Fig. 20.33) is located between the ulnar aspect of the lunate and the radial aspect of the triquetrum. Its structure and histology is similar to the adjacent SLI ligament, having dorsal, proximal, and volar ligament subregions[2]; however, the thicker region is volar as opposed to the thicker, dorsal portion of the SLI ligament.[31] Although the volar portion is thicker and has twice the failure

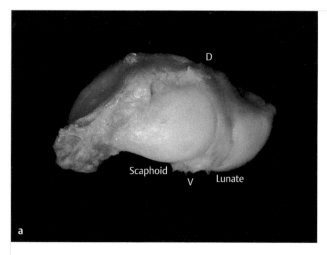
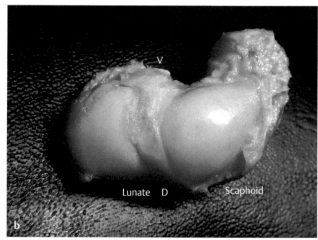
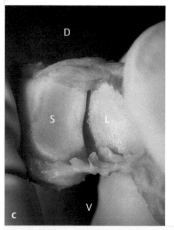
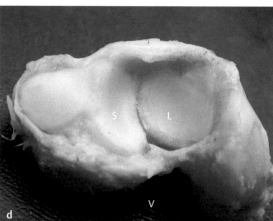
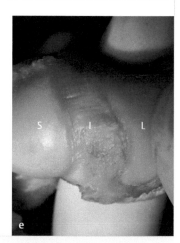

Fig. 20.32 (a–e) Dorsal, Interosseous and Volar Scapholunate Ligaments and the motion between the scaphoid and lunate when these ligaments are intact. D: dorsal, I: interosseous, V: volar.

force, Ritt el al found that biomechanically the dorsal subregion was more important in rotational and proximal–distal stability. The volar portion was found to contribute more in distraction of lunate and triquetrum but was not statistically significant. This anatomical difference is hypothesized to balance the lunate between the scaphoid and triquetrum when flexion and extension moments are encountered by the SLI and LTI ligaments, respectively.[31] Just as the SLI is important in preventing DISI, the LTI ligament helps prevent the volar variety of carpal instability (VISI).[32,33] Horii et al showed that sectioning the LTI (dorsal and volar) alone did not result in significant kinematic alteration whereas when DRC and DIC sectioning was added, static VISI deformity reulted.[20] LTI ligament incompetence can result from isolated trauma, perilunate dislocation, or ulnocarpal impingement with a positive ulnar variance, as well as from normal aging and inflammatory arthritis.[15,17,31,34] Recognizing the foregoing injury patterns and their close association with the LTI ligament is key, for early intervention will help prevent progressive carpal instability.

20.12 Scaphotriquetral Ligament

This ligament was first named by Gunther in 1841,[35] and Porier[36] supported these findings in 1908. This ligament went largely unreferenced until 1994, by Sennwald et al.[6] Sennwald et al sectioned 15 adult and 10 fetal cadaveric wrists and found

all to contain the the palmar scaphotriquetral ligament. The triquetral portion is located between the LTI and the TC ligaments. These fibers were found to be much thicker and more robust than the small fan like fibers that insert onto the scaphoid. These thin fan like fibers were found to interdigitate with those of the RSC, which may be obscured if careful attention is not taken during dissection.[6] The ST fibers run dorsal to the RSC ligament and course transversely, connecting the scaphoid to the triquetrum (▶ Fig. 20.32, 20.34). As the ST passes over the capitate, the ligament is separated by a synovial fold, for which no direct attachment was reported by Sennwald et al. Functionally, it is hypothesized to act as a sling to support the capitate, similar to the RSC ligament. Biomechanically, the ligament becomes taut in extension and lax in flexion; however, no change in length or tension is found with radial or ulnar deviation.[6] The ST ligament may also serve to help stabilize the transverse carpal arch,[6,37] but its function and biomechanical importance is only postulated and is not objectively supported in the literature.

20.13 Scaphotrapeziotrapezoidal Ligament

The STT ligament has been described as a portion of a larger ligamentous complex and provides biomechanical support to the STT joint (▶ Fig. 20.35).[38]

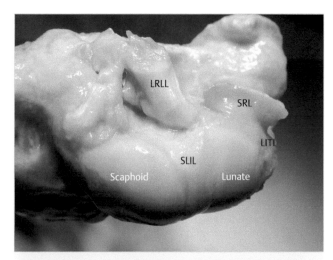

Fig. 20.33 Palmar view of the wrist joint showing the scapholunate interosseous ligament (SLIL) and the lunotriquetral interosseous ligament (LTIL) and the palmar carpal ligaments: Long radiolunate ligament (LRLL) and Short radiolunate ligament (SRL).

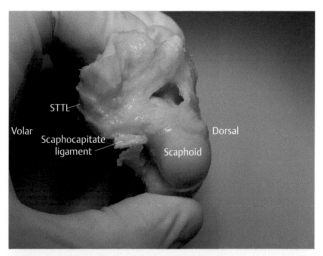

Fig. 20.35 The scaphotrapeziotrapezoidal ligament.

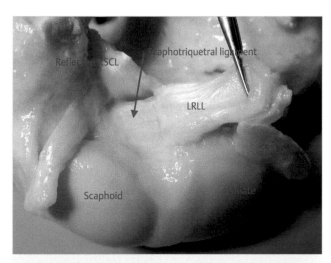

Fig. 20.34 The palmar scaphotriquetral ligament. The RSC ligament and the LRL ligament have been elevated (left wrist). RSCL: radioscaphocapitate ligament, LRLL: long radiolunate ligament, SRLL: short radiolunate ligament.

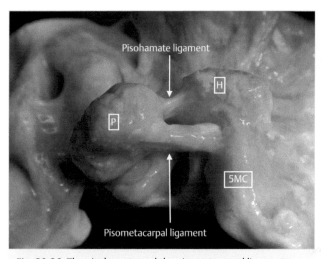

Fig. 20.36 The pisohamate and the pisometacarpal ligaments. P; pisiform, H; hamate, 5MC: Fifth metacarpal.

It has separate scapho trapezial and a scapho trapezoid components that interdigitate with other volar capsular and ligamentous structures.

20.14 Soft-Tissue Attachments of the Pisiform

The pisiform is a sesamoid in the flexor carpi ulnaris (FCU) tendon.

The soft-tissue attachments to the pisiform include the FCU, extensor retinaculum, abductor digiti minimi, transverse carpal ligament, ulnar collateral ligament, TFC complex, pisohamate ligament, pisometacarpal ligament, and pisotriquetral joint fibrous capsule (▶Fig 20.36).[39]

References

1. Berger RA, Garcia-Elias M. General anatomy of the wrist. In: An KN, Berger RA, Cooney WB, eds. Biomechanics of the Wrist Joint. New York, NY: Springer; 1991
2. Berger RA. The anatomy of the ligaments of the wrist and distal radioulnar joints. Clin Orthop Relat Res 2001;(383):32–40
3. Taleisnik J. The ligaments of the wrist. J Hand Surg Am 1976;1(2):110–118
4. Berger RA, Landsmeer JM. The palmar radiocarpal ligaments: a study of adult and fetal human wrist joints. J Hand Surg Am 1990;15(6):847–854
5. Cooney WP. The Wrist, Diagnosis and Operative Treatment: Ligament Anatomy. 2nd ed. Rochester, MN: Lippincott Williams & Wilkins; 2010
6. Sennwald GR, Zdravkovic V, Oberlin C. The anatomy of the palmar scaphotriquetral ligament. J Bone Joint Surg Br 1994;76(1):147–149
7. Garcia-Elias M. Carpal instability. In: Wolfe SH, ed. Green's Operative Hand Surgery. 6th ed. Philadelphia, PA: Elsevier Churchill Livingston; 2011:465–522

8. Hixson ML, Stewart C. Microvascular anatomy of the radioscapholunate ligament of the wrist. J Hand Surg Am 1990;15(2):279–282

9. Berger RA, Kauer JM, Landsmeer JM. Radioscapholunate ligament: a gross anatomic and histologic study of fetal and adult wrists. J Hand Surg Am 1991;16(2):350–355

10. Landsmeer J. Atlas of Anatomy of the Hand. New York, NY: Churchill Livingstone; 1976

11. Berger RA, Blair WF. The radioscapholunate ligament: a gross and histologic description. Anat Rec 1984;210(2):393–405

12. Buck-Gramcko D. Denervation of the wrist joint. J Hand Surg Am 1977;2(1):54–61

13. Dellon AL, Mackinnon SE, Daneshvar A. Terminal branch of anterior interosseous nerve as source of wrist pain. J Hand Surg [Br] 1984;9(3):316–322

14. Vekris MD, Mataliotakis GI, Beris AE. The scapholunate interosseous ligament afferent proprioceptive pathway: a human in vivo experimental study. J Hand Surg Am 2011;36(1):37–46

15. Mayfield JK, Johnson RP, Kilcoyne RK. Carpal dislocations: pathomechanics and progressive perilunar instability. J Hand Surg Am 1980;5(3):226–241

16. Mizuseki T, Ikuta Y. The dorsal carpal ligaments: their anatomy and function. J Hand Surg [Br] 1989;14(1):91–98

17. Viegas SF, Patterson RM, Peterson PD, et al. Ulnar-sided perilunate instability: an anatomic and biomechanic study. J Hand Surg Am 1990;15(2):268–278

18. Linscheid RL. Kinematic considerations of the wrist. Clin Orthop Relat Res 1986;(202):27–39

19. Elsaidi GA, Ruch DS, Kuzma GR, Smith BP. Dorsal wrist ligament insertions stabilize the scapholunate interval: cadaver study. Clin Orthop Relat Res 2004;(425):152–157

20. Horii E, Garcia-Elias M, An KN, et al. A kinematic study of lunotriquetral dissociations. J Hand Surg Am 1991;16(2):355–362

21. Viegas SF, Yamaguchi S, Boyd NL, Patterson RM. The dorsal ligaments of the wrist: anatomy, mechanical properties, and function. J Hand Surg Am 1999;24(3):456–468

22. Slater RR Jr, Szabo RM, Bay BK, Laubach J. Dorsal intercarpal ligament capsulodesis for scapholunate dissociation: biomechanical analysis in a cadaver model. J Hand Surg Am 1999;24(2):232–239

23. Viegas S. Ligamentous repair following acute scapholunate dissociation. In: Gelberman R, ed. Master Techniques in Orthopaedic Surgery: The Wrist. New York, NY: Lippincott-Raven; 2000

24. Smith DK. Dorsal carpal ligaments of the wrist: normal appearance on multiplanar reconstructions of three-dimensional Fourier transform MR imaging. AJR Am J Roentgenol 1993;161(1):119–125

25. Viegas SF. The dorsal ligaments of the wrist. Hand Clin 2001;17(1):65–75, vi

26. Berger RA. The ligaments of the wrist. A current overview of anatomy with considerations of their potential functions. Hand Clin 1997;13(1):63–82

27. Berger RA. The gross and histologic anatomy of the scapholunate interosseous ligament. J Hand Surg Am 1996;21(2):170–178

28. Ruby LK, An KN, Linscheid RL, Cooney WP III, Chao EY. The effect of scapholunate ligament section on scapholunate motion. J Hand Surg Am 1987;12(5 Pt 1):767–771

29. Short WH, Werner FW, Green JK, Masaoka S. Biomechanical evaluation of the ligamentous stabilizers of the scaphoid and lunate: Part II. J Hand Surg Am 2005;30(1):24–34

30. Meade TD, Schneider LH, Cherry K. Radiographic analysis of selective ligament sectioning at the carpal scaphoid: a cadaver study. J Hand Surg Am 1990;15(6):855–862

31. Ritt MJPF, Bishop AT, Berger RA, Linscheid RL, Berglund LJ, An KN. Lunotriquetral ligament properties: a comparison of three anatomic subregions. J Hand Surg Am 1998;23(3):425–431

32. Linscheid RL, Dobyns JH, Beckenbaugh RD, Cooney WP III, Wood MB. Instability patterns of the wrist. J Hand Surg Am 1983;8(5 Pt 2):682–686

33. Linscheid RL, Dobyns JH, Beabout JW, Bryan RS. Traumatic instability of the wrist. Diagnosis, classification, and pathomechanics. J Bone Joint Surg Am 1972;54(8):1612–1632

34. Taleisnik J. Current concepts review. Carpal instability. J Bone Joint Surg Am 1988;70(8):1262–1268

35. Gunther, G. Das Handgelenk in mechanischer, anatomischer und chirurgischer Beziehung. Johann August Meissner; 1841:61–64

36. Porier PCA. Abreege d' anatomie. Masson et Cie; 1908

37. Garcia-Elias M, An KN, Cooney WP III, Linscheid RL, Chao EY. Stability of the transverse carpal arch: an experimental study. J Hand Surg Am 1989;14(2 Pt 1):277–282

38. Drewniany JJ, Palmer AK, Flatt AE. The scaphotrapezial ligament complex: an anatomic and biomechanical study. J Hand Surg Am 1985;10(4):492–498

39. Pevny T, Rayan GM, Egle D. Ligamentous and tendinous support of the pisiform, anatomic and biomechanical study. J Hand Surg Am 1995;20(2):299–304

21 Vascularity of the Distal Radius and Carpus

Joost I. P. Willems and Allen T. Bishop

21.1 Introduction

The gross vascular anatomy of the distal radius and carpus was first described over 200 years ago by Von Haller and subsequently by Tiedeman and Henle.[1–3] Due to improvements in tissue processing and visualization techniques, several publications have been written over the past three decades that describe the vascularity of the distal radius and carpus in greater detail. Other than providing us with better understanding of bone pathology, this knowledge has also enabled the development of pedicled vascularized bone grafts useful in treating carpal nonunion or avascular necrosis.

In this chapter, we review the current literature on the extraosseous and intraosseous vascularity of the distal radius and carpus, providing some examples of the vascularized pedicled bone grafts that are used today.

21.2 Vascular Anatomy of the Distal Radius

21.2.1 Extraosseous Vascularity

Dorsal Radius

The distal dorsal radius has a robust and consistent blood supply provided by a series of longitudinal extraosseous vessels originating from the anterior interosseous and radial arteries. The anterior interosseous artery divides into anterior and posterior divisions proximal to the distal radioulnar (DRU) joint. The primary source of orthograde blood flow to the distal dorsal radius is provided by the posterior division, together with the radial artery. They also supply nutrition to soft tissues, creating the possibility of raising a composite pedicled flap that includes the posterior interosseous nerve, skin, and muscle.[4]

Branches from the major longitudinal forearm vessels ultimately supply nutrient arteries to the distal dorsal radius. The dorsal vessels are best described by their location in relationship to the extensor compartments of the wrist and the extensor retinaculum. They provide a consistent group of nutrient arteries to the distal radius. Of importance, all have distal anastomotic connections. Two of the vessels are superficial in location, lying on the dorsal surface of the extensor retinaculum between the 1st and 2nd and the 2nd and 3rd dorsal compartments. At these locations, the retinaculum is adherent to an underlying bony tubercle separating their respective compartments, allowing nutrient vessels to penetrate bone. Because of their location, they have been named the 1,2 and 2,3 intercompartmental supraretinacular arteries (1,2 and 2,3 ICSRA)[5] (▶Fig. 21.1).

Two deep vessels also provide nutrient vessels to the dorsal distal radius. They lie on the surface of the radius in the floor or against the wall of the 4th and 5th dorsal compartments. They are consequently named the 4th and 5th extensor compartment arteries (4th and 5th ECA)[5] (▶Fig. 21.1).

The 1,2 ICSRA originates from the radial artery approximately 5 cm proximal to the radiocarpal joint, passing beneath the brachioradialis muscle and tendon to lie on the dorsal surface of the extensor retinaculum. Distally, it passes beneath the tendons of the first extensor compartment to enter the anatomic snuffbox and anastomose to the radial artery in most cases or occasionally to a radial branch supplying the scaphoid.[6] This distal anastomotic connection is the "ascending irrigating branch" described previously.[4] It is the smallest the four vessels (mean internal diameter of 0.30 mm). Like all the vessels, it is accompanied by venae comitantes[7] (▶Fig. 21.1, ▶Fig. 21.2, and ▶Fig. 21.3; ▶Table 21.1 and ▶Table 21.2).

Its position superficial to the retinaculum and directly on the bony tubercle between the first and second extensor compartments makes its dissection and use as a vascularized pedicled graft to the scaphoid fairly straight forward. However, its arc of rotation is short, its nutrient artery branches are small in number and caliber, and the vessel itself is occasionally absent. These factors may significantly limit its usefulness in carpal bones other than the scaphoid and, of course, in any patient if absent. In some individuals, a more proximal branch of the 1,2 ICSRA enters the floor of the 2nd compartment, ending as a large nutrient vessel (2nd EC branch of the 1,2 ICSRA). A graft centered on this branch results in a pedicle long enough to reach the lunate.[5]

The 2,3 ICSRA originates proximally from the anterior interosseous artery or the posterior division of the anterior interosseous artery (▶Fig. 21.1 and ▶Fig. 21.4; ▶Table 21.1 and ▶Table 21.2). It runs superficial to the extensor retinaculum directly on the dorsal radial tubercle (Lister's tubercle) to anastomose with the dorsal intercarpal arch (dICa) and, in some cases, the dorsal radiocarpal arch (dRCa) and/or the 4th ECA. It has a mean internal diameter of 0.35 mm. The number, location, and size of its nutrient branches are shown in ▶Table 21.2. These nutrient branches often penetrate deep into cancellous bone. One large proximal branch enters the radius in the floor of the 2nd extensor compartment (2nd EC branch of the 2,3 ICSRA). Like the 1,2 ICSRA, the 2,3 ICSRA may be based as a retrograde pedicle for a vascularized bone graft.[5] that its mid axial dorsal position provides an arc of rotation that may reach the entire proximal carpal row, the pedicle overlies the wrist joint capsule at the site of most capsulotomy incisions. Its dissection and mobilization, which must be done prior to inspection of the carpus, is more difficult than for the more marginally located 1,2 ICSRA and 5th ECA. Therefore, the use of this pedicle has been largely abandoned in most clinical practice.

The 4th ECA (▶Fig. 21.1 and ▶Fig. 21.3) lies directly adjacent to the posterior interosseous nerve on the radial aspect of the 4th extensor compartment. In a minority of cases, the vessel may be found within the 3,4 septum for most of its course. Proximally, this artery originates from the posterior division of the anterior interosseous artery or its 5th extensor compartment branch. It anastomoses distal to the radius with the dICa and, in most cases, to the dRCa. Connections to the neighboring 2,3 ICSRA and/or the 5th ECA are common. It has a mean internal

251

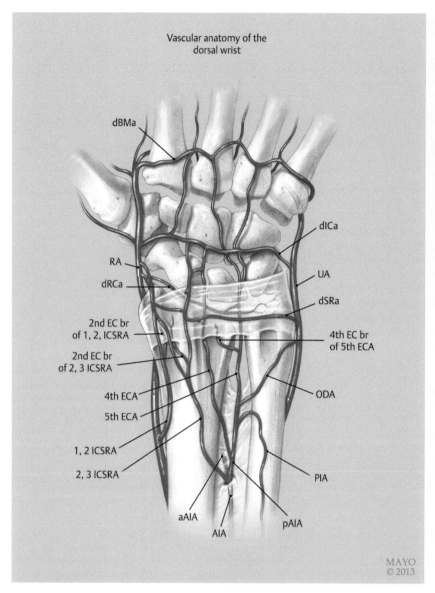

Vascular anatomy of the
dorsal wrist

Fig. 21.1 Schematic view of the dorsal arterial supply of the wrist. dBMa = dorsal basal metacarpal arch, dICa = dorsal intercarpal arch, dRCa = dorsal radiocarpal arch, EC br = extensor compartmental branch, RA = radial artery, dSRa = dorsal supraretinacular artery, ECA = extra compartment artery, UA = ulnar artery, ODA = oblique dorsal artery, pAIA = posterior division of the anterior interosseous artery, aAIA = anterior division of the anterior interosseous artery, PIA = posterior interosseous artery, AIA = anterior interosseous artery. From Sheetz KK, Bishop AT, Berger RA. The arterial blood supply of the distal radius and ulna and its potential use in vascularized pedicled bone grafts. J Hand Surg. 1995;20A:902–14. Used with permission of Mayo Foundation for Medical Education and Research, all rights reserved.

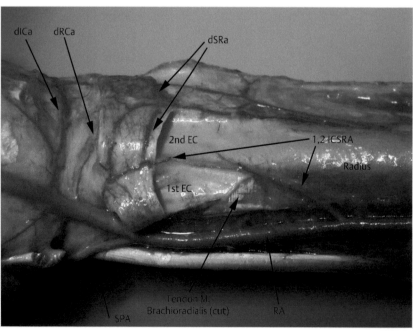

Fig. 21.2 Dorsolateral view of the wrist with the 1,2 ICSRA clearly visible. Extensor muscles removed. ICSRA = intercompartmental supraretinacular artery, dICa = dorsal intercarpal arch, dRCa = dorsal radiocarpal arch, SPA = superficial palmar artery, RA = radial artery, dSRa = dorsal supraretinacular artery, EC = extensor compartment.

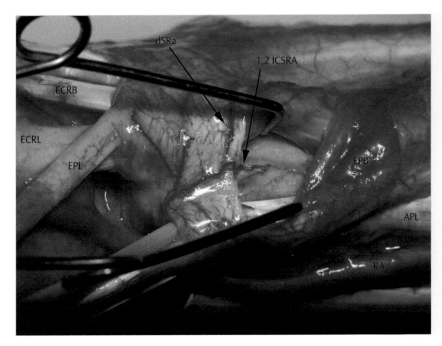

Fig. 21.3 Detailed view of the 1,2 ICSRA following its course between the muscles of the first and second compartment. ICSRA = intercompartmental supraretinacular artery, dSRa = dorsal supraretinacular artery, ECRB = extensor carpi radialis brevis, ECRL = extensor carpi radialis longus, EPB = extensor pollicis brevis, APL = abductor pollicis longus, RA = radial artery.

Table 21.1 Extraosseous vessel characteristics distal radius vessels

Artery	Artery present (%)	Internal diameter mean(range) (mm)	Provides nutrient arteries to bone Y/N
Radial artery	100	2.48 (1.71–3.09)	N
Ulnar artery	100	2.30 (1.49–3.05)	N
Posterior interosseous artery	100	0.48 (0.25–0.65)	N
Anterior interosseous artery	100	1.28 (0.57–1.63)	N
Anterior division AIA	100	0.89 (0.61–1.20)	N
Posterior division AIA	100	0.71 (0.20–1.18)	N
1,2 ICSRA	94	0.30 (0.14–0.58)	Y
2nd EC br of 1,2 ICSRA	56	0.16 (0.14–0.19)	Y
2,3 ICSRA	100	0.35 (0.14–0.55)	Y
2nd EC br of 2,3 ICSRA	91	0.17	Y
4th ECA	100	0.38 (0.28–0.72)	Y
5th ECA	100	0.49 (0.27–0.76)	N
4th EC br of 5th ECA	39	0.15 (0.11–0.19)	Y
dICa	100	0.68 (0.43–1.47)	N
dRCa	100	0.36 (0.20–0.84)	Y
dSRa	100	0.37 (0.12–0.98)	N
ODA distal ulna	100	0.32 (0.08–0.67)	Y
pMeta	100	0.50 (0.30–0.74)	Y
rPCa	100	0.47 (0.19–0.76)	Y
uPCa	100	0.41 (0.24–0.55)	Y

Extraosseous vessel characteristics. ICSRA = intercompartmental supraretinacular artery, EC = extensor compartment, br = branch, ECA = extensor compartment artery, dICa = dorsal intercarpal arch, dRCa = dorsal radiocarpal arch, dSRa = dorsal supraretinacular arch, ODA distal ulna = oblique dorsal artery of the distal ulna, pMeta = palmar metaphyseal arch, rPCa = radial branch of palmar carpal arch, uPCa = ulnar branch of palmar carpal arch. Reprinted from Sheetz KK, Bishop AT, Berger RA, The arterial blood supply of the distal radius and ulna and its potential use in vascularized pedicled bone grafts , J Hand Surg, Vol 20A, 902–14, Copyright (1995), with permission from Elsevier.

Table 21.2 Nutrient artery characteristics

Artery supplying nutrient arteries	# of nutrient arteries [mean (range)]	Nutrient artery internal diameter (mm) [mean (range)]	Distance from nutrient artery penetration to RC joint (mm) [mean (range)]	% of nutrient arteries that penetrate cancellous bone (%)
1,2 ICSRA	3.2 (0–9)	<0.10 (<0.05–0.15)	15 (4–26)	6
2nd EC br of 1,2 ICSRA	1 (1)	0.16 (0.14–0.19)	21 (17–28)	57
2,3 IC SRA	1.8 (0–5)	0.11 (0.07–0.19)	13 (3–24)	22
2nd EC br of 2,3 ICSRA	1.4 (1–4)	0.19 (0.09–0.28)	18 (14–32)	48
4th ECA	3.2 (1–6)	0.16 (0.07–0.29)	11 (3–19)	45
4th EC br of 5th ECA	1.2 (1–2)	0.15 (0.15)	10 (6–12)	43
dRCa	2.6 (0–7)	0.18 (0.14–0.29)	4 (1–12)	79
pMeta	2.0 (0–5)	<0.10 (<0.05 0.20)	12 (10–34)	20
rPCa	6.0 (2–10)	0.15 (0.04–0.33)	6 (1–15)	70
uPCa	3.7 (0–8)	0.20 (0.10–0.40)	12 (1–31)	37

Nutrient artery characteristics. ICSRA = intercompartmental supraretinacular artery, EC = extensor compartment, br = branch, ECA = extensor compartment artery, dRCa = dorsal radiocarpal arch, pMeta = palmar metaphyseal arch, rPCa = radial branch of palmar carpal arch, uPCa = ulnar branch of palmar carpal arch. Reprinted from Sheetz KK, Bishop AT, Berger RA, The arterial blood supply of the distal radius and ulna and its potential use in vascularized pedicled bone grafts, J Hand Surg, Vol 20A, 902–14, Copyright (1995), with permission from Elsevier.

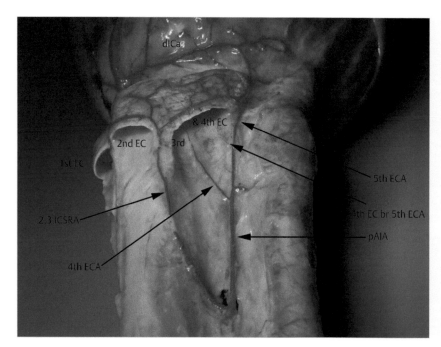

Fig. 21.4 Dorsal oblique view of the wrist showing dorsal arterial patterns. Extensor muscles removed and 5th and 6th extensor compartments exposed. dICa = dorsal intercarpal arch, EC = extensor compartment, ECA = extensor compartment artery, br = branch of the, ICSRA = intercompartmental supraretinacular artery, pAIA = posterior division of the anterior interosseous artery.

diameter of 0.38 mm. The 4th ECA is the source of numerous nutrient vessels to the floor of the 4th compartment that frequently penetrate cancellous bone (►Table 21.1). The vessels entering more distally tend to supply primarily cortical bone, whereas those more proximal are more likely to penetrate cancellous bone.[5]

The 5th ECA is generally the largest of all the dorsal vessels (mean 0.49 mm internal diameter) (►Fig. 21.1 and ►Fig. 21.4; ►Table 21.1). It is located in the radial floor of the 5th extensor compartment, passing mostly through the 4,5 septum in one-third of specimens.[5] This vessel is supplied proximally by

the posterior division of the anterior interosseous artery and anastomoses distally with the dICa. It may also make distal connections with the 4th ECA, the dRCa, the 2,3 ICSRA, and/or the oblique dorsal artery of the distal ulna. Only 39% of the 5th ECAs in the study of Sheetz et al had a branch that supplied 1 or 2 nutrient vessels to the floor of the 4th compartment (4th EC branch of 5th ECA).[5] It is therefore most useful as a large conduit of retrograde flow from the intercarpal arch to other vessels with more consistent nutrient branches. Its large diameter and multiple anastomoses allow creation of a vascular pedicle that can reach almost anywhere in the hand, for example, when retrograde flow through the 5th ECA supplies orthograde (proximal to distal) blood supply to a radial bone graft centered over the 4th ECA (5 + 4 ECA pedicle). Experimental studies in the canine distal radius have demonstrated that similar reverse-flow pedicle bone grafts have measurable flow immediately after elevation and have marked hyperemia when reevaluated after 2 weeks.[8,9]

A series of arches across the dorsum of the hand and wrist provide distal anastomoses with these intercompartmental and compartmental arteries. These include the dICa, dRCa, and dorsal supraretinacular arch (dSRa). The dICa contributes blood supply to the distal ulna and radius only indirectly, through connecting arteries. It is an important part of several potential grafts because of its anastomotic connections. The arch can be used as a source of retrograde arterial flow allowing proximal vessel ligation and graft mobilization. The dRCa contributes significantly to the dorsal distal radius via small nutrient arteries. These nutrient branches enter bone just proximal to the radiocarpal joint and proceed perpendicularly to supply cancellous bone in the extreme distal end of the metaphysis. Its close proximity to the radius and its location on or deep to the superficial joint capsule limits its potential use as a source of retrograde arterial flow due to a short arc of rotation and difficult dissection. The dSRa provides anastomoses between the arteries running parallel to the radial and ulnar diaphyses. It is not a single artery but rather is an anastomotic network of small vessels connecting the dorsal arteries. Because of its small caliber vessels, it is not of use in providing retrograde bone graft pedicle blood flow[5] (▶Fig. 21.1, ▶Fig. 21.2, ▶Fig. 21.3, ▶Fig. 21.4, and ▶Fig. 21.5; ▶Table 21.1 and ▶Table 21.2).

In the passage on carpal extraosseous vascularity, the dICa and dRCa is described in further detail.

Palmar Radius

The nutrient vasculature of the distal palmar radius is supplied by branches of three arteries: the ulnar artery, the radial artery, and the anterior division of the anterior interosseous artery. The anterior division of the anterior interosseous artery provides the majority of the periosteal and endosteal vasculature of the distal palmar radius and ulna, which consists of small nutrient arteries branching laterally and medially every 1 to 2 cm.[10–12]

The palmar carpal arch (PCa), in reality, is a dual arch providing the palmar metaphyses of radius and ulna with blood supply via the anterior division of the anterior interosseous artery, the radial artery and the ulnar artery.[5,12] The point of origin of the two halves of the arch has been named the "area of arterial convergence"[13] or the "T-shaped point,"[12] lying proximal and lateral to the DRU joint. The radial branch of the PCa (rPCa) runs immediately proximal to the radiocarpal joint and distal to the pronator quadratus muscle to meet the radial artery which also contributes orthograde flow to the arch. The ulnar branch (uPCa) is generally smaller in diameter, with additional inflow provided from the ulnar artery. Characteristics of these arteries are shown in ▶Table 21.1 and ▶Table 21.2 (▶Fig. 21.6, ▶Fig. 21.7, and ▶Fig. 21.8).

A second arch is seen more proximally at the metaphyseal level, termed the palmar metaphyseal arch (pMeta), formed by a branch from the anterior division of the anterior interosseous artery (96%) or from the anterior interosseous itself (4%), which anastomoses distally with the radial artery in all cases and in 57% of cases also sent a branch to the rPCa[5] (▶Fig. 21.6; ▶Table 21.1 and ▶Table 21.2). It runs through the pronator quadratus muscle supplying nutrient vessels to the muscle as well as to the palmar aspect of the metaphyseal radius often penetrating cancellous bone, which makes this a region of interest for pedicled muscle–bone grafts.[5,14,15]

Palmar radius grafts have been thoroughly described in literature, based upon a pronator quadratus pedicle or the PCa.[13,15–25] Flow through the pedicle may be based on the anterior interosseous artery, harvesting the graft from the lateral aspect of the palmar radius, or on the terminal palmar metaphyseal or PCa of the radial artery, when the bone is harvested from the medial palmar radius.[5] Inclusion and therefore dissection of the PCa may place important palmar carpal ligaments at risk,

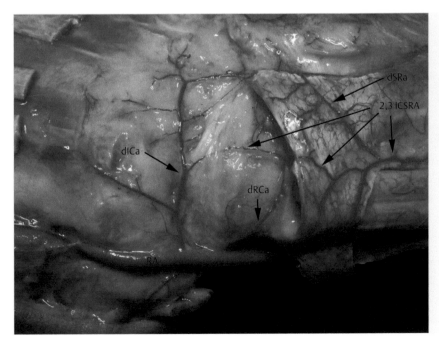

Fig. 21.5 Detailed view of the distal anastomosis of the 2,3 ICSRA with the dorsal intercarpal arch. Extensor muscle tendons of 1ˢᵗ, 2ⁿᵈ, 3ʳᵈ and 4ᵗʰ extensor compartments removed. Extensor muscles of 5ᵗʰ extensor compartment removed and 5ᵗʰ compartment exposed. ICSRA = intercompartmental supraretinacular artery, dSRa = dorsal supraretinacular artery, dICa = dorsal intercarpal arch, dRCa = dorsal radiocarpal arch, RA = radial artery.

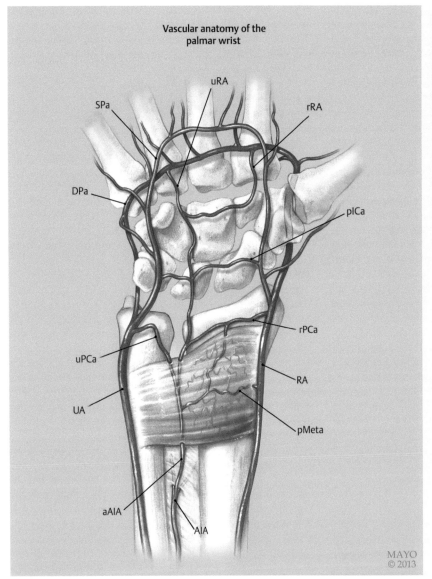

Vascular anatomy of the palmar wrist

Fig. 21.6 Schematic view of the palmar arterial supply of the wrist. SPa = superficial palmar arch, DPa = deep palmar arch, uRA = ulnar recurrent artery, rRA = radial recurrent artery, pICa = palmar intercarpal arch, uPCa = ulnar branch of palmar carpal arch, rPCa = radial branch of palmar carpal arch, UA = ulnar artery, pMeta = palmar metaphyseal arch, aAIA = anterior division of the anterior interosseous artery, RA = radial artery, AIA = anterior interosseous artery. From Sheetz KK, Bishop AT, Berger RA. The arterial blood supply of the distal radius and ulna and its potential use in vascularized pedicled bone grafts. J Hand Surg. 1995;20A:902–14. Used with permission of Mayo Foundation for Medical Education and Research, all rights reserved.

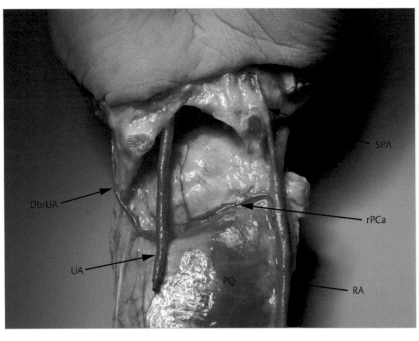

Fig. 21.7 Palmar view of the wrist showing the radial and ulnar artery and the radial branch of the palmar carpal arch. Flexor muscles removed. SPA = superficial palmar artery, DbrUA = dorsal carpal branch of the ulnar artery, pPCa = radial branch of the palmar carpal arch, uPCa = ulnar branch of the palmar carpal arch, UA = ulnar artery, RA = radial artery, PQ = pronator quadratus muscle.

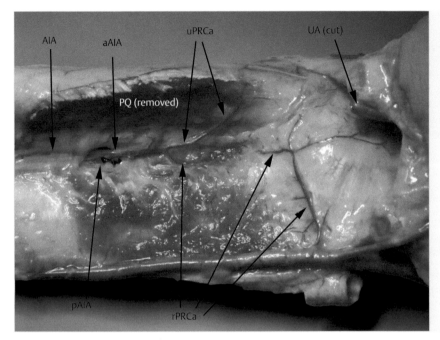

Fig. 21.8 Palmar view of the wrist showing the anterior interosseous artery with its divisions. Flexor muscles, ulnar artery and pronator quadratus muscle removed. AIA = anterior interosseous artery, aAIA = anterior division of the AIA, pAIA = posterior division of the AIA, uPCa = ulnar branch of the palmar carpal artery, rPCa = radial branch of the palmar carpal artery, UA = ulnar artery.

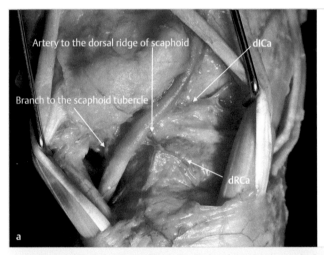
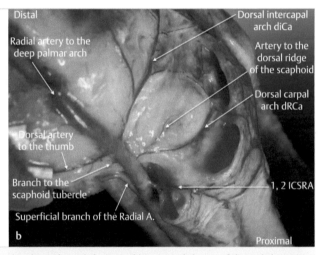

Fig. 21.9 (a) Detailed view of dorsal carpal and scaphoid vascular branches from the radial artery. (b) Dorsoradial view of the radial artery and its branches at the level of the wrist in the most common seen configuration.

and the nutrient supply of the more proximal pMeta within the pronator quadratus muscle is small and highly variable in location.[5] These grafts are further limited by the need for carpal exposure through important radiocarpal ligaments. This limits exposure and may risk radiocarpal instability postoperatively. Nevertheless, excellent clinical results have been reported with this flap.[17]

21.2.2 Intraosseous Vascularity

As described in a study by Lamas et al, the intraosseous blood supply of the distal radius can be subdivided into three main vascular systems: the epiphyseal, metaphyseal, and the diaphyseal. The epiphyseal blood supply is provided palmarly by the PCa via the radial and the anterior interosseous artery and dorsally from the dorsal extraosseous vessels described previously. Multiple nutrient vessels enter the epiphysis through many nutrient foramina located at the wrist capsular attachments, both dorsally and palmarly, as well as the radial styloid, Lister's tubercle, and the sigmoid notch.[26]

The distal metaphyseal vascular supply of the radius and ulna is provided mainly by multiple periosteal and endosteal branches of the anterior division of the anterior interosseous artery and from the metaphyseal arch, embedded in the dorsal aspect of the pronator quadratus muscle, as described earlier.[5,10–12] These nutrient vessels penetrate the cortex on numerous locations and their terminal branches anastomose with the terminal branches of the medullary arterioles at both ends of the medullary cavity.[26]

The diaphyseal supply of the radius is provided mainly by numerous endosteal and periosteal branches arising from the anterior interosseous artery and occasionally accompanied by a direct branch from the radial artery. The distal diaphysis is supplied by a nutrient artery originating from the anterior division of the anterior interosseous artery, which penetrates the cortex and divides into ascending and descending branches of the medullary artery. These then subdivide and provide the entire diaphyseal endosteum with arterioles.[10,26]

21.3 Vascular Anatomy of the Carpus

21.3.1 Extraosseous Vascularity

Extraosseous blood supply to the carpus is provided by the ulnar artery, the radial artery, and three pairs of transverse arches.[27] These are, from proximal to distal, the dorsal and palmar radiocarpal arches, the dorsal and palmar intercarpal arches, and the dorsal basal metacarpal and deep palmar arches (▶Fig. 21.1, ▶Fig. 21.2, ▶Fig. 21.3, ▶Fig. 21.4, ▶Fig. 21.5, ▶Fig. 21.6, and ▶Fig. 21.7; ▶Table 21.1 and ▶Table 21.2).

Dorsal

The dRCa is the second largest dorsal arch, with a mean diameter of 0.36 mm, and it supplies the distal radial metaphysis and the dorsum of the lunate and triquetrum. It receives contributions from the radial artery and at least two additional sources such as the dICa (67%), 4th ECA (59%), 2,3 ICSRA (52%), 1,2 ICSRA (52%), and the 5th ECA (23%)[5] (▶Fig. 21.1 and ▶Fig. 21.5).

The dICa is the largest dorsal arch with a mean diameter of 0.68 mm and provides the major blood supply to the distal carpal row and contributes to the vascularity of the triquetrum and lunate. It receives contributions from the ulnar, radial, and 5th ECA and frequently anastomoses with the 2,3 ICSRA (94%), the 4th ECA (94%), the dRCa (67%), and occasionally with the 1,2 ICSRA (19%)[5] (▶Fig. 21.1 and ▶Fig. 21.5).

The dorsal basal metacarpal arch (dBMa) is the smallest dorsal arch, located at the base of the metacarpals. It comprises a series of vascular retia; its presence is the most variable among the dorsal arches. It is complete in 27%, absent in 27%, and present in its radial aspect alone in 46% of specimens. It is supplied by perforating arteries from the second, third, and fourth interosseous spaces. It supplies the carpus only indirectly, through several small anastomosing vessels to the intercarpal arch[27] (▶Fig. 21.1).

Palmar

The PCa is the most proximal palmar arch located just proximal to the radiocarpal joint. It is consistently present and receives contributions from the ulnar, radial, and anterior division of the anterior interosseous artery. It supplies the palmar surface of the lunate and triquetrum.[28]

The palmar intercarpal arch (pICa) is located between the proximal and distal carpal rows. It is present in only 53% of cases and receives contributions from the ulnar, radial, and anterior interosseous arteries in 75% of specimens and from the ulnar and radial arteries alone in 25% of specimens. It is a relatively small and inconsistent arch and is a minor contributor of nutrient vessels to the carpus.[28]

The deep palmar arch (DPa) is a more consistent arch located at the level of the metacarpal bases, just distal to the carpometacarpal joints. The radial side comes from the deep palmar branch of the radial artery in all cases. The ulnar side of the arch is supplied by the inferior deep branch of the ulnar artery in 44% of cases, the superior deep branch of the ulnar artery in 33% of cases, or both deep branches of the ulnar artery in 20% of cases.[29] The arch gives rise to the palmar metacarpal arteries, perforating vessels to the dorsal metacarpal arch, and ulnar and radial recurrent arteries. The ulnar recurrent artery originates between the bases of the long and ring metacarpals and courses within the ligamentous groove between the capitate and the hamate supplying both bones. The radial recurrent artery originates just lateral to the base of the index metacarpal and anastomoses with the ulnar recurrent artery in 45% of cases. In 27% of cases, an accessory ulnar recurrent artery was present which supplied the medial aspect of the hook of the hamate. Both recurrent arteries are present in 100% of cases and are the primary blood supply to the distal carpal row.[27,29,30]

21.3.2 Intraosseous Vascularity

Three major patterns of blood supply have been described in the carpal bones[31] (▶Table 21.3). *Group 1* includes bones in which vessels enter on only one surface or supply a large area without additional anastomotic supply. The capitate, the scaphoid, and 4 to 20% of all lunates are in this group, which may have a relatively large risk for avascular necrosis (AVN). *Group 2* bones have at least two distinct areas of vessel entry, but lack intraosseous anastomoses in all or a significant portion of the bone. The trapezoid and hamate are placed into this group. Bones with at least two surfaces receiving nutrient arteries, no large areas of bone dependent on a single vessel, and consistent intraosseous anastomoses constitute *group 3*. The trapezium, triquetrum, pisiform, and 80 to 96% of the lunate are in this group. The trapezium probably has the richest internal blood supply of any carpal bone.

Scaphoid

The scaphoid is largely covered by articular cartilage, with limited areas where nutrient vessels may enter the bone. These include a narrow, oblique dorsal ridge where the capsular ligaments attach and a small area palmarly at the scaphoid tubercle.[32–34] Generally, a single dorsal nutrient vessel supplies the proximal 70% of the bone, originating from the radial artery directly in 70% of cases, from the dICa in 23%, and from branches of both arteries in 7% of cases (▶Fig. 21.9a and b). Usually a dorsal nutrient artery penetrates bone at the level of the waist, with an occasional nutrient artery entering more proximally or distally. The vessels divide within bone into several branches running palmarly and proximally to supply the proximal pole.

Table 21.3 Groups by vascular characteristics of carpal bones

Group 1	Scaphoid Capitate Lunate 4–20%	• Large areas dependent on single IO vessel • No IO anastomosis • Risk of AVN higher following fracture
Group 2	Trapezoid Hamate	• No large areas dependent on single vessel • Lack IO anastomosis in all or most • At least two areas of vessel entry
Group 3	Trapezium Triquetrum Pisiform Lunate 80–96%	• No large areas dependent on single vessel • Consistent IO anastomoses • At least two areas of vessel entry

The three groups of normal carpal bones characterized by their type of blood supply, according to Panagis et al [27]. IO = intraosseous, AVN = avascular necrosis.

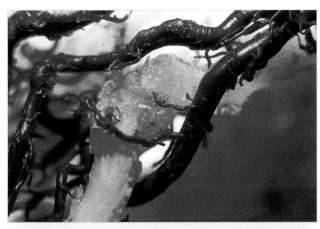

Fig. 21.10 Extraosseous vascular supply of the scaphoid. (from Zancolli EA, Cozzi EP: Atlas of Surgical Anatomy of the Hand. Churchill Livingstone, New York, 1992.)

Several small vessels enter the palmar tubercle, arising from the radial artery in 75% of cases and from the superficial palmar artery in 25% of cases[32] (▶Fig. 21.10). After entering the tubercle, the palmar vessels divide into several branches to supply the distal 20 to 30% of the scaphoid. The scaphoid is a group 1 bone, using the classification described by Panagis et al.[31] That is, large areas of the bone are dependent on a single vessel and there are no intraosseous anastomoses.[32,33] The limited vascular supply therefore makes the scaphoid more vulnerable to nonunion and AVN than carpal bones having more robust circulatory patterns.

Lunate

The lunate receives its palmar blood supply from branches of the pICa, the PCa, or communicating branches from the anterior interosseous artery and the ulnar recurrent artery. Dorsal blood supply is provided by branches of the dRCa, the dICa, or from a branch of the distal part of the 4th or 5th ECA. The literature suggests that 8 to 20% of lunates may have a single palmar or dorsal blood supply (group 1) and therefore be vulnerable to development of AVN by disruption of extraosseous vessels alone. The other 80 to 92% of lunates have a consistent dorsal and palmar blood supply with an intraosseous anastomosis (group 3). This extensive extrinsic blood supply and/or robust intraosseous connections therefore require considerable disruption of extraosseous and/or intraosseous vasculature if AVN is to develop.[27,28,31,35–37]

Of the group 3 lunates, the intraosseous blood supply follows three different patterns, formed in the shape of the letters Y, I, and X[35] (▶Fig. 21.11). The Y configuration is the most common and occurs in 59% of cases with the base of the Y either on the palmar or on the dorsal side. The I configuration is seen in about one-third of all cases (31%) and the X configuration in 10% of studied cases. The proximal pole of the lunate has the lowest rate of perfusion, making this an area of higher risk for nonunion or AVN.

Triquetrum

The triquetrum is considered a type 3 vascularized carpal bone. It receives its nutrient vessels from branches from the ulnar artery, the dICa, and the pICa. Two to four nutrient arteries enter the dorsal ridge, running from its medial to lateral aspect, and supply the dorsal 60% of bone, which is the dominant blood supply in 60% of specimens. Twenty percent of specimens had a palmar dominant blood supply and 20% an equal contribution. On the palmar aspect, proximal and distal to its articulation with the pisiform, one or two nutrient arteries enter the triquetrum. These vessels anastomose with each other and provide the remaining 40% of blood supply. Eighty-six percent of 25 specimens studied had significant intraosseous anastomoses.[27,28,31] AVN of the triquetrum is not described in literature to date.

Pisiform

The pisiform typically is a group 3 vascularized carpal bone. It receives its blood supply from the ulnar artery via its deep palmar and dorsal carpal branches.[36,38] The dorsal carpal branch is the major source of nutrition, with at least two descending branches entering the proximal tip of the bone in the area of the attachment of the flexor carpi ulnaris. After traversing the cortex, nutrient arteries usually divide into multiple branches. Two or more dorsal branches run parallel beneath the articular surface of the facet. One or two palmar branches run along the palmar cortex and anastomose with the dorsal branches.[31]

At the distal end, one to three vessels enter close to the articular facet. After traversing the cortex, they too divide into multiple branches, travel parallel to the articular facet, and eventually anastomose with the proximal intraosseous arteries. Multiple anastomoses create an arterial ring deep to the facet.[31]

This consistent and robust vascularization allows elevation of a pedicled pisiform graft, which may be used to replace the

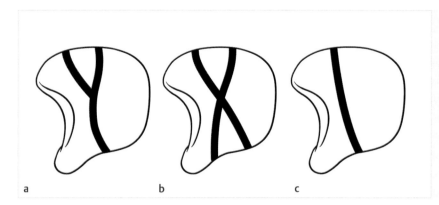

Fig. 21.11 (a–c) Schematic view of group 3 lunates showing the three different patterns of intraosseous vascular supply: Y, X and I. From Gelberman RH, Bauman TD, Menon J, Akeson WH. The vascularity of the lunate bone and Kienbock's disease. J Hand Surg Surg 5:276, 1980. Used with permission. Copyright Elsevier.

lunate[20,21,25,39,40] or, when placed as a decorticated graft within the lunate, to revascularize it.[40–43]

Although vascularization of the pisiform seems adequate, literature shows several case reports of idiopathic AVN of the pisiform.[44,45]

Hamate

Blood supply to the hamate is provided by the dICa, the ulnar recurrent artery, and the ulnar artery. It has three nonarticular surfaces where vessels enter: the dorsal, the palmar, and the medial surface through the hook of the hamate. Three to five vessels penetrate the dorsal triangular surface which supply the dorsal 30 to 40% of the bone. The palmar surface is also triangular and is perforated by usually one large vessel that enters through the radial base of the hook. In the bone it then branches and anastomoses with the dorsal vessels in 50% of specimens studied.[28,31,46]

The hook of the hamate is consistently provided by one to two small vessels entering through the medial base and the tip of the hook. In most cases, these vessels anastomosed but failed to anastomose with the vessels supplying the body of the hamate. Fractures at the hook base therefore are considered more prone to nonunion.[28,31,47]

Few reports in literature describe cases of AVN in the hamate, which in most cases is secondary to a prior traumatic event.[46,48–50]

Capitate

The capitate receives its blood supply from branches of the dICa and the dBMa and from anastomoses between the ulnar recurrent artery and the pICa. Nutrient foramina are located on the palmar and dorsal nonarticular surfaces. Dorsally, the surface allows for ligamentous attachment and is usually penetrated by two to four nutrient vessels along the distal two-thirds of the surface. Occasionally, small vessels enter more proximally, at the neck of the capitate. After entering the bone, the dorsal vessels course palmarly, proximally, and ulnarly, providing blood supply for the capitate head in 67% of cases studied. At the palmar side, the adductor pollicis muscle attaches and one to three vessels enter the distal half of the capitate, slightly more proximal than the dorsal foramina. In 33% of cases studied, the head of the capitate was entirely supplied by these branches. In only 30% of specimens there are significant anastomoses between dorsal and palmar blood supply.[28,31,36]

Due to the anatomy of the intraosseous vessels, fractures of the capitate neck are at high risk of nonunion and consequent secondary AVN of the head. Being placed in group 1, this is a relatively common problem and usually part of a greater arc pattern of perilunate instability. This includes the association of capitate and scaphoid fractures, termed "naviculocapitate syndrome."[51–56] Idiopathic AVN of the capitate is quite rare. Jönsson was the first to describe a case of idiopathic AVN of the capitate in 1942.[57] A review of the literature in 2002 identified only three such cases.[58] Several others resulting from nontraumatic causes, such as Gaucher's disease, steroid use, and gout, have been reported.[59–65] Most of the truly idiopathic cases have occurred in young women.[66] Other secondary causes are thought to be prior repetitive microtrauma or pressure on the palmar side.[56]

Trapezoid

Trapezoid blood supply is provided by branches from the dorsal radiocarpal, the intercarpal, and the basal metacarpal arches and the radial recurrent artery. Nutrient vessels enter the bone through the palmar and dorsal nonarticular surfaces. Dorsal vessels provide primary blood supply to the trapezoid in the form of three or four small nutrient vessels. After entering the subchondral bone, these vessels supply the dorsal 70% of the bone. Palmar blood supply is provided by one or two small nutrient vessels that enter the narrow, flat, and small nonarticular surface. They provide vascular supply to the remaining palmar 30% of bone. No anastomoses are seen between the palmar and dorsal vessels; therefore, the trapezoid is classified as a group 2 bone.[30,67]

Several cases have been reported on AVN of the trapezoid. A traumatic dislocation precipitated AVN in two reported cases.[68,69] Sturzenegger reported a case of idiopathic, nontraumatic AVN of the trapezoid,[70] and D'Agostino reported a rare case of bilateral AVN of the trapezoid, most likely caused by repetitive microtrauma.[71]

Trapezium

The trapezium receives its blood supply from distal branches of the radial artery. There are three nonarticular surfaces where nutrient vessels enter the bone. The dorsoradial and lateral surfaces are sites for ligamentous attachment; the palmar tubercle serves as the origin site of the thenar muscles. Dorsoradially, one to three vessels traverse the cortex to supply the entire dorsal part of the bone. Palmarly, one to three vessels enter the middle part of the bone to anastomose intraosseously with the dorsal vessels. Laterally, three to six small vessels penetrate the surface and anastomose with the dorsal and palmar vessels. Dorsal blood supply is dominant, and frequent anastomoses are seen among all three systems.[28,31,36]

The trapezium is therefore placed in group 3, and its extensive vascular supply makes idiopathic AVN of the trapezium unlikely. Indeed, no such case exists in the literature to date. Garcia-López et al described AVN as a secondary problem after a high-impact force trauma.[72] Another case also reported the osteonecrosis to be secondary to prior injury that possibly disrupted the blood supply.[73]

21.4 Vascularized Bone Grafts

Vascularized bone grafts may be applied to the carpus to aid or accelerate fracture healing, replace bone deficiency, or aid in direct revascularization of ischemic bone. Most commonly, and with increasing frequency, vascularized grafts are applied to treat scaphoid fractures and pseudarthroses, and for cases of AVN such as Kienbock's or Preiser's disease.

References

1. Haller Av, ed. Fasciculus VI. Gottingae. In: Vandenhoek A, ed. Incones anotomicae; 1753
2. Tiedeman F, ed. Manual of Angiology, translated by Robert Knox. Stewart Ma, ed. Edinburgh 1831
3. Henle J, ed. Handbuch der systematischen anatomie des menschen. Braunschweig1868. Vieweg, ed; No. 3
4. Zaidemberg C, Siebert JW, Angrigiani C. A new vascularized bone graft for scaphoid nonunion. J Hand Surg Am 1991;16(3):474–478
5. Sheetz KK, Bishop AT, Berger RA. The arterial blood supply of the distal radius and ulna and its potential use in vascularized pedicled bone grafts. J Hand Surg Am 1995;20(6):902–914
6. Waitayawinyu T, Robertson C, Chin SH, Schlenker JD, Pettrone S, Trumble TE. The detailed anatomy of the 1,2 intercompartmental supraretinacular artery for vascularized bone grafting of scaphoid nonunions. J Hand Surg Am 2008;33(2):168–174
7. Lin SD, Lai CS, Chiu CC. Venous drainage in the reverse forearm flap. Plast Reconstr Surg 1984;74(4):508–512
8. Tu YK, Bishop AT, Kato T, Adams ML, Wood MB. Experimental carpal reverse-flow pedicle vascularized bone grafts. Part I: the anatomical basis of vascularized pedicle bone grafts based on the canine distal radius and ulna. J Hand Surg Am 2000;25(1):34–45
9. Tu YK, Bishop AT, Kato T, Adams ML, Wood MB. Experimental carpal reverse-flow pedicle vascularized bone grafts. Part II: bone blood flow measurement by radioactive-labeled microspheres in a canine model. J Hand Surg Am 2000;25(1):46–54
10. Menck J, Schreiber HW, Hertz T, Bürgel N. [Angioarchitecture of the ulna and radius and their practical relevance]. Langenbecks Arch Chir 1994;379(2):70–75
11. Pagliei A, Brunelli F, Gilbert A. Anterior interosseous artery: anatomic bases of pedicled bone-grafts. Surg Radiol Anat 1991;13(2):152–154
12. Haerle M, Schaller HE, Mathoulin C. Vascular anatomy of the palmar surfaces of the distal radius and ulna: its relevance to pedi-

13. cled bone grafts at the distal palmar forearm. J Hand Surg [Br] 2003;28(2):131–136
14. Kuhlmann JN, Mimoun M, Boabighi A, Baux S. Vascularized bone graft pedicled on the volar carpal artery for non-union of the scaphoid. J Hand Surg [Br] 1987;12(2):203–210
15. Braun RM. Viable pedicle bone grafting in the wrist. In: Urbaniak JR, ed. Microsurgery for Major Limb Reconstruction. St. Louis, MO: C.V. Mosby; 1987:220–229
16. Kawai H, Yamamoto K. Pronator quadratus pedicled bone graft for old scaphoid fractures. J Bone Joint Surg Br 1988;70(5):829–831
17. Braun RM. Proximal pedicle bone grafting in the forearm and proximal carpal row. Orthop Trans. 1983;7(1):35
18. Mathoulin C, Haerle M. Vascularized bone graft from the palmar carpal artery for treatment of scaphoid nonunion. J Hand Surg [Br] 1998;23(3):318–323
19. Chacha PB. Vascularised pedicular bone grafts. Int Orthop 1984;8(2):117–138
20. Guimberteau JC, Panconi B. Recalcitrant non-union of the scaphoid treated with a vascularized bone graft based on the ulnar artery. J Bone Joint Surg Am 1990;72(1):88–97
21. Heymans R, Adelmann E, Koebke J. Anatomical bases of the pediculated pisiform transplant and the intercarpal fusion by Graner in Kienböck's disease. Surg Radiol Anat 1992;14(3):195–201
22. Heymans R, Koebke J. The pedicled pisiform transposition in Kienböck's disease. An anatomical and functional analysis. Handchir Mikrochir Plast Chir 1993;25(4):199–203
23. Kuhlmann JN, Guérin-Surville H, Boabighi A. Vascularisation of the carpus, a systematic study. Surg Radiol Anat 1988;10(1):21–28
24. Leung PC, Hung LK. Use of pronator quadratus bone flap in bony reconstruction around the wrist. J Hand Surg Am 1990;15(4):637–640
25. Roy-Camille R. Fractures et pseudarthroses du scaphoide moyen utilisation d'un gretion pedicule. Actualites de Chirugie Orthopedique Raymond Poincare. 1965;4:197–214
26. Saffar P. Replacement du semi-lunaire par le pisiforme: description d'une nouvelle technique pour le traitement de la maladie de Kienbock. Ann Chir Main 1982;1982(1):276–279
27. Lamas C, Llusà M, Méndez A, Proubasta I, Carrera A, Forcada P. Intraosseous vascularity of the distal radius: anatomy and clinical implications in distal radius fractures. Hand (NY) 2009;4(4):418–423
28. Gelberman RH, Panagis JS, Taleisnik J, Baumgaertner M. The arterial anatomy of the human carpus. Part I: the extraosseous vascularity. J Hand Surg Am 1983;8(4):367–375
29. Gelberman RH, ed. Vascularity of the carpus. 2nd ed. WB Saunders; 1997. D.M. L, ed. The Wrist and Its Disorders
30. Gellman H, Botte MJ, Shankwiler J, Gelberman RH. Arterial patterns of the deep and superficial palmar arches. Clin Orthop Relat Res 2001; (383):41–46
31. Freedman DM, Botte MJ, Gelberman RH. Vascularity of the carpus [see comment]. Clin Orthop Relat Res 2001; (383):47–59
32. Panagis JS, Gelberman RH, Taleisnik J, Baumgaertner M. The arterial anatomy of the human carpus. Part II: the intraosseous vascularity. J Hand Surg Am 1983;8(4):375–382
33. Gelberman RH, Menon J. The vascularity of the scaphoid bone. J Hand Surg Am 1980;5(5):508–513
34. Taleisnik J, Kelly PJ. The extraosseous and intraosseous blood supply of the scaphoid bone. J Bone Joint Surg Am 1966;48(6):1125–1137
35. Barber H, ed. The intraosseous arterial anatomy of the human carpus. 5th ed. Orthopaedics; 1972

35. Gelberman RH, Bauman TD, Menon J, Akeson WH. The vascularity of the lunate bone and Kienböck's disease. J Hand Surg Am 1980;5(3):272–278

36. Gelberman RH, Gross MS. The vascularity of the wrist. Identification of arterial patterns at risk. Clin Orthop Relat Res 1986;(202):40–49

37. Williams CS, Gelberman RH. Vascularity of the lunate. Anatomic studies and implications for the development of osteonecrosis. Hand Clin 1993;9(3):391–398

38. Mestdagh H, Houcke M, Mairesse JL, Vilette B, Depreux R. Vascular anatomy of the pisiformis bone. Ann Chir Main 1984;3(2):145–148

39. Erbs G, Böhm E. Long-term results of pisiform bone transposition in lunate necrosis. Handchir Mikrochir Plast Chir 1984;16(2):85–89

40. Godina M. Preferential use of end-to-side arterial anastomoses in free flap transfers. Plast Reconstr Surg 1979;64(5):673–682

41. Bochud RC, Büchler U. Kienböck's disease, early stage 3—height reconstruction and core revascularization of the lunate. J Hand Surg [Br] 1994;19(4):466–478

42. Beck E. Die Verpflanzung des Os pisiforme am Gefässstiel zur Behandlung der Lunatummalazie. Handchirurgie 1971;3(2):64–67

43. Martini AK. Results of vascular pedicled bone transposition in advanced necrosis of the lunate bone. Handchir Mikrochir Plast Chir 1987;19(6):318–321

44. Match RM. Nonspecific avascular necrosis of the pisiform bone: a case report. J Hand Surg Am 1980;5(4):341–342

45. Oláh J. Bilaterale aseptische Nekrose des Os pisiforme. Z Orthop Ihre Grenzgeb 1968;104(4):590–591

46. Van Demark RE, Parke WW. Avascular necrosis of the hamate: a case report with reference to the hamate blood supply. J Hand Surg Am 1992;17(6):1086–1090

47. Failla JM. Hook of hamate vascularity: vulnerability to osteonecrosis and nonunion. J Hand Surg Am 1993;18(6):1075–1079

48. Telfer JR, Evans DM, Bingham JB. Avascular necrosis of the hamate. J Hand Surg [Br] 1994;19(3):389–392

49. De Smet L. Avascular necrosis of multiple carpal bones. A case report. Chir Main 1999;18(3):202–204

50. Mazis GA, Sakellariou VI, Kokkalis ZT. Avascular necrosis of the hamate treated with capitohamate and lunatohamate intercarpal fusion. Orthopedics 2012;35(3):e444–e447

51. Steffens K, Luce S, Koob E. Unusual course of scapho-capitate syndrome. Handchir Mikrochir Plast Chir 1994;26(1):12–14

52. Sawant M, Miller J. Scaphocapitate syndrome in an adolescent. J Hand Surg Am 2000;25(6):1096–1099

53. Newman JH, Watt I. Avascular necrosis of the capitate and dorsal dorsi-flexion instability. Hand 1980;12(2):176–178

54. Mazur K, Stevanovic M, Schnall SB, Hannani K, Zionts LE. Scapho-capitate syndrome in a child associated with a distal radius and ulna fracture. J Orthop Trauma 1997;11(3):230–232

55. Kumar A, Thomas AP. Scapho-capitate fracture syndrome. A case report. Acta Orthop Belg 2001;67(2):185–189

56. Ye BJ, Kim JI, Lee HJ, Jung KY. A case of avascular necrosis of the capitate bone in a pallet car driver. J Occup Health 2009;51(5):451–453

57. Jönsson G. Aseptic bone necrosis of the os capitum (os magnum). Acta Radiol 1942;1942(23):562–564

58. Niesten JA, Verhaar JA. Idiopathic avascular necrosis of the capitate—a case report and a review of the literature. Hand Surg 2002;7(1):159–161

59. De Smet L, Aerts P, Walraevens M, Fabry G. Avascular necrosis of the carpal scaphoid: Preiser's disease: report of 6 cases and review of the literature. [Review] [20 refs] Acta Orthop Belg 1993;59(2):139–142

60. Kato H, Ogino T, Minami A. Steroid-induced avascular necrosis of the capitate. A case report. Handchir Mikrochir Plast Chir 1991;23(1):15–17

61. Kutty S, Curtin J. Idiopathic avascular necrosis of the capitate. J Hand Surg [Br] 1995;20(3):402–404

62. Arcalis Arce A, Pedemonte Jansana JP, Massons Albareda JM. Idiopathic necrosis of the capitate. Acta Orthop Belg 1996;62(1):46–48

63. Niesten JA, Verhaar JA. Idiopathic avascular necrosis of the capitate—a case report and a review of the literature. Hand Surg 2002;7(1):159–161

64. Wounlund J, Lohmann M. Aseptic necrosis of the capitate secondary to Gaucher's disease: a case report. J Hand Surg [Br] 1989;14(3):336–337

65. Prommersberger KJ, van Schoonhoven J, Lanz U. [Aseptic necrosis of the capitate: a rare cause for wrist pain. Case report and review of the literature]. Handchir Mikrochir Plast Chir 2000;32(2):123–128

66. Lapinsky AS, Mack GR. Avascular necrosis of the capitate: a case report. J Hand Surg Am 1992;17(6):1090–1092

67. Panagis JS, Gelberman RH, Taleisnik J, Baumgaertner M. The arterial anatomy of the human carpus. Part II: the intraosseous vascularity. J Hand Surg Am 1983;8(4):375–382

68. Stein AH Jr. Dorsal dislocation of the lesser multangular bone. J Bone Joint Surg Am 1971;53(2):377–379

69. Dunkerton M, Singer M. Dislocation of the index metacarpal and trapezoid bones. J Hand Surg [Br] 1985;10(3):377–378

70. Sturzenegger M, Mencarelli F. Avascular necrosis of the trapezoid bone. J Hand Surg [Br] 1998;23(4):550–551

71. D'Agostino P, Townley WA, Roulot E. Bilateral avascular necrosis of the trapezoid. J Hand Surg Am 2011;36(10):1678–1680

72. García-López A, Cardoso Z, Ortega L. Avascular necrosis of trapezium bone: a case report. J Hand Surg Am 2002;27(4):704–706

73. Zafra M, Carpintero P, Cansino D. Osteonecrosis of the trapezium treated with a vascularized distal radius bone graft. J Hand Surg Am 2004;29(6):1098–1101

22 Interosseous Vascularity of the Carpus

Mohamed Morsy, Nick A. van Alphen, and Steven L. Moran

22.1 Introduction

The blood supply to the carpal bones plays an important role in bone development, remodeling, and healing. The interosseous arterial network to each carpal bone is capable of transporting important hormones and growth factors, allowing for ossification during development, and it also stimulates bone healing in times of trauma.[1] Evidence of a vascular ingrowth into the lunate bone is seen as early as 14 weeks of fetal gestation. This early vascular ingrowth leads to the process of endochondral ossification.[2] Subsequently, each of the developing carpal bone anlages is penetrated by isolated arterial buds which terminate in sinusoidal formations. Ossification begins near the center of each carpal bone, with the exception of the distal eccentric ossification center of the scaphoid. The vascular buds progressively retreat and are replaced with a series of nutrient trunks, which, in most cases, enter through opposing surfaces and anastomose within the bone.[3]

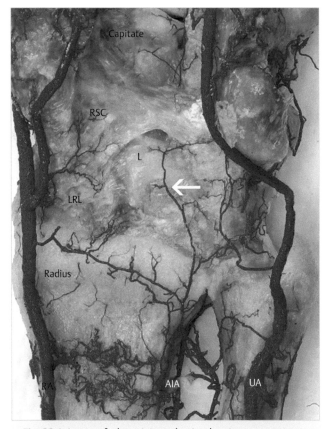

Fig. 22.1 Image of a latex-injected wrist showing extraosseous arterial system penetrating volar wrist capsule to contribute to the interosseous vascular blood supply. Note vessel entering volar surface of lunate (*arrow*). RA, radial artery, AIA, anterior interosseous artery, UA, ulnar artery, LRL, long radiolunate ligament, L, lunate bone, RSC, radioscaphocapitate ligament. (Copyright Mayo Clinic.)

The extrinsic blood supply to the carpal bones is provided through anastomosis between a dorsal transverse and palmar transverse carpal arterial arcade; this *extraosseous* system originates from the radial, ulnar, and anterior interosseous arteries. The anatomic details of this extraosseous vascular system are discussed elsewhere within the text. The extraosseous arteries penetrate the carpal bones through nutrient foramina, where they go on to form the intraosseous arterial system within each carpal bone (▶ Fig. 22.1). In long bones, the blood supply to the bone comprises a combination of periosteal, nutrient, epiphyseal, and metaphyseal vessels. Vessels usually enter through noncartilaginous areas of ligamentous attachment.[4,5] In the carpus, many of the bones have a large surface area covered with articular cartilage (such as the scaphoid and lunate), thus limiting the area for blood vessel in growth.

The study of the interosseous blood supply of the carpus has been limited by technology. Early studies with long bones used India ink injections to evaluate the interosseous system.[6] This was followed by the use of the Spalteholz technique, in which barium sulfate is injected into the vasculature of the bone. The bone is then sequentially decalcified, dehydrated, and sectioned. Specimens are then made transparent by placing them in Spalteholz fluid.[3,7]

In the late 1970s and early 1980s, building on the work of Crock and others, Gelberman and colleagues produced several landmark papers which sought to evaluate the complexities and intricacies of the interosseous blood supply by performing a series of experiments utilizing a modification of the Spalteholz technique.[3,8,9] From this work it was shown that carpal bones can be categorized into three groups based on the location and number of intraosseous vessels (▶ Table 22.1).[5] Abnormalities or damage to the intraosseous blood supply can lead to bone dysmorphology and osteonecrosis.[10,11] Carpal bones found in group I, the scaphoid, capitate, and a percentage of lunates, are more prone to avascular necrosis due to the dependence of a major portion of the bone on a single vessel lacking intraosseous anastomosis with other nutrient arteries.[5,9,12]

Since the time of these publications, there has been substantial advancement in imaging technology with both magnetic resonance imaging (MRI) and micro-computed tomography (micro-CT). Although studies utilizing the Spalteholz technique have stood the test of time, they provide primarily

Table 22.1 Classification of carpal bones by intraosseous vascular anatomy[5]

Group 1; perforators or nutrient branches penetrating on one bony surface, or a large portion of the bone is supplied by a single perforator	Scaphoid, capitate, and minority of lunate bones
Group 2; at least two perforators, but lacks intraosseous anastomosis	Trapezoid, hamate
Group 3; at least two perforators with intraosseous anastomosis	Trapezium, triquetrum, pisiform, and majority of lunate bones

two-dimensional imaging. To overcome these shortcomings, more recent studies have used micro-CT techniques to visualize the intraosseous vascular network.[13,14] This technology can provide accurate three-dimensional information that was not possible with more classic techniques. The image resolution of micro-CT can allow for imaging of structures of 1 to 2 μm. In addition, newer low-viscosity radiopaque substances can fill the interosseous microvasculature. Using this technology, measurements can also be made that were not previously possible, such as of vessel diameter, length, and volume. All this can be obtained without alteration of the internal bony architecture that can occur with the previous decalcification techniques.[15,16] This new information can be utilized to update our understanding of avascular necrosis and its etiology, as well as to describe safe zones for surgical intervention and instrumentation of these bones. A more thorough understanding of the intricacies of the carpal bone vascular system may have widespread ramifications on bone pathology, fracture fixation, and surgical intervention. This chapter briefly reviews the latest advances and discoveries related to intraosseous vascular anatomy of the lunate, capitate, and scaphoid, as well as the impact they may have on clinical practice.

22.2 The Lunate

The lunate lies at the center of the proximal row and plays an important biomechanical and clinical role in carpal kinematics.[17] It acts as a pillar for the lunate–capitate column and as a major stabilizer of the proximal row. The arterial blood supply to the lunate is derived from either volar or dorsal nutrient vessels with intraosseous anastomoses.[5,8,18-21] These vessels enter near the short radiolunate ligament palmarly and dorsally through the attachments of the radiocarpal ligament. Although traumatic fracture of the lunate is uncommon, the lunate is the

second most common carpal bone to undergo avascular necrosis, a process referred to as Kienbock's disease.[22,23]

Gelberman and colleagues identified three patterns for the interosseous anastomosis of the nutrient vessels within the lunate. These are described according the their shape as they pass through the bone as the letters Y (occurring in 59% of specimens), X (occurring in 10% of specimens), and I (occurring in 31% of specimens; ▶Fig. 22.2).[8] It has been shown that up to 20% of the lunates are dependent solely on either a volar or a dorsal nutrient system, potentially making them more prone to avascular necrosis if this single nutrient system were to be damaged.[5,8,22,24,25]

In a recently published study using micro-CT imaging, Van Alphen and colleagues further examined the intraosseous vascular patterns of the lunate bone. They noted that all specimens could be classified according to the previously described Y, X, and I classification scheme. In addition, these patterns were found to occur in similar distributions as those reported by Gelberman and colleagues[8,14] (▶Fig. 22.3). The vascular pattern seen within each specimen was not found to be associated with the presence or absence of a hamate facet on the lunate.[14] The presence or absence of a hamate facet has been postulated as a factor contributing to the development of Kienbock's disease[26,27]

With more accurate measurement of the number, diameter, and total cross-sectional area of the interosseous vessels, Van Alphen also found that the nutrient vessels from the volar and dorsal sides were comparable in diameter and cross-sectional area; however, some specimens had only a volar vessel (no dorsal nutrient vessel) as the lunates' sole source of interosseous blood supply. There were no specimens identified where there was a sole dorsal blood supply.[14] Lunates with an isolated single volar vessel may be at risk for traumatic or iatrogenic injury, which could have an impact on the development

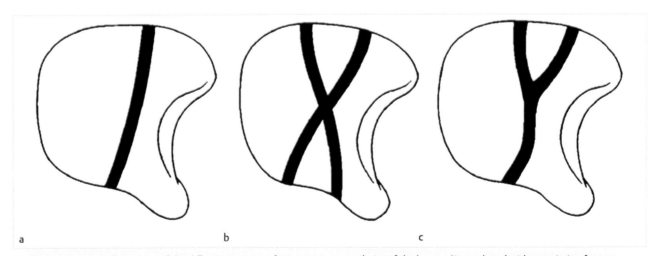

a   b   c

Fig. 22.2 (a–c) An illustration of the different patterns of intraosseous vascularity of the lunate. (Reproduced with permission from Gelberman RH, Bauman TD, Menon J, Akeson, WA. The vascularity of the lunate bone and Kienbock's disease. *J Hand Surg* 1980;5:276.)

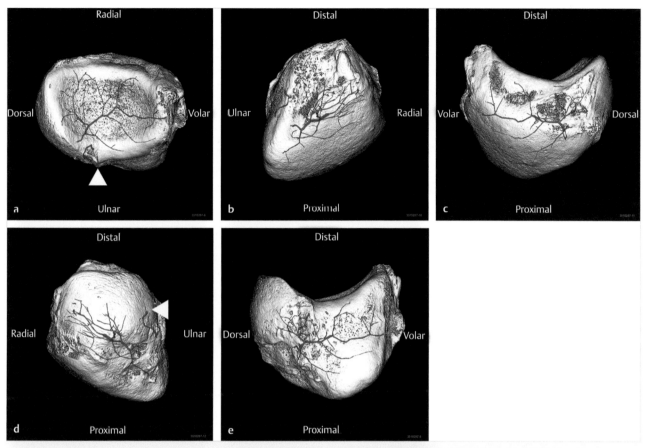

Fig. 22.3 Multiple images of a lunate cadaveric specimen imaged with micro-CT and rendered in three dimensions following vascular injection. The red structure correlates with the path of the nutrient artery. This lunate fits within the general "I"-type intraosseous vascular pattern. The various views seen include distal (**a**), volar (**b**), radial (**c**), dorsal (**d**), and ulnar (**e**). Note the dorsal and volar locations of main nutrient foramina. *White arrow* points to accessory nutrient vessel which has no perceivable anastomosis to main central arterial system. (Copyright Mayo Clinic.)

of localized bone ischemia and future ability to respond to trauma.

Iatrogenic avascular necrosis of the lunate and scaphoid has been described in the literature.[28–31] Based on the previous findings, a dorsal approach would have the lowest chance of irreversible injury to the lunates blood supply, as no specimen was noted to have an isolated dorsal blood supply to the lunate.[14] Van Alpehen goes on to describe safe zones for surgical fixation and intervention on the lunate. These sites may favor hardware placement, as they are areas with a lower likelihood of injuring a dominant nutrient vessel (▶ Fig. 22.4).[14] Volar approaches to the lunate, for ligament reconstruction or perilunate injury, may result in localized ischemia in a subset of patients with an absent dorsal nutrient vessel.

22.3 Capitate

The capitate has been traditionally considered one of the carpal bones at high risk for posttraumatic avascular necrosis.[5,22,32–40]

Risk of avascular necrosis has been attributed to the retrograde intraosseous vascular pattern of the capitate, which is similar to the mechanism of avascular necrosis seen in the proximal pole of the scaphoid following waist fractures.[41–44] Previous studies have demonstrated that nutrient vessels enter the capitate from its volar and dorsal surfaces at the nonarticular distal portion, forming two separate networks that anastomose only in 30% of capitates. These vessels travel proximally, supplying the proximal articular portion of the bone.[4,5,22,40]

In a recent study of 10 cadaveric capitates evaluated using micro-CT, 70% of specimens had evidence for a nutrient vessel entering proximal to the capitate waist (▶ Fig. 22.5).[13] In the same study, the average fracture line in 22 capitate fracture patients was plotted and compared with the vessel entry points. The study demonstrated that 90% of capitates should theoretically have at least one vessel entering proximal to the fracture line (▶ Fig. 22.6). These findings are supported by a recent clinical studies reporting the absence of avascular necrosis of the proximal capitate following fracture, even in cases of delayed nonunions; this study was limited to cases of primary capitate fracture

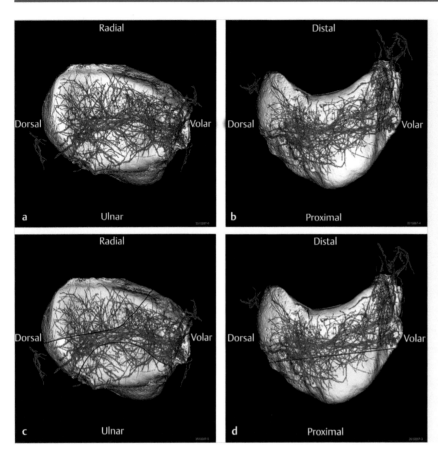

Fig. 22.4 (a,b) The advancement of CT technology allows one to overlap the vascular architecture from different specimens. This allows one to produce a composite view of where the majority of the intraosseous blood supply lies in relation to the dorsal and volar surface of the bone. Surgical safe zones can then be assigned to areas which avoid these "high-traffic" areas for the nutrient vessels. **(c,d)** Demonstration of the safe zones for surgical intervention (*yellow areas*) in the lunate on a distal view of a lunate bone with vasculature of all specimens superimposed to create a vessel density map. (Reproduced with permission from van Alphen NA, Morsy M, Laungani AT, et al. A three-dimensional micro-computed tomographic study of the intraosseous lunate vasculature: implications for surgical intervention and the development of avascular necrosis. Plast Recon Surg 2016;138(5):869e–878e.)

and could not comment on the etiology or incidence of capitate avascular necrosis seen secondarily where the mechanism of injury was unknown.[45] Moreover, avascular necrosis has not been described as a complication following the capitate-shortening procedure done for Kienbock's disease, which suggests adequate blood supply to the proximal pole in a large majority of patients.[46–48] Although the results of these studies cannot completely abolish the possibility of posttraumatic avascular necrosis of the capitate in cases of delayed nonunion, it could indicate that the risk is much less than historically believed.

22.4 Scaphoid

The scaphoid is the most common carpal bone to be fractured, accounting for up to 90% of carpal bone fractures.[49,50] Blood supply of the scaphoid has been classically described as retrograde entering at the dorsal ridge. This retrograde blood supply is thought to be responsible for the occurrence of posttraumatic avascular necrosis of the proximal pole in cases of scaphoid fracture.[9,51]

In a recent study, utilizing micro-CT technology, scaphoid specimens were scanned and 3D renderings reconstructed (▶Fig. 22.7). The retrograde nature of the intraosseous vascularity was confirmed, although a number of specimens had evidence of vessels entering the scaphoid volarly at the nonarticular portion of the waist, to join and supplement the intraosseous vascular system (▶Fig. 22.8). This vessel has not been described in previous studies.[52] Another novel finding was that in some specimens, smaller caliber vessels were identified entering the scaphoid's proximal pole at the scapholunate ligament attachment (▶Fig. 22.9).[52] While a direct clinical correlation was not possible with this study, these findings may explain why some scaphoid waist and proximal pole fractures are capable of healing even after a delay in management.[53]

Most operative scaphoid fractures are now managed with the placement of headless compression screws. Morsy and colleagues sought to examine the impact of compression screw insertion on the intraosseous vascularity. Scaphoid screws may be placed centrally or eccentrically down the long axis of the bone. The course of the screw is determined by surgical approach (volar vs. dorsal) and by location of the fracture. Using

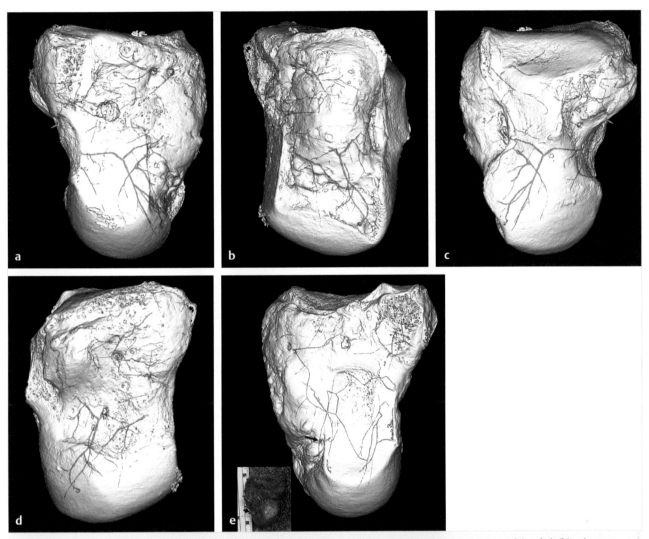

Fig. 22.5 3D rendering of a scanned capitate with the intraosseous vascular pattern apparent in various views; (**a**) radial, (**b**) volar, (**c**) ulnar, (**d**) dorsal and (**e**) Inset image of capitate specimen with arrow pointing to vessel entering directly into proximal pole from volar aspect of the specimen. The 3-D rendered specimen following micro-CT reconstruction shows nutrient vessels in the proximal pole and in the distal portion of the capitate. (Reproduction from Kadar A, Morsy M, Sur YJ, Laungani AT, Akdag O, Moran SL. The Vascular Anatomy of the Capitate: New Discoveries Using Micro-Computed Tomography Imaging. J. Hand Surg 2017;42(2):78–86.)

computer modeling, various screw axes were examined to see what percentage of nutrient vessels would be affected by screw trajectory. The study found that the true central axis had the least detrimental effect on the internal blood supply. This was closely followed by the antegrade insertion axis, while the retrograde insertion axis had the highest likelihood of injuring in vascular axis of the scaphoid (▶ Fig. 22.10).[52] This suggests that antegrade screw insertion may be a safer technique with less potential detrimental effect on the intraosseous vascularity.

As technology continues to advance, we believe that someday there will be a means of real-time evaluation of carpal bone vascularity; thus one could identify early evidence of avascular necrosis, identify scaphoid fractures which would benefit from vascularized bone grafts, and limit the potential for blood vessel injury following hardware placement. Until that time, surgeons will need to rely on their knowledge of anatomy and remember the most common patterns of carpal blood flow in order to minimize nutrient vessel injury and maximize carpal bone healing potential.

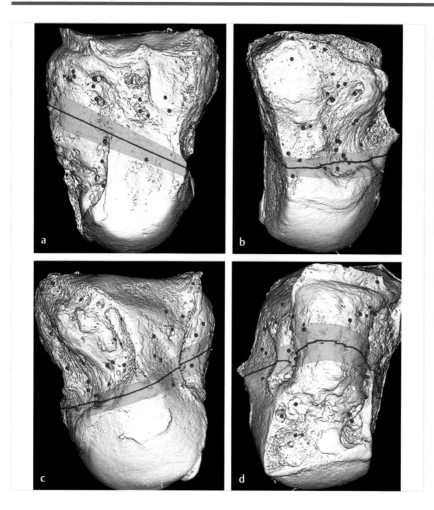

Fig. 22.6 (a–d) Vessel entry points (*red circles*) from 10 capitate specimens projected on a single capitate where the average fracture line of a series of 22 capitate fractures (*blue line*) and its 95% confidence interval (*light blue shaded surface*) were plotted. The image shows that most capitate fractures have some blood supply to the proximal pole. This may explain why avascular necrosis of the capitate head is so rare and why more complications are not reported following capitate shortening procedures. (Reproduction from Kadar A, Morsy M, Sur YJ, Laungani AT, Akdag O, Moran SL. The vascular anatomy of the capitate: new discoveries using micro-computed tomography imaging. J Hand Surg 2017;42(2):78–86.)

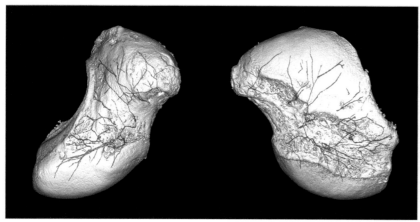

Fig. 22.7 A three-dimensional reconstruction of a scanned scaphoid specimen showing the intraosseous vascular tree. (Copyright Mayo Clinic.)

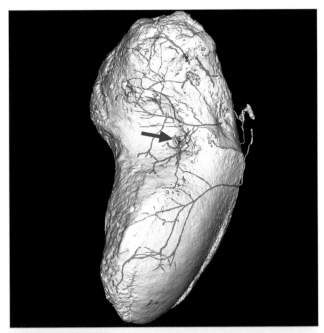

Fig. 22.8 A volar view of a scaphoid specimen showing a nutrient vessel entering the bone at the nonarticular volar waist (*blue arrow*). (Copyright Mayo Clinic.)

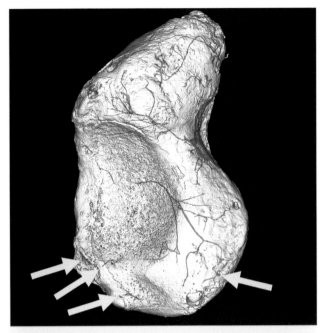

Fig. 22.9 Minute vessels entering a scaphoid specimen at the scapholunate ligament attachment (*yellow arrows*). (Copyright Mayo Clinic.)

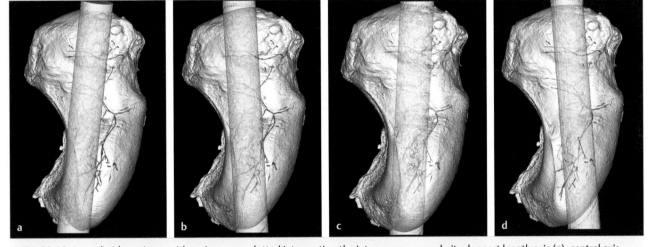

Fig. 22.10 A scaphoid specimen with various axes plotted intersecting the intraosseous vascularity; longest length axis (**a**), central axis (**b**), retrograde axis (**c**), antegrade axis (**d**). (Copyright Mayo Clinic.)

References

1. Tomlinson RE, Silva MJ. Skeletal blood flow in bone repair and maintenance. Bone Res 2013;1(4):311–322

2. Hita-Contreras F, Martínez-Amat A, Ortiz R, et al. Development and morphogenesis of human wrist joint during embryonic and early fetal period. J Anat 2012;220(6):580–590

3. Crock HV, Chari PR, Crock MC. The Blood Supply of the Wrist and Hand Bones in Man. Vol 1. Philadelphia, PA: W.B. Saunders Co.; 1981

4. Grettve S. Arterial anatomy of the carpal bones. Acta Anat (Basel) 1955;25(2-4):331–345

5. Panagis JS, Gelberman RH, Taleisnik J, Baumgaertner M. The arterial anatomy of the human carpus. Part II: The intraosseous vascularity. J Hand Surg Am 1983;8(4):375–382

6. Trias A, Fery A. Cortical circulation of long bones. J Bone Joint Surg Am 1979;61(7):1052–1059

7. Spalteholz W. Ueber das Durchsichtigmachen von menschlichen und tierischen Präparaten; nebst Anhang: Ueber Knochenfärburg. Leipzig: S. Hirzel; 1911

8. Gelberman RH, Bauman TD, Menon J, Akeson WH. The vascularity of the lunate bone and Kienböck's disease. J Hand Surg Am 1980;5(3):272–278

9. Gelberman RH, Menon J. The vascularity of the scaphoid bone. J Hand Surg Am 1980;5(5):508–513

10. Chan WP, Liu YJ, Huang GS, et al. Relationship of idiopathic osteonecrosis of the femoral head to perfusion changes in the proximal femur by dynamic contrast-enhanced MRI. AJR Am J Roentgenol 2011;196(3):637–643

11. Filipowska J, Tomaszewski KA, Niedźwiedzki Ł, Walocha JA, Niedźwiedzki T. The role of vasculature in bone development, regeneration and proper systemic functioning. Angiogenesis 2017;20(3):291–302

12. Taleisnik J, Kelly PJ. The extraosseous and intraosseous blood supply of the scaphoid bone. J Bone Joint Surg Am 1966;48(6):1125–1137

13. Kadar A, Morsy M, Sur YJ, Laungani AT, Akdag O, Moran SL. The vascular anatomy of the capitate: new discoveries using micro-computed tomography imaging. J Hand Surg Am 2017; 42(2):78–86

14. van Alphen NA, Morsy M, Laungani AT, et al. A three-dimensional micro-computed tomographic study of the intraosseous lunate vasculature: implications for surgical intervention and the development of avascular necrosis. Plast Reconstr Surg 2016;138(5):869e–878e

15. Jorgensen SM, Demirkaya O, Ritman EL. Three-dimensional imaging of vasculature and parenchyma in intact rodent organs with X-ray micro-CT. Am J Physiol 1998;275(3 Pt 2):H1103–H1114

16. Kline TL, Zamir M, Ritman EL. Accuracy of microvascular measurements obtained from micro-CT images. Ann Biomed Eng 2010;38(9):2851–2864

17. Linscheid RL, Dobyns JH, Beabout JW, Bryan RS. Traumatic instability of the wrist. Diagnosis, classification, and pathomechanics. J Bone Joint Surg Am 1972;54(8):1612–1632

18. Dubey PP, Chauhan NK, Siddiqui MS, Verma AK. Study of vascular supply of lunate and consideration applied to Kienböck disease. Hand Surg 2011;16(1):9–13

19. Lamas C, Carrera A, Proubasta I, Llusà M, Majó J, Mir X. The anatomy and vascularity of the lunate: considerations applied to Kienböck's disease. Chir Main 2007;26(1):13–20

20. Lee ML. The intraosseous arterial pattern of the carpal lunate bone and its relation to avascular necrosis. Acta Orthop Scand 1963;33:43–55

21. Stahl F. On Lunatomalacia (Kienböck's disease): a clinical and roentgenological study, especially on its pathogenesis and late results of immobilization treatment. Acta Chir Scand 1947;95(Suppl 126):3–133

22. Gelberman RH, Gross MS. The vascularity of the wrist. Identification of arterial patterns at risk. Clin Orthop Relat Res 1986; (202):40–49

23. Irisarri C. Aetiology of Kienböck's disease. J Hand Surg [Br] 2004;29(3):281–287

24. Gelberman RH, Panagis JS, Taleisnik J, Baumgaertner M. The arterial anatomy of the human carpus. Part I: The extraosseous vascularity. J Hand Surg Am 1983;8(4):367–375

25. Williams CS, Gelberman RH. Vascularity of the lunate. Anatomic studies and implications for the development of osteonecrosis. Hand Clin 1993;9(3):391–398

26. Rhee PC, Jones DB, Moran SL, Shin AY. The effect of lunate morphology in Kienböck disease. J Hand Surg Am 2015;40(4): 738–744

27. Viegas SF, Wagner K, Patterson R, Peterson P. Medial (hamate) facet of the lunate. J Hand Surg Am 1990;15(4):564–571

28. Berschback JC, Kalainov DM, Bednar MS. Osteonecrosis of the scaphoid after scapholunate interosseous ligament repair and dorsal capsulodesis: case report. J Hand Surg Am 2010;35(5): 732–735

29. De Smet L, Sciot R, Degreef I. Avascular necrosis of the scaphoid after three-ligament tenodesis for scapholunate dissociation: case report. J Hand Surg Am 2011;36(4):587–590

30. Fok MW, Fernandez DL. Chronic scapholunate instability treated with temporary screw fixation. J Hand Surg Am 2015;40(4): 752–758

31. Vitale MA, Shin AY. Avascular necrosis of the scaphoid following a scapholunate screw: a case report. Hand (N Y) 2013;8(1): 110–114

32. Bolton-Maggs BG, Helal BH, Revell PA. Bilateral avascular necrosis of the capitate. A case report and a review of the literature. J Bone Joint Surg Br 1984;66(4):557–559

33. Ichchou L, Amine B, Hajjaj-Hassouni N. Idiopathic avascular necrosis of the capitate bone: a new case report. Clin Rheumatol 2008;27(Suppl 2):S47–S50

34. Kato H, Ogino T, Minami A. Steroid-induced avascular necrosis of the capitate. A case report. Handchirurgie, Mikrochirurgie, plastische Chirurgie: Organ der Deutschsprachigen Arbeitsgemeinschaft fur Handchirurgie. Organ der Deutschsprachigen Arbeitsgemeinschaft fur Mikrochirurgie der Peripheren Nerven und Gefasse 1991;23(1):15–17

35. Kutty S, Curtin J. Idiopathic avascular necrosis of the capitate. J Hand Surg [Br] 1995;20(3):402–404

36. Niesten JA, Verhaar JA. Idiopathic avascular necrosis of the capitate—a case report and a review of the literature. Hand Surg 2002;7(1):159–161

37. Peters SJ, Degreef I, De Smet L. Avascular necrosis of the capitate: report of six cases and review of the literature. J Hand Surg Eur Vol 2015;40(5):520–525

38. Rahme H. Idiopathic avascular necrosis of the capitate bone—case report. Hand 1983;15(3):274–275

39. Resnik CS, Gelberman RH, Resnick D. Transscaphoid, transscaphitate, perilunate fracture dislocation (scaphocapitate syndrome). Skeletal Radiol 1983;9(3):192–194

40. Vander Grend R, Dell PC, Glowczewskie F, Leslie B, Ruby LK. Intraosseous blood supply of the capitate and its correlation with aseptic necrosis. J Hand Surg Am 1984;9(5):677–683

41. Botte MJ, Pacelli LL, Gelberman RH. Vascularity and osteonecrosis of the wrist. Orthop Clin North Am 2004;35(3):405–421, xi

42. Freeman BH, Hay EL. Nonunion of the capitate: a case report. J Hand Surg Am 1985;10(2):187–190

43. Rand JA, Linscheid RL, Dobyns JH. Capitate fractures: a long-term follow-up. Clin Orth Rel Res. 1982:209–216

44. Yoshihara M, Sakai A, Toba N, Okimoto N, Shimokobe T, Nakamura T. Nonunion of the isolated capitate waist fracture. J Orthop Sci 2002;7(5):578–580

45. Kadar A, Morsy M, Sur YJ, Akdag O, Moran SL. Capitate fractures: a review of 53 patients. J Hand Surg Am 2016;41(10): e359–e366

46. Rabarin F, Saint Cast Y, Cesari B, Raimbeau G, Fouque PA. [Capitate osteotomy in Kienböck's disease in twelve cases. Clinical and radiological results at five years follow-up]. Chir Main 2010;29(2): 67–71

47. Afshar A. Lunate revascularization after capitate shortening osteotomy in Kienböck's disease. J Hand Surg Am 2010;35(12): 1943–1946

48. Citlak A, Akgun U, Bulut T, Tahta M, Dirim Mete B, Sener M. Partial capitate shortening for Kienböck's disease. J Hand Surg Eur Vol 2015;40(9):957–960

49. Hove LM. Epidemiology of scaphoid fractures in Bergen, Norway. Scand J Plast Reconstr Surg Hand Surg 1999;33(4): 423–426

50. Leslie IJ, Dickson RA. The fractured carpal scaphoid. Natural history and factors influencing outcome. J Bone Joint Surg Br 1981; 3-B(2):225–230

51. Gelberman RH, Wolock BS, Siegel DB. Fractures and non-unions of the carpal scaphoid. J Bone Joint Surg Am 1989;71(10): 1560–1565

52. Morsy M, Kadar A, Moran SL. Micro-CT study of the intraosseous vascularity of the scaphoid. Paper presented at: American Association for Hand Surgery; January, 2017; Kona, Hawaii

53. Brogan DM, Moran SL, Shin AY. Outcomes of open reduction and internal fixation of acute proximal pole scaphoid fractures. Hand (N Y) 2015;10(2):227–232

23 Function of the Wrist Joint

Marc Garcia-Elias

23.1 Introduction

The hand gives meaning to the upper extremity. Without a hand, the upper limb is like a crane without a hook at the end of the cable. For the hand to be functional, however, the proximal articulations must be both mobile and stable.[1] If the upper limb has poor mobility, the hand cannot be placed where it is required. If the proximal articulations lack stability, the hand will give way when attempting to grip, pinch, or lift an object. Thus to understand upper limb function, one must investigate both how the upper limb joints move (kinematics) and how they sustain load without yielding (kinetics).[2,3]

The wrist has often been regarded as the least important articulation of the upper extremity—a joint that can be eliminated without creating much functional impairment. Certainly, the implications of having a stiff wrist are not as substantial as having the shoulder or the elbow arthrodesed. This, however, should not be taken to the extreme of considering the wrist as a disposable joint. When specifically asked for, patients with a fused wrist admit serious difficulties with many activities of daily living, such as turning a door knob, washing one's back, dusting lower surfaces, rotating the steering wheel, or beating an egg.[4,5] The wrist provides precision, delicacy, and effectiveness to most hand actions. The wrist allows adjusting the position of the hand in ways that are not conceivable without the carpus. Furthermore, without a wrist capable of throwing stones with accuracy, the early chimpanzees would have not been able to defend themselves from faster predators, and probably human evolution would have not been the same.[6] Indeed, the wrist is not an irrelevant articulation that can be eliminated without paying a functional penalty.

The wrist is a complex composite joint. To explain its function, several mechanical models have been suggested: the wrist as two interconnected rows (proximal and distal), as a system of three interdependent columns (lateral, central, and medial), or as a ring of four linked units (distal row, scaphoid, lunate, and triquetrum).[3] Unsurprisingly, none of these models has been able to explain all the intricate mechanisms of the joint, which, according to many authors, is one of the most complex in the human body.[3,7,8]

Aside from placing the hand in the best possible position to manipulate objects, the wrist is also responsible of controlling the moment arms of most extrinsic tendons of the hand.[9,10,11] This is achieved by means of pulleys. Palmarly, the carpal tunnel, acting as a pulley, keeps the flexor tendons as close as possible to the center of rotation of the joint in order to minimize their moment arms. Dorsally, six osteofibrous compartments prevent the extensor tendons from subluxing medially or laterally during wrist flexion, or from displacing dorsally during wrist extension. Controlling proper positioning of these tendons relative to the radius is another important task assigned to the wrist that cannot be underestimated.

For the wrist joint to function properly, it must have: (1) normally shaped joint surfaces with adequate orientation to guide carpal bone motion (▶ Fig. 23.1a–d), (2) a system of ligaments providing primary mechanical stability (▶ Fig. 23.2a, b), (3) a network of intracapsular mechanoreceptors supplying unconscious proprioceptive information from inside the joint, and (4) finely tuned reflexes ensuring proper neuromuscular control of carpal alignment.[7,8] To discuss these issues, this chapter has been divided into two sections. The first section discusses carpal bone motion (kinematics), and the second analyzes force transmission across the carpus, wrist proprioception, and the mechanisms of wrist stabilization (kinetics).

23.2 Wrist Kinematics

As already stated, to manipulate an object, the hand needs to be placed in the best possible position to reach that object; this is mainly achieved by the shoulder, the elbow, and the forearm articulations. Once close to the object, the wrist is in charge of making the final adjustments in hand positioning to maximize finger efficiency. If the wrist is stiff, the hand cannot be adjusted as per the requirement for a precise and effective hand performance. Wrist mobility, therefore, is important to achieve adequate hand function.

Most descriptions of the kinematic behavior of the carpal bones have been based on observations made on cadaver or on in vivo determinations using stepwise, statically acquired CT scans of wrists from normal individuals.[12-19] Despite all efforts spent in these regards, we still have incomplete understanding of carpal kinematics. There are two main reasons explaining this: first, because there is not one but rather a spectrum of different, yet all normal, carpal behaviors;[12,15,16] second, because the current techniques for measuring individual carpal motion are too cumbersome and time-consuming to allow collection of data from a large number of wrists. Indeed, we lack information about the incidence and relevance of the different patterns of carpal kinematics.[14] Fortunately, a new method to assess joint motion has been recently introduced. It is the so-called four-dimensional dynamic tomography (▶ Fig. 23.3).[20,21] This novel technology permits obtaining high-quality three-dimensional (3D) images of moving bones, in just a few minutes, with acceptable levels of radiation. Doubtless, in the near future, it will be easy for the clinician to measure individual carpal bone motion with high precision and little cost. This will allow more accurate assessment of problems (carpal dyskinematics) for which we still have little to offer.

Wrist motion may occur as a result of an external force inducing passive rotation of the carpal bones, or it may be the consequence of active contraction of the muscles crossing the articulation. This chapter will mostly concentrate on the latter. When the wrist moves, there is an interaction and accumulation of motions at different levels of the joint. Global wrist motion cannot be understood without a detailed analysis

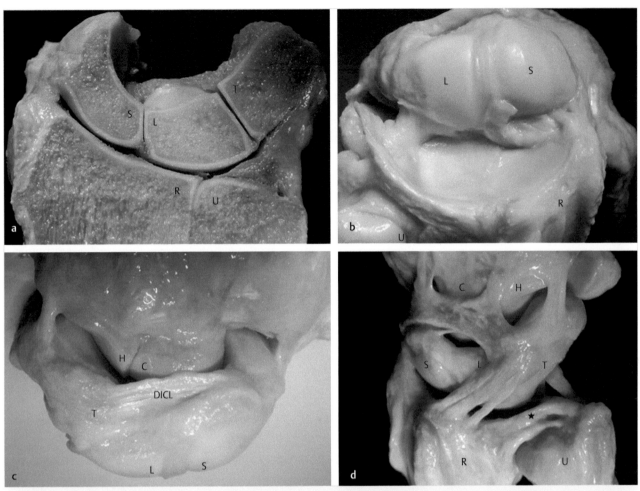

Fig. 23.1 Anatomical preparations showing the proximal row as an intercalated segment between the two forearm bones and the distal row. (**a**) Coronal section of the carpus (distal row excluded) with the volar half of the radiocarpal articulation exposed. (**b**) The radiocarpal joint has been widely opened to show the proximal convexities of the scaphoid and lunate, connected by the scapholunate fibrocartilaginous membrane, and the two slightly concave facets of the distal radius to accommodate these two bones. (**c**) Dorsal view of the midcarpal joint. Note the dorsal intercarpal ligament (1) (DICL) acting as a labrum that deepens the scapholunate distal socket, thus preventing dorsal subluxation of the capitate. (**d**) Dorsal view of the radiocarpal and midcarpal joint. C, capitate; H, hamate; L, lunate; R, radius; S, scaphoid; T, triquetrum; U, ulna; *, triangular fibrocartilage.

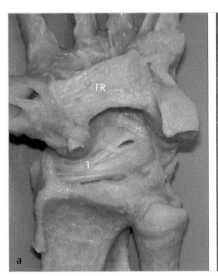

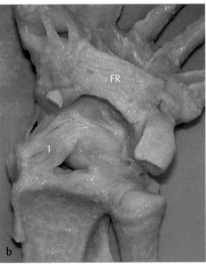

Fig. 23.2 Volar view of the radiocarpal ligaments (*1*) and how their arrangement changes as the wrist rotates from radial deviation (**a**) to ulnar deviation (**b**). In radial deviation they act as a hammock on which the flexing scaphoid rests; while in ulnar deviation they become taut preventing the carpus from sliding ulnarly. The flexor retinaculum (*FR*), by contrast, changes little with wrist motion.

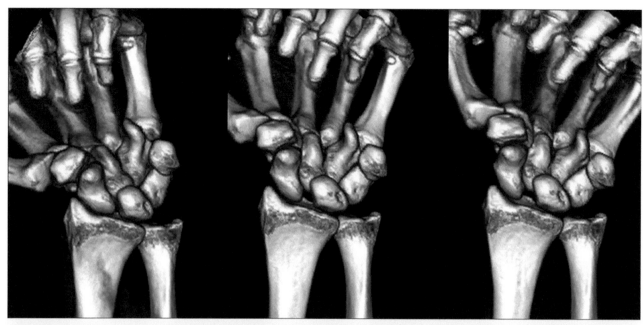

Fig. 23.3 Three static images of a wrist with partial scapholunate dissociation obtained with a "four-dimensional" dynamic computed tomography. This novel technology allows obtaining multiple three-dimensional representations of the moving carpus (in this case, as it moves along the dart-throwing plane). Once integrated in a video, these images provide excellent kinematic evidence of this patient's problem.

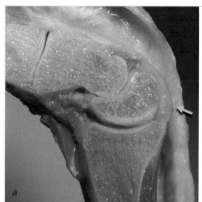
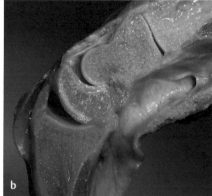

Fig. 23.4 Wrist motion is the result of interaction and accumulation of motions occurring at the different levels of this composite joint. This sagittal section of the central column of a cadaver wrist was artificially set in two positions—flexion (**a**) and extension (**b**)—to demonstrate the two levels of motion—radiolunate and lunocapitate. Note that the lunate is more constrained palmarly, by the short radiolunate ligament (*arrow*), than dorsally, by the more elastic capsule.

Table 23.1 Individual carpal bone rotation (average Eulerian angles) relative to the radius during wrist movements

	Wrist flexion 60°	Wrist extension 60°	Wrist radial deviation 15°	Wrist ulnar deviation 30°
Scaphoid (n: 22)	Flx 40°, UD 8°	Ext 52°, UD 4°	RD 4°, Flex 8°	Ext 17°, UD 14°, Pron 7°
Lunate (n: 22)	Flx 23°, UD 11°	Ext 30°, UD 4°	RD 2°, Flex 7°	Ext 22°, UD 15°, Pron 4°
Triquetrum (n: 22)	Flx 30°, UD 10°	Ext 39°	RD 5°, Flex 4°	Ext 17°, UD 18°
Trapezium (n: 13)	Flx 54°, UD 3°	Ext 59°	RD 14°, Sup 5°	UD 32°, Flx 10°, Pron 16°
Capitate (n: 22)	Flx 63°, UD 3°	Ext 60°	RD 15°, Sup 4°	UD 31°, Flx 6°, Pron 12°

Abbreviations: Ext, extension; Flx, flexion; Pron, pronation; RD, radial deviation; Sup, supination; UD, ulnar deviation.
Source: Per the kinematic study by Kobayashi et al.[13]

of the kinematic behavior of all its elements (▶Fig. 23.4a, b). Individual carpal bone motion is usually described as a combination of rotations along three orthogonal planes (sagittal, frontal, and transverse), taking the distal radius as a reference (▶Table 23.1).[13,15,19] Rotation along the sagittal plane determines flexion–extension (yaw angle), the frontal plane determines radial–ulnar deviation (pitch angle), and the transverse plane determines pronation–supination (roll angle). Until recently, it was believed that only the first and second types of rotation (flexion–extension and radial–ulnar deviation) could be actively produced by the tendons crossing the wrist. It was thought that intracarpal pronosupination was a passive rotation, possible

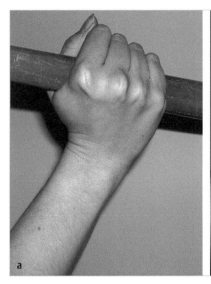
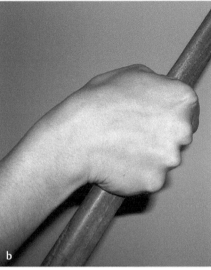

Fig. 23.5 The so-called dart-thrower's motion is the most commonly used wrist rotation in most activities of daily living. It involves moving the wrist from an extended radially deviated position (**a**) to a flexed ulnarly deviated position (**b**).

only if the wrist was not loaded. Now it is known that not only the forearm muscles may actively rotate the distal row up to an average 19° pronation and 23° supination but also that such a rotation is the key to understanding the neuromuscular stabilization of the carpus.[22,23]

Because the wrist is not a single-axis joint with collateral ligaments guiding a unidirectional arc of motion, the unconstrained wrist seldom rotates in a pure flexion–extension or radial–ulnar deviation mode. In fact, most activities of daily living (using a hammer, fishing, bouncing a ball, or lifting heavy objects) involve an oblique type of wrist motion, from extension-radial deviation to flexion–ulnar deviation; it is the so-called dart-throwing plane of motion (▶Fig. 23.5).[17,19,24] What follows is a description of the behavior of the carpal bones when the wrist moves along the more commonly used planes of motion.

23.2.1 Flexion–Extension

Flexion of the wrist is defined as a rotation that approximates the palm to the anterior aspect of the forearm. The transverse axis along which this rotation occurs is located about the proximal part of the head of the capitate near the lunate and is parallel to the palmar aspect of the distal radial metaphysis. Extension of the wrist is also a rotation about this axis but in the opposite direction: the dorsum of the hand approximates the dorsal aspect of the forearm. Any tendon crossing the wrist palmar to this axis is likely to induce wrist flexion, while extension may result from the action of any tendon dorsal to this axis.[25] This includes all wrist motor tendons (flexor carpi radialis [FCR], flexor carpi ulnaris [FCU], palmaris longus [PL], extensor carpi radialis brevis and longus [ECRB-L], and extensor carpi ulnaris [ECU]) and all finger and thumb extrinsic tendons. The efficacy of these muscles in producing flexion or extension of the wrist is directly proportional to the distance between the tendon and the axis of rotation (moment arm). The average maximal active flexion and extension in normal wrists is 59 and 79°, respectively.[26] This range varies substantially from one individual to another, being wider among hyperlax individuals.[27]

The distal row is a very rigid structure formed by four bones (trapezium, trapezoid, capitate, and hamate) solidly interconnected to each other by strong and stout interosseous ligaments

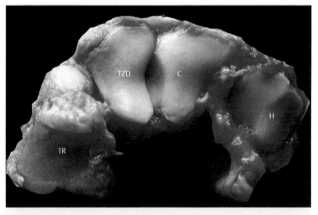

Fig. 23.6 Distal articular surfaces of a disarticulated carpometacarpal joint. The bones of the distal carpal row fit together like stones in an arch, and they are so strongly bound to each other that they may be thought of as one functional unit. C, capitate; H, hamate; TR, trapezium; TZD, trapezoid.

(▶Fig. 23.6).[28] During wrist flexion–extension, little intercarpal motion exists between the four bones; they all move synergistically, in the same direction, as if they were one functional unit.[13–15]

The proximal carpal row has no tendon insertions. All wrist motor tendons are inserted onto the distal row or at the base of the metacarpals. The pisiform has a tendon insertion, but it is not a true proximal row bone but rather a sesamoid to enhance the mechanical advantage of the FCU. Consequently, when one of these muscles contracts only the distal row starts moving. The proximal row does not rotate until a certain level of tension develops in the midcarpal crossing ligaments; this tension generates eccentric compressive forces in the midcarpal joint, forcing the proximal bones to move (▶Fig. 23.7). Indeed, it takes some time between the contraction of muscles and the movement of proximal row. During that period, there is only motion at the midcarpal joint. In other words, most actions around the neutral position are done without moving the radiocarpal joint.

Unlike the distal row, the bones of the proximal carpal row are less strongly bound to one another. Marked differences in

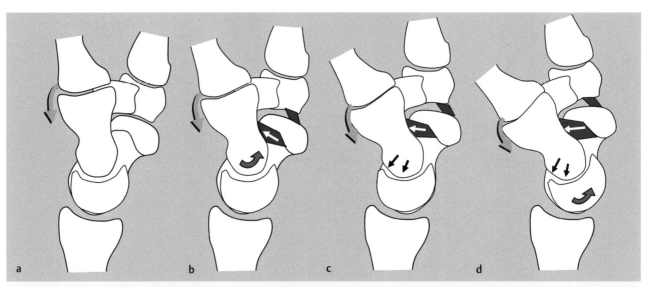

Fig. 23.7 Schematic representation of how muscle forces initiate wrist motion. (**a**) Except for the flexor carpi ulnaris that inserts into the pisiform, there are no tendons inserted in the proximal row. When these muscles contract (*green arrow*), motion starts always at the distal row. (**b**) As the distal row moves (*red arrow*), tension develops at the midcarpal crossing ligaments (*white arrow*). (**c**) The more the midcarpal joint rotates, the higher the eccentric compressive forces will be (*black arrows*). (**d**) As a result of the development of articular compressive loads and increased tension in the ligaments, the proximal row starts moving (*red arrow*). The midcarpal joint, therefore, starts moving earlier and for a wider range than the radiocarpal row. When the wrist rotates about its central position, there is only motion at the midcarpal joint; the radiocarpal joint moves only at the extremes of wrist motion.

the magnitude of rotation exist between the scaphoid, lunate, and triquetrum (►Fig. 23.8a–c). As found by Kobayashi et al,[13] for a total 120° of wrist flexion–extension, the scaphoid rotates an average of 92°, while the lunate rotates 53°, and the triquetrum 69° (►Table 23.1). Such differences in bone rotation are the consequence of the different radii of curvatures of their proximal poles: with smaller radii of curvature, the scaphoid needs to rotate more than the lunate to get to the wrist maximal range.

It is commonly believed that the axis of rotation of the scaphoid relative to the lunate is located at the center of curvature of the two bones. This is not so. As demonstrated in different studies,[13,19] there is an instantaneous axis of scapholunate (SL) rotation, slightly oblique, located very close to the dorsal SL ligament (►Fig. 23.8c). In fact, scaphoid and lunate rotate not as two wheels sharing a central axis but rather about a dorsal eccentric axis, implying a "scissor like" type of rotation. If the dorsal SL ligament is so stout and strong, it is because, as a hinge, it must resist important torsions. In contrast, the palmar SL ligament is elastic, long, and oblique in order to allow larger rotation to the scaphoid (►Fig. 23.9).

The axis of flexion–extension of the lunotriquetral (LTq) joint appears to be more centrally located. On average the triquetrum rotates 16° more than the lunate, but this is small compared with the 39° average rotation exhibited by the SL joint as the wrist moves from maximal flexion to maximal extension.[13]

The contribution of the radiocarpal and midcarpal joints to the overall wrist flexion–extension varies substantially from one column to another. In the central column, about 31% of the overall flexion and 66% of extension occurs at the proximal radiolunate joint, while the rest occurs at the lunocapitate interval.[14] In the lateral column, the radioscaphoid joint

contributes 62% of the overall flexion and 86% of the extension, while the rest occurs at the scapho–trapezial–trapezoidal (STT) joint.[14]

23.2.2 Radial–Ulnar Deviation

Ulnar deviation (adduction) is defined as a rotation of the wrist in which the ulnar border of the hand approximates to the medial border of the forearm. The axis mediating this rotation is located at about the center of the head of the capitate and is perpendicular to the axis of flexion–extension. Radial deviation (abduction) is also a rotation about this axis, but in the opposite direction: the thumb approximates the radial border of the forearm. Any tendon crossing the wrist radial to that axis is likely to induce radial deviation, while any ulnarly located tendon is a potential ulnar-deviating muscle.[25] The average maximal range of active radial–ulnar deviation is 21 and 38°, respectively.[26]

As mentioned for flexion–extension, the distal row bones shift together during radioulnar deviation. The scaphoid, lunate, and triquetrum are less tightly bound to each other and exhibit different amounts of rotation. From a flexed position in radial deviation to an extended position in ulnar deviation, they all move synergistically, but the lunate moves less than the scaphoid or the triquetrum. Obviously, this implies the presence of substantial intrinsic rotation at the SL joint (average 10°) and at the LTq joint (14°; ►Table 23.1).[29]

Recent studies have disclosed the existence of a spectrum of carpal bone behaviors during wrist radial–ulnar deviation: while some wrists show basically a flexion–extension type of rotation, in some others the lateral-to-medial deviation component predominates.[12,30] The wrists with a predominant flexion–extension, the so-called column-type wrists,

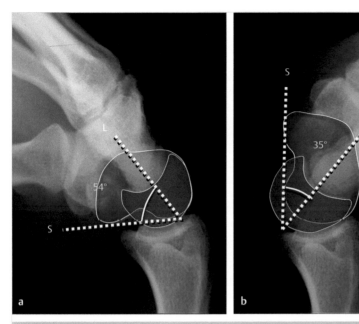

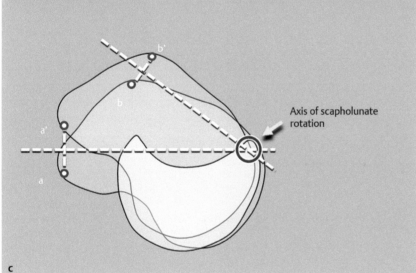

Fig. 23.8 As the wrist rotates along the sagittal plane from full flexion (**a**) to full extension (**b**), the scaphoid (*S*) rotates more than the lunate (*L*). Good evidence of this may be found by comparing the scapholunate angle in both positions. In this particular example, the scaphoid rotates 19° more than the lunate. (**c**) By superimposing the outlines of the scaphoid and lunate, and applying the method of Reuleaux to identify the location of the axis of scapholunate rotation, it is clear that this axis is located not at the center of curvature of these bones, as commonly assumed, but rather at the dorsal corner of the lunate. Indeed, the scaphoid rotates about the dorsal scapholunate ligament, which is used as a hinge.

tend to be more lax than the wrists with a predominant lateromedial scaphoid translation, the so-called row-type wrists (▶Fig. 23.10a, b).[30] Furthermore, most wrists with a double distal facet, one for the capitate, another for the hamate (lunate type II), appear to behave as "column" wrists, while the ones with a lunate type I are predominantly the "row wrists."[16] The implications of such differential behaviors, however, are yet to be established.

23.2.3 "Dart-Throwing" Motion

Since the early 20th century it has been known that the unconstrained wrist seldom moves along the sagittal or frontal planes; it actually moves along oblique planes. Particularly active is the so-called dart-throwing (DT) plane of motion, an oblique plane that brings the wrist from an extended radial deviated position to a flexed ulnar-deviated position (▶Fig. 23.5).[24] Recent laboratory

work has confirmed these observations by demonstrating that the mechanical axis of the wrist and the DT plane of motion have a similar obliquity, different from that of the anatomical (frontal and sagittal) axes of rotation (▶Fig. 23.11).[17,19] Indeed, the wrist tends to move along the DT plane when performing most activities of daily living.

The obliquity of the DT plane, however, is not the same for all wrists; each individual has unique DT plane of motion.[24] A number of anatomic and physiologic factors determine this obliquity: (1) most scaphoids have an obliquely oriented ridge on its distal surface that acts as a rail to the STT joint, (2) in the transverse plane, the scaphocapitate (SC) articulation has an oblique orientation inducing the distal row to move along the DT plane of motion, (3) the SL distal concavity is not spherical but ovoid, its major axis oriented along the axis of DT motion, (4) the two ligaments controlling midcarpal rotation (SC and STT) are inserted along the axis of DT rotation, indicating a role as collateral ligaments, and (5) of all muscles acting on the

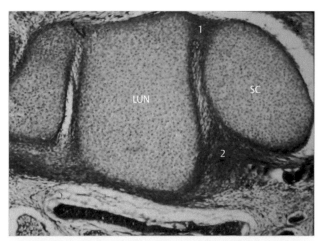

Fig. 23.9 Transverse section of the wrist of a 90 mm CR fetal specimen from the Domènech-Mateu collection (Bellaterra, Spain), demonstrating the dorsal (*1*) and palmar (*2*) scapholunate ligament connections between lunate (LUN) and scaphoid (SC). Note that the dorsal ligament is short, thick, and transversely set to support its role as a hinge about which the scaphoid rotates. The palmar ligament, by contrast, is longer, obliquely set, and less dense than the dorsal ligament, allowing a scissoring type of scapholunate rotation. (Masson's trichrome staining; x20)

midcarpal joint, the ones with the greatest mechanical advantage (FCU and ECRB-L) are located at the two ends of the DT rotation. Indeed, by moving along the DT plane the wrist spends less energy than along any other plane.

The contribution of the radiocarpal joint to the DT motion is minimal. It consists of only few degrees of lateral-to-medial deviation. During DT rotation, the proximal row bones do not exhibit the out-of-plane rotation seen in radioulnar deviations: the scaphoid does not flex in radial deviation, and it does not extend in ulnar deviation. In other words, when the wrist moves along the DT plane, only the midcarpal joint moves, not the radiocarpal joint (▶ Fig. 23.12a, b).[17,19,24]

One of the keys to understand the paucity of movements of the proximal row during DT rotation can be found by studying the behavior of the STT ligament. If the wrist deviates radially along the frontal plane, the scaphoid is likely to rotate into flexion in order to allow the trapezium to approximate to the radial styloid. The STT ligament is only taut at the extreme of radial deviation, when the scaphoid is maximally flexed. However, if at the same time when the wrist radially deviates there is a concomitant extension of the distal row, the trapezium slides down the dorsal slope of the scaphoid, thus pulling the scaphoid into extension via the STT ligaments. The balance between the scaphoid flexion tendency induced by the radially deviating

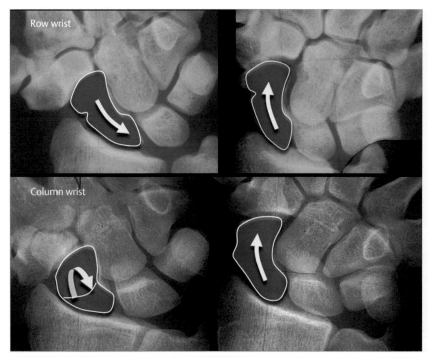

Fig. 23.10 During radioulnar inclination, most scaphoids exhibit a predominant flexion–extension type of rotation; when that happens, the wrist is qualified as a "column-type" wrist.[12] Less commonly, the scaphoid does not rotate along the sagittal plane but rather predominantly translates lateromedially; it is the so-called row-type of wrist. Obviously, between the two extremes, there is a spectrum of carpal behaviors, all normal.

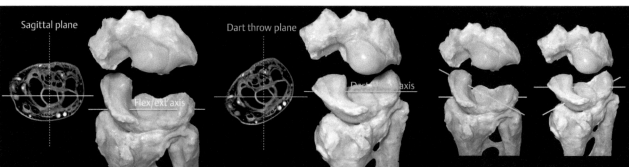

Fig. 23.11 Dart throw plane and axis and the sagittal plane and axis.

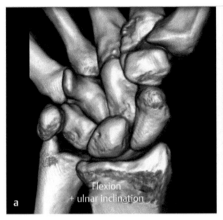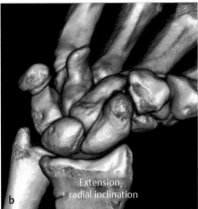

Fig. 23.12 Three-dimensional images obtained from a normal individual using dynamic tomography. The images where acquired while the wrist was performing a "dart-throwing" rotation, from a flexed ulnar deviated position (**a**) to an extended radially deviated position (**b**). Note that the proximal row does not extend or flex but rather only slightly translates along the frontal plane. Truly, "dart-throwing" implies very little radiocarpal rotation and maximal midcarpal activity.

Flexion + ulnar inclination

Extension + radial inclination

trapezium and the tensile forces exerted by the STT ligament is what explains why the scaphoid remains in neutral position during extension–radial deviation motion. Similarly, if the wrist ulnarly deviates along the frontal plane, tension on the STT ligament is likely to increase, thus inducing scaphoid extension. Such tendency is eliminated if the ulnar deviating wrist also rotates into flexion, in which case the STT ligament becomes loose. The fact that DT rotation occurs mostly in the midcarpal joint explains why some forms of radio–scaphoid–lunate stiffness, partial fusions included, are functionally so well tolerated. Indeed, with a stiff radiocarpal joint, one may cope effectively with most activities of daily living, especially those requiring only rotation along the DT plane.

23.3 Wrist Kinetics

Most tasks done by the hand generate forces that need to be transferred proximally. A wrist is said to be stable when it is able to transfer such centripetal forces, from distal to proximal, without losing its normal anatomical relationships. Albeit certain wrist positions are better prepared to bear loads than others,[11] the stable wrist does not need to be placed in one particular position to grasp, push, or pull an object. Regardless of the position, a stable wrist is always able to develop self-locking strategies to convert the carpus into a solid block through which forces can be transferred properly. To better understand those strategies, it is important to consider, first, the magnitude of forces crossing the wrist and, second, how are they distributed among the different carpal articulations.

23.3.1 Magnitude and Distribution of Forces across the Wrist

During most hand activities, the wrist sustains considerable compressive and shear stress.[31] Such loads are the consequence of external forces being applied to the hand but are also the result of contraction of the different muscles crossing the joint, plus the reaction forces induced by the different stabilizing ligaments. According to An et al,[31] the amount of compressive forces crossing each carpometacarpal joint may be as high as 1.5 to 4.2 times the applied force at the tip of the corresponding fingers. By adding all loads being transmitted onto the distal carpal row, we may estimate that the wrist resists loads up to 14 times the applied force at the tip of the fingers. Based on this, if we are capable of gripping a dynamometer with up to 30 to 40 kg force, the wrist probably

is resisting compressive forces of up to 300 kg or more. In 2007, Rikli et al[32] introduced a capacitive pressure sensor device in the radioulnocarpal joint of one healthy volunteer, under local anesthesia. The device allowed real-time determination of intra-articular forces in different active positions of the wrist. In neutral pronosupination, the radius resisted a total force of 107 N in flexion, 31 N in neutral position, and 197 N in extension.

Once in the wrist, the axial forces do not randomly distribute among the different joints but rather follow specific paths depending upon the direction and point of application of the external loads, the position of the wrist, and the orientation and shape of the articular surfaces. In global terms, most of the load is transferred across the scaphoid and lunate into the radius.

According to the most recent study by Majima et al,[33] in neutral position, about 59% of the load borne by the distal row is transferred from the capitate into the scaphoid and lunate, while 29% of the loads are being transferred across the STT joint, and 12% goes across the triquetrum–hamate joint. At a more proximal level, the forces distribute as follows: radioscaphoid joint, 52%; radiolunate joint, 42%; and ulnolunate joint 6% (▶Fig. 23.13). These percentages vary with wrist position, the radiolunate fossa being more loaded with ulnar deviation but the scaphoid resisting more load with radial deviation. When the wrist is pushing an unyielding object in its most extended position, the scaphoid column becomes the center of load transmission with a radioscaphoid joint bearing 62% of all the load; this may explain why it is in this position that most scaphoid fractures occur.[33]

23.3.2 Primary Ligament Stabilization of the Carpus

When a force is applied to an object, this will translate and/or rotate depending upon the magnitude, direction, and point of application of that force. The carpal bones are not an exception; when axially loaded, they all exhibit a tendency to displace in specific directions.[3,34] The amount and direction of such displacements are determined by the magnitude of the force being applied, the shape and inclination of the articular surfaces holding each bone, and the resistance presented by the ligaments binding each articulation. Of course, motion stops when balance is reached between compressive forces and ligament tensions. What follows is a description of the most consistent patterns of carpal displacement observed in the carpus

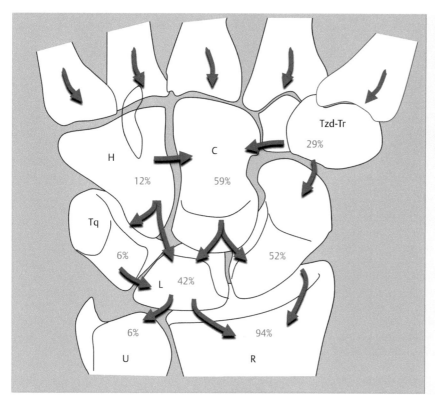

Fig. 23.13 Once in the carpus, all axial forces distribute following quite consistent patterns. The percentages indicated in this Figure were calculated by Majima et al,[33] using a three-dimensional rigid body spring model for the wrist in neutral position. The role of the scaphoid becomes more prominent when the wrist is loaded in a more functional extended position. C, capitate; H, hamate; L, lunate; R, radius; Tr, trapezium; Tzd, trapezoid; Tq, triquetrum; U, ulna; S, scaphoid.

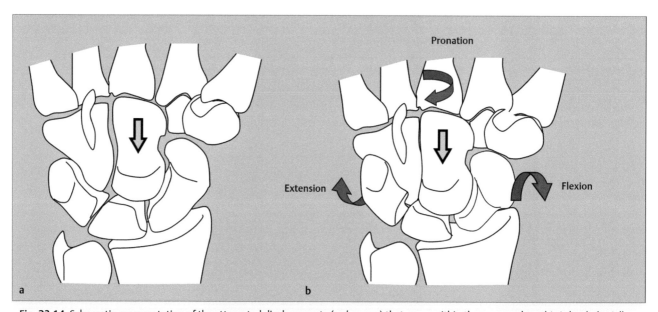

Fig. 23.14 Schematic representation of the attempted displacements (*red arrows*) that occur within the carpus when this is loaded axially (*green arrow*). (**a**) Wrist unloaded, (**b**) wrist loaded. The scaphoid tends to flex, the triquetrum to extend, and the distal row to pronate.

when an axial load is applied from distal to proximal across the carpometacarpal joint.

Because of its oblique orientation relative to the long axis of the forearm, the axially loaded scaphoid tends to rotate always into flexion and pronation.[23,34] If the SC and STT ligaments are intact, the pronation moment exhibited by the scaphoid is transmitted to the distal row. The more the distal row pronates, the more the hamate displaces dorsally; with this, the palmar triquetrum–capitate–hamate ligament (the

so-called ulnar leg of the arcuate ligament) becomes taut and pulls the triquetrum into extension (▶ Fig. 23.14). The proximal row, therefore, is subjected to two opposite moments: a flexion moment generated by the scaphoid and an extension moment produced by the triquetrum–hamate–capitate (ulnar arcuate) ligament. If both the palmar and dorsal SL and LTq ligaments are intact, the two opposite moments generate increasing torques at both SL and LTq levels resulting in a stable cooptation of these joints. In this regard, the proximal row has been compared to a spring with two prongs directed in opposite directions.[3] The more you load the spring, the more compact the spring becomes, and more stable the overall structure is.

Comparing the wrist to a spring is useful because it provides an easy-to-understand picture of how the two proximal row moments counteract to each other. Unfortunately, it is an oversimplified model that does not explain how the distal row is prevented from rotating into excessive pronation or how the carpal condyle resists the tendency to slide down the ulnarly inclined distal radial articulation. What follows is a description of a more complete model with which to explain the primary ligament stabilization of the carpus. The model has two parts: (1) the spiral stabilization of the midcarpal joint, and (2) the sling stabilization of the radiocarpal joint.

Spiral Stabilization of the Midcarpal Joint

Several ligaments, acting together, are necessary to avoid excessive flexion of the scaphoid, extension of the triquetrum, and pronation of the distal row: it is the so-called anti-pronation ligamentous complex (APLC). With a spiral configuration around the scapholunocapitate articulation, the APLC is set to constrain this joint pronation but also to control both the scaphoid and triquetrum stance (▶Fig. 23.15a). From proximal to distal, the APLC is formed by (1) the long radiolunate ligament, (2) the palmar LTq ligament, (3) the dorsal LTq ligament, (4) the dorsal SL ligament, (5) the dorsal intercarpal ligament, and (6) the volar SC ligament (▶Fig. 23.15b, c). Additional support to the APLC may be provided by the radioscaphocapitate ligament, particularly when the wrist is in ulnar deviation. When the APLC is intact, not only is the pronation tendency of the distal row controlled, but also the two opposite moments of the proximal row (scaphoid flexion vs. triquetral extension) are readily

constrained by ligaments belonging to the APLC: the scaphoid cannot flex beyond normal when the dorsal SL and palmar SC ligaments are intact; the triquetrum cannot extend if the palmar and dorsal LTq ligaments act together.

Based on this, if the APLC is torn only in one place, the carpus may still be stable; the rest of the APLC may act as an indirect secondary stabilizer. By contrast, if there is a two-level injury, instability is almost unavoidable. A typical example of a two-level APLC rupture is when both the dorsal SL and palmar SC ligaments are ruptured; in those circumstances the unconstrained scaphoid cannot maintain its stance and collapses into an abnormally flexed and pronated posture (the so-called rotatory subluxation of the scaphoid), while the lunate and triquetrum are pulled by the distal row into an abnormal extension, known as a "dorsal intercalated segment instability."[3,34] If it is not the scaphoid inserted ligaments but the LTq ligaments that failed, the scaphoid and lunate tend to adopt an abnormal flexed posture ("volar intercalated segment instability"), while the triquetrum remains solidly linked to the distal row.

Sling Stabilization of the Radiocarpal Joint

The so-called carpal condyle, formed by the proximal convexities of the scaphoid, lunate, and triquetrum, articulates to an ulnarly and palmarly inclined antebrachial glenoid, formed by the distal articular surface of the radius and the triangular fibrocartilage. When loaded, the carpal condyle has an inherent tendency to slide down ulnarly and palmarly.[3] This tendency is effectively constrained by a ligament sling formed by both palmar and dorsal radiocarpal ligaments whose oblique orientation is ideal to resist such ulnar and palmar translation vectors. Failure of these obliquely oriented ligaments tends to result in a very dysfunctional ulnar and palmar translocation of the carpus relative to the radius.

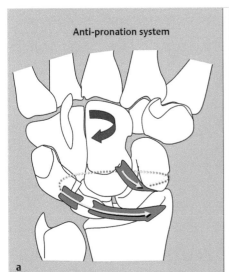 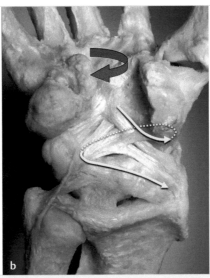 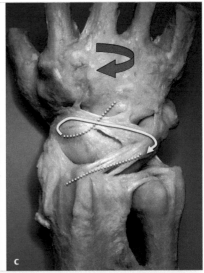

Fig. 23.15 When the wrist is axially loaded, the distal row tends to pronate (*red arrow*). (**a**) To avoid this pronation to reach unacceptable limits of joint congruency, there is an anti-pronation system of ligaments (*yellow arrows*), including the palmar radiolunotriquetral, the dorsal lunotriquetral, the dorsal scapholunate, the dorsal intercarpal, and the palmar scaphocapitate ligaments. (**b**) Volar view of a dissected specimen demonstrating the spiral arrangement of ligaments involved in this anti-pronation system. (**c**) The same specimen, viewed from the dorsum.

23.3.3 Secondary Neuromuscular Stabilization of the Carpus

Ligaments are the first to detect and react against excessive bone displacement, but they are not the only stabilizers. If they were, they would not last long, because ligaments are not strong enough to resist the amount of traction involved in carpal stabilization. The dorsal SL ligament, for instance, has the greatest yield strength of all the components of the SL interosseous, yet it fails at an average of only 260 N. The palmar SL ligament fails at 118 N and the proximal membrane at 63 N.[35] The palmar LTq ligament is thicker and stronger than the dorsal ligament, but still it fails at an average 301 N, while the dorsal LTq ligament disrupts at 121 N.[29] Since these ligaments are weak, one would expect to see more ligament injuries. Particularly in certain sports, such as gymnastics, where gymnasts pirouette on the air and fall from substantial height on their wrists, one would expect ligaments to be frequently injured. However, there are not many ligament injuries, because ligaments are protected by muscles. Truly, muscles are the ultimate stabilizers.[8,22,23] Subsequent text presents a review of the neuromuscular mechanisms of joint stabilization.

Wrist Proprioception

Wrist proprioception, understood as the conscious and unconscious perception of what occurs within the wrist capsule, is the first subject we need to review to comprehend the entire process of muscle stabilization.[7,8] Here only a summary is given, as it will be discussed in greater detail in another chapter of this book.

When a carpal ligament is about to disrupt, the mechanoreceptors contained in that ligament detect the presence of unusually growing tension and react by sending a warning message to the spinal cord. That message triggers efferent (motor) stimuli to specific muscles whose contraction will prevent further ligament damage. Needless to say, the faster the muscle response the less substantial the injury will be. If the time elapsed between ligament aggression and muscle response, the so-called latency time, is abnormally long, the ligament will suffer more extensive damage.

In the past few years, several attempts have been made to identify and characterize mechanoreceptors within the wrist ligaments. In 1997, Petrie and coworkers were the first to show Golgi organs, Pacinian and Ruffini corpuscles, and nerve endings within the course of three palmar wrist ligaments.[36] Recently, several investigators have used immunohistochemical methods to identify, qualify, and quantify mechanoreceptors in the carpal ligaments.[37–39] Not all carpal ligaments were found to contain equal amounts of sensory corpuscles. From very densely innervated ligaments to ligaments with almost no innervation, a spectrum of possibilities was found.[37] Furthermore, the ligaments with fewer amounts of receptors were the ones with highest yield strength, while the most sensory innervated ligaments had the least dense arrangement of collagen fibers. In other words, there are mechanically important ligaments, acting like cables holding bones in place, and sensorially important ligaments that mostly have a sensorial role.[37] Interestingly, most ligaments inserted into the triquetrum are richly innervated, with plenty of receptors. Whether that means that the triquetrum plays a key role in the detection of abnormal

loading in the wrist is a hypothesis worth considering in future studies.

Hagert et al went a step further.[40] Using ultrasound guidance, a fine wire electrode was inserted into the dorsal SL ligament of normal volunteers. After electrically stimulating that ligament, the electromyographic activity of specific forearm muscles was recorded in different wrist positions. For the first time ever, this investigation provided evidence of wrist ligamento-muscular reflexes, with early reactions being interpreted as a primary joint protective function, while later cocontractions probably indicating a more elaborate supraspinal control of wrist stability. Activity changes were not restricted to one muscle for each wrist position. Combined reactions were the rule, and not all the reactions were in terms of muscle stimulation. Sometimes there were negative reactions; that is, muscle inhibition. The ECU, for instance, always reacted negatively when the wrist was tested in ulnar deviation, as if its contraction could worsen the SL problem. Interestingly enough, when the posterior interosseous nerve was anesthetized in those volunteers, all this muscle response was eliminated.[8] Denervating the joint, therefore, might not alter the conscious perception of joint position, but it certainly alters the unconscious proprioception necessary to modulate muscle protection of the joint.[7,8] In order to understand why this happens, it is important to investigate the effects of muscle contraction in carpal alignment.

Effects of Global Muscle Contraction on Carpal Bone Alignment

Salvà-Coll et al,[22,23] using 3D motion tracking sensors in a cadaver model, analyzed the effects of isometric tendon loading on carpal bone alignment. Even though the forearm bones were blocked in neutral pronosupination, some muscles induced pronation to the distal row, while others induced supination. The reason some muscles are intracarpal supinators or pronators can be found by observing the location of their corresponding tendons at the level of the distal radius and at their distal insertion (▶ Fig. 23.16). The ECU muscle, for instance, is a strong pronator because its tendon, from a dorsal location at the level of the ulna, has an oblique direction toward its insertion at the medial corner of the fifth metacarpal (▶ Fig. 23.17). The APL muscle, by contrast, is a strong intracarpal supinator, because its distal tendon changes direction from a dorsal location at the level of the radius to an anterolateral distal insertion.

When all muscles are loaded proportionally to their physiologic cross-sectional area, the distal row always supinates.[23] As already noted, however, the natural tendency of the distal carpal row is to rotate into pronation. By inducing the opposite type of rotation, the muscles prevent the wrist from following its natural tendency into pronation. Indeed, muscles play an important role in controlling the overall carpal alignment.

Effects of Individual Muscle Contraction on Carpal Bone Alignment

As already stated, when the wrist is axially loaded by an external force, the distal row pronates. Capitate pronation induces tension in the SC ligament, thus forcing the scaphoid into pronation. The more the scaphoid pronates, the more tension is generated in the dorsal SL ligament. Consequently, if the SL ligaments are torn, pronation would increase the SL gap and

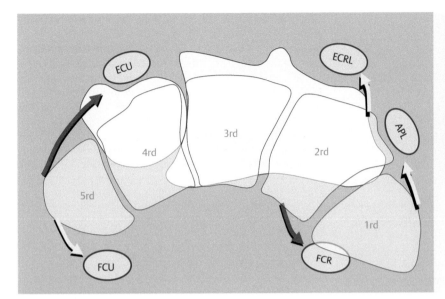

Fig. 23.16 Muscles are active carpal stabilizers. Their role is based on their ability to resist intracarpal pronation (ECRL, APL, and FCU; *yellow arrows*) or supination (ECU and FCR; *red arrows*). That ability is proportional to the obliquity of the tendon when it crosses the carpus. The APL, for instance, is a strong intracarpal supinator because it is dorsally located at the level of the radius, but it inserts at the anterolateral corner of the base of the first metacarpal. Consequently, isometric contraction of the APL is bound to supinate the metacarpal unit.

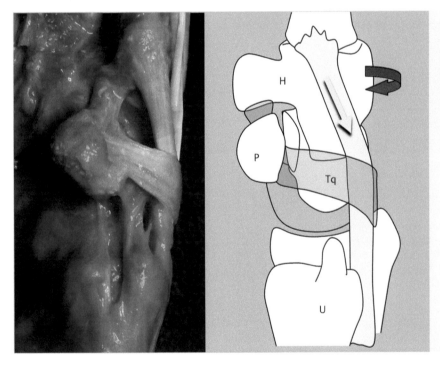

Fig. 23.17 The ECU (*yellow arrow*) is a strong intracarpal pronator because it is dorsally located at the level of the ulna, but it insets at the anteromedial corner of the fifth metacarpal. In this regard, the ECU is an antagonist of the APL. H, hamate; P, pisiform; Tq, triquetrum; U, ulna.

make the instability worse. According to the experiments by Salvà-Coll et al,[23] the ECU is a strong pronator, and therefore, an SL joint destabilizer. Certainly, after a dorsal SL ligament repair, contraction of the ECU may affect negatively by pulling the sutures apart. It is no wonder that Hagert et al[39] found that stimulation of the SL ligament muscle resulted in the inhibition of the ECU muscle. Indeed, the ECU is an SL-destabilizing muscle. This muscle is the only one that can make worse the symptoms of an SL deficient wrist.

According to Salvà-Coll et al,[22,23] there are three muscles that consistently cause supination to the distal row: the ECRL, the APL, and the FCU (▶ Fig. 23.15). Interestingly enough, these muscles are the ones inducing a DT type of rotation, a rotation that should be emphasized in patients with an SL deficient wrist but not in patients with a LTq instability. In the latter, the intracarpal pronation capability of the ECU should probably be considered.

The FCR has long been believed to be a dynamic scaphoid stabilizer.[3] This assumption was based on the fact that the tendon uses the scaphoid as a pulley to increase its mechanical advantage. Because it angles around the scaphoid tuberosity, any contraction was said to generate a dorsally directed vector that would extend the scaphoid.[3] Recent studies, however, have proved this not to be completely true.[22] Regardless of the wrist position, contraction of the FCR muscle always generates flexion and supination to the scaphoid. The positive effects of strengthening the FCR in SL deficient wrists, therefore, are linked not to its scaphoid flexion capability but rather to its supination capability. By supinating the scaphoid, the SL gap is closed.[22] In short, all muscle strengthening protocols for treating patients who have dynamic SL instability should enhance the efficacy of the scaphoid supinators (dart-thrower's and FCR) while protecting the wrist against the ECU. Certainly more research is needed to complete our knowledge in this regard.

References

1. The Anatomy and Biomechanics Committee of the International Federation of Societies for Surgery of the Hand. Definition of carpal instability. J Hand Surg Am 1999;24(4):866–867

2. Kijima Y, Viegas SF. Wrist anatomy and biomechanics. J Hand Surg Am 2009;34(8):1555–1563

3. Garcia-Elias M. Carpal instability. In: Wolfe S, Hotchkiss R, Pederson W, Kozin S. Green's Operative Hand Surgery, Vol. 1. 6th ed. Philadelphia, PA: Elsevier Churchill Livingstone, 2011:465–521

4. Adey L, Ring D, Jupiter JB. Health status after total wrist arthrodesis for posttraumatic arthritis. J Hand Surg Am 2005;30(5):932–936

5. Nelson DL. Functional wrist motion. Hand Clin 1997;13(1):83–92

6. Rohde RS, Crisco JJ, Wolfe SW. The advantage of throwing the first stone: how understanding the evolutionary demands of Homo sapiens is helping us understand carpal motion. J Am Acad Orthop Surg 2010;18(1):51–58

7. Riemann BL, Lephart SM. The sensorimotor system, part I: the physiologic basis of functional joint stability. J Athl Train 2002;37(1):71–79

8. Hagert E. Proprioception of the wrist joint: a review of current concepts and possible implications on the rehabilitation of the wrist. J Hand Ther 2010;23(1):2–17

9. Netscher D, Lee M, Thornby J, Polsen C. The effect of division of the transverse carpal ligament on flexor tendon excursion. J Hand Surg Am 1997;22(6):1016–1024

10. Li ZM. The influence of wrist position on individual finger forces during forceful grip. J Hand Surg Am 2002;27(5):886–896

11. Iwamoto A, Morris RP, Andersen C, Patterson RM, Viegas SF. An anatomic and biomechanic study of the wrist extensor retinaculum septa and tendon compartments. J Hand Surg Am 2006;31(6):896–903

12. Craigen MA, Stanley JK. Wrist kinematics. Row, column or both? J Hand Surg [Br] 1995;20(2):165–170

13. Kobayashi M, Berger RA, Nagy L, et al. Normal kinematics of carpal bones: a three-dimensional analysis of carpal bone motion relative to the radius. J Biomech 1997;30(8):787–793

14. Moojen TM, Snel JG, Ritt MJ, Venema HW, Kauer JM, Bos KE. In vivo analysis of carpal kinematics and comparative review of the literature. J Hand Surg Am 2003;28(1):81–87

15. Feipel V, Rooze M. Three-dimensional motion patterns of the carpal bones: an in vivo study using three-dimensional computed tomography and clinical applications. Surg Radiol Anat 1999;21(2):125–131

16. Galley I, Bain GI, McLean JM. Influence of lunate type on scaphoid kinematics. J Hand Surg Am 2007;32(6):842–847

17. Werner FW, Green JK, Short WH, Masaoka S. Scaphoid and lunate motion during a wrist dart throw motion. J Hand Surg Am 2004;29(3):418–422

18. Kaufmann R, Pfaeffle J, Blankenhorn B, Stabile K, Robertson D, Goitz R. Kinematics of the midcarpal and radiocarpal joints in radioulnar deviation: an in vitro study. J Hand Surg Am 2005;30(5):937–942

19. Crisco JJ, Coburn JC, Moore DC, Akelman E, Weiss AP, Wolfe SW. In vivo radiocarpal kinematics and the dart thrower's motion. J Bone Joint Surg Am 2005;87(12):2729–2740

20. Leng S, Zhao K, Qu M, An KN, Berger R, McCollough CH. Dynamic CT technique for assessment of wrist joint instabilities. Med Phys 2011;38(Suppl 1):S50–S56

21. Halpenny D, Courtney K, Torreggiani WC. Dynamic four-dimensional 320 section CT and carpal bone injury—a description of a novel technique to diagnose scapholunate instability. Clin Radiol 2012;67(2):185–187

22. Salvà-Coll G, Garcia-Elias M, Llusá-Pérez M, Rodríguez-Baeza A. The role of the flexor carpi radialis muscle in scapholunate instability. J Hand Surg Am 2011;36(1):31–36

23. Salvà-Coll G, Garcia-Elias M, Leon-Lopez MT, Llusa-Perez M, Rodríguez-Baeza A. Effects of forearm muscles on carpal stability. J Hand Surg Eur Vol 2011;36(7):553–559

24. Moritomo H, Apergis EP, Herzberg G, Werner FW, Wolfe SW, Garcia-Elias M. 2007 IFSSH committee report of wrist biomechanics committee: biomechanics of the so-called dart-throwing motion of the wrist. J Hand Surg Am 2007;32(9):1447–1453

25. Brand PW, Hollister A. Mechanics of individual muscles at individual joints. In: Brand PW, Hollister A. Clinical Mechanics of the Hand. 2nd ed. St. Louis, MO: Mosby Year Book; 1993:254–352

26. Ryu JY, Cooney WP III, Askew LJ, An KN, Chao EY. Functional ranges of motion of the wrist joint. J Hand Surg Am 1991;16(3):409–419

27. Remvig L, Jensen DV, Ward RC. Epidemiology of general joint hypermobility and basis for the proposed criteria for benign joint hypermobility syndrome: review of the literature. J Rheumatol 2007;34(4):804–809

28. Garcia-Elias M, An KN, Cooney WP III, Linscheid RL, Chao EY. Stability of the transverse carpal arch: an experimental study. J Hand Surg Am 1989;14(2 Pt 1):277–282

29. Ritt MJ, Linscheid RL, Cooney WP III, Berger RA, An KN. The lunotriquetral joint: kinematic effects of sequential ligament sectioning, ligament repair, and arthrodesis. J Hand Surg Am 1998;23(3):432–445

30. Garcia-Elias M, Ribe M, Rodriguez J, Cots M, Casas J. Influence of joint laxity on scaphoid kinematics. J Hand Surg [Br] 1995;20(3):379–382

31. An KN, Chao EY, Cooney WP, Linscheid RL. Forces in the normal and abnormal hand. J Orthop Res 1985;3(2):202–211

32. Rikli DA, Honigmann P, Babst R, Cristalli A, Morlock MM, Mittlmeier T. Intra-articular pressure measurement in the radioulnocarpal joint using a novel sensor: in vitro and in vivo results. J Hand Surg Am 2007;32(1):67–75

33. Majima M, Horii E, Matsuki H, Hirata H, Genda E. Load transmission through the wrist in the extended position. J Hand Surg Am 2008;33(2):182–188

34. Garcia-Elias M. Kinetic analysis of carpal stability during grip. Hand Clin 1997;13(1):151–158

35. Berger RA, Imeada T, Berglund L, An KN. Constraint and material properties of the subregions of the scapholunate interosseous ligament. J Hand Surg Am 1999;24(5):953–962

36. Petrie S, Collins J, Solomonow M, Wink C, Chuinard R. Mechanoreceptors in the palmar wrist ligaments. J Bone Joint Surg Br 1997;79(3):494–496

37. Hagert E, Garcia-Elias M, Forsgren S, Ljung BO. Immunohistochemical analysis of wrist ligament innervation in relation to their structural composition. J Hand Surg Am 2007;32(1):30–36

38. Lin YT, Berger RA, Berger EJ, et al. Nerve endings of the wrist joint: a preliminary report of the dorsal radiocarpal ligament. J Orthop Res 2006;24(6):1225–1230

39. Mataliotakis G, Doukas M, Kostas I, Lykissas M, Batistatou A, Beris A. Sensory innervation of the subregions of the scapholunate interosseous ligament in relation to their structural composition. J Hand Surg Am 2009;34(8):1413–1421

40. Hagert E, Persson JK, Werner M, Ljung BO. Evidence of wrist proprioceptive reflexes elicited after stimulation of the scapholunate interosseous ligament. J Hand Surg Am 2009;34(4):642–651

24 Anatomy of the Distal Radioulnar Joint

Makoto Tamai

24.1 The Distal Radioulnar Joint (The *Mobile* DRUJ)

The distal radioulnar joint (DRUJ) is an articulation between the ulnar head and the sigmoid notch of the distal radius (▶ Fig. 24.1). The DRUJ functions as a pivot joint allowing the radius to rotate around the ulna within a range of movement restricted by soft tissues that connect the radius and the ulna and also those surrounding this joint. The stability of the DRUJ is provided by a combination of cartilage-to-cartilage contact between the sigmoid notch and the ulnar head, and the soft-tissue stabilizers.[1] The triangular fibrocartilage complex (TFCC), the interosseous membrane of forearm, and the extensor retinaculum work as static stabilizers of the DRUJ.[2,3,4,5] The extensor carpi ulnaris (ECU) tendon and the pronator quadratus muscle work as dynamic stabilizers of this joint.[6,7,8] These dynamic stabilizers work independently or cooperatively according to the changing kinematics during forearm rotation.

Comparative anatomical studies of the wrist joint revealed that the mobile DRUJ is one of the major dominant traits inherited in hominoids from the common ancient ancestor of humans and anthropoid apes. This unique anatomical feature might have been advantageous to their life in the trees, especially for locomotive brachiation.[9] It is considered that the mobility of the DRUJ, along with the prehensile thumb, are hallmarks of humans, and helped in handling tools, in using weapons to defeat enemies, and improved survival in lethal environments. The mobile DRUJ

also helped creativity, with improved upper extremity function being more useful to the imagination of the larger more capable brain that evolved.[10]

The characteristics of the human mobile DRUJ that differentiate it from the animal DRUJ with limited mobility include (1) the formation of diarthrotic DRUJ, (2) the absence of ulnocarpal articulation, and (3) the presence of TFCC.[9] In contrast with the syndesmotic DRUJ of most animals, the sigmoid notch of the distal radius forms a synovial joint with the ulnar head. Another major modification is that the distal end of the ulna no longer articulates with the triquetrum and the pisiform, and is reduced in size significantly to became the ulnar styloid process. Thus the human wrist has wider deviation in the coronal (radioulnar) plane and sufficient forearm rotation.

24.2 The Extensor Retinaculum

After removing the skin and subcutaneous tissue around the wrist joint, the extensor retinaculum, consisting of a supratendinous layer and an infratendinous layer, can be observed as a thickening of the antebrachial fascia. (▶ Fig. 24.2).[11] The fibers of the extensor retinaculum arise from the radiopalmar edge of the distal radius, run ulnarly parallel to the fibers of dorsal radiotriquetral ligament, skim the ulnar styloid distally, and end on the ulnar aspect of the pisiform. There are six dorsal compartments of the extensor retinaculum for the extensor tendons, divided by five septae. The 5th dorsal compartment exists between the supratendinous layer and the infratendinous layer of the extensor retinaculum that covers the dorsoradial portion of the DRUJ. The ECU tendon has its own synovial sheath that attaches on the dorsal aspect of the ulnar head under the extensor retinaculum to balance stability of the ECU and mobility of the DRUJ

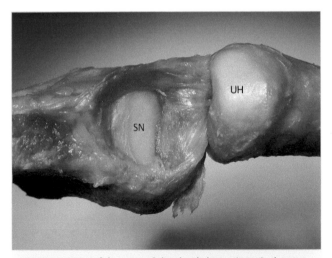

Fig. 24.1 View of the opened distal radial joint (DRUJ), showing both the sigmoid notch (SN) of the radius, and the ulnar head (UH) matching articular surface, with the joint hinging open on the TFCC. The radius is seen from medially, looking directly at the sigmoid notch, with the proximal radius to the left. The ulnar head has been hinged away from the sigmoid notch, hinging on the TFCC, with the proximal ulna to the right. The TFCC radial attachments are seen just to the right of the sigmoid notch, with the ulnar TFCC attachments just to the left of the ulnar head, with the articular disc viewed from proximal, exposed by the ulnar head hinging away from the sigmoid notch.

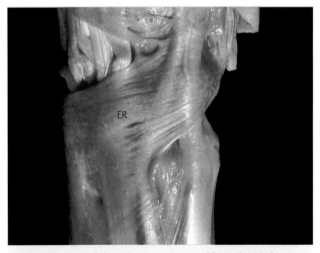

Fig. 24.2 View of the right wrist, as viewed from dorsal ulnar aspect. The fibers of the extensor retinaculum (ER) connect the radio-palmar edge of the radius and the ulnar aspect of the pisiform. The ER forms six dorsal compartments, as pulleys for the extensor tendons.

during forearm rotation. The ECU tendon sheath is considered a duplication of infratendinous layer of the extensor retinaculum (▶ Fig. 24.3).

The posterior (dorsal) groove on the ulnar head and the posterior aspect of the ulnar styloid process are the place for the ECU tendon sheath to attach. The tendon sheath is a structure that consists of a tubular membranous body and a relatively thick fibrous floor, formed between the supra- and infratendinous extensor retinaculum. This structure can be divided into three parts. In the proximal portion, where the floor of the sheath strongly attaches on the ulnar head, the exterior of the sheath is covered by only thin antebrachial fascia. In the middle portion, between the ulnar head and triquetrum, the floor attaches on the dorsal aspect of the ulnar collateral ligament. Though the exterior of the membranous wall is covered with thick supratendinous retinaculum, these two are separated by loose connective tissue and the ECU tendon sheath is permitted a radioulnar translation under the retinaculum. In the distal portion dorsal to the triquetrum, the floor unites with the infratendinous retinaculum and attaches strongly on to the triquetrum. The membranous sheath also merges with the supratendinous retinaculum and permits little movement of the ECU tendon. Removal of both layers of extensor retinaculum except the ECU tendon sheath between the 5th dorsal compartment and the pisiform allows better observation of the TFCC (▶ Fig. 24.4).

24.3 The Triangular Fibrocartilage Complex (TFCC)

The TFCC, as a term to indicate the ligamentous complex on the ulnar side of the wrist, was introduced by Palmer and Warner in 1981.[12] It was a structural concept to define the classification of the injuries within this complex. They selected following six structures that have close relation in anatomy as structural components of TFCC: (1) articular disc, (2) meniscus homologue, (3) radioulnar ligaments, (4) palmar ulnocarpal ligaments, (5) ulnar collateral ligament, and (6) ECU tendon sheath

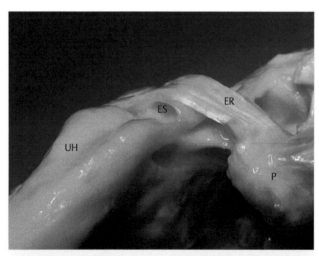

Fig. 24.3 View of right ulnar wrist, with ulna viewed from posterior, and hand viewed from ulnar. with palmar aspect of hand at bottom. The 6th dorsal compartment holds the extensor carpi ulnaris (ECU) tendon sheath (ES) that attaches on the dorsal aspect of the ulnar head (UH). The extensor retinaculum (ER) attaches on the ulnar aspect of the pisiform (P).

(▶ Fig. 24.5). The articular disc, or the "triangular fibrocartilage," is located ulnarly, continuing from the sigmoid notch of the radius (▶ Fig. 24.6). It has two smooth concave facets articulating with the ulnar head proximally and the carpal bones distally. The meniscus homologue, named to indicate the "homologous structure of ape meniscus in the human wrist joint," is observed

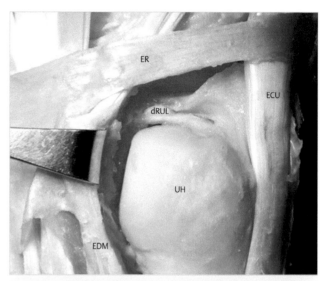

Fig. 24.4 View of right wrist, from dorsal ulnar aspect. The proximal part of the extensor retinaculum and the dorsal wrist capsule between the 5th and the 6th dorsal compartments have been removed, leaving the distal portion of the extensor retinaculum (ER) intact. The extensor digiti minimi (EDM) tendon and the ECU tendon are exposed. The dorsal fascicles of the radioulnar ligament (dRUL) can be seen as a part of the TFCC. UH: ulnar head.

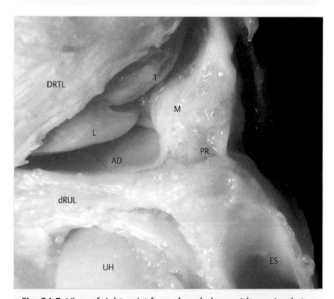

Fig. 24.5 View of right wrist from dorsal ulnar, with proximal at bottom. The extensor retinaculum and dorsal wrist capsule. The extensor retinaculum and dorsal wrist capsule ulnar to proximal portion of the dorsal radiotriquetral ligament (DRTL) are removed to show the components of TFCC. The articular disc (AD) that merges with the dorsal fascicles of radioulnar ligament (dRUL) is located between ulnar head (UH) and carpal bones, lunate (L) and triquetrum (T). On the periphery of the AD, the meniscus homologue (M) and the prestyloid recess (PR) are confirmed. The fibrous floor of the ECU tendon sheath (ES) corresponds the dorsal wall of the TFCC (removed).

protruding from the dorsal and palmar joint capsule.[9,13] At the ulnarmost corner of the articular disc, between the dorsal and palmar lamellae of meniscus homologue, is a dimple named the "prestyloid recess," the cavity of which is usually occupied by synovial villi. Normally, there is no communication between DRUJ and radiocarpal joint cavity unless there is tear or perforation of the TFC or disruption of TFCC.

The radioulnar ligaments, the palmar ulnocarpal ligaments, the ulnar collateral ligament, and the ECU tendon sheath are considered stabilizing structures of TFCC that support the articular disc and the meniscus homologue. The radioulnar ligaments that connect distal radius and ulna are observed at the dorsal and palmar portions of the articular disc after removing loose connective tissue of joint capsule and other external components of TFCC (▶Fig. 24.7 and ▶Fig. 24.8). The dorsal fascicle of the radioulnar ligament arises from the dorsal rim of the sigmoid notch and runs ulnarly uniting with the dorsal margin of the articular disc. The palmar fascicle arises from the palmar rim of the sigmoid notch and widely from the palmar rim of the lunate facet of the radius. These two fascicles merge at the ulnar apex of the articular disc, then divide into proximal (deep) and distal (superficial) layers, attaching on the fovea of the ulnar head and the ulnar styloid process, respectively (▶Fig. 24.9). This arrangement of the ligaments permits swing motion of the radius around the ulna (▶Fig. 24.10).

The palmar ulnocarpal ligaments connect the ulnar head and the carpus (▶Fig. 24.11). They include three ligament fascicles: (1) the *ulnolunate ligament* that connects the ulna and the palmar aspect of the lunate, proximal to the attachment of the lunotriquetral ligament; (2) the *ulnotriquetral ligament* that connects the ulna and the palmar aspect of the triquetrum, proximal to the pisotriquetral joint facet; and (3) the *ulnocapitate ligament* that connects the ulna and the palmar aspect of the capitate along with the fibers of triquetrocapitate ligament. The ulnocapitate ligament was clearly confirmed by gross anatomical dissections (▶Fig. 24.12). The proximal portion of the ulnocarpal ligaments interdigitate with the fibers of tongue like "distal extension" of the palmar radioulnar ligament (Palmar Distal Extension, PDE) (the term was suggested by Julio Taleisnik, MD in a personal communication) and attach on the base of the ulnar styloid process. The "distal extension" covers

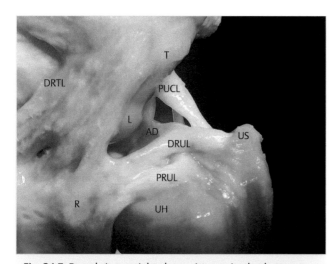

Fig. 24.6 View of right wrist from distal, with dorsal at right and the radial styloid at the bottom. The TFCC is observed from the perspective of the radiocarpal joint. All carpal bones are removed. The articular disc (AD) forms an articular surface for the carpal bones, smoothly continuing from the lunate facet of the radius (R). The meniscus homologue (M) protrudes from dorsal and palmar capsule. On the most ulnar corner of the AD, the prestyloid recess (PR) is seen. The "distal extension" of the palmar radioulnar ligament (PDE) covers the volar aspect of the short radiolunate ligament (SRLL) that connect the volar rim of the lunate facet and the palmar proximal portion of the lunate. ER: extensor retinaculum, DRTL: dorsal radio triquetral ligament.

Fig. 24.7 Dorsal view or right ulnar wrist, proximal at bottom. The articular disc (AD) is supported by the radioulnar ligament that consists of proximal radioulnar ligament (PRUL) and distal radioulnar ligament (DRUL). The palmar ulnocarpal ligaments (PUCL) appear to be a single bundle. R: radius, L: lunate, T: triquetrum, UH: ulnar head, US: ulnar styloid, and DTRL: dorsal radio triquetral ligament.

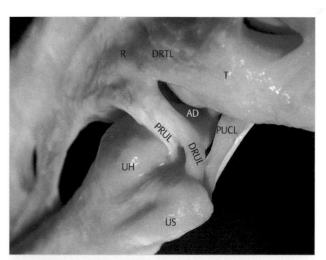

Fig. 24.8 Dorsal view of the right wrist, showing the internal structures of the TFCC, with the ulnar head (UH) at the bottom of the picture, proximal at lower left, and the radius (R) at upper left. The proximal radioulnar ligament (PRUL) attaches on the fovea of the ulnar head (UH). The distal radioulnar ligament (DRUL) attaches on the middle of the ulnar styloid process (US). The palmar ulnocarpal ligaments (PUCL) attach on the base of the US. T: triquetral, DRTL: dorsal radio triquetral ligament, and AD: articular disc.

the palmar aspect of the short radiolunate ligament that connects the palmar rim of the radius and palmar proximal portion of the lunate, and its most distal portion loosely attaches on the palmar aspect of the lunate (▶ Fig. 24.13). The ulnar styloid process, a cone-shaped bony protrusion located on the ulnar head, provides space for several structural elements of the TFCC to attach (▶ Fig. 24.14). When the DRUJ is observed in neutral position of the forearm, the ulnar collateral ligament is seen to attach to the ulnar styloid proximally and the triquetrum distally. The distal (superficial) radioulnar ligament attaches on the radial (medial) aspect of the ulnar styloid process. The "distal extensions" of the palmar radioulnar ligament and the palmar ulnocarpal ligaments attach on the proximal portion of the

radial aspect of the styloid process. In other words, the "distal extensions" of palmar radioulnar ligament, the palmar ulnocarpal ligaments, and the ulnar collateral ligament surround the distal (superficial) radioulnar ligament and attach together on the broad area of the ulnar styloid process. There exists a cavity surrounded by these ligaments that connects the radiocarpal

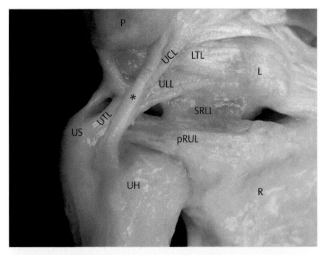

Fig. 24.11 View of right wrist from palmar, with proximal at bottom, radius (R) at lower right, and ulnar head (UH) at lower left. The palmar ulnocarpal ligaments include three ligament fascicles: ulno lunate ligament (ULL), ulnotriquetral ligament (UTL), and ulnocapitate ligament (UCL). The ULL connects the ulna and anterior aspect of the lunate (L), between the insertions of short radiolunate ligament (SRLL) and lunotriquetral ligament (LTL). The UTL connects the ulna and the anterior aspect of the triquetrum, proximal to the pisotriquetral articular facet. The UCL connects the ulna and the palmar aspect of the capitate. The palmar fascicles of the radioulnar ligament (pRUL) attach widely on the volar rim of the distal radius. An unknown bundle that connect the palmar aspect of the ulna and radial portion of the triquetrum was left uncut on this specimen (*). This was not a capsular ligament. US: ulnar styloid.

Fig. 24.9 View of the right radiocarpal joint from distal, with all the carpal bones removed, showing the TFCC, with the radius (R) right, and the ulnar head (UH), left. The distal radioulnar ligament (DRUL) merges with the articular disc (AD) and attaches on the ulnar styloid process (US). The dorsal fascicle (dPRUL) and palmar fascicle (pPRUL) of proximal radioulnar ligament can be confirmed proximal to the DRUL. TFCC: the triangular fibrocartilage complex.

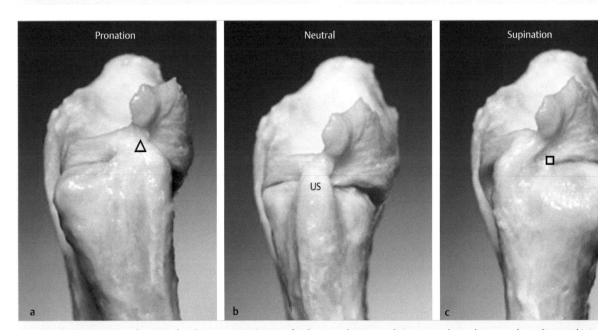

Fig. 24.10 (a: Pronation; b: Neutral and c: Supination) View of right wrist showing radius at top, ulna at bottom, the radiocarpal joint, and TFCC. The distal radioulnar ligament (△) that attaches on the ulnar styloid process (US) shows a swing motion during rotation of the forearm. In contrast, the proximal radioulnar ligament (□) that attaches on the fovea keeps nearly isometric configuration during pronosupination. TFCC: the triangular fibrocartilage complex.

joint and the tip of the ulnar styloid process. This cavity corresponds to the prestyloid recess (▶Fig. 24.6). The volar wall of the recess has a thin membranous portion between the ulnotriquetral ligament and the ulnar collateral ligament. This was recognized as an oval window, the result of anatomical dissection of the joint capsule, to remove as much areolar tissue and visualize the hidden capsular ligaments (▶Fig. 24.12). These findings suggested that the ulnar collateral ligament that connects the ulnar styloid process and the triquetrum can be recognized as a part of the ulnotriquetral ligament that consists of two fascicles separated by the anterior thin membranous portion. The ulnar insertions of the "distal extension" of palmar radioulnar ligament, the palmar ulnocarpal ligaments, the ulnar collateral ligament, and the distal (superficial) radioulnar ligament (DRUL) are separated from that of the proximal (deep) radioulnar ligament (PRUL) by vascular loose connective tissue.[9,14,21] There may exist variations in size of the opening space occupied by this tissue (▶Fig. 24.15). In some specimens, the opening is widely spread and the two ligament insertions are definite. Other specimens show a narrow opening where the insertions are in close approximation. These differences might be affected by the variations of this part, i.e., the thickness of the vascular areolar tissue, the length of the ulnar styloid process, or the ulnar variance during the development of DRUJ.

24.4 Discussion

Although much has been published regarding anatomy, biomechanics, pathologies, and treatments of the DRUJ and its disorders, a few points impede the understanding of this small joint. These include difficulty in visualization of anatomical structures and existence of significant variations of anatomy as well as of different terminologies.

The detailed anatomy of this area has attracted the attention of hand surgeons, especially during the past three decades, and the terminology has evolved without international consensus. As a result, many different terms are used to indicate the same structure. It is quite likely that such confusion arises due to differences in research methods and a lack of consensus on the histological definition of connective tissues, especially regarding the ligaments.

A skeletal ligament is defined as a "strong band of parallel collagen bundles" that can contain few elastic fibers among the collagen fibers. The capsular ligament is regarded as a "cord-like thickening of the fibrous capsule." A ligament works as a stabilizer of a joint by connecting two bones together. Although the fibrils of the collagenous fibers do not branch individually, groups of them may separate and give

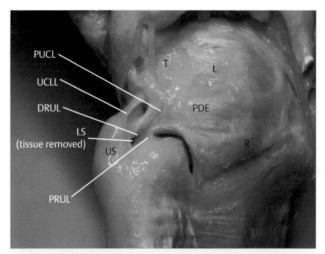

Fig. 24.12 View or right palmar ulnar wrist, with proximal at bottom, and radius (R) at right. The fibers of ulnolunate ligament (ULL), ulnotriquetral ligament (UTL) and ulnocapitate ligament (UCL) interdigitate with the fibers of "distal extension" of palmar radioulnar ligament (PDE) and attach proximally on the base of the ulnar styloid process (US). The ulnar collateral ligament (UCLL) that connects the ulnar styloid process and the ulnar aspect of the triquetrum is separated from UTL by an oval window (☆). pRUL: proximal radioulnar ligament.

Fig. 24.14 Palmar view of right wrist with proximal at bottom. The "distal extension" of the palmar radioulnar ligament (PDE), palmar ulnocarpal ligaments (PUCL), and the ulnar collateral ligament (UCLL) surround the distal radioulnar ligament (DRUL) and attach on the ulnar styloid process (US). These attachments are separated from that of the proximal radioulnar ligament (PRUL) by vascular loose connective tissue that was removed.
T: triquetrum, L: lunate, R: radius, LS: Ligamentum Subcruentum.

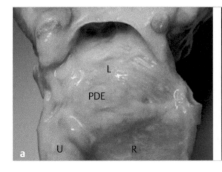
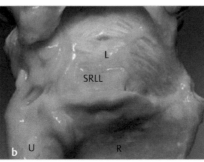

Fig. 24.13 Two views of palmar right carpus, with proximal at bottom. (a) The fibers of "distal extension" of the palmar radioulnar ligament (PDE) connect the volar rim of the distal radius (R) and ulna (U). Its distal portion loosely attaches on the palmar aspect of the lunate (L). (b) When the PDE is detached from the lunate and flipped proximally, the short radiolunate ligament (SRLL) can be exposed.

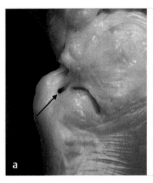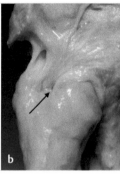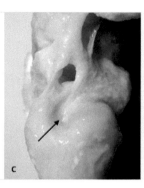

Fig. 24.15 Views of the right carpus from palmar, of three different specimens. The ulnar insertions of the "distal extension" of the palmar radioulnar ligament, palmar ulnocarpal ligaments, ulnar collateral ligament, and distal radioulnar ligament (DRUL) are separated from that of the proximal radioulnar ligament (PRUL). The samples show the variations: (**a**) wide opening type; (**b**) narrow opening type; and (**c**) no opening type.

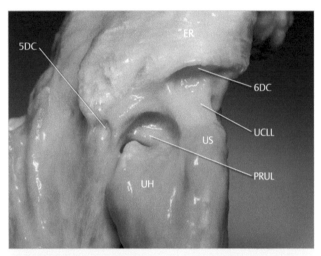

Fig. 24.16 View of the right carpus from dorsal ulnar, with proximal at bottom. The ulnar collateral ligament (UCLL) connects the ulnar styloid process (US) and the triquetrum, forming the distal and dorsal walls of the TFCC. The ECU tendon sheath (removed) loosely attaches on the dorsal aspect of the UCLL. 5DC: 5th dorsal compartment, 6DC: 6th dorsal compartment, UH: ulnar head, PRUL: proximal radioulnar ligament, and ER: extensor retinaculum.

a branched appearance. In other words, a bundle of connective tissue that mainly consists of regularly arranged collagen fibers and binds bones together can be considered as a ligament regardless of its appearance or strength. Histological verification of the ligament bundle and its bony insertions is fundamental. Although there is no formally described rule in anatomical terminology regarding capsular ligaments of the wrist joint, it is suggested to name a ligament listing the names of bones that the ligament attaches, in order from proximal to distal and from radial to ulnar side. Application of the name of the discoverer or use of any adjectives that do not describe the specific characteristics of a structure, should be avoided. Care should be taken with a selection of general terms, like modifiers that define the positional relations of anatomical structures. All relations should be anatomically absolute. For example, the terms, "superficial" and "deep" can only be used to indicate the relationship in depth between surface and core of a body part. By this reason, these modifiers should not be used to distinguish the proximal and distal layers of the radioulnar ligament.

There are controversies regarding DRUJ anatomy, including the validity of the ulnar collateral ligament and the short radiolunate ligament, consistency of the ulnocapitate ligament,

and location of the ulnar attachments of the ulnocarpal ligaments.[15,16,17] The existence of the ulnar collateral ligament has been confirmed by many researchers and was incorporated into the six components of the TFCC.[12] Although it is actually not a distinct fascicle and looks more like a thickening of the joint capsule, there is no reason to exclude this consistent structure from the ligaments of the wrist joint (▶Fig. 24.16).[17,18,19] The structure called the short radiolunate ligament is observed between the palmar rim of the lunate facet of the radius and the palmar proximal portion of the lunate (Berger and Landsmeer 1990), dorsal to the "distal extension" of the palmar radioulnar ligament (▶Fig. 24.13). The characteristics of the short radiolunate ligament, with its yellowish semitranslucent appearance and great elasticity, seems quite different from other capsular ligaments of the wrist joint. This structure might be a remnant of the ligament that possibly had an important role in quadrupedalism.

The anatomy of ulnocarpal ligaments, including the exact location of their ulnar attachments and relationships with the radioulnar ligament, are also subjects of discussion (▶Fig. 24.11, ▶Fig. 24.12, and ▶Fig. 24.14).[21,22,23] The ulnar-sided capsular ligaments are hardly separable because they lost their separate identity by merging with the anterior margin of the articular disc.[13] Although each of the ligaments is not significant compared with the radiocarpal ligaments, they interdigitate and construct a large ligamentous complex that connects the ulna and the radius or the ulna and the carpus. The different recognitions of the construction might be affected by differences in study method, such as of histology versus gross anatomy. A two-dimensional histological study is limited in its ability to organize a three-dimensional structure. On the contrary, a fine anatomical dissection with a clear isolation of each structure is helpful to understand the construction, though doing so can be challenging because some structures are fused to each other and others are buried in a thick layer of loose connective tissue. A gross anatomical dissection with removal of as much areolar tissue and separation of each structure may result in an alteration of morphology or relationships with surrounding structures from their original form. This might be a reason that, as far as I know, no clear photograph of this part has been shown in past publications.

The many morphological variations of structures around this joint may be one of the factors that make understanding of the DRUJ difficult. The variations can be seen in the shape of the sigmoid notch and the ulnar head, the length of the ulna relative to the radius (ulnar variance), the height of the ulnar styloid process, the presence or absence of cartilage coverage of the ulnar styloid process, the thickness of the articular disc, the shape and size of the meniscus homologue, the shape and size of the prestyloid recess, and the presence or absence of the lunula (a bony nodule that rarely exists in the meniscus homologue).[4,9,22,24,254,9,22,24,25] Some of those variations may produce inconsistency in the biomechanical features of the DRUJ.

When looking at the unique anatomy of DRUJ, the following questions always spring to my mind: Even though the mobility of the DRUJ has brought great benefits to human life, was this a perfect solution to permit forearm rotation? Although we tend to understand anatomy by its function, are all structures around DRUJ really functional? Since anatomy is a result of morphogenesis, answers to these questions might be obtained through research into phylogenesis and ontogenesis. Observations of morphogenesis and comparisons of anatomy among the primates by the pioneers in the past half-century have offered hints for understanding the complicated construction of the DRUJ.[9,16,26] The mobile human DRUJ was inherited from our ancestors. This more recently obtained functional component in the evolutional history of mammals might not be a property that those ancestors desired, even if this trait happened to provide a functional benefit for modern human activities. Our ancestors obtained the trait to enable forearm rotation by chance, as a result of modification of anatomy about the distal ulna.

During the development of human wrist joint, an articulation between the ulna and triquetrum was observed in a 30 mm crown–rump–length fetus.[26] The anlage of a part of ulna that corresponds to the original ulnar head stops developing earlier than other parts and remains as a tiny ulnar styloid process. This results in withdrawal of the ulnocarpal articulation. An anlage of the articular disc is formed between the newly created ulnar head and the carpus to partition the radiocarpal joint and the DRUJ.[19] The ligaments attaching on the ulnar head and the styloid process are pulled distally or radially, according to the development of the carpal bones and radius, and form a ligamentous construction that corresponds to the exterior framework that surrounds the articular disc. It is speculated that the prestyloid recess was created as a result of a prolongation of the radiocarpal joint cavity due to the exclusion of the ulna from the wrist joint.

Although the articular disc, meniscus homologue, and palmar capsular ligaments were marked in 64 to 120 mm crown–rump–length fetus, the radioulnar ligament was not well observed as an isolated structure in histological studies of fetuses.[16,18,19,26] It is generally accepted that the fascicles of the radioulnar ligament can be divided into proximal (deep) and distal (superficial) layers.[8,21,22] A possible explanation for these complex structures is that the proximal and distal layers of radioulnar ligament are derived from two different origins, with the distal layer derived from radiocarpal joint capsule and the proximal layer from DRUJ capsule. Mechanical stress between the ulnar head and the carpus might promote transformation of the anlage of the articular disc into fibrocartilage and as a result unite the two capsular ligament layers. This can provide a reasonable explanation for why radioulnar ligaments are integrated into the articular disc and why the two insertions of the radioulnar ligaments are separated by vascular areolar tissue (ligamentum subcruentum).

Those who find the complexity of the DRUJ to be a significant barrier to understanding its anatomy, might start by learning its history of transformation during phylogenesis or ontogenesis. The morphology of human DRUJ was not a product of modification from nonmobile DRUJ in order to achieve a purposive evolution, and not every structure about the DRUJ seems to have its specific function. It is assumed that the reason the DRUJ holds many anatomical variations and is responsible for a variety of clinical disorders is that the joint was not perfectly optimized for its function. However, it is needless to say that knowledge of the detailed anatomy of the DRUJ is essential to correctly assess the results of biomechanical studies and consider appropriate treatment methods for disorders of this joint. To systematize knowledge and further develop derivative applications into clinical uses, standardization of newly obtained knowledge and correction of past descriptions is necessary. Lack of consensus on anatomical terms is a problem that should be resolved in the near future.

References

1. Hagert E, Hagert CG. Understanding stability of the distal radioulnar joint through an understanding of its anatomy. Hand Clin. 2010 Nov;26(4):459–66
2. Gofton WT, Gordon KD, Dunning CE, Johnson JA, King GJ. Soft-tissue stabilizers of the distal radioulnar joint: an in vitro kinematic study. J Hand Surg Am. 2004 May;29(3):423-31
3. Kihara H, Short WH, Werner FW, Fortino MD, Palmer AK. The stabilizing mechanism of the distal radioulnar joint during pronation and supination. J Hand Surg Am. 1995 Nov;20(6):930-6
4. Palmer AK, Glisson RR, Werner FW. Relationship between ulnar variance and triangular fibrocartilage complex thickness. J Hand Surg Am. 1984 Sep;9(5):681-2
5. Ward LD, Ambrose CG, Masson MV, Levaro F. The role of the distal radioulnar ligaments, interosseous membrane, and joint capsule in distal radioulnar joint stability. J Hand Surg Am. 2000 Mar;25(2):341-51
6. Garcia-Elias M, Hagert E. Surgical approaches to the distal radioulnar joint. Hand Clin. 2010 Nov;26(4):477-83
7. Gordon KD, Dunning CE, Johnson JA, King GJ. Influence of the pronator quadratus and supinator muscle load on DRUJ stability. J Hand Surg Am. 2003 Nov;28(6):943-50
8. Kleinman WB. Stability of the distal radioulna joint: biomechanics, pathophysiology, physical diagnosis, and restoration of function what we have learned in 25 years. J Hand Surg Am. 2007 Sep;32(7):1086-106
9. Lewis OJ. Evolutionary change in the primate wrist and inferior radio-ulnar joints. Anat Rec. 1965 Mar;151:275-85
10. Almquist EE. Evolution of the distal radioulnar joint. Clin Orthop Relat Res. 1992 Feb;(275):5-13
11. Taleisnik J, Gelberman RH, Miller BW, Szabo RM. The extensor retinaculum of the wrist. J Hand Surg Am. 1984 Jul;9(4):495-501
12. Palmer AK, Werner FW. The triangular fibrocartilage complex of the wrist--anatomy and function. J Hand Surg Am. 1981 Mar;6(2):153-62
13. Lewis OJ, Hamshere RJ, Bucknill TM. The anatomy of the wrist joint. J Anat. 1970 May;106(3):539-52
14. Chidgey LK. Histologic anatomy of the triangular fibrocartilage. Hand Clin. 1991 May;7(2):249-62
15. Berger RA, Landsmeer JM. The palmar radiocarpal ligaments: a study of adult and fetal human wrist joints. J Hand Surg Am. 1990 Nov;15(6):847-54
16. Lewis OJ. The development of the human wrist joint during the fetal period. Anat Rec. 1970 Mar;166(3):499-515
17. Taleisnik J. The ligaments of the wrist. J Hand Surg Am. 1976 Sep;1(2):110-8

18. Hogikyan JV, Louis DS. Embryologic development and variations in the anatomy of the ulnocarpal ligamentous complex. J Hand Surg Am. 1992 Jul;17(4):719-23

19. Mérida-Velasco JA, Garcia-Garcia JD, Espín-Ferra J, Sánchez-Montesinos I. Development of the human wrist joint ligaments. Anat Rec. 1996 May;245(1):114-21

20. Berger RA, Landsmeer JM. The palmar radiocarpal ligaments: a study of adult and fetal human wrist joints. J Hand Surg Am. 1990 Nov;15(6):847-54

21. Berger RA. The anatomy of the ligaments of the wrist and distal radioulnar joints. Clin Orthop Relat Res. 2001 Feb;(383):32-40

22. Ishii S, Palmer AK, Werner FW, Short WH, Fortino MD. An anatomic study of the ligamentous structure of the triangular fibrocartilage complex. J Hand Surg Am. 1998 Nov;23(6):977-85

23. Garcia-Elias M. Soft-tissue anatomy and relationships about the distal ulna. Hand Clin. 1998 May;14(2):165-76

24. Mikic ZD. Detailed anatomy of the articular disc of the distal radioulnar joint. Clin Orthop Relat Res. 1989 Aug;(245):123-32

25. Palmer AK, Glisson RR, Werner FW. Ulnar variance determination. J Hand Surg Am. 1982 Jul;7(4):376-9

26. Whillis J. The development of synovial joints. J Anat. 1940 Jan;74(Pt 2):277-83

25 Function of the Distal Radioulnar Joint

William B. Kleinman

The distal radioulnar joint (DRUJ) is the foundation for a moving relationship between radius and ulna through their full arc of forearm pronosupination. Biomechanics of healthy, human forearm pronosupination allow the hand to be *put or placed in space* (▶Fig. 25.1). Perhaps this is an oversimplification of a more complicated interrelationship among the forearm, elbow, and shoulder; but the contribution of stable, painless forearm rotation to function of the entire upper limb cannot be overstated.

The purpose of this chapter is to provide the reader with a clear understanding of the details of DRUJ anatomy and biomechanics—of how the DRUJ functions. We hope that the readers

will gain a clear understanding not only of the fine details of DRUJ anatomy, but of the distal forearm biomechanics that allow stable, painless pronosupination through a 180° arc, repetitively and regularly under considerable load (▶Fig. 25.2).

The DRUJ is responsible for two critical functions. The first is to provide a diarthrodial joint platform for rotation of the distal radius around a fixed and stable distal ulna. This arc of rotation is generated from full supination, where both bones of the forearm are essentially parallel and the interosseous space is at its widest breadth, to full pronation, where the radius crosses the ulna from lateral to medial, narrowing the interosseous space to its smallest dimension. The second function of the DRUJ is

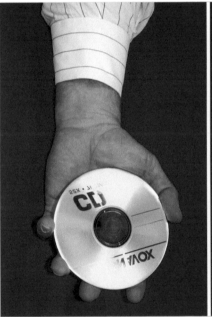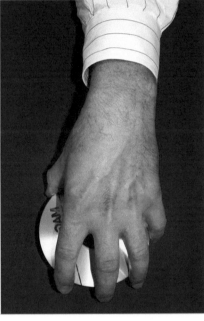

Fig. 25.1 Enabling the hand to be *put or placed* in space is the primary function of a healthy arc of forearm prono-supination.

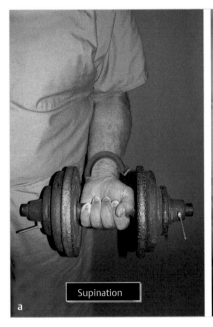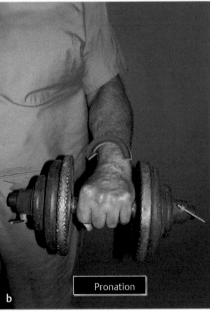

Supination

Pronation

a b

Fig. 25.2 (a, b) The joint reaction force (JRF) passing between sigmoid fossa and ulna seat can exceed many times body weight, even in the extremes of supinaton and pronation, where <10% of the fossa is in contact with the seat.

to provide the mechanism that allows the transfer of load from the hand, through this diarthrodial joint from radius to ulna (sigmoid fossa through the seat of the distal ulna), and up the ulna for transmission to the ginglymus ulnotrochlear joint of the elbow. In other words, the DRUJ allows the hand not only to be *put or placed in space* with precision but also to perform work and load transfer with stability and painlessness. Without healthy DRUJ function, forearm pronosupination and forearm load bearing would be profoundly compromised, significantly impacting the function of the entire upper limb.

The longitudinal axis of the forearm for this full, functional arc of pronosupination passes proximally through the center of the radial head at the radio capitellar joint and distally through the fovea of the distal ulna. The fovea is a well-vascularized bony recess, or sulcus, between the hyaline cartilage-covered pole of the distal ulna and the base of the ulna styloid (▶ Fig. 25.3). The pole is the bony platform of the distal ulna that receives direct load-transfer from the medial carpus, through the articular disc of the triangular fibrocartilage (TFC), onto the distal ulna itself. Proximally, the ulna is attached to the trochlear of the distal humerus as a hinged, diarthrodial, ginglymus elbow joint. The ulnotrochlear joint participates only in elbow flexion

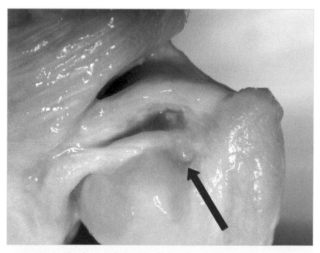

Fig. 25.3 The fovea of the distal ulna (arrow) is a well-vascularized sulcus between the base of the ulna styloid and the hyaline cartilage-covered pole of the distal ulna. This site is the origin of the deep fibers of the triangular fibrocartilage (*Ligamentum subcruentum*).

and extension; it does not contribute to rotation of the forearm. The mechanics of forearm rotation only involve movement of the radius around a fixed ulna (▶ Fig. 25.4). The ulna flexes and extends in a single plane at the elbow; the radius rotates around the fixed ulna in the forearm.

Affixed to the lateral border of the olecranon process is the annular ligament that holds the radial head securely at the proximal radioulnar joint (PRUJ) (Fig. 25.5). The annular ligament encircles and constrains the radial head, allowing rotation of the head around the longitudinal axis of forearm; the axis passes directly through the head's center. The annular ligament holds the rotating radial head securely against the fixed, nonrotating ulna at the diarthrodial PRUJ. The ulna *only* flexes and extends on the humerus; with respect to forearm rotation, it is fixed. Therefore, movement of the radius relative to a fixed ulna generates the entire arc of prono-supination. In order to generate a full 180° arc of pronosupination (understanding that the proximal radial head is held securely by the annular ligament and *only* allowed to spin around the longitudinal axis of the forearm) the radius must roll from a position where both forearm bones are parallel to a position where the radius crosses the ulna (▶ Fig. 25.6). In the bipedal human condition, supination puts the hand "palm up," with the two forearm bones paralleling each other and the interosseous space at its maximum breadth. Full pronation puts the hand "palm down," with the radius crossing the ulna, collapsing the interosseous space to its narrowest breadth. The transition from parallel to crossed forearm bones decreases the apparent length of the radius relative to the ulna, resulting in **ulna-plus variance** in full pronation. As a result of increasing ulna variance in pronation, load on the TFC proportionally increases. Full forearm supination draws the radius back into parallel alignment with the ulna, thus relieving pressure on the TFC as the apparent length of the radius increases, resulting in **ulna-minus variance**.

DRUJ design provides healthy articular hyaline cartilage on the surfaces of both the sigmoid fossa and the adjacent distal ulna seat. This relationship is stabilized through a healthy arc of pronosupination by intrinsic (within the DRUJ) and extrinsic (outside the DRUJ) soft-tissue stabilizers that guide the radius through its physiologic arc of forearm rotation, actively driven by the forearm muscles of supination and pronation. Since rotation of the forearm from full supination to full pronation results in a change from ulna-minus variance to ulna-plus variance as the radius rolls across the ulna, the principal axis of load

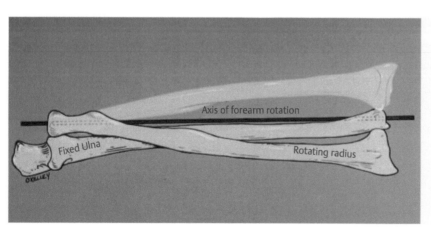

Fig. 25.4 The longitudinal axis of rotation of the forearm (red line) passes through the head of the radius proximally and through the fovea of the ulna distally.

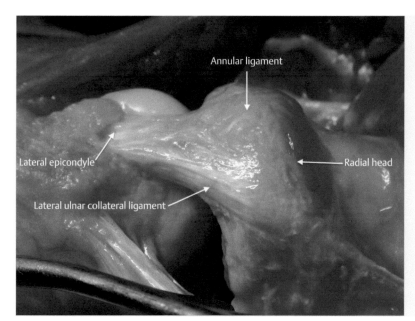

Fig. 25.5 The annular ligament arises from the lateral border of the olecranon, at the ginglymus ulno-trochlear joint. It encircles the radial head, allowing head rotation around the longitudinal axis of the rotating forearm.

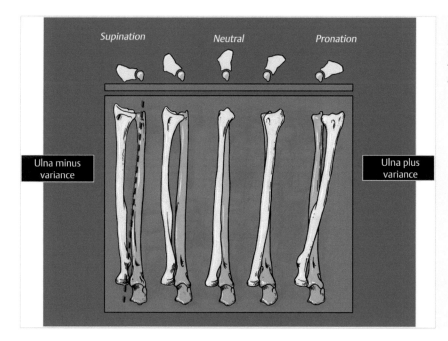

Fig. 25.6 As the radius rotates from full supination to full pronation around a fixed ulna, the radio-carpal unit shortens relative to the ulna, resulting in ulna-positive variance in the pronated position.

bearing[a] at the DRUJ cannot simply track transversely across the articular surface of the sigmoid fossa. Rather, the tracking line for DRUJ load bearing extends from proximal–proximal (PP) in full supination to dorsal–distal (DD) in full pronation (▶Fig. 25.7). The reader should note the transverse orientation of the sigmoid fossa in this figure. It is the larger anteroposterior dimension of the rectangular configuration of the sigmoid fossa that allows it enough surface area to rotate around the fixed ulna seat (which is covered 270° by hyaline cartilage). Rotation of the radius around the fixed ulna occurs simultaneous with oblique translation of the principal axis of load bearing at the DRUJ from dorsal–distal in supination to volar–proximal in pronation. The principal axis of radius-to-ulna load transmission at the DRUJ has plenty of room to track obliquely across the sigmoid fossa through the full arc of healthy forearm pronosupination, simply because of the adequate dimension of the fossa.

Extrinsic stabilizers of the two-bone relationship at the DRUJ include: the extensor carpi ulnaris (ECU) tendon; the VIth dorsal compartment fibro-osseous subsheath of the ECU; the two heads of the pronator quadratus (PQ); and the interosseous ligament (IOL; ▶Fig. 25.8). Recent descriptions of thickened fibers of the most distal portion of the interosseous membrane (IOM) of the forearm—adjacent to the proximal portion of the DRUJ

---

[a]The "principal axis of load bearing" is an engineering term used to describe the imaginary center of a cluster of surface contact points where two surfaces come together under load. As the surfaces move relative to each other, the principal axis of load bearing will track across the sigmoid fossa, along an imaginary line. In the case of the DRUJ, physiologic rotation and translation of the sigmoid fossa on the ulna seat create an oblique line from volar-proximal in supination to dorsal-distal in pronation, because of the relative radius shortening as it crosses the fixed ulna in pronation.

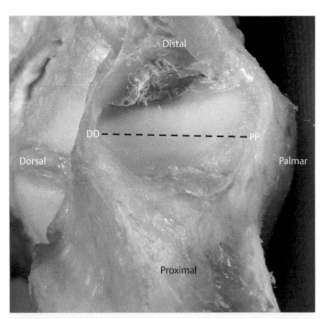

Fig. 25.7 The principal axis of load-bearing (see text) tracks across the sigmoid fossa from proximal/palmar (PP) in supination to distal/dorsal (DD) in pronation.

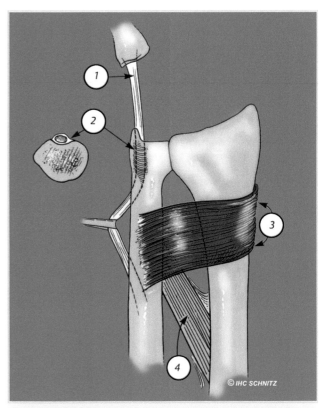

Fig. 25.8 Extrinsic stabilizers of the inherently unstable DRUJ include: (1) the tendon of the Extensor carpi ulnaris; (2) the VIth dorsal compartment subsheath; (3) the superficial and deep heads of the Pronator quadratus; and (4) the Interosseous ligament of the forearm. Even when considered together as a group, the extrinsic DRUJ stabilizers are relatively ineffective in physiologically maintaining DRUJ stability through the arc of pronation/supination under load (see text).

capsule—suggest that this area of the IOM may provide some additional extrinsic DRUJ support.[1,2]

The intrinsic TFC and its components, however, are the primary and principal stabilizers of DRUJ mechanics through the full arc of forearm pronosupination (▸Fig. 25.9). In order to fully appreciate the details of anatomy of the TFC, one must first understand the *nonconstrained* nature of the articulating surfaces of the DRUJ. Af Ekenstam and Hagert[3] demonstrated more than 25 years ago that the radii of curvature of the sigmoid fossa of the distal radius and the seat of the ulna are not concentric. The radius of curvature of the fossa is significantly greater than that of the ulna seat (▸Fig. 25.10). In contrast to the constrained nature of the femoral head and the pelvic acetabulum, the seat of the ulna does not fit into an inherently stable, constrained socket at the medial surface of the distal radius. Rather, the DRUJ more closely resembles the relationship between the humeral head and the glenoid, requiring additional stabilizers to ensure normal biomechanics and prevent joint subluxation or dislocation. In the shoulder, stability of glenohumeral joint is provided by the musculotendinous shroud that forms the rotator cuff, and secondarily by the glenoid labrum and the glenohumeral capsule. At the DRUJ, the complex anatomy of the TFC provides primary joint stability, assisted by extracapsular soft-tissue stabilizers and the DRUJ capsule.[4]

In their 1985 published cadaver dissections, af Ekenstam and Hagert[3] demonstrated that in full supination the radius (with its attached carpus and hand) rotates and *translates* across the sigmoid fossa. Hence in full supination < 10% of the *volar* sigmoid fossa still remains in contact with the cartilage surface of the seat of the ulna, as the radius literally rolls off the ulna seat.

Conversely, in full pronation < 10% of the *dorsal* sigmoid fossa still remains in contact with the edge of the ulna seat. The dissections of af Ekenstam and Hagert (in which they excised the central, articular disc of the TFC) suggest that

only **deep** fibers of the TFC—those taking their origin from the fovea of the ulna—are responsible for exerting a "check-rein" effect on the rotating/translating radius, thereby preventing super-physiologic translation, a state in which the radio–ulna relationship would become unstable. In full supination, this checkrein effect of the TFC component (from the af Ekenstam/Hagert dissections) comes from deep, dorsal fibers originating from the fovea. Conversely, the checkrein effect precluding super-physiologic translation in pronation is the volar, deep portion of the TFC originating from the fovea. It was af Ekenstam's and Hagert's belief that only the deep portion of the TFC is principally responsible for rotational/translational stability of the DRUJ.

Six years later, in 1991, Schuind et al[5] published conflicting data from the Mayo Clinic Biomechanics Laboratory, based on stereophotogrammetric computer studies using phosphorescent markers on the *surface* of cadaver TFCs, loaded through a full arc of pronosupination. The group's data suggest increased importance of the **superficial** fibers of the TFC as forearm rotational stabilizers: the superficial volar fibers in supination, and the superficial dorsal fibers in pronation. These conclusions contradicted the findings of af Ekenstam and Hagert 6 years earlier.

The opinions of these two camps of thought were academically and clinically controversial until Hagert published a short,

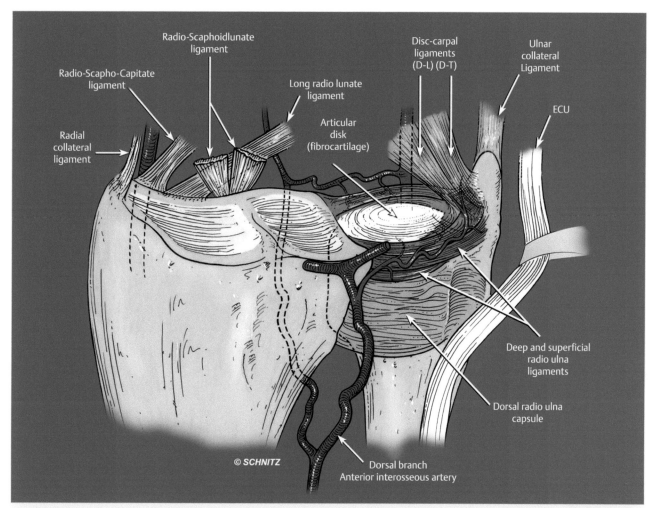

Fig. 25.9 The primary intrinsic stabilizer of the DRUJ is the triangular fibrocartilage (TFC). The TFC complex consists of superficial (green) and deep (blue) radio-ulna fibers, the two disk-carpal ligaments (disk-lunate and disk-triquetral), and the central articular disk (white). The articular disk is responsible for transferring load from the medial carpus to the pole of the distal ulna. The vascularized, peripheral radio-ulna ligaments (green and blue) are nourished by dorsal and palmar branches of the posterior interosseous artery, and are responsible for guiding the radiocarpal unit around the seat of the ulna.

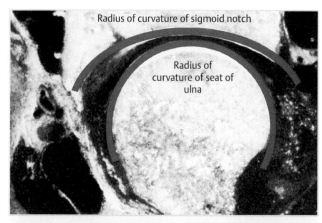

Fig. 25.10 Transverse section through the DRUJ: the radius-of-curvature of the sigmoid fossa is greater than the radius-of-curvature of the seat of the ulna, leading to inherent instability of the DRUJ through its arc of prono-supination. Rotation of the forearm around a longitudinal axis of rotation (see Fig. 25.4) is manifest at the DRUJ by rotation and translation of the sigmoid fossa against the ulna seat. (From af Ekenstam F, Hagert CG: Anatomical studies on the geometry and stability of the distal radioulnar joint. Scan J Plast Reconstr Surg. 1985;19:17–25).

remarkable paper in 1994,[6] explaining how *both* groups of investigators were correct. (▶Fig. 25.11) is reproduced directly from Hagert's original work; (▶Fig. 25.12 and ▶Fig. 25.13) represent my interpretation of Hagert's thesis. Indeed, as Af Ekenstam and Hagert suggested in their 1985 work, supination of the forearm results in rotation and translation of the sigmoid fossa on the fixed seat of the ulna, the extent of which is limited by the checkrein effect of the **deep dorsal** fibers of the TFC, originating from the fovea of the ulna. This origin is quite lateral relative to the origin of the superficial TFC fibers, which have their origin much more medial on the ulna styloid itself. Cadaver dissections in (▶Fig. 25.14 and ▶Fig. 25.15) nicely demonstrate the origins and insertions of the superficial fibers of the TFC: (A) originating of the ulna styloid, and the deep fibers and (B) originating from the fovea. Throughout the articles I have published on this subject over the past 10 years, I have referred to the deep fibers of the vascularized, peripheral fibrous portion of the TFC (B in ▶Fig. 25.14 and ▶Fig. 25.15) as the ligamentum subcruentum.

Af Ekenstam and Hagert are correct in their interpretation of TFC biomechanics. But Schuind et al are correct as well. Superficial, vascularized fibers of the TFC (superficial radioulnar ligaments) also tighten during pronosupination. As the **dorsal** ligamentum subcruentum tightens in full

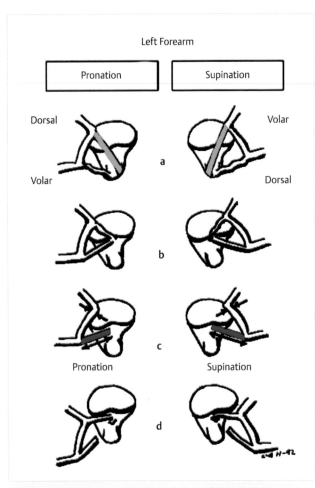

Left Forearm

Pronation | Supination

Dorsal | Volar

Volar | Dorsal

a

b

c

Pronation | Supination

d

Fig. 25.11 Reproduction of Hagert's 1994 work illustrating the effectiveness of the deep fibers of the TFC in controlling distal radio-ulna rotation, and the relative ineffectiveness of the superficial fibers. The critical factor is the angle-of-attack of the *Ligamentum subcruentum* from the fovea of the ulna to the radius. (From Hagert CG: Distal radius fracture and the distal radioulnar joint—anatomical considerations. Handchir Mikrochir Plast Chir. 1994;26:22-26).

supination, the **volar** superficial fibers tighten as well. Which of the two components is more crucial for DRUJ stability in full supination? (▶ Fig. 25.12 and ▶ Fig. 25.13) are my attempt to illustrate how, in the extremes of supination and pronation, there is so much translation of the sigmoid fossa on the seat of the ulna that the entire head of the ulna literally herniates out from under cover of the superficial component of the TFC. Even though in full forearm supination the superficial volar fibers of the TFC are taut, the position of the ulna head relative to the origin and insertion of the superficial volar fibers renders them relatively ineffective as checkreins against super-physiologic translation of the fossa relative to the seat. In contrast, the dorsal, deep ligamentum subcruentum is crucial in preventing super-physiologic rotation and translation in supination.

Conversely, in full pronation, the ulna head slips dorsally from under cover of most of the TFC, rendering the **volar** superficial component ineffective as a checkrein, even though it tightens (as demonstrated by Schuind et al). The **volar** ligamentum subcruentum becomes the principal checkrein against super-physiologic rotation and translation of the radius on the ulna in full pronation.

Hagert's 1994 thesis[6] is explained by the two artistic renderings seen in (▶ Fig. 25.12 and ▶ Fig. 25.13). These figures show the relative demands on the two connective tissue portions of the ligamentum subcruentum when subjected to excessive loads in full supination and full pronation. The differences in how the superficial and deep components of the vascularized portion of the TFC behave in stabilizing the forearm through its arc of pronosupination is based entirely on the tensile angles at which the four components are oriented from their origins to their insertions. (▶ Fig. 25.12 and ▶ Fig. 25.13) clarify these biomechanics.

The cadaver dissection in ▶ Fig. 25.15 demonstrates the **acute** angle of attack of the two components (volar and dorsal) of the superficial radio–ulna portion of the TFC from the ulna styloid to the medial border of the radius (**A**). Also demonstrated is the more **obtuse** angle of attack of the deeper ligamentum subcruentum (**B**). Using the "buckboard analogy" I first published in the *Journal of Hand Surgery* in

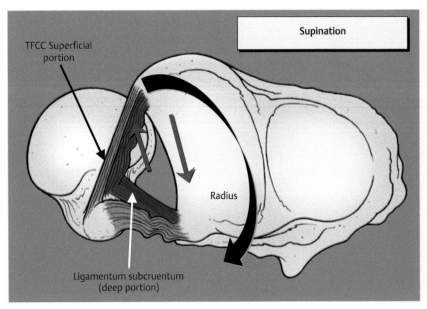

TFCC Superficial portion

Supination

Radius

Ligamentum subcruentum (deep portion)

Fig. 25.12 Illustration of tightening of the dorsal fibers of the deep *Ligamentum subcruentum* (blue) as the radius rotates and translates dorsally off the seat of the ulna in supination. The head of the ulna translates along the sigmoid fossa, and herniates out from under cover of the tightening superficial volar TFC fibers, rendering these (green) fibers ineffective in controlling DRUJ mechanics.

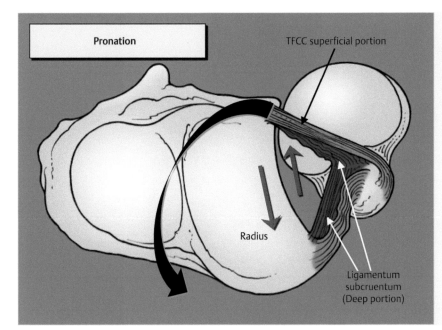

Fig. 25.13 An illustration of tightening of the volar fibers of the *Ligamentum subcruentum* as the radius rotates and translates palmarly off the seat of the ulna in pronation. The head of the ulna translates along the sigmoid fossa and herniates out from under cover of tightening superficial dorsal TFC fibers, rendering these fibers relatively ineffective in controlling DRUJ mechanics.

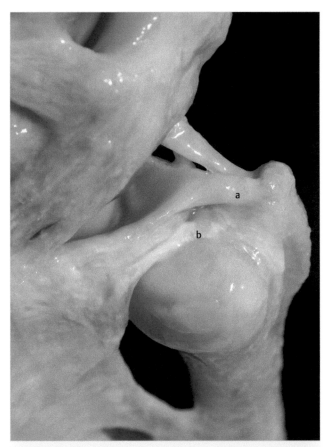

Fig. 25.14 Cadaver dissection of the distal radio-ulna relationship demonstrating the origin of *superficial*, vascularized peripheral fibers of the TFC originating from the ulna styloid (a), and *deep* fibers of the TFC (*Ligamentum subcruentum*) originating from the fovea, lateral to the base of the styloid.

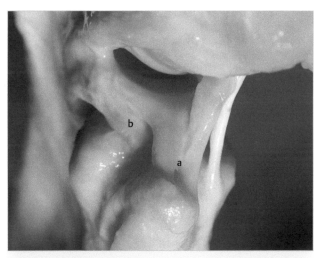

Fig. 25.15 Fibers of the *superficial* TFC insert on the medial radius at an acute angle (a); fibers of the *Ligamentum subcruentum* (deep TFC) insert at an obtuse angle (b).

2007[7] (▶Fig. 25.16, ▶Fig. 25.17, and Fig. 25.18), one begins to understand how the anatomy of the more obtuse fiber angle of the deep ligamentum subcruentum makes the volar and

dorsal deep TFC components much more mechanically effective as checkreins against hyper physiologic translation of the sigmoid fossa on the ulna seat. The radius/carpus/hand unit is analogous to the team of four horses, rotating and translating as they whip the trailing buckboard around behind it. If we think of the buckboard itself as the fixed ulna and of the rotating/translating radius as the team of four horses, the seated buckboard driver (representing the origins of the radio–ulna fibers of the TFC) has the best control of his team of horses though those reins that attach to the *outside* harnesses of the two outside horses. The driver's mechanical advantage for controlling the entire team is most effective when the reins are attached as widely apart as possible to the two outside horses. I have drawn these more mechanically advantageous reins in blue, since they mimic the more mechanically advantageous blue fibers of the ligamentum subcruentum (▶Fig. 25.18) in preventing super-physiologic rotation and translation of the radius sigmoid fossa off the ulna seat. The more lateral origin

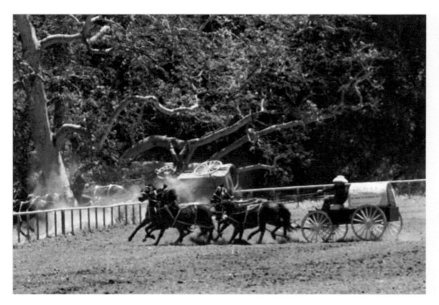

Fig. 25.16 Photo of a buckboard inserted for those readers not familiar with this means of transportation, not seen today in most urban environments. (Courtesy: Hill Hastings II, M.D.)

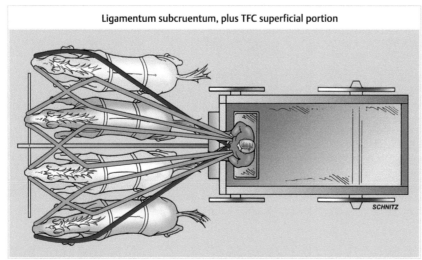

Ligamentum subcruentum, plus TFC superficial portion

Fig. 25.17 The narrower angle-of-attack of green reins on the central horses of the team makes them less effective in controlling the team. These acutely-angled central reins mimick the acute angle-of-attack of the less effective, green-colored fibers of the TFC (superficial, and originating from the ulna styloid).

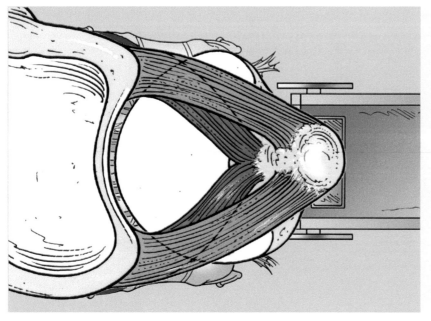

Fig. 25.18 Using the buckboard analogy, the more mechanically-advantageous, obtuse angle-of-attack of the *Ligamentum subcruentum* on the medial radius can be easily appreciated as the principle stabilizer of DRUJ rotation/translation.

of the ligamentum subcruentum from the ulna fovea establishes its obtuse angle of attack on the medial radius (dorsal and palmar). The ligamentum subcruentum, therefore, is a more mechanically advantageous stabilizer of the DRUJ than the superficial TFC fibers. ►Fig. 25.17 shows that even though the green reins that are attached to the two central horses of the team of four can be tightened by the buckboard driver, these reins (imitating the superficial fibers of the TFC) are less effective in controlling rotation and translation of the team because of their acute angle of attack on the two central horses. The analogy to the ineffectiveness of the angle of attack of the superficial fibers on the radius is clear (►Fig. 25.19). Adding to this the anatomic/biomechanical fact that in full supination or pronation < 10% of the articular surfaces of the ulna seat and

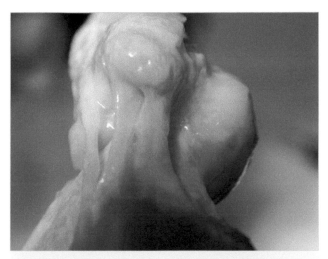

Fig. 25.19 Cadaver view of the *superficial fibers* of the TFC, originating from the ulna styloid. This dissection is viewed in a transverse orientation, looking distal to proximal. The acute angle-of-attack on the medial radius is clearly demonstrated.

sigmoid fossa are in contact with each other, with the ulna head herniating out from under cover of the superficial fibers of the TFC, we can now understand why the ligamentum subcruentum is the more crucial intrinsic stabilizer of DRUJ pronosupination (►Fig. 25.20 and ►Fig. 25.21).

In addition to the vascularized superficial fibers and the ligamentum subcruentum, the TFC complex itself consists of a central fibrocartilage articular disc, responsible for load transmission from the medial side of the carpus directly onto the pole of the distal ulna (►Fig. 25.9). The articular disc is nourished by synovial fluid washings; it contains essentially no blood supply, unlike the well-vascularized superficial and deep radioulnar ligaments that stabilize physiologic DRUJ rotation and translation.[8] The articular disc of the TFC does not participate in stabilizing the biomechanically sound two-bone forearm relationship through its pronosupination arc.

Additional components of the TFC that participate as stabilizers of the DRUJ are the two disccarpal ligaments. These ligaments arise along the **volar** margin of the radioulnar ligaments of the TFC already described in detail and insert as two distinct ligaments on the **volar** lunate and **volar** triquetrum. The origin of these secondary TFC stabilizers of the DRUJ was defined in two elegant independent embryological studies, by Garcia-Elias and Domenech-Mateu[9] and by Hogikyan and Louis.[10] These authors were able to demonstrate, by careful dissections and photomicrographs, that connective tissue (vascularized TFC tissue)—rather than the ulna bone itself—was the site of origin of these two important components of the TFC (►Fig. 25.22 and ►Fig. 25.23). The disc–carpal ligaments stabilize the volar medial carpus (lunate and triquetrum) to the volar ulna. Their orientation reduces the propensity for the radio–carpal unit to subluxate volarly off the seat of the ulna (i.e., functioning as checkreins to help prevent dorsal ulna subluxation/dislocation). The disc–carpal ligaments of the TFC should not be confused with the more superficial, thin, and vestigial ulnocarpal ligament

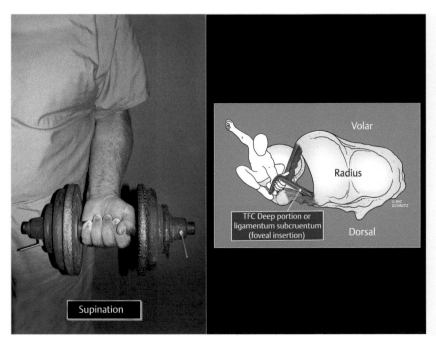

Supination

Fig. 25.20 The dorsal *Ligamentum subcruentum* is the principal stabilizer of the rotating/translating distal radius in full, loaded supination. While the volar *superficial fibers* also tighten, translation of the sigmoid fossa off the non-rotating ulna seat renders these fibers less effective than the *Ligamentum subcruentum* as stabilizing DRUJ check-reins (see text).

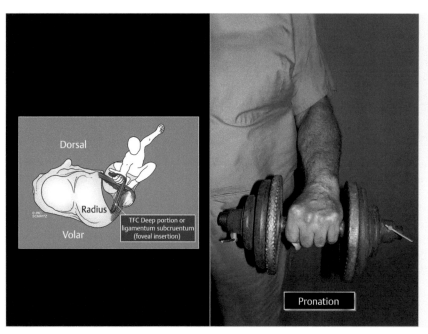

Fig. 25.21 In full pronation, the volar component of the *Ligamentum subcruentum* is the principal check-rein against super-physiologic translation of the sigmoid fossa on the ulna seat (see text). The dorsal superficial component also tightens, but is relatively ineffective as a check-rein because of the position of the distal ulna pole relative to the angle-of-attack of the superficial fibers on the medial radius.

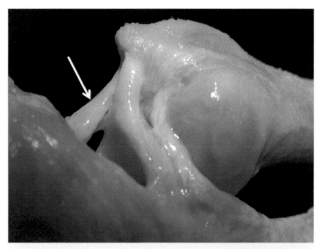

Fig. 25.22 The two disk-carpal ligaments (arrow) originate from the volar margin of the TFC (disk-lunate and disk-triquetral) and insert on the volar margin of the lunate and triquetrum, respectively. These ligaments are an important part of the TFC complex, and provide crucial support of the ulno-carpal relationship.

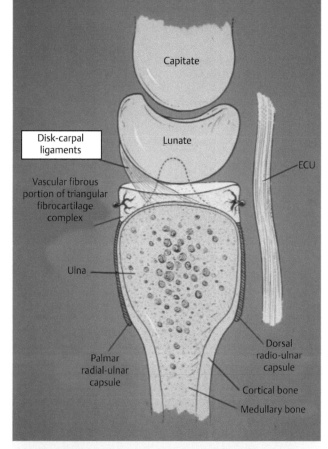

Fig. 25.23 Blood supply to the peripheral TFC enters from volar and dorsal, and penetrates ~40% of the antero-posterior dimension in adults (20% volar, 20% dorsal). It is because of this rich native vascularity along the important stabilizing components of the TFC that many direct reconstructive procedures in this area can heal well. Primary contributors to TFC peripheral circulation are the volar and dorsal branches of the anterior interosseous artery.

(ulnocapitate) (▶ Fig. 25.24), which has not been defined as contributing to DRUJ rotational stability.

Humans are bipedal animals. Our hands are usually working in front of us, with elbow flexion neutralizing the force of gravity on our hand–forearm unit. Most of our activities of daily living take place with our forearms in neutral rotation. ▶ Fig. 25.25 demonstrates this usual work attitude in X-ray form, showing how the ulna is hinged at the ginglymus ulnotrochlear joint only for flexion/extension, with the radius/carpus/hand unit sitting balanced on top of the ulna. Gravity pulls the unit (and whatever is in the hand) toward the floor. This anatomic arrangement establishes the ulna seat of the DRUJ as the fulcrum for forearm mechanics. In neutral forearm rotation, with the radius perfectly balanced atop the fixed, nonrotating ulna, all peripheral, vascularized radioulnar ligaments of the TFC are **lax**. Neutral rotation is the only position where both the superficial fibers and ligamentum subcruentum fibers of the TFC are not under tension; nor are they functioning as checkreins against super-physiologic rotation/translation of the forearm. As the forearm rotates either into supination or pronation, specific components of the TFC described above will tighten. But in neutral rotation, muscle tone of the forearm is enough to maintain balance without any static checkrein effect by the components of the TFC.

Applying elementary principles of physics, in equilibrium (static forearm in neutral, no rotation), the length from the hand to a DRUJ fulcrum, defined by the seat of the ulna (L), times the weight of the hand and anything held in it (F), establishes a *moment arm* distal to the DRUJ. In **equilibrium**, this *moment arm* must equal a proximal *moment arm,* defined by the length of the entire forearm from DRUJ to the elbow (L') times the restraining force of the annular ligament on the radial head (F') (▶Fig. 25.25). The load borne by the ulna seat is the joint reaction force (JRF) of the DRUJ, equaling the sum of the

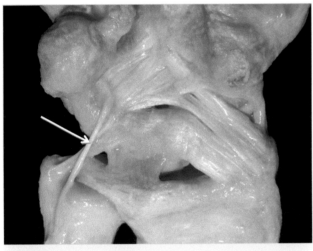

Fig. 25.24 Cadaver dissection clearly demonstrating all the volar support ligaments of the DRUJ and carpus. The arrow points to the ulno-carpal (ulno-capitate) ligament, superficial to the two crucial disk-carpal ligaments which attach the volar TFC to the lunate and triquetrum.

moments on both the distal and proximal sides of the ulna seat fulcrum. It is easy to appreciate from this model the enormity of load bearing potential at the DRUJ. The JRF can easily exceed multiple times body weight without any component of forearm rotation.

Remember that in neutral or zero rotation, the dorsal and volar radioulnar ligaments are lax. TFC laxity is *only* seen in this position. Once forearm rotation is initiated from the neutral position, some parts of the vascularized peripheral fibers of the TFC begin to tighten. Consider the tensile strength of the fibrous connective tissue required to maintain DRUJ stability in the extremes of supination and pronation. Elegant histological sections performed by Chidgey et al in 1991[11] demonstrate fibrocyte alignment of the connective tissues of the superficial and deep components of the vascularized periphery of the TFC. At the extremes of supination and pronation, where < 10% of the sigmoid fossa is in contact with the ulna seat, the radioulnar ligaments can be under tremendous load in stabilizing the DRUJ—particularly when the DRUJ JRF is high (▶Fig. 25.21 and ▶Fig. 25.22). Chidgey et al, in their cadaver TFC sections, showed at a cellular level the significance of orientation of connective tissue fibers in both the superficial and deep components of the TFC (i.e., the superficial dorsal and volar fibers, and the dorsal and volar ligamentum subcruentum). Cellular alignment is a requirement for maximizing load-bearing capacity of these checkrein ligaments. The cellular orientation physiologically favors the extraordinary demands for tensile strength in this tissue. Only with longitudinal fiber orientation in the radioulnar ligaments can they serve as effective checkreins against DRUJ instability. In supination under load (▶Fig. 25.20), and under conditions of static equilibrium (no rotational movement), the *moment arm* distal to the DRUJ must still equal the *moment arm* proximal to the DRUJ. This fact is defined by the physical state of equilibrium. In this position, the principal checkrein keeping the radius/carpus/hand unit from being pulled by gravity off the fixed, nonrotating ulna is the **dorsal** ligamentum subcruentum. In full pronation (▶Fig. 25.22), only the **volar** ligamentum subcruentum keeps the radius/carpus/hand unit from being pulled off the ulna seat by the gravitational force on the loaded hand. At the extremes of pronosupination, the superficial fibers of the vascularized periphery of the TFC are less critical than the deep components in preventing DRUJ instability and subluxation (▶Fig. 25.19).

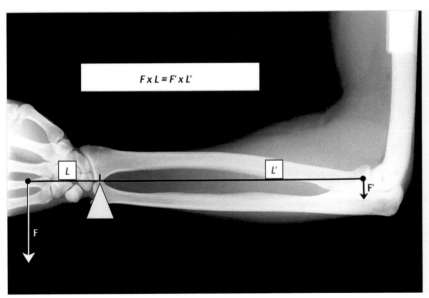

$$F \times L \equiv F' \times L'$$

Fig. 25.25 In equilibrium, the moments on the distal and proximal sides of the ulna seat fulcrum are - by physical definition - equal. Load in the hand (F) times the distance of this load from the ulna seat fulcrum (L) must equal the length of the forearm from the fulcrum to the elbow (L') times the resistance of displacement provided by the constraining annular ligament at the radial head (F').

The dorsal ligamentum subcruentum blocks super-physiologic translation of the DRUJ in supination; the volar ligamentum subcruentum prevents super-physiologic translation in pronation. The superficial radioulnar ligaments (cadaver dissection (▶Fig. 25.14, ▶Fig. 25.15, and ▶Fig. 25.19) participate in stabilizing the DRUJ by holding the two bones together at the articular surface, but the ligamentum subcruentum prevents radius translation of the notch beyond the final 10% contact area between articular surfaces at the extremes of supination and pronation.

DRUJ function anatomy is complex, but the intrinsic and extrinsic factors that provide stability of this diarthrodial joint through a physiologic arc of DRUJ pronosupination are even more complex. Health of all the components is critical in providing the human forearm with a full arc of painless, stable motion under load.

Suggested Reading

Ishii S, Palmer AK, Werner FW, Short WH, and Fortino MD. An Anatomic Study of the Ligamentous Structure of the Triangular Fibrocartilage Complex. J Hand Surg 1998; 23A:977–985

Kleinman WB. Stability of the Distal Radioulna Joint: Biomechanics, Pathophysiology, Physical Diagnosis, and Restoration of Function; What We Have Learned in 25 Years. Review Article—invited journal publication. J Hand Surg September 2007;32A(7):1086–1106

Kleinman WB. Stability Of The Distal Radio-Ulna Joint: Biomechanics, Pathophysiology, Physical Diagnosis, and Restoration of Function. In: Slutsky, Principles and Practice of Wrist Surgery; 2010, 5;41–58

Kleinman WB. Stability Of The Distal Radio-Ulna Joint. Slutsky and Osterman, Fractures and Injuries Of The Distal Radius and the Carpus: The Cutting Edge. Elsevier, 2009. Slutsky and Osterman. 25:261–274

Kleinman WB, Graham TJ. Distal ulnar injury and dysfunction. In: Peimer CA (ed). Surgery of the Hand and Upper Extremity. New York: McGraw-Hill, 1996, pp. 667–710

Kleinman WB. Distal Radius Instability and Stiffness: Common complications of Distal Radius Fractures - Hand Clinics May 2010: Vol:26 Number 2:245–264

Kleinman WB. Distal ulnar injury and dysfunction: part 1. Indiana Hand Center Newsletter 2(1): 7-17, 1995

Kleinman WB. Distal ulnar injury and dysfunction: part 2. Indiana Hand Center Newsletter 2(2):6-14, 1996

Kleinman WB. DRUJ contracture release. Techniques in Hand and Upper Extremity Surgery, 3(1):13-22, 1999

Kleinman WB. Distal Radio-Ulna Joint Capsulectomy for Post-Traumatic Limitation of Forearm Rotation.. Master Techniques in Orthopaedic Surgery: The Wrist 3rd Edition. Richard H. Gelberman, M.D. 2010. 36:411-428

References

1. Arimitsu S, Moritomo H, Kitamura T, et al. The Stabilizing Effect of the Distal Interosseous Membrane on the Distal Radioulnar Joint in an Ulnar Shortening Procedure: A Biomechanical Study. J Bone Joint Surg Am. 2011;93:2022–2030
2. Kitamura T, Moritomo H, Sayuri A, et al. The Biomechanical Effect of the Distal Interosseous Membrane on Distal Radioulnar Joint Stability: A Preliminary Anatomic Study. J Hand Surg. 2011;36A:1626–1630
3. Af Ekenstam F, Hagert CG. Anatomical studies on the geometry and stability of the distal radio ulnar joint. Scand J Plast Reconstr Surg 1985;19:17–25
4. Kleinman WB, Graham TJ. The distal radioulnar joint capsule: clinical anatomy and role in posttraumatic limitation of forearm rotation. J Hand Surg 23A:588–599, 1998
5. Schuind F, An KN, Berglund L, Rey R, Cooney WP, Linscheid RL, Chao EYS. The distal radioulnar ligaments: a biomechanical study. J Hand Surg 1991;16A:1106–1114
6. Hagert CG. Distal radius fracture and the distal radioulnar joint—anatomical considerations. Handchir Mikrochir Plast Chir 1994;26:22–26
7. Kleinman WB. Stability of the Distal Radioulna Joint: Biomechanics, Pathophysiology, Physical Diagnosis, and Restoration of Function; What We Have Learned in 25 Years. Review Article—invited journal publication. J Hand Surg. September 2007;32A(7):1086–1106
8. Bednar MS, Arnoczky SP, Weiland AJ. The microvasculature of the triangular fibrocartilage complex: its clinical significance. J Hand Surg 1991;16A:1101–1105
9. Garcia-Elias M and Domenech-mateu J. Anatomy of the ulnocarpal ligaments. Presentation at the 46th Annual Meeting of the American Society for Surgery of the Hand, 1991
10. Hogikyan JV, and Louis DS. Embryologic development and variations in the anatomy of the ulnocarpal ligament complex. J Hand Surg 1992:17A; 719–723
11. Chidgey LK, Dell PC, Bittar ES, Spanier SS. Histologic anatomy of the triangular fibrocartilage. J Hand Surg 1991;16A:1084–1100

26 Hand Fascia, Retinacula, and Microvacuoles

Duncan A. McGrouther, Jason K. F. Wong, and Jean-Claude Guimberteau

The term "fascia" has been applied to a large number of very different tissues within the human body and in particular to specialized connective tissue structures in the hand.

These range from organized ligamentous formations such as the longitudinal bands of the palmar fascia, whose aligned type I collagen fibers are visible to the naked eye as parallel silvery bundles or the loose packing tissues that surround all of the moving structures within the hand. In other parts of the body the terms "superficial" and "deep" fascia are often used but these have little application in the hand and fingers.

Fascia provides a number of important roles that can broadly be considered as providing either mechanical function or frictionless gliding motion. The fascial continuum can be considered as a fibrous skeleton or framework channelling and guiding the course of a variety of longitudinal anatomical components as they pass through the palm to the digits. The mechanical, that is *retinacular*, roles of individual fascial structures include transmission of loads, acting as anchors for the skin, binding together mobile structures thus restraining unwanted motion, tethering, or limiting motion. Overall Benjamin[1] has considered the role of fascia as optimizing the transfer of muscle force.

The most defined connective tissue structures, i.e., tendons and ligaments, are well known and named individually, but the more delicate connective tissue structures also have important functional roles. Furthermore, they have very different specializations on the palmar and dorsal surfaces. The palm is adapted for padding and anchorage whereas the dorsum is particularly developed for gliding. The terms "palmar fascia" or "palmar aponeurosis" deserve special mention as they have often been used clinically as a generic term for all fascia in the hand. These terms are best reserved for the well-developed planes of longitudinal and transverse ligamentous fibers in the central part of the palm (▶ Fig. 26.1). The longitudinal fibers represent the distal fascial bundles of palmaris longus when it is present (the fibers are present even when the muscle is absent).

These fibers, clinically known as "pretendinous", are arranged in bundles corresponding to the four digital rays; in addition, there is a variable bundle crossing the thenar eminence toward the radial side of the thumb. This structural arrangement was well known to early anatomists and surgeons (Albinus[2]; Weitbrecht[3]; Dupuytren[4]; many early works have been translated by Stack[5] in his book *The Palmar Fascia*).

The thin fascial coverings over the thenar and hypothenar muscles have sometimes been considered as lateral and medial parts of the palmar aponeurosis, but these are much thinner and more flexible than the central part. Much has been written about palmar spaces (Chapter 33), particularly in relation to the accumulation of pus in infections,[6] but there are many potential spaces and it is difficult to identify their margins when operating on sepsis.

The fascial structures of the hand are all in continuity; the term continuum is often applied, although certain individual components are well defined. Their structure can best be understood by considering their different functional roles.

26.1 Channelling of Structures in Transit Between Forearm and Digits

When visualized in cross-section, the hand comprises a series of compartments that channel tendons, nerves, and blood vessels. The separating longitudinal septa, illustrated in transverse section as a honeycomb structure by Bojsen-Møller and Schmidt[7] (▶ Fig. 26.2), act as spacers between the tendons and neurovascular bundles of the individual digital rays. Fascial septa between the flexor tendons in the palm were described by Legueu and Juvara[8] that seem to be quite filmy structures in the proximal palm and may be merged with the annular pulleys

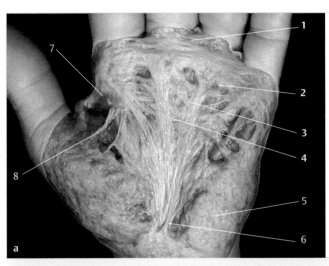
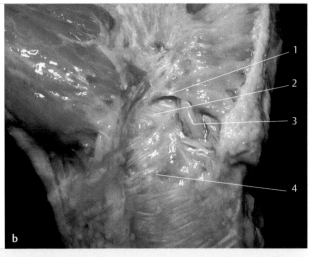

Fig. 26.1 (a) Palmar Fascial Ligaments. (1) Transverse fibres of natatory ligament (2) Distal palmar fat pad (3) Longitudinal fibres of palmar fascia (4) Transverse fibres of palmar aponeurosis (5) Hypothenar fat pad (6) Fibres in continuity with Palmaris Longus (7) Distal commissural ligament of first web space, part of natatory ligament system. (8) Proximal commissural ligament **(b)** Flexor retinaculum after removal of Palmaris Longus. (1) Proximal entry of Guyon's Canal which lies superficial to the Flexor retinaculum (2) Flexor retinaculum (3) Ulnar artery and nerve (4) Deep fascia of forearm

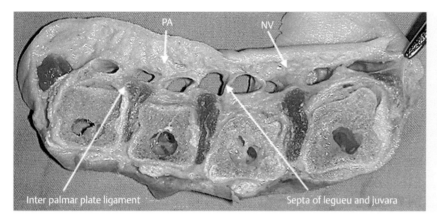

Fig. 26.2 Transverse section of palm at the level of the heads of the metacarpal bones. The flexor tendons, lumbrical muscles and interossei have been removed to show the 'honeycomb' structure of the palmar fascial continuum. PA: palmar aponeurosis. NV: neurovascular bundle overlying lumbrical compartment. (Dissection and Photograph Courtesy of Ghazi M. Rayan M.D.)

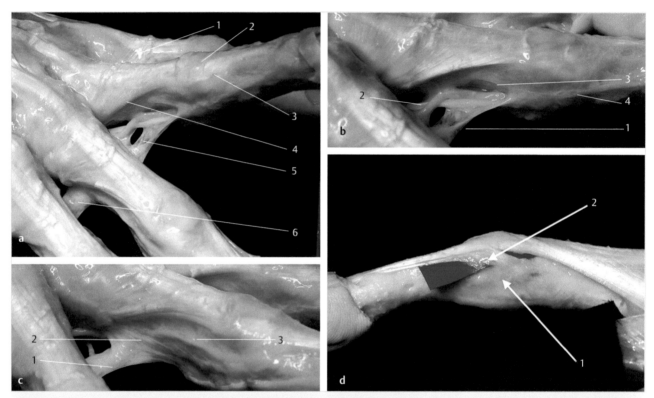

Fig. 26.3 Dorsum of web space showing the effect of different directions of tension on the lateral digital sheet of fascia. (**a**) Prominence of the distal continuation of the arcuate fibres of the natatory ligament 1) Transverse retinacular fibres at MPJ of little finger 2) Landsmeer's transverse retinacular ligament at PIP joint. The oblique retinacular ligament lies deep to this fascial plane 3) This line of tension in the fascia is probably the basis of descriptions of the retrovascular band or lateral digital sheet 4) Lateral tendon of extensor hood 5) Arcuate fibres of natatory ligament curving around web space 6) Transverse fibres of natatory ligament. (**b**) to show spiral cord 1) Arcuate fibres of natatory ligament 2) Digital nerve 3) Fibres extending distally from layer 2) of the longitudinal fibres of the palmar fascia pass to the web spaces either around the neurovascular bundle (**c,d**) or deep to it as shown here to join the lateral digital sheet. (**c**) Dorsum of web space to show retrovascular band 1) Arcuate fibres of natatory ligament 2) Lateral digital sheet 3) Spiral fibres from layer 2 of longitudinal fibres of palmar aponeurosis radiating towards lateral digital sheet. (**d**) Retinacular ligaments at the PIPjoint 1) Landsmeer's transverse retinacular ligament 2) Landsmeer's oblique retinacular ligament

of the flexor sheath distally. This is one of a number of areas where there are diferent interpretations of the fascial structure depending on the anatomical preparation and tissue dissection technique.

26.2 Restraint of Unwanted Motion

The channels are thickened and have a retinacular role, forming sheaths with specialized annular pulleys where tendons must change direction around a concave surface so as to prevent tendon springing away from the underlying skeleton. These pulleys allow

the direction of pull in a tendon to change as it rounds a corner, and in doing so the pulley must itself apply a considerable lateral load on the tendon. It must, therefore, have considerable strength and a system of lubrication to prevent frictional resistance to gliding. The pulley in such areas has a more cartilaginous matrix specialization and a different surface morphology. The flexor and extensor retinacula at the wrist have a similar function.

The term "retinaculum" (meaning that which retains or keeps in place) is not restricted to sheaths but is also used for various retaining ligaments of the extensor apparatus in the digits that keep it in place over convex surfaces (▶Fig. 26.3). In this instance, the retinacular ligaments form not pulleys but guy ropes, sufficiently long to allow the extensor apparatus to glide backward and forward.

26.3 Transmission of Loads

When compressive loading is applied to the hand, shock absorption is into the loculi of fat contained within defined fibrous boundaries in palm and digital pulp, such that the shape of each loculus can change when external pressure is applied but not its volume (▶ Fig. 26.1 and ▶ Fig. 26.4).

Thus, the compliance or deformability of the fascial boundaries between fat compartments determines the amount of shock absorption. The clinical term "turgor" is a measure of this anatomical property together with the vascular supply, since the local blood, and extracellular fluid, volume also has a major influence on tissue compliance. The palm septae has a shock absorber function in addition to the subcutaneous fat loculi, which is due to the larger honeycomb fibrous compartments between skin and skeleton described above (▶ Fig. 26.2). No plane of fascia, therefore, has a simple mechanical role; all are involved in distortion of the tissues but whether the tissue is compressed or pulled, the individual collagen bundles are placed under tensional strain; the different fiber orientations in the fascia reflect the various directional vectors of loading. The soft padded parts of the hand are able to conform to the contours of objects being grasped, allowing better interpretation of sensation and better grip.

On a macroscopic scale, the palm of the hand must resist not only compression but tensile loading. Tendons and ligaments are structures particularly suitable for resisting such forces but many parts of the fascial continuum also have a major function in resisting "pulling" forces such as the anchorage system of the palm.

26.4 Anchorage

Skin is retained by fascial ligaments in an ingenious system that allows the hand to flex while retaining the skin in position. The skin folds at palmar and digital creases but there are few deep anchoring fibers located exactly at the point of folding; it is the skin on either side of the crease lines that has the best developed deep anchorage ligaments, perpendicular to the plane of the palm, allowing the unanchored skin between to fold in a repetitive pattern; the palmar creases have been described as skin "joints" which are apparent from early stages of intrauterine development.

A particularly well-developed anchorage system is the insertion of the longitudinal (pretendinous) fibers of the palmar aponeurosis, which represents the distal continuation of palmaris longus. These fibers are well developed even when

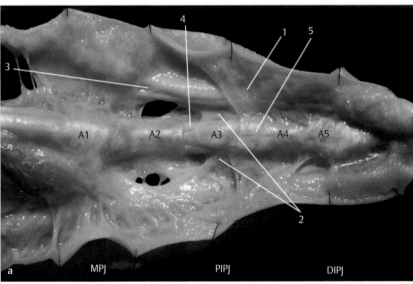

Fig. 26.4 (a) Palmar dissection of digit to show Cleland's and Grayson's ligaments.
(1) Grayson's ligament
(2) Cleland's ligaments – these fibers extending from PIP region to lateral digital sheet overlying the proximal phalanx
(3) Neurovascular bundle
(4) FDS
(5) FDP
(b) Diagram of the volar aspect of th efinger showing Grayson's and Cleland's ligaments and their relationship to the neurovascular bundles. (Copyright Kleinert Institute, Louisville, KY).
(1) Grayson's Ligament.
(2) Cleland's Ligaments.
(3) Neurovascular bundle.
(4) Longitudinal fibers of the palmar fascia.
(5) Transverse (Skoog) fibers of the palmar fascia.
(6) Natatory igament.

the tendon is absent, in which case the fibers may merge with other fascial systems in the region of the flexor retinaculum or receive an insertion from flexor carpi ulnaris.[9] This is the fiber system principally involved in Dupuytren's Contracture and knowledge of its detail will facilitate surgical dissection. There are three distal insertions which can be considered in layers (►Fig. 26.5). The most superficial longitudinal fibers insert into the dermis of the distal palm, distal to the distal palmar crease, rather than in to the creases per se. This arrangement resists horizontal shearing force in gripping tasks such as holding a golf club, in which it prevents distal skin slippage or degloving of the palm on striking the golf ball. The characteristic blisters on the palms of those unaccustomed to such sports map out the sites of the skin anchorage points. The readers can demonstrate this anchorage system on their own hand by flexing the palm until the skin of the distal palm folds loosely. This loose skin can then be pinched by the thumb and forefinger of the other hand. An attempt to pull the skin distally will reveal the anchoring longitudinal fibers of the palmar aponeurosis.

There are two deeper types of anchorage of the longitudinal fibers (►Fig. 26.5d). Layer 2 consists of fibers that bifurcate on either side of the A1 flexor tendon sheath pass underneath the superficial transverse metacarpal ligament (natatory ligament) and deep to the neurovascular bundles toward the digits. When this fascial system becomes involved in Dupuytren's Contracture, it forms a spiral cord as the encircled neurovascular bundle can be displaced, making it vulnerable to surgical injury. The deepest longitudinal fibers (layer 3) pass around the sides of the flexor sheath and metacarpophalangeal (MP) joint to merge with a number of ligamentous structures eventually reaching the retinacular fibers that retain the extensor apparatus over the MP joints (McGrouther 1990, Zancolli 1979). Thus, the longitudinal fibers of the palmar fascia have wide insertions into skin and fascia in the distal hand.

The skin anchorage sytem in the digits is more complex but the overall pattern is arranged to anchor the skin to the axis region of the interphalangeal (IP) joints thus preventing sliding (degloving) of the skin on digital flexion. Cleland's ligaments are oblique anchors which tether the skin of proximal and middle segments of the digits to the region of the proximal IP joints (►Fig. 26.4 and ►Fig. 26.6). There is a particularly well-developed band arising from fascial structures overlying the lateral aspect of the proximal interphalangeal (PIP) joint which then passes distally to reach the lateral digital subcutaneous region in the middle segment of the digit. It is not possible to define a point origin or insertion as there is a fascial continuum merging proximally with flexor sheath and continuous with fascia over the lateral band of the extensor tendon. Distally there is a loose network of lateral subcutaneous fascia, the lateral digital sheet, which can form bands in a number of directions depending on the direction of tension on this structure (►Fig. 26.3). This rather imprecise anatomy has led to a variety of different anatomical descriptions with some controversy as to whether certain structures exist as defined structures (such as the retrovascular band and lateral digital sheet) or merely

as tension lines in a three-dimensional (3D) network of fibers. Cleland's ligaments are however easily defined, and a second bundle passes proximally from the PIP joint region to the lateral skin area over the proximal segment of the digit (►Fig. 26.4). A similar pair of ligaments orientated proximally and distally radiates from the distal interphalangeal (DIP) joint region. Cleland's ligaments lie posterior to the neurovascular bundles, whereas Grayson's ligaments are skin-retaining ligaments anterior to the bundles (►Fig. 26.4).[12,13,14,15]

26.5 Binding Role

The deep transversely orientated fascial structures have a role in maintaining the transverse arch of the hand by "binding" the skeletal structures or the tendon sheaths. The flexor retinaculum is one of such structures and more distally the deep transverse metacarpal ligament (►Fig. 26.2), which runs from one MP joint volar plate to another thus crossing the hand.[3,11] The next more superficial layer is that of the transverse fibers of the palmar aponeurosis (►Fig. 26.5), clinically often termed as Skoog's fibers as he advised their retention in Dupuytren's fasciectomy operations. These lie immediately deep (posterior in anatomical terms) to the longitudinal fibers, and form tunnels over the neurovascular bundles and flexor tendons.[8,16] They have been considered to form part of the flexor tendon pulley system.[17] The most superficial transverse fibers lying just beneath the web skin (►Fig. 26.1) have the Nomina Anatomica designation "superficial transverse metacarpal ligaments," but the German description Schwimmband,[18] or natatory (swimming) ligament, better describes their position at the margins of the interdigital webs.

26.6 Limiting or Tethering Role

The natatory system has two components namely transverse fibers crossing the palm and arcuate fibers curving around the webs. They seem to reinforce the skin and limit web abduction. Joint motion is limited by ligamentous action, but also in some cases by skin tightness. In the interdigital webs, the skin is generally reinforced by fascial ligamentous fibers running just beneath the dermis and in a direction that resists the stretch (►Fig. 26.5c). They are well developed in the thumb web.[19]

Other structures that limit motion are joint capsules, and specific joint ligaments such as the checkrein ligaments at the PIP joints (►Fig. 26.7). The relative mechanical strength of such structures determines the pattern of injury. One example is forced separation of the thumb and index, usually due to a fall on the outstretched hand, from a rather less glamorous event than those mentioned in textbooks, skiing (USA) or gamekeepers thumb from wringing rabbit's necks (UK). The abducting force is resisted by the natatory ligament in the first web space (also termed distal commissural ligament; ►Fig. 26.1), the proximal commissural ligament (thenar continuation of the transverse fibers of the palmar aponeurosis), and last but not

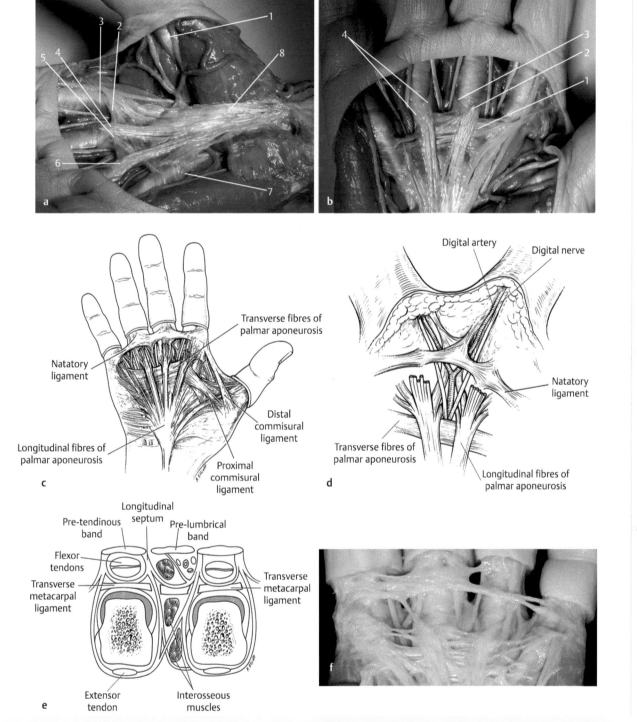

Fig. 26.5 (a) Longitudinal fibres of palmar fascia. (1) Flexor pollicis longus (2) Transverse fibers of the palmar aponeurosis (3) A1 pulley of flexor tendon sheath (4) Longitudinal (pretendinous) fibers of palmar fascia terminating in dermis distal to distal palmar crease (layer1) (5) Longitudinal fibers passing deeply on either side of flexor sheath and MPJ (layer3) (6) Longitudinal fibers passing deep to the neurovascular bundle forming a 'spiral band'. (It is in fact a thin filmy layer in the normal hand). It is this layer of fibers (layer2) which can contract in Dupuytren's Disease displacing the neurovascular bundle. (7) Deep septal fibres described by Legueu and Juvara (8) Longitudinal fibers of palmar fascia. (b) Three distal attachments of longitudinal fibers (1) Transverse fibers of palmar aponeurosis (2) Longitudinal fibers terminating in skin (layer1) (3) Longitudinal fibers passing deeply around MPJ's (layer3) (4) Longitudinal fibers bifurcating and passing distally deep to neurovascular bundles to reach the lateral digital sheet. (c) Plan of the longitudinal and transvers fibers of the palmar aponeurosis. (d) Detail of distal course of longitudinal fibers. (e) The deepest longitudinal fibers pass around the sides of the flexor sheaths and MP joints to reach the retinacular fibers which retain the extensor expansion over the MP joints. (f) Natatory ligaments and the relationship to the neurovascular bundles.

309

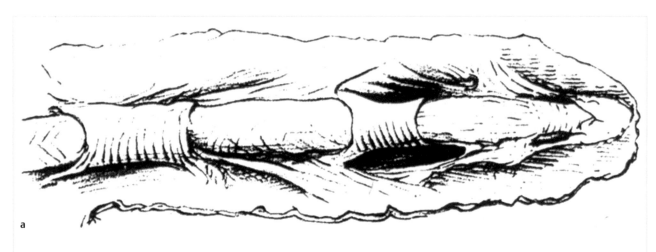

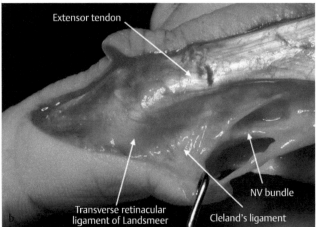

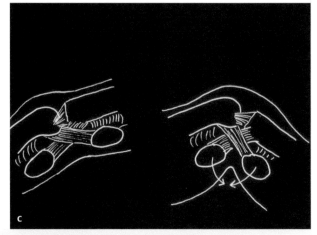

Fig. 26.6. Dynamic motion of Cleland's ligaments on PIPJ flexion (**a**) Cleland's original illustration of skin retaining ligaments. (**b**) Ligamentous structures at the PIP joint viewed from posteriorly with skin traction (1) Part of Landsmeer's transverse retinacular fibres (2) Cleland's ligaments passing from the PIP region to skin distally. (**c**) Diagrammatic representation of the different orientation of Cleland's ligaments on PIP flexion.

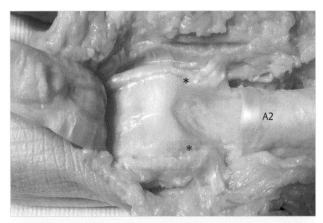

Fig. 26.7 Check Rein Ligaments inserting on the volar surface of the proximal phalanx inside the mouth of the A2 pulley (*).

26.7 Framework for Muscle Origins and Insertions

Many of the small muscles of the hand arise from the "fascial skeleton," at least in part (e.g., abductor pollicis brevis from the flexor retinaculum). Other muscles insert into it (palmaris longus). The fascial framework can therefore be visualized as a harness by which the muscles act on the underlying bony skeleton. For example, the MP joint is surrounded by a ring of fascial and ligamentous structures by which the joint is moved, there being no insertions of long flexor or extensor muscles into the proximal phalanx.

26.8 Vascular Protection and Pumping Action

The delicate blood vessels of the hand are protected from pressure by surrounding them with a cuff of tough fascia or a fatty pad. When the hand is compressed, as in gripping, the relatively incompressible fascial structures act as a venous pumping

least all of the collateral ligaments of all of the joints of thumb and index. The weakest point of this entire chain is the distal attachment of the ulnar collateral ligament of the thumb MP joint, as all hand surgeons know.

mechanism to assist return of blood from the limb.[20] On the dorsum, by contrast, there are large capacitance veins in gliding skin. The fascia around these veins is loose areolar tissue, which allows venous dilatation, an important component of thermoregulation.

26.9 Lubricating Role
26.9.1 The Microvacuolar System

It is important to understand how connective tissue sliding works, as many structures glide considerable distances under the surface of the skin. During finger flexion, the flexor tendons at the level of the palm move approximately 35 mm with little skin movement, and yet they retain their blood supply.[21,22] Traditionally, this motion has been largely attributed to loose areolar tissue, superficial fascia, or loose connective tissue without clear definition of the mechanism.[23] Mayer[24] described the different connective tissue layers surrounding tendon which are specialized into paratenon (outside sheaths), mesotenon (in sheaths), bursae, and specialized sheaths.

Mayer appreciated that mesotenon in tendon sheaths was an incomplete layer; there is gliding tissue on the posterior surface of flexor tendons in synovial sheaths but a fluid film on the anterior surface which is in contact with the pulley system.

Unlike the organized condensed fascia for force transmission, there is a different type of fascia, the "microvacuolar collagenous dynamic absorbing system (MCDAS)" or "microvacuolar system" for short, which provides lubrication and allows almost frictionless musculotendinous movement. From in vivo video microscopic examination of the flexor tendons, Guimberteau[25,26] has mapped the tendon sliding system in zones I to V. Single connective tissue strands are assembled into a 3D framework of what appear in two dimensions to be deformable polygonal

structures (▶ Fig. 26.8). Some of the fibers are adherent at crossing points while others are unattached and droplets of fluid adhering to the fibers may facilitate relative motion. In three dimensions these polyhedral structures surround actual or potential spaces, i.e., "microvacuoles." The microvacuolar system is assembled in to a dynamic 3D structure best described as a random fractal pattern rather than a geometric pattern. When dissecting a tissue plane with surgical retraction, the connective tissue strands become aligned disguising the normal microvacuolar arrangement.

The fibrils of the vacuoles provide a supporting framework for branching blood vessels which by their tortuous course through the microvacuolar system have sufficient length to allow the backward and forward gliding of tendon (▶ Fig. 26.9)

As the tendon slides longitudinally, the polyhedral shape of the microvacuoles renders them capable of multidirectional expansion, compression, and deformation in a fashion similar to a 3D wire frame model, and due to their elasticity, distraction of the fibers is also possible. These tiny dynamic structures are constantly changing shape and position on movement which, with each deformation, cause neighboring microvacuoles to change shape.

In the flexor tendon sheath, the flexor digitorum profundus (FDP) and flexor digitorum superficialis (FDS) are restricted in their excursion by joint movement and the vincular vessels have enough length to adjust to the full range of tendon excursion. In all zones, the sliding system has sufficient dynamic deformation and available vessel length to accommodate the necessary tendon excursion.

In zones I and II, the tendon is intrasynovial and passes through a specialized flexor tendon sheath with blood vessels lying within the dorsal vincula.[27] These vincula have different structures but all contain blood vessels which have two fixed points—one near the skeleton and the other on the

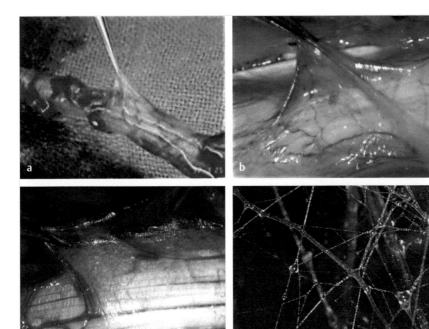

Fig. 26.8 Distraction of the microvascular system (**a**) Flexor carpi radialis vascular unit. (**b**) Radial distraction of the microvacuolar system showing vascular channels. (**c**) Radial distraction of the microvacuolar system showing microvacuoles. (**d**) Fibrous hydrated matrix showing polyhedral arrangement. (From J.C. Guimberteau, CL. Verdan, and H Kleinert: News ideas in hand flexor tendon surgery. The sliding system, vascularized island tendons transfers. Aquitaine Domaine Forestier 2001. 210p.)

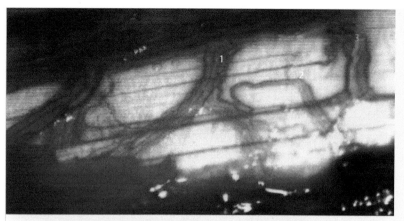
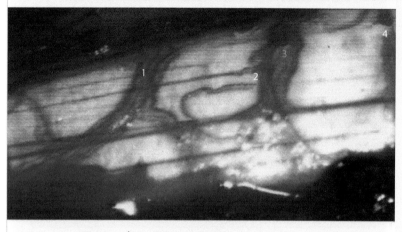
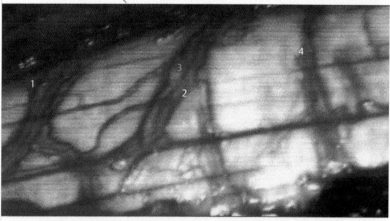
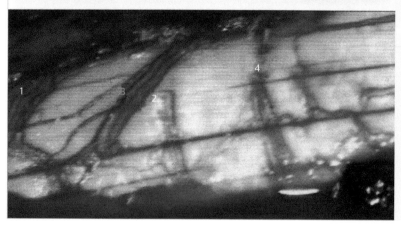

Fig. 26.9 The microvacuolar system over the flexor carpi radialis. Images show the tendon being pulled into flexion with time lapse images every 2 seconds between frames. Transverse vascular channels have been numbered 1, 2, 3, and 4 for ease of identification and tracking. Note how the sliding layers slide at different rates during flexion indicating different deformation. (From J.C. Guimberteau, CL. Verdan, and H Kleinert: News ideas in hand flexor tendon surgery. The sliding system, vascularized island tendons transfers. Aquitaine Domaine Forestier 2001. 210p.)

tendon surface. These vessels move to and fro, like a windscreen wiper, as the tendon slides proximally or distally. The blood vessels enter the dorsum of the flexor digitorum tendons and there is no microvacuolar system on the palmar surface (▶Fig. 26.10).

In zone III and also in zone V, the extrasynovial flexor tendons have a sliding system arrangement with fibers forming multiple microvacuoles between the tendon and surrounding structures. The fibers form random polyhedral compartments, with branching fibers and longitudinal fibers running from tendon to the periphery. The tendon surface is connected by the microvacuolar system to the surrounding tissues. The microvacuolar system in extrasynovial tendon was what Mayer[24] described as "paratenon" (▶Fig. 26.11).

In zone IV, the flexor tendons are connected to one another by a microvacuolar sliding system. Within the carpal tunnel there are only a few loose filmy attachments dorsally and the

tendons have no connections with the flexor retinaculum. A multitude of small blood vessels lie within the dorsal filmy attachments and enter the tendons dorsally (▶Fig. 26.12).

In extrasynovial zones, the ultrastructural appearance of the tendon surface shows multiple collagenous strands from the microvacuolar system connected to the tendon surface. The microvacuolar system appears as a series of polyhedral microvacuoles with highly variable shapes and sizes.[28] It contains high levels of proteoglycan (70%) only 23% type I and III collagen with some type IV and V collagen, and 4% lipid. In comparison, tendon and deep fascia is composed of 60% type I collagen with some type III and V collagen. Only 0.5 to 3.5% of tendon is proteoglycan.[29]

A basic 3D model demonstrates how the skin is in continuity with the underlying tendon through the microvacuolar system (▶Fig. 26.13). The forward and backward excursion of the modeled system demonstrates how the underlying

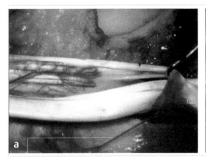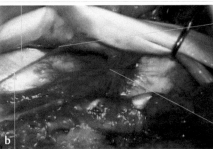

Fig. 26.10 Flexor tendons in Zone II. **(a)** Many dorsal blood vessels seen entering the FDS tendon (arrow). **(b)** On retraction the vinculum brevis (right arrow) and vinculum longum (left arrow) enter the tendon. There is no blood supply or sliding system on the palmar surface. (From J.C. Guimberteau, CL. Verdan, and H Kleinert: News ideas in hand flexor tendon surgery. The sliding system, vascularized island tendons transfers. Aquitaine Domaine Forestier 2001. 210p.)

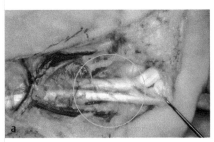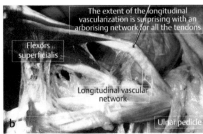

Fig. 26.11 Typical microvacuolar system arrangement. **(a)** Start of sliding system at the A1 pulley at the border between Zone II and III. Microvacuolar system and associated vasculature seen around the tendon. **(b)** Zone V proximal to the carpal tunnel. Multiple collagenous interconnections between the tendons of FDS and FDP housing blood vessels, typical of type 1 microvacuolar system. (From J.C. Guimberteau, CL. Verdan, and H Kleinert: News ideas in hand flexor tendon surgery. The sliding system, vascularized island tendons transfers. Aquitaine Domaine Forestier 2001. 210p.)

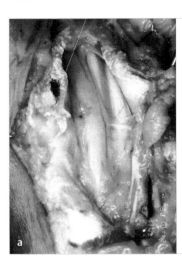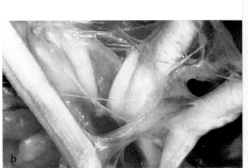

Fig. 26.12 Microvacuolar system in the carpal tunnel. **(a)** The FDS and FDP tendons glide with no collagenous connections with the palmar aspect of the tunnel shown with the carpal ligament removed (CL). **(b)** The FDS and FDP tendons are interconnected by the microvacuolar system within the tunnel. (From J.C. Guimberteau, CL. Verdan, and H Kleinert: News ideas in hand flexor tendon surgery. The sliding system, vascularized island tendons transfers. Aquitaine Domaine Forestier 2001. 210p.)

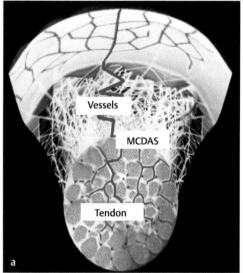
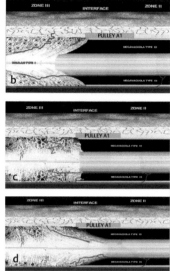

Fig. 26.13 Three-dimensional model of continuity. (**a**) Between the skin and tendon provided by the sliding system which is also able to sustain independent movement. (**b**) At the level of the Zone II/ Zone III interface as the tendon flexes, the microvacuolar system deforms producing the cul de sac. (**c**) In a relaxed state the interface conforms. (**d**) As the tendon is extended the microvacuolar system deforms. In all positions of tendon excursion the skin moves slightly. (From J.C. Guimberteau, CL. Verdan, and H Kleinert: News ideas in hand flexor tendon surgery. The sliding system, vascularized island tendons transfers. Aquitaine Domaine Forestier 2001. 210p.)

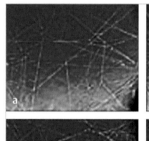
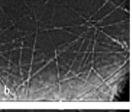
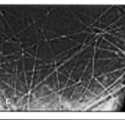
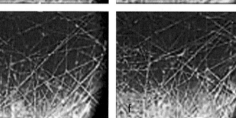

Fig. 26.14 (a–f) Deformation of the microvacuolar system during flexor tendon motion. Computer modeling sequences of polyhedral framework deforming. Note fibres splitting, deforming and reforming, a feature made possible by fibrous composition and fluid cohesion. (From J.C. Guimberteau, CL. Verdan, and H Kleinert: News ideas in hand flexor tendon surgery. The sliding system, vascularized island tendons transfers. Aquitaine Domaine Forestier 2001. 210p.)

tendon moves without causing any deformation of the overlying skin. This arrangement and its surrounding interactions reach an interface at the A1 pulley with the flexor sheath arrangement. Proximally, its arrangement changes within the carpal tunnel. In addition to the fibers deforming, contracting, and expanding, the fibers split and reform (▶Fig. 26.14). It is possible to define five types of sliding system arrangements. These are as follows:

- Type 1: typical microvacuolar system with a deformable matrix surrounding the tendon and blood vessels (▶Fig. 26.15a).
- Type 2: typical microvacuolar system with one surface adjacent to a synovial filled space, for example, next to a bursa (▶Fig. 26.15b).
- Type 3: specialized synovial sheath with specialized dominant vincular blood supply (▶Fig. 26.15c).
- Type 4: absent microvacuolar system with only intratendinous blood supply (▶Fig. 26.15d).
- Type 5: a mixture of type 1 and type 3, for example, within the carpal tunnel where the tendons are interconnected by a type 1 arrangement but the tendons as a unit are surrounded by a specialized sheath with a dorsal blood supply (▶Fig. 26.15e).

Based on this classification, the flexor zones of the hand can be simplified into:
- Zone I/II with a type 3 microvacuolar system, part of zone II has a type 4 circulation.
- Zone III/V with a type 1 microvacuolar system.
- Zone IV with a type 5 microvacuolar system.

Overall, the sliding system is a space filled with a filmy vascularized collagenous network that connects the dermal tissues and tendon/dense fascia/muscle, but allows them to function independently.

The microvacuoles help the tissues to withstand compression and expansion, and form and reform due to the chaotic fiber arrangement and the hydrophilic extracellular matrix. Cells within these tissues are also interconnected and form a body-wide organ, sensing deformations of these tissues.[30,31]

Ultrasound and cadaveric studies have shown that three levels of sliding tissue separated by a fine membrane exist in many body sites.[28] The most superficial of these layers has the greatest fat content while the intermediate layer harbors the large veins and nerves. The deepest of the layers has the greatest degree of glide and may be connected to tendons or deep fascia. This can be demonstrated by observing the dorsum of the hand where finger flexion allows the translation of the extensor tendons under the veins and skin, and pinching of the skin leaves the position of the veins and tendon unaltered.[32]

The microvacuolar system explains the way in which different interconnected layers move differentially. The high proteoglycan content explains its unique gliding characteristics and also explains why it can only be reliably demonstrated in living or fresh tissues. Proteoglycans and their subcompositions of glycoaminoglycans (GAG) are strongly negatively charged,[33] and hence are capable of drawing in water molecules.[34]

The high GAG content with its viscoelastic properties behaves like a gel, allowing tissue distortion. Dehydration makes this network difficult to assess in the laboratory; however, mathematical computer models allow its function to be understood.[35] The microvacuolar system provides lubrication, absorbs shear stresses, contains water, and houses blood vessels, nerves, and lymphatics. It fills the spaces or potential spaces between defined structures and enables vascular continuity between tissues. This arrangement is found wherever movement of adjacent tissues against each other is needed. In hand surgery, understanding and using the vascular territories of the microvacuolar system has been valuable in restoring function in heavily scarred fingers.[25] When this sliding system is removed, for example, in cases where the radial forearm flap is harvested and the donor defect skin grafted, cosmetic and functional results are poor.[36] As it forms the gliding tissue between the dense fascial structures of the hand, edema and fibrosis within this tissue will cause stiffness and contracture of digits. Loss of tissue turgor in aging, although associated with loss of elastic tissue, may also be related to changes in the microvacuolar system. Indeed, volumetric rejuvenation of the dorsum of the hand focuses on the restoration of fat in these atrophied areas.[37] The adipofascial cross finger flap and the fascial flap are surgical examples of the microvacuolar system being used to reconstruct defects.

26.9.2 Flexor Tendon Sheaths

The fibrous sheaths of the flexor tendons are specialized parts of the palmar fascial continuum. Each finger has an osseoaponeurotic tunnel extending from midpalm to the distal phalanx, and there is a tunnel for flexor pollicis longus from the metacarpal to distal phalanx. The proximal border is to some extent a matter of definition, as the transverse fibers of the palmar aponeurosis may be considered to be a part of the pulley system. The structure of the sheath will be described elsewhere but consists basically of arcuate fibers arching anteriorly over the tendons where the sheath is required to be stiff, overlying bone or at the centres of joints, where a bucket-handle of arcuate fibers is a mechanically favorable arrangement. In contrast, at places where the sheath is required to fold to permit joint flexion, there is an arrangement of cruciate fibers supporting a thin synovial membrane to provide a sealed lubrication system containing synovial fluid. There is a filmy outer covering of fascia overlying the sheath permitting frictionless gliding between the sheath and surrounding structures on digital flexion. A tubular filmy fascial layer proximal to the A1 pulleys in

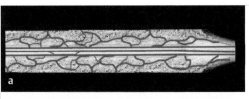

▶ **Type I**
Typical sliding system with MCDAS surrounding the tendon in zones without exterior stress. Zones III-V.

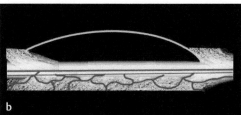

▶ **Type II**
Sliding system under stress
MCDAS involves a MEGAVACUOLA but is conserved with blood supply in preserved areas
FS IV and V[th] in zone IV

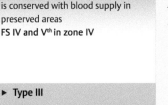

▶ **Type III**
MCDAS has almost completely evolved in a MEGAVACUOLA conserving only vincula for blood supply.
Zones I and III
Flexor pollicis longus

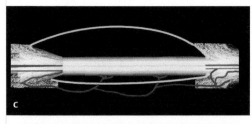

▶ **Type IV**
Last step
MCDAS is completely transformed in a MEGAVACUOLA with different and more convenient physical arrangement
Extensor pollicis longus

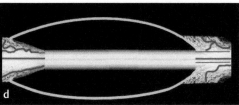

Fig. 26.15 Classification of microvacuolar systems in the hand. (**a**) Type 1—typical microvacuolar sliding system. (**b**) Type 2—typical microvacuolar sliding system with one surface opposed to a synovial environment. (**c**) Type 3 synovial environment with contribution from specialized blood supply. (**d**) Type 4—synovial environment with purely intratendinous blood supply. (From J.C. Guimberteau, CL. Verdan, and H Kleinert: News ideas in hand flexor tendon surgery. The sliding system, vascularized island tendons transfers. Aquitaine Domaine Forestier 2001. 210p.)

(Continued)

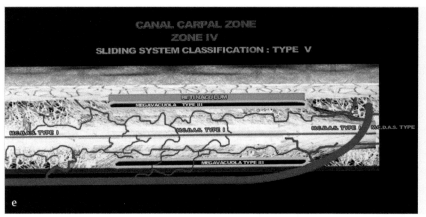

Fig. 26.15 (*Continued*) (**e**) Type 5—combination of both Type I and Type III. (From J.C. Guimberteau, CL. Verdan, and H Kleinert: News ideas in hand flexor tendon surgery. The sliding system, vascularized island tendons transfers. Aquitaine Domaine Forestier 2001. 210p.)

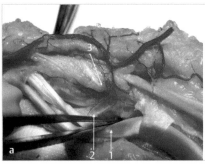

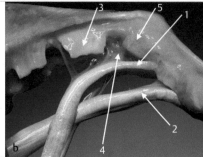

Fig. 26.16 Vinculum brevium at PIP joint. (**a**) Fascial cone of vinculum at neck of proximal phalanx covering over check rein ligaments and in continuity with Cleland's ligaments (1) FDS retracted (2) Short vinculum (3) Cleland's ligament (**b**) Vincula brevia and its relation to the FDS at the PIP joint level. (1) FDS (2) FDP (3) A2 pulley (4) vincula brevia (5) PIP joint.

index, middle, and ring fingers reflects on to the tendon surfaces providing a watertight seal for the intrasynovial fluid film The little finger has a continuity with the flexor sheath in front of the wrist. The thumb has a similar arrangement. The parietal synovial membrane is reflected onto the surface of the flexor tendon, forming a visceral synovium. This "membrane" appears to be a microvacuolar system posteriorly but on the anterior surface of the flexor tendon where it is pressed upon by the pulleys or in the FDS area where FDS grips the FDP (▶ Fig. 26.10),[38] the surface of the tendons appears to be a monolayer of specialized cells. Considerable uncertainties remain about the cell biology of the various "synovial" cell populations within the flexor tendon sheaths.

The A2 arcuate pulley overlies the middle third of the proximal phalanx and is the strongest pulley. Its distal edge is well developed and in sagittal cross-section it is seen that there is a pouch or recess of synovium superficial to the free edge of the pulley fibers so that the free edge forms a lip protruding into the synovial space.[39,40] During flexion, the cruciate fibers become orientated more transversely in the digits and the edges of adjacent annular pulleys approximate to form, in full flexion, a continuous tunnel of transversely orientated fibers.

The phenomenon of tendon gliding within a fibrous sheath requires a very specialized arrangement of vascular supply. Folds of synovial membrane, containing a loose plexus of fascial fibers, carry blood vessels to the tendons at certain defined points. These folds, termed vincula tendinum (singular: vinculum tendinum, plural vincula) are of two kinds. Vincula brevia (singular: vinculum brevium), of which there are two in each finger, are attached to the deep surfaces of the tendons near to their insertions. There is thus one vinculum brevium

attaching FDP to the region of the DIP joint, and a more proximal vinculum deep to FDS at the PIP joint (▶ Fig. 26.16). These short vincula are more than just blood vessels, they are cones of connective tissue which are deformable fascial microvacuolar systems. The short vinculum at the PIP joint arises at the neck of the proximal phalanx forming a cone between the checkrein ligaments (▶ Fig. 26.16). The vincula longa are filiform, and usually two are attached to each superficial tendon, one to each deep tendon. These long vincula are little more than blood vessels with a thickened adventitia.[41,42]

The extensor apparatus in the digit has a microvacuolar system on both deep and superficial aspects with a number of retinacula in addition (▶ Fig. 26.3) and vertical skin anchors maintaining the dorsal skin wrinkle pattern.[43] There is fairly general agreement about a transverse system of fibers, usually attributed to Landsmeer,[44] at the PIP joint level helping to locate the extensor apparatus over the joint, yet allowing lateral movement of the lateral slips of the extensor tendon (▶ Fig. 26.3d). What is more controversial is the oblique retinacular ligament of Landsmeer, which is difficult to dissect as a true ligament and it may be largely a tension band in a 3D fascial continuum extending from the A2 flexor sheath region at its proximal end to merge distally with the lateral slip of the extensor apparatus (▶ Fig. 26.3d). It is easier to demonstrate the function of this tissue in the living hand (DIP flexion is limited when the PIP joint is held in extension, but as the PIP joint flexes this allows both IP joints to flex simultaneously) than its actual origin and insertion on anatomical dissection. As there is only a limited amount of excursion of the extensor apparatus,[11] it is particularly vulnerable to adhesion following trauma, a pathological process still not understood.

References

1. Benjamin M. The fascia of the limbs and back – a review. J Anat. 2009; 214:1–18

2. Albinus B.S. Historia Musculorum Hominis. Leidae Batavorum. Bibliotheque Chirurg, Paris; 1734

3. Weitbrecht I. Syndesmologia sive Historia Ligamentorum. Corpoaris Humani Petropoli. Faculte de Medicine de Paris; 1742

4. Dupuytren G. De la retraction des doigts par suite d'une affection de l'aponeurose palmaire. Journal universel et Hebdomadaire de medicine et de chirurgie practiques de des institutions medicales. 1831; 25.5.349–365

5. Stack H.G. The palmar fascia. London, Churchill Livingstone; 1973

6. Kanavel A.B. Infections of the hand. London, Bailliere Tindall and Cox; 1925

7. Bojsen-Moller F., Schmidt L. The palmar aponeurosis and the central spaces of the hand. J Anat. 1974;117:55–68

8. Legeu F., Juvara E. Des aponeuroses de la paume de la main. Bull Soc anat de Paris. 1892;6:383–400

9. Fahrer M. The proximal end of the palmar aponeurosis. The Hand. 1980;12:33–38

10. McGrouther D.A. The palm. In McFarlane R.M., McGrouther D.A., Flint M.H (eds). Dupytren's Disease. Vol 5, Edinburgh, London, Melbourne, New York; Churchill Livingstone; 1990:127–135

11. Zancolli E.A., Structural and dynamic of bases of hand surgery. Philadelphia and Toronto, Lippincott; 1979

12. Cleland J. On the cutaneous ligaments of the phalanges. JAnat and Physiol. 1878;12:526–7

13. Grayson M. The cutaneous ligaments of the digits. J Anatomy. 1941;75:164-165

14. Milford L.W. Retaining ligaments of the digits of the hand. Philadelphia, Saunders; 1968

15. McFarlane R.M. Pattern of the diseased fascia in the fingers in Dupytren's contracture. Plastic and Reconstructive Surgery. 1974; 54:31–43

16. Skoog T. The transverse elements of the palmar aponeurosis in Dupytren's contracture. Scand J Plast Reconstr Surg. 1967; 1:51

17. Manske P.R., Lesker P.A. Palmar aponeurosis pulley. Journal of Hand Surgery. 1983;8:259–263

18. Grapow G. Die Anatomie und Physiologische Bedeutung der Palmaraponeurose. Archiv für Anatomie und Physiologie. Anat Abt. 1887; 143:2–3

19. De Frenne H. A. Les structures aponeurotiques au niveau de la premiere commissure. Annales de Chirurgie. 1977;31:1017–1019

20. Simons P., Coleridge Smith P., Lees W.R., McGrouther D.A. Venous pumps of the hand. J Hand Surg Br. 1996; 21(5):595–9

21. McGrouther D.A., Ahmed M.R. Flexor tendon excursions in 'no-man's land'. Hand. 1981;13:129–41

22. Wehbe M.A., Hunter J.M. Flexor tendon gliding in the hand. Part I. In vivo excursions. J Hand Surg Am. 1985;10:570–74

23. Ragan C. The physiology of the connective tissue (loose areolar). Annu Rev Physiol. 1952;14:51–72

24. Mayer L. The physiological method of tendon transplantation. Surg Gynecol Obstet. 1916;22:182–97

25. Guimberteau J.C., Panconi B., Boileau R. Mesovascularized island flexor tendon: new concepts and techniques for flexor tendon salvage surgery. Plast Reconstr Surg. 1993;92:888–903

26. Guimberteau J.C., Sentucq-Rigall J., Panconi B., Boileau R., Mouton P., Bakhach J. Introduction to the knowledge of subcutaneous sliding system in humans. Ann Chir Plast Esthet. 2005:50(1):19–34

27. Ochiai N., Matsui T., Miyaji N., et al. Vascular anatomy of flexor tendons. I. Vincular system and blood supply of the profundus tendon in the digital sheath. J Hand Surg Am. 1979;4:321–30

28. bu-Hijleh M.F., Roshier A.L., Al-Shboul Q., et al. The membranous layer of superficial fascia: evidence for its widespread distribution in the body. Surg Radiol Anat. 2006; 28:606–19

29. Wang J.H. Mechanobiology of tendon. J Biomech. 2006; 39: 1563–82

30. Ingber D.E. Tensegrity: the architectural basis of cellular mechanotransduction. Annu Rev Physiol. 1997;59:575–99

31. Langevin H.M., Cornbrooks C.J., Taatjes D.J. Fibroblasts form a body-wide cellular network. Histochem Cell Biol. 2004;122:7–15

32. Bidic S.M., Hatef D.A, Rohrich R.J. Dorsal hand anatomy relevant to volumetric rejuvenation. Plast Reconstr Surg. 2010;126(1):163–8

33. Yanagishita M. Function of proteoglycans in the extracellular matrix. Acta Pathol Jpn. 1993:43:283–93

34. Stern R., Maibach H.I. Hyaluronan in skin: aspects of aging and its pharmacologic modulation. Clin Dermatol. 2008;26:106–22

35. Chaudhry H., Schleip R., Ji Z., et al. Three-dimensional mathematical model for deformation of human fasciae in manual therapy. J Am Osteopath Assoc. 2008;108:379–90

36. Wong C.H, Lin J.Y, Wei F.C. The bottom-up approach to the suprafascial harvest of the radial forearm flap. Am J Surg. 2008; 196:e60–4

37. Coleman S.R. Hand rejuvenation with structural fat grafting. Plast Reconstr Surg. 2002;110:1731–44

38. Wahlbeehm E.T., McGrouther D.A., An anatomical study of the mechanical interactions of flexor digitorum superficialis and profoundus and the flexor tendon sheath in zone 2. J Hand Surg Br. 1995;20:269–80

39. Lundborg G., Myrhage R. The vascularization and structure of the human digital tendon sheath as related to flexor tendon function. An angiographic and histological study. Scand J Plast Reconstr Surg. 1977;11:195–203.

40. Jones M.M., Amis A.A. The fibrous flexor sheaths of the fingers. J Anat. 1988;156:185–96

41. Leffert R.D., Weiss C. Athanasoulis C.A. The vincula; with particular reference to their vessels and nerves. J Bone Joint Surg A. 1974: 56: 1191–8

42. Armenta E, Fisher J. Anatomy of flexor pollicis longus vinculum system. J Hand Surg Am. 1984; 9:210–2.

43. Law P., McGrouther D.A. The dorsal wrinkle ligaments of the proximal interphalangeal joint. J Hand Surg Br. 1984;9:271–5

44. Landsmeer J.M. The anatomy of the dorsal aponeurosis of the human finger and its functional significance. Anat Rec. 1949; 104:31–44

27 Thumb

Russell A. Shatford, Antony Hazel, and James M. Kleinert

27.1 Osteology

The skeleton of the radial side of the hand includes the trapezium, first metacarpal, and two phalanges—the proximal phalanx and the distal phalanx (▶Fig. 27.1). The thumb carpometacarpal (CMC) joint has very little inherent bony stability and relies on a complex network of ligaments. The thumb CMC joint is a complex joint, capable of perpendicular motions of flexion–extension, abduction–adduction, and rotation. For the complete description of the thumb CMC joint, please see Chapter 34 that is specifically devoted to this joint.

The thumb metacarpophalangeal (MCP) joint (▶Fig. 27.2) is considered a condyloid joint though the condyles of the first metacarpal are less spherical than the other metacarpals. This less spherical shape limits lateral movement. The MCP joint is capable of flexion–extension, abduction–adduction, and rotation. Flexion ranges from 5 to 100°, with 53° being average. The radial condyle projects slightly more than the ulnar condyle, which results in pronation with flexion.[1]

The proper and accessory collateral ligaments[2] of the MCP originate from the metacarpal head (▶Fig. 27.2). The ulnar collateral ligament (UCL) originates on the first metacarpal, approximately 4.2 mm from the dorsal surface, 5.3 mm from the articular surface, and 7 mm from the volar surface. The proper UCL inserts on the base of the proximal phalanx, approximately 9.2 mm from the dorsal surface, 3.4 mm from the articular surface, and 2.8 mm from the volar surface. The UCL is also joined by the insertion of the adductor pollicis (AP) (▶Fig. 27.3). The UCL is critical in stabilizing key pinch (▶Fig. 27.4a, b). The radial collateral ligament (RCL) originates on the metacarpal head, approximately 3.5 mm from the dorsal surface, 3.3 mm from the articular surface, and 8.1 mm from the volar surface, while the insertion of the proper RCL is 7.2 mm from the dorsal surface, 2.6 mm from the articular surface, and 2.8 mm from the volar surface (▶Fig. 27.5a, b).[3] The RCL is joined by the abductor pollicis brevis (APB) muscle at its insertion. The accessory collateral ligaments insert into the volar plate (▶Fig. 27.6).[4] The volar plate resists MCP joint hyperextension, originating at the

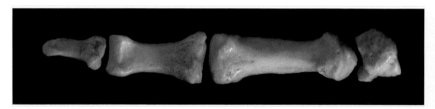

Fig. 27.1 Thumb osteology. Volar view of right thumb. From *right* to *left* the bones are as follows: trapezium, first metacarpal, proximal phalanx, and distal phalanx. The groove in the trapezium that accommodates the flexor carpi radialis can be seen at the *bottom right* of the photograph.

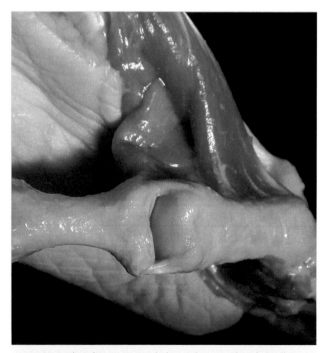

Fig. 27.2 Thumb metacarpophalangeal joint with radial collateral ligament (*bottom*) and ulnar collateral ligament (*top*).

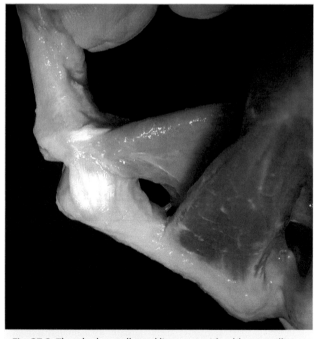

Fig. 27.3 Thumb ulnar collateral ligament with adductor pollicis insertion. The adductor pollicis is inserting into the ulnar collateral ligament. The first dorsal interosseous muscle lateral head is originating from the first metacarpal.

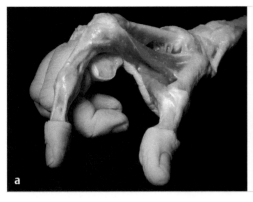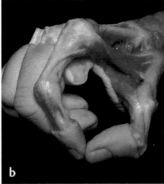

Fig. 27.4 The relationship between thumb and index finger during pinch. (**a**) In this figure the thumb and index finger interphalangeal joints are fully extended. The first dorsal interosseous muscle is dorsal to the adductor pollicis. (**b**) Here, the interphalangeal joints are flexed. In pinch, the first dorsal interosseous and adductor pollicis are contracted.

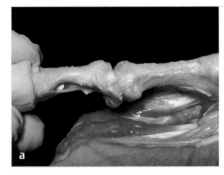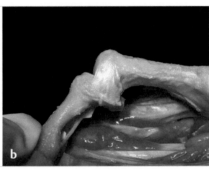

Fig. 27.5 Radial collateral ligament of the thumb metacarpophalangeal joint in extension (**a**) and flexion (**b**).

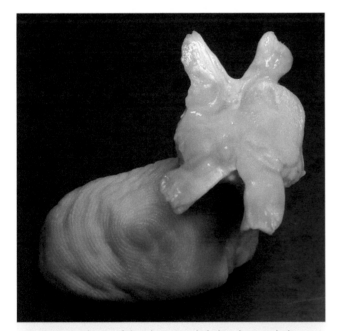

Fig. 27.6 Axial view of thumb proximal phalanx base with the volar plate to the left of the joint. The proper collateral ligaments can be seen inserting into the proximal phalanx base, while the accessory collateral ligaments can be seen inserting into the volar plate.

volar neck of the first metacarpal and inserting into the base of proximal phalanx. The volar plate also contains the sesamoid bones.[5] The MCP joint capsule inserts into the dorsal base of the proximal phalanx and provides some indirect joint stability. In MCP extension, the volar plate and accessory collateral can resist ulnar and radial deviation, even in the absence of the

proper collateral. Therefore, resistance testing of the proper collateral is performed with the MCP flexed. Complete laxity of the MCP in extension requires incompetence of both the proper and accessory collateral ligaments.

The thumb interphalangeal (IP) joint is a trochlear joint that acts as a hinge.[1] The thumb proximal phalanx has two condyles, with an intercondylar notch in between that engages with the median ridge of the distal phalanx base, which provides some relative stability. The IP joint is further stabilized by the collateral ligaments and volar plate, and the insertions of the flexor pollicis longus (FPL) and extensor pollicis longus (EPL) tendons, at the volar and dorsal base of the distal phalanx, respectively.[6] Range of motion of the IP joint is from approximately 20° extension beyond neutral, to 80° flexion.

27.2 Myology

Thumb motion is achieved through a coordination of intrinsic and extrinsic muscles. The muscles can be defined as having a primary or secondary function, based on electromyographic data.[6]

The intrinsic musculature of the thumb includes the APB, flexor pollicis brevis (FPB), opponens pollicis (OP), and adductor pollicis (AP) (▶Fig. 27.7a, b).

The APB originates from the flexor retinaculum (FR) of the wrist, flexor carpi radialis tendon sheath, trapezium, and scaphoid. The APB inserts into the radial base of the proximal phalanx, MCP joint capsule, and radial sesamoid (▶Fig. 27.7c). The APB is usually innervated by the median nerve (95%) or the ulnar nerve (2.5%) or both (2.5%). The APB muscle's actions include abduction and flexion of the thumb metacarpal, extension of the thumb IP joint, and ulnar deviation of the MCP joint.[5]

The FPB originates from the FR and inserts into the MCP joint capsule and also the radial sesamoid (▶Fig. 27.7d, f). The

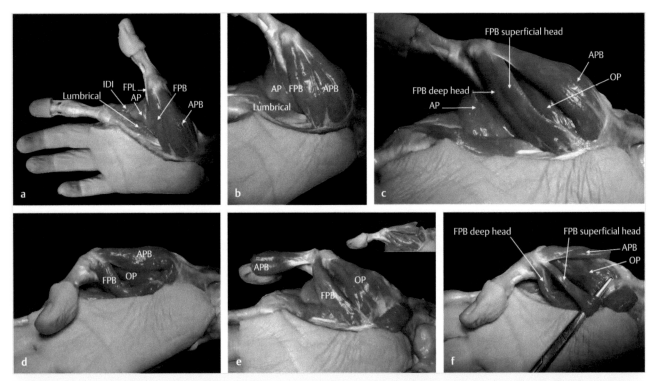

Fig. 27.7 Thenar musculature: (a) overview, (b) detail view. From proximal to distal, the muscle mass volar to the flexor pollicis longus (FPL) tendon includes both the abductor pollicis brevis (APB, proximally) and flexor pollicis brevis (FPB, distally), with subtle separation at their origin, and separation distally by a tendinous portion, shown in more detail in the next figure. The opponens pollicis (OP) is not seen, as it is deep to the APB. Distal and dorsal to the FPL, the adductor pollicis (AP) courses from its origin, on the third metacarpal, to its insertion at the ulnar side of the thumb. The thumb pulleys are discussed later, but the first annular pulley can be seen at the level of the APB and FPB insertion, the variable annular pulley just distal to the first annular pulley, and the oblique pulley coursing from proximal ulnar to radial distal. Just distal and ulnar to the AP lies the first lumbrical, with its unipennate origin from the flexor digitorum profundus of the index, exiting the carpal tunnel, along with other digital flexor tendons. (c) This figure demonstrates the distinction between the APB (proximal and radial) and the FPB (distal and ulnar), with the OP deep, showing between the APB and FPB. (d) The actions of the FPB during thumb metacarpophalangeal joint flexion, with the muscle lax during passive flexion, are shown. (e) The APB muscle has been divided (inset) and reflected to reveal the OP muscle. (f) The FPB is separated into superficial head (elevated with scissor) and deep head, distal, and ulnar.

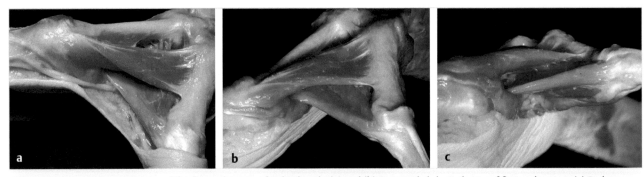

Fig. 27.8 Progressive axial views of the first web space of right thumb. (a) and (b) Pronated abducted view of first web space; (c) End on view of first web space. The first dorsal interosseous muscle (lying dorsal to the adductor pollicis muscle) arises from the first and second metacarpals, with the major head arising from the ulnar aspect of the thumb metacarpal and the minor head arising from the radial aspect of the second metacarpal. The first dorsal interosseous muscle inserts primarily on the radial aspect of the index proximal phalanx, acting mainly as an abductor of the index metacarpophalangeal joint.

superficial head is classically innervated by the median nerve while the deep head is innervated by the ulnar nerve. The FPB muscle's functions include MCP joint flexion, IP joint extension, and thumb pronation.

The OP originates from the FR, trapezium, and thumb CMC joint and inserts into the distal volar radial aspect of the first metacarpal (►Fig. 27.7e). The OP muscle is usually innervated by the median nerve (83%), less frequently by the ulnar nerve (10%), and, very rarely, by dual innervation (7%).[5] The OP muscle's functions include flexion and pronation of the thumb metacarpal.

The AP originates from the long finger metacarpal and inserts into the ulnar aspect of the thumb proximal phalanx base, dorsal–extensor complex, and ulnar sesamoid (►Fig. 27.8a–c). The AP innervation arises from the ulnar nerve. The AP adducts the thumb metacarpal, flexes the MCP joint, and extends the thumb IP joint.

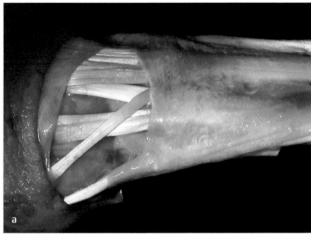

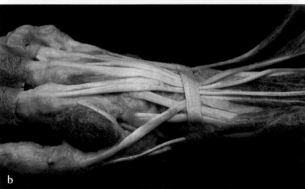

Fig. 27.9 Wrist extensor tendons seen with (a) and without (b) the overlying fascia. The extensor pollicis longus tendon angles at approximately 45° around Lister's tubercle, passes superficial to the second compartment, and, along with the extensor pollicis brevis from the first compartment, overlies the dorsum of the thumb metacarpal.

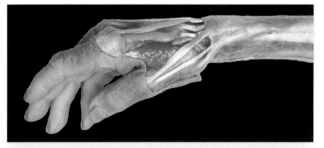

Fig. 27.10 Lateral projection of wrist. The extensor pollicis longus and extensor pollicis brevis (EPB) overlie the first metacarpal. The extensor pollicis longus tendon lies ulnar and dorsal to the EPB tendon, and the EPB tendon lies dorsal to the abductor pollicis longus, with the EPB of highly variable size.

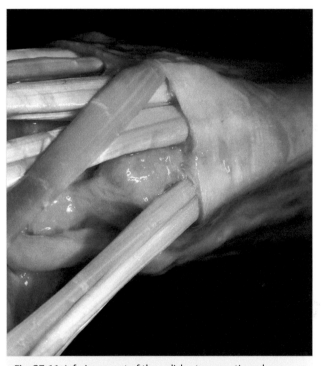

Fig. 27.11 Inferior aspect of the radial extensor retinaculum, including the first dorsal compartment. The extensor pollicis brevis (EPB) tendon is seen exiting the first dorsal compartment pulley dorsal to the abductor pollicis longus tendon (at *bottom*). The extensor pollicis longus (EPL) tendon can be seen crossing superficial to the second compartment tendons (extensor carpi radialis longus and brevis). The radial artery is seen deep to the abductor pollicis longus, EPB, and EPL.

The extrinsic musculature consists of the extensor pollicis brevis (EPB), EPL, abductor pollicis longus (APL), and FPL.

The main thumb extensors are the EPB and EPL muscles (▶Fig. 27.9a, b). The APL muscle also has some contribution to thumb extension as seen with electromyographic analysis.[6]

The EPB originates from the radius and interosseous membrane. The EPB tendon lies within the first dorsal compartment at the wrist along with the APL tendon, whose muscle originates from the radius, interosseous membrane, and ulna on the dorsum of the forearm (▶Fig. 27.10). The EPB tendon classically inserts into the proximal portion of the dorsum of the thumb proximal phalanx. The actions of the EPB are to extend the thumb MCP joint and abduct the thumb CMC joint. The EPB muscle also contributes to wrist radial deviation. Variations of the EPB tendon include multiple tendon slips, fusion with the APL tendon, insertion on the extensor hood or distal phalanx, and absence (5%).[7,8] The EPB lies dorsal to the APL within the first dorsal compartment pulley at the radial styloid (▶Fig. 27.11). The EPB normally shares a single compartment with the APL, but the EPB can have its own separate compartment, or sub-compartment, which is associated with an increased incidence of de Quervain's tenosynovitis, as well as an increased prevalence of distal insertion on the extensor hood or distal phalanx (▶Fig. 27.12a, b).[8]

The EPL muscle arises in the dorsal forearm, from the interosseous membrane and ulna. The EPL tendon courses alone within the third dorsal extensor compartment, changing direction at Lister's tubercle (▶Fig. 27.12a–h). The EPL joins the dorsal aponeurosis and continues distally to insert on the dorsal distal phalanx base. The EPL muscle's actions are to extend the IP joint and also extend the MCP joint of the thumb. The EPL also retropulses and adducts the thumb at the CMC joint.

Dorsal to the metacarpal region, the EPL and EPB tendons form interconnections (▶Fig. 27.13a, b). Proximal to the MCP joint, the dorsal aponeurosis is formed with contributions from

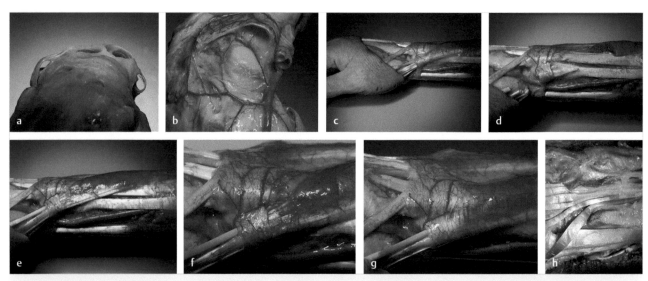

Fizg. 27.12 **(a)** Axial view of the dorsal compartments and extensor retinaculum, viewed from distal, with the first dorsal compartment on the *right*, the second dorsal compartment on the *top right*, the third dorsal compartment as the round oblique pulley almost within the second compartment, the 4th compartment at the *top*, the 5th compartment collapsed and not well seen, and the sixth compartment at the *left*. On the right, the first dorsal compartment is seen with a well-defined small dorsal channel through which the extensor pollicis brevis (EPB) passes (*top*) and with the larger volar channel for the abductor pollicis longus (APL) (*bottom*). **(b)** On the far *right*, the first dorsal compartment is also seen just dorsal to the radial artery, but this time with separate compartments for the APL (volar) and EPB (dorsal), separated by a complete septum. **(c)** The radial wrist (dorsal top, distal left), showing first and third dorsal compartments. **(d)** The radial wrist with the APL and EPB divided, showing the first dorsal compartment dorsal to the dorsal branch of the radial artery, with the artery passing deep to the APL, EPB, and extensor pollicis longus (EPL), to dive between the two heads of the first dorsal interosseous. The insertion of the brachioradialis forms part of the floor of the first dorsal compartment. **(e, f)** The APL and EPB tendons intact, without their investing fascia, but with the first dorsal compartment pulley intact. The APL muscle is volar, with its more proximal muscle belly, and the EPB is dorsal with its more distal muscle belly. **(g)** The muscles shown with the investing fascia still intact proximally, and the blood supply to the retinaculum. **(h)** Dorsal view of the wrist (distal right, radial bottom) showing Lister's tubercle, and the EPL, with the EPL running nearly longitudinally proximal to Lister's tubercle, then changing direction at Lister's tubercle, angling radial and distal, distal to Lister's tubercle.

the thenar muscular epimysium and longitudinal fibers of both extensor tendons. There are some transverse fibers from the AP muscle that continue in the MCP joint region to dorsally envelop the EPL tendon as a rough fibrous bundle, combining with contributions of fibers of APB and FPB muscles.[9]

The APL inserts primarily into the radial side of the base of the first metacarpal (▶ Fig. 27.14a, b). There are often multiple additional slips of the tendon insertion, including into the trapezium, dorsal aponeurosis, thenar musculature, and flexor retinaculum. As many as 14 separate APL slips have been reported.[10] The APL muscle abducts the thumb at the CMC and also radially deviates the wrist. The EPB, APL, and EPL muscles are all innervated by the posterior interosseous nerve.

The FPL is a unipennate muscle with bundles of muscle fibers 40 to 50 mm long when the thumb is extended. Approximately 100 to 130 mm of tendon lies on muscle surface, and the tendon extends a similar distance beyond the musculotendinous junction to reach the insertion (▶ Fig 27.15).[11] With the wrist in neutral position, the FPL tendon curves around the trapezium to reach its insertion, but the course is straight with the wrist in ulnar deviation. For isometric thumb flexion, the FPL acts primarily. For isometric adduction, the FPL muscle acts secondarily.[6]

Classically, three constant pulleys were identified constraining the FPL tendon (▶ Fig. 27.16a, b). The first "annular pulley" (A1) is located at the level of the MCP joint with dimensions

of 7 to 9 mm in width and 0.5 mm thickness (▶ Fig. 27.17). Proximally, two-thirds of the A1 attaches to the volar plate at the MCP joint. Distally, one-third of the A1 attaches to the base of the proximal phalanx. The second "oblique" pulley lies obliquely volar to the proximal phalanx and is 9 to 11 mm wide and 0.6 to 0.75 mm thick (▶ Fig. 27.18). The orientation of the oblique pulley is ulnar proximal to radial distal. The proximal ulnar portion is associated closely with the AP tendon insertion. During pulley release for "trigger thumb," the oblique pulley is at less risk for inadvertent release with radial, rather than ulnar, release of the A1 pulley. The third pulley, the "annular 2" (A2), is located just proximal to the FPL insertion and centered over the volar plate of the IP joint (▶ Fig. 27.18). The A2 pulley is approximately 8 to 10 mm wide and 0.25 mm thick.[12]

Cadaver dissections have suggested that the classic pulley description is incomplete. More commonly, there is an additional pulley, appearing as though the oblique pulley split at its ulnar origin and contributed another pulley between the classic A1 pulley and the oblique pulley. Although this additional pulley appears to be an offshoot or splitting of the oblique pulley, the additional pulley has been labeled the "variable transverse," or Av pulley, even though one of the most common patterns for the Av pulley is as a second oblique pulley. The Av pulley may be absent (7%), transverse distal to the A1 (39%), oblique (39%), or transverse and fused to the A1 (16%), but in all instances the Av

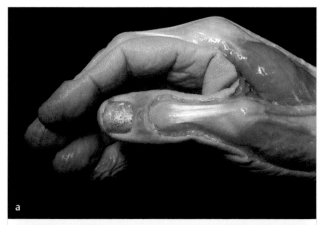

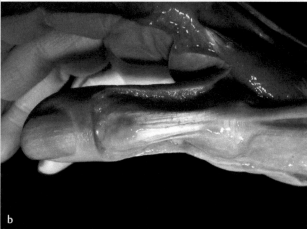

Fig. 27.13 Dorsal view of thumb with exposure of proximal phalanx and first metacarpal. The extensor pollicis brevis (EPB) is volar and radial to the extensor pollicis longus (EPL) tendon, and interconnections between the two tendons are present at the metacarpophalangeal joint. The EPL tendon has a broad insertion into the distal phalanx. (a) The EPB can be seen to insert on the proximal phalanx dorsal base, while the EPL continues distally to insert on the distal phalanx dorsal base. (b) The EPB can be seen to have fibers that continue distally to insert on the distal phalanx dorsal base.

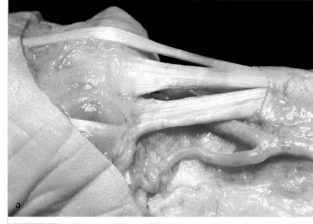

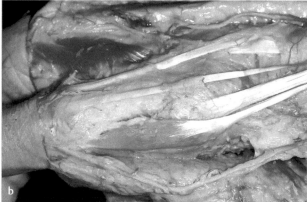

Fig. 27.14 View of radial wrist (distal left, dorsal top), showing insertion of the abductor pollicis longus (APL, multiple slips) with the extensor pollicis brevis (EPB, dorsal and smaller in diameter in this specimen) continuing distally. (a) Two slips of the APL tendon are seen inserting into the base of the first metacarpal and passing directly over the radial artery. (b) The dorsal slip of the APL inserts into the first metacarpal while the volar slip inserts into the thenar musculature (*bottom*), while the EPB, lying just dorsal to the APL insertion into the first metacarpal base, continues distally, and the extensor pollicis longus lying more dorsal and ulnar, is seen crossing superficial to the second dorsal compartment proximally and continuing distally.

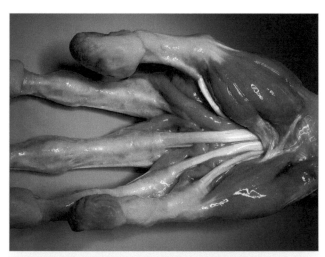

Fig. 27.15 Volar view of hand. The flexor pollicis longus muscle emerges from the carpal tunnel and passes along the thenar musculature to insert on the volar distal phalanx.

pulley lies between the classic A1 and classic oblique pulleys.[13] Even these four thumb pulley patterns are not comprehensive, and further variation is shown with a complete cruciate pulley at the oblique position (▶Fig. 27.18).

27.3 Arteries

The thumb is unique to the digits of the hand, because the thumb possesses a redundant robust dual blood supply from both volar and dorsal arteries. In the classic description, the radial artery and its branches supply the thumb. The radial artery gives off the volar branch, which contributes to the palmar arch and can directly supply the volar radial digital artery to the thumb (▶Fig. 27.19). The main radial artery passes through the floor of the anatomic snuff box deep to the tendons of the first and third extensor compartments, the APL/EPB, and EPL (▶Fig. 27.20). The radial artery gives rise to the princeps pollicis artery deep to the first dorsal interosseous (FDI) muscle, at the base of first metacarpal (▶Fig. 27.21)[14].

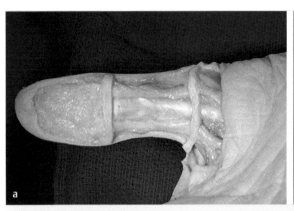
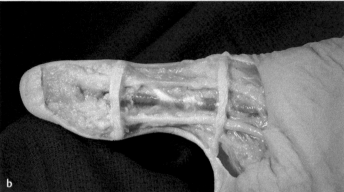

Fig. 27.16 Pulley system of thumb with tendon in place (**a**) and then removed and replaced with a red spacer (**b**) to highlight pulleys. The A1 pulley in this specimen lies deep to the palmar digital crease and can be seen extending proximal and distal to the skin of the palmar digital crease that was left in situ. A relatively substantial oblique pulley is seen, approximately midway between the palmar digital crease, and the interphalangeal joint crease. The A2 pulley is relatively diaphanous in this specimen, but lies just proximal to the interphalangeal joint crease. Between the A1 pulley and oblique, lies a second transverse pulley, the variable transverse pulley. In this specimen, the oblique pulley has some minor cruciate fibers in addition to the main oblique fibers.

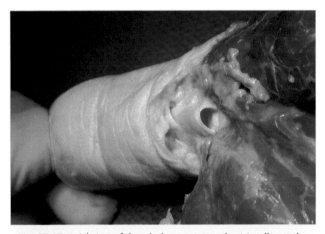

Fig. 27.17 Axial view of thumb demonstrates the A1 pulley at the level of the metacarpophalangeal joint, viewed proximally.

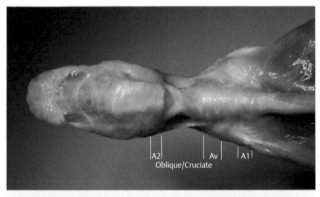

Fig. 27.18 Volar view of the thumb demonstrating the pulley system. The A1 pulley can be seen at the level of the MP joint and distal to the A1 is a transverse Av pulley. Between the A1 and A2 pulleys, lies a well-defined cruciate pulley, instead of the classic oblique pulley.

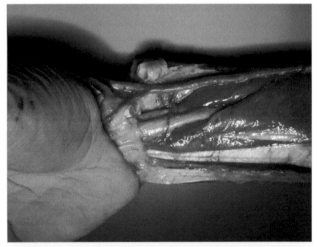

Fig. 27.19 Volar aspect of wrist. The volar branch of the radial artery can be seen arising at the level of the first dorsal compartment pulley and coursing volarly to contribute to the palmar arch. The main radial artery continues dorsally and distally.

The volar branch of the radial artery can supply the volar vascularity either directly or indirectly through the superficial palmar arch (▶Fig. 27.19). The princeps pollicis artery is also sometimes called the first dorsal metacarpal artery and gives off an ulnar branch that serves as the arterial supply of the first dorsal metacarpal artery flap. The princeps pollicis artery runs along the diaphysis of the first metacarpal and then reaches the thumb MCP joint. The princeps pollicis artery then bifurcates giving rise to the volar digital arteries at the volar aspect of the MCP joint, with the radial palmar digital artery supplied by a branch that passes deep to the FPL, to reach the radial side of the thumb. (▶Fig. 27.23a–c).[14]

The dorsal digital vessels arise proximal to the MCP joint. The ulnar dorsal digital artery to the thumb arises from the princeps pollicis artery along the first metacarpal. The radial dorsal digital artery originates from the radial artery at the thumb CMC joint and runs parallel to the EPL tendon (▶Fig. 27.24a, b).

In actuality, there is considerable variation in the thumb arterial supply within studies and between studies, and there is

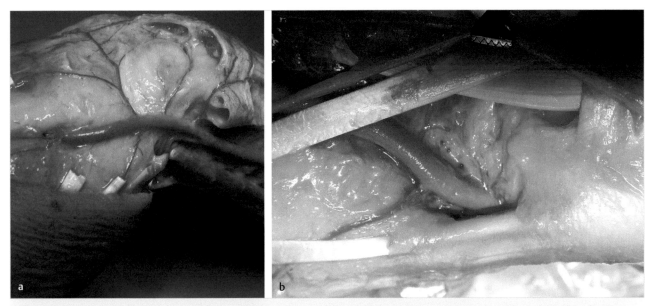

Fig. 27.20 (a) View of radial artery coursing dorsally. First, second, and third dorsal compartments are seen with tendons excised. A separate compartment for the extensor pollicis brevis can be seen within the first dorsal compartment. (b) The radial artery passes deep to the abductor pollicis longus and extensor pollicis brevis tendons, into the anatomic snuffbox, giving off branches to the scaphoid and the first metacarpal, and then passing deep to the EPL before diving between the two heads of the first dorsal interosseous muscle.

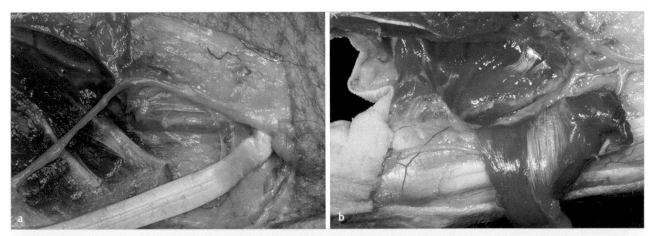

Fig. 27.21 Princeps pollicis artery. (a) The radial artery is seen dorsally, in the interspace between the first and second metacarpal bases, providing a dorsal radial branch to the second metacarpal and a radial dorsal branch ulnar to the first metacarpal, before diving between the two heads of the first dorsal interosseous muscle. (b) The first dorsal interosseous muscle lateral head has been divided and reflected radially, revealing the princeps pollicis artery continuing distally along the ulnar aspect of the first metacarpal. (RA: radial artery; PPA: princeps pollicis sartery).

variation in the nomenclature between studies. But basically, any artery on the radial side of the hand, may be providing the arterial supply to one or more of the thumb digital vessels. Potential sources of thumb digital arterial supply include: princeps pollicis artery, superficial palmar branch of radial artery; superficial palmar arch; or deep palmar arch. (a branch arising from the palmar arch is sometimes called the first palmar metacarpal artery). (▶Fig. 27.19). (▶Fig. 27.22a, b). The difference between what might be called a princeps pollicis artery supplying the thumb, and what might be called a first palmar metacarpal artery arising

from the deep arch, is subjective. There are also anastomoses between the various systems, where a digital vessel may have more than one source of arterial inflow, sometimes without clear dominance, making descriptions more complicated.

The digital vessels are more consistent than the vessels that supply them. In a review by Miletin et al., the thumb ulnar palmar digital artery is present 99.63%, the thumb radial palmar digital artery 99.26%, the thumb ulnar dorsal digital artery 88.39%, and the thumb radial dorsal digital artery 70.38%.[15]

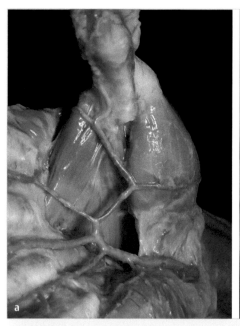
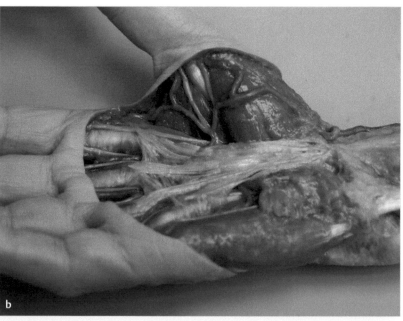

Fig. 27.22 Variations of the digital arteries to the thumb from superficial palmar arch. (**a**) The volar branch of the radial artery does not directly supply the volar radial digital artery of the thumb. (**b**) The volar branch of the radial artery directly supplies the volar radial digital artery or the thumb. The superficial radial artery contributes to the superficial arch. A common branch gives rise to the thumb ulnar proper digital artery and the radial proper digital artery to the index finger.

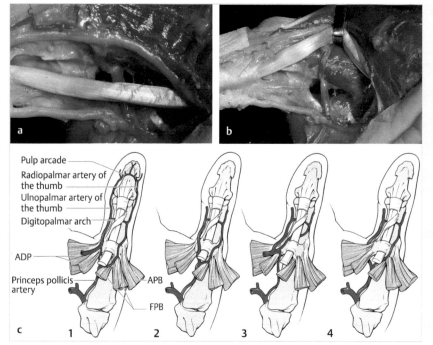

Fig. 27.23 (**a**) Volar aspect of thumb with flexor pollicis longus skeletonized (distal left, radial top). (**b**) The volar radial digital artery, formed from a branch of the first metacarpal artery and a branch of the princeps pollicis artery, crosses from ulnar to radial deep to the flexor pollicis at the thumb metacarpophalangeal joint. (**c**) Variations of the branches of the princeps pollicis artery. (From Schmidt H-M, Lanz U. Surgical Anatomy of the Hand. Thieme; 2004.)

27.4 Veins

The dorsal venous system begins with small veins at the distal aspect of the nail sulcus and eponychial fold. These small veins coalesce into four to eight larger veins at the level of the IP joint. As the veins progress proximally to the level of the MCP joint, there are two to three veins with diameter of 1 to 1.5 mm.[16] On the volar aspect within the pulp, one to two veins with diameter greater than 0.5 mm are present. As the volar veins progress proximal to the IP joint, the veins take

a more dorsal course and have communicating branches with the dorsal system.

On the ulnar aspect of the thumb, the veins take an oblique course from the volar aspect to the dorsum more distally and then take a more longitudinal course and remain on the ulnar aspect while going into the first web space. On the radial aspect, there are multiple communicating branches between the dorsal and volar veins, with a large communicating vein often present at the level of the IP joint, with a diameter of up to 1.5 mm.[16]

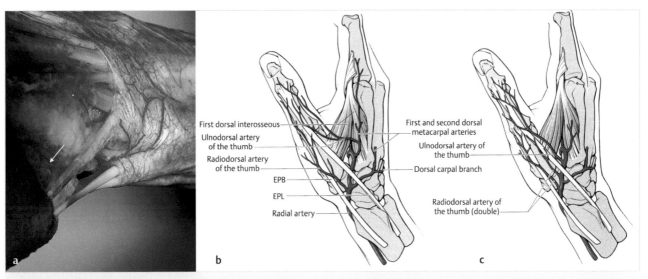

Fig. 27.24 (**a, b**) Dorsal radial view of wrist with extensor pollicis longus and first dorsal compartment tendons visible. Deep to the tendons, the dorsal branch of the radial artery is seen (*arrow*) with distal branches supplying the thumb as dorsal digital branches. (**c**) Variations of radiodorsal artery. (From Schmidt H-M, Lanz U. Surgical Anatomy of the Hand. Thieme; 2004.)

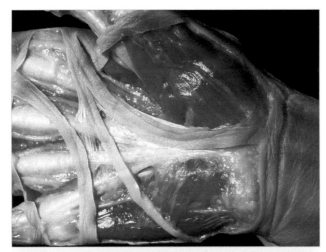

Fig. 27.25 Volar view of hand with skin creases left intact for reference. The motor branch of the median nerve is seen entering the thenar musculature transversely, just radial to the thenar crease, in line with the radial border of the long finger.

27.5 Nerves

Multiple nerves contribute to the innervation of the thumb for both motor and sensory function. Motor function to the thumb involves all three nerves to the hand. The radial nerve, via the posterior interosseous nerve, innervates the extrinsic dorsal forearm muscles: the APL, EPB, and EPL. The median nerve via the anterior interosseous nerve innervates the FPL. The median recurrent motor branch innervates the APB, OP, and FPB superficial head. The ulnar nerve innervates the AP, FPB deep head, and FDI. There is variability in innervation of the thenar musculature with potential ulnar contribution. One example is through the Riche-Cannieu connection between the ulnar and median nerves in the palm. Of the thenar musculature, the APB is least likely to have a major innervation contribution from the ulnar nerve.[17]

The thenar or recurrent motor branch of the median nerve has been extensively studied because of its clinical relevance for practitioners who perform carpal tunnel release. In anatomic study, the recurrent motor branch was seen to originate from the median nerve at or beyond the distal edge of the FR most commonly (▶ Fig. 27.25), with few specimens having origin proximal to the distal edge of the FR (▶ Fig. 27.26a, b). The nerve in most cases took an extraligamentous path and then would course radially and proximally forming a 30 to 40° angle with the median nerve. In some individuals, the recurrent motor branch courses through the FR and has a similar path to the thenar musculature. The recurrent motor branch most commonly has three terminal branches, with a branch to the abductor pollicis, the OP, and the FPB (superficial head). There are some variations regarding the terminal branching. Some variations seen include three terminal branches with no branches to FPB and four terminal branches with one to flexor, two to abductor, and one to opponens. An accessory thenar nerve can be seen in some individuals arising from the first common digital nerve or the radial proper digital nerve. This accessory thenar branch innervates the FPB.[18]

Sensory innervation of the thumb is from the radial and median nerves. However, while the ulnar nerve does not contribute any cutaneous sensory innervation to the thumb, the ulnar motor nerve contains a high proportion of sensory fibers, which presumably provide sensory feedback from the ulnar innervated intrinsic muscles, with proprioceptive information.

The superficial branch of the radial nerve (SBRN) provides sensation to the dorsum of thumb. The SBRN arises at the level of the lateral humeral epicondyle, continues deep to the brachioradialis, and emerges between the extensor carpi radialis longus tendon and the brachioradialis. The SBRN becomes subcutaneous approximately 9 cm proximal to the radial styloid and divides into two branches—palmar and dorsal (▶ Fig. 27.27). The branches pass distally radial to Lister's tubercle and sometimes include a branch superficial to the first dorsal compartment (▶ Fig. 27.28a, b). The major palmar branch continues distal to become the dorsoradial digital nerve

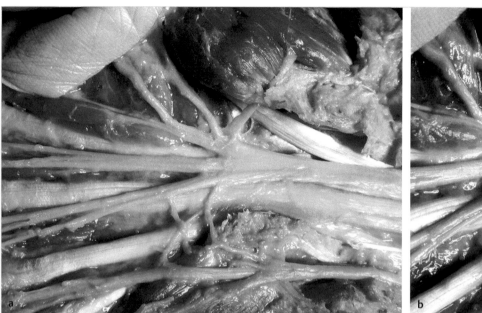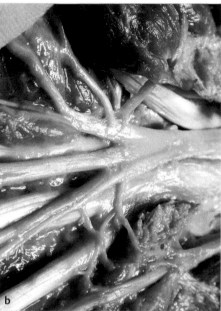

Fig. 27.26 (a, b) Volar view of the median nerve with the transverse carpal ligament resected. The motor branch passes volar to the flexor pollicis longus tendon, to enter the thenar musculature. There is a common digital nerve, arising just distal to the motor branch from the median nerve, innervating the ulnar aspect of the thumb and radial aspect of index finger.

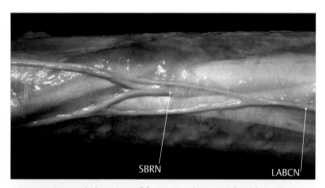

Fig. 27.27 Radial aspect of forearm. The superficial branch of the radial nerve (SBRN) emerges from deep to the brachioradialis tendon, becomes superficial between the brachioradialis and the extensor carpi radialis longus, then continues superficial to the first dorsal compartment, with a volar branch that provides the dorsal radial innervation of the thumb and a dorsal branch that provides the dorsal ulnar sensation of the thumb, as well as the dorsal radial hand. In this specimen, in addition to the SBRN, which is seen becoming superficial in the middle of the photograph, there are contributions from the lateral antebrachial cutaneous nerve (LABCN), which bifurcates proximal to the SBRN emerging, in this case contributing to form a plexus with the dorsal and volar branches of the SBRN.

of the thumb. Interconnections may be present between the branches of SBRN and lateral antebrachial cutaneous nerve. The major dorsal branch of the SBRN continues and branches into the dorsoulnar digital nerve to the thumb and branches to the dorsal proximal aspect of the index and middle fingers.[19]

Mackinnon and Dellon[20] investigated the overlap pattern between the lateral antebrachial cutaneous nerve (LABCN) and the superficial branch of the radial nerve (SBRN) both clinically and anatomically. They found that partial and complete overlap between the two nerves in 75% of cases whereas in 25% the two nerves innervated separate territories.

Anatomic variations can also be seen with sensory innervation of the volar aspect of the thumb. Three main variations have been seen of the terminal branch of the median nerve to the radial aspect of the hand. The first is a proper digital nerve to the radial thumb and a common digital nerve to the first web space that divides into terminal branches supplying the ulnar aspect of the thumb and radial side of the index finger (▶ Fig. 27.29a, b). Another variation is a common digital nerve to the thumb and radial digital nerve to the index finger (▶ Fig. 27.30). A third variation consists of a proper digital nerve to the radial thumb, ulnar thumb, and radial aspect of the index finger.[21] Additional variation can arise from nerves rejoining distally, forming neural plexi.[22] In addition, rare variations have been reported clinically,

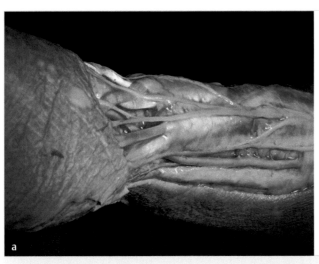
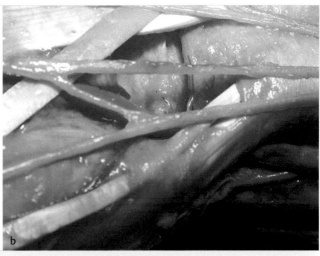

Fig. 27.28 (a) Dorsal radial aspect of the forearm (distal left, dorsal top). The superficial branch of the radial nerve branch bifurcates to form the dorsal and volar branches. The volar branch forms the radial sensory nerve to the thumb. The dorsal branch gives off multiple subsequent branches supplying sensation to the dorsal ulnar aspect of dorsal thumb, dorsal proximal index, dorsal long, and radial dorsal aspect of ring finger. (b) At the level of the anatomic snuffbox, in this specimen, there is a contribution from the proper dorsal ulnar digital nerve to the thumb, back to the dorsal branch of the superficial branch of the radial nerve to the dorsum of the index finger.

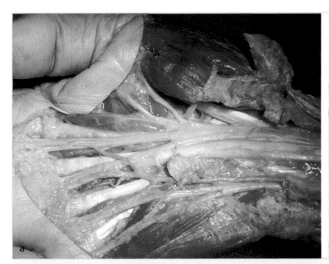
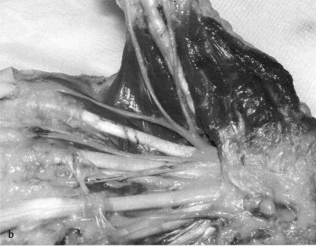

Fig. 27.29 Volar view of thumb with the volar digital nerves of the thumb. (a) The thumb volar radial digital nerve branches first, then the thumb volar ulnar digital nerve and radial aspect of index finger, as the proper volar radial digital nerve. (b) This figure shows the innervation more distally, with the proper volar radial sensory nerve of the thumb arising first, then a common digital nerve bifurcating into the volar ulnar digital nerve to the thumb, and the volar radial digital nerve to the index.

where an injury to a dorsal radial sensory branch resulted in numbness of the normally median innervated thumb pad.[17]

In conclusion, the preceding anatomic description is intended to present a common anatomic presentation. However, anatomic variations are infinite, and structures frequently differ from the above descriptions in minor ways, and sometimes even in major ways.

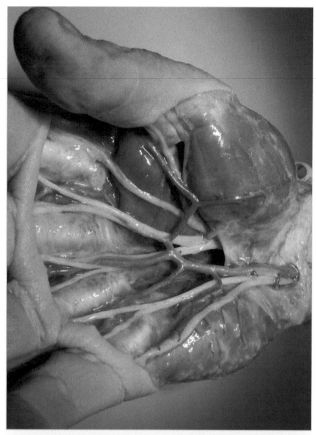

Fig. 27.30 Variation in the branching pattern of the thumb digital nerves. A common digital nerve to the thumb gives rise to the proper volar thumb radial and volar ulnar digital branches. A separate proper radial digital nerve to the index finger is present.

References

1. Emerson ET, Krizek TJ, Greenwald DP. Anatomy, physiology, and functional restoration of the thumb. Ann Plast Surg 1996;36(2):180–191

2. Craig SM. Anatomy of the joints of the fingers. Hand Clin 1992;8(4):693–700

3. Carlson MG, Warner KK, Meyers KN, Hearns KA, Kok PL. Anatomy of the thumb metacarpophalangeal ulnar and radial collateral ligaments. J Hand Surg Am 2012;37(10):2021–2026

4. Imaeda T, An KN, Cooney WP III. Functional anatomy and biomechanics of the thumb. Hand Clin 1992;8(1):9–15

5. Leversedge FJ. Anatomy and pathomechanics of the thumb. Hand Clin 2008;24(3):219–229

6. Cooney WP III, An KN, Daube JR, Askew LJ. Electromyographic analysis of the thumb: a study of isometric forces in pinch and grasp. J Hand Surg Am 1985;10(2):202–210

7. von Schroeder HP, Botte MJ. Anatomy and functional significance of the long extensors to the fingers and thumb. Clin Orthop Relat Res 2001; (383):74–83

8. Alemohammad AM, Yazaki N, Morris RP, Buford WL, Viegas SF. Thumb interphalangeal joint extension by the extensor pollicis brevis: association with a subcompartment and de Quervain's disease. J Hand Surg Am 2009;34(4):719–723

9. Bade H, Krolak C, Koebke J. Fibrous architecture of the dorsal aponeurosis of the thumb. Anat Rec 1995;243(4):524–530

11. Rack PM, Ross HF. The tendon of flexor pollicis longus: its effects on the muscular control of force and position at the human thumb. J Physiol 1984;351:99–110

12. Doyle JR, Blythe WF. Anatomy of the flexor tendon sheath and pulleys of the thumb. J Hand Surg Am 1977;2(2):149–151

13. Schubert MF, Shah VS, Craig CL, Zeller JL. Varied anatomy of the thumb pulley system: implications for successful trigger thumb release. J Hand Surg Am 2012;37(11):2278–2285

14. Ramírez AR, Gonzalez SM. Arteries of the thumb: description of anatomical variations and review of the literature. Plast Reconstr Surg 2012;129(3):468e–476e

15. Miletin J, Sukop A, Baca V, Kachlik D., Arterial supply of the thumb: Systemic review. Clin Anat. 2017 Oct;30(7):9637–973

16. Matloub HS, Strathy KM, Sanger JR, Yousif NJ. Venous anatomy of the thumb. J Hand Surg Am 1991;16(6):1063–1069

17. Falconer D, Spinner M. Anatomic variations in the motor and sensory supply of the thumb. Clin Orthop Relat Res 1985;(195):83–96

18. Mumford J, Morecraft R, Blair WF. Anatomy of the thenar branch of the median nerve. J Hand Surg Am 1987;12(3):361–365

19. Abrams RA, Brown RA, Botte MJ. The superficial branch of the radial nerve: an anatomic study with surgical implications. J Hand Surg Am 1992;17(6):1037–1041

20. Mackinnon SE and Dellon AL: The overlap pattern of the lateral antebrachial cutaneous nerve and the superficial branch of the radial nerve. J Hand Surg Am 1985;10(4):522–526

21. Jolley BJ, Stern PJ, Starling T. Patterns of median nerve sensory innervation to the thumb and index finger: an anatomic study. J Hand Surg Am 1997;22(2):228–231

22. Bas H, Kleinert JM. Anatomic variations in sensory innervation of the hand and digits. J Hand Surg Am 1999;24(6):1171–1184

28 The Flexor Tendons and the Flexor Sheath

Sandeep Jacob Sebastin and Beng Hai Lim

The forearm flexor muscles (flexor–pronator group) are present in the anterior (volar) compartment of the forearm. Most of them originate from the medial epicondyle of the humerus (common flexor origin). They include eight muscles that may be divided into three distinct functional groups: (1) muscles that rotate the radius on the ulna (pronator teres [PT] and pronator quadratus [PQ]); (2) muscles that flex the wrist (flexor carpi radialis [FCR], palmaris longus [PL], and flexor carpi ulnaris [FCU]); and (3) muscles that flex the digits (flexor digitorum superficialis [FDS], flexor digitorum profundus [FDP], and flexor pollicis longus [FPL]).[1] Anatomically, these eight muscles are arranged in three distinct layers or compartments. The superficial compartment includes (radial to ulnar) PT, FCR, PL, and FCU. The intermediate compartment includes the FDS, and the deep compartment includes the FPL, FDP, and the PQ.[2]

In general, the term *flexor tendon* refers to the tendinous portions of the wrist (FCR, PL, and FCU) and digital flexors (FDS, FPL, and FDP). They extend from the musculotendinous junction in the midforearm to their respective bony insertions. The flexor sheath refers to the specialized tissue that covers the digital flexor tendons (FDS, FPL, and FDP). This sheath allows the tendons to glide and turn around a corner to produce smooth and efficient flexion of the digits.[2] The arrangement of the flexor tendons and the flexor sheaths changes as they proceed from the distal forearm to the digits. This chapter will discuss the gross and functional anatomy of the flexor tendons and the flexor sheath with specific reference to clinical correlations.

28.1 Flexor Tendons

There are 12 flexor tendons. They include the tendons of the three wrist flexors (FCR, PL, and FCU) (▶ Fig 28.1), the thumb flexor (FPL), and four tendons each for the finger flexors (FDS and FDP).

28.1.1 Flexor Carpi Radialis

Etymology: Flexor is derived from the Latin word *flexus*, meaning "bent" (thus flexor indicates "that which bends," or "bending"). Carpi is derived from Latin word *carpalis* and the Greek word *karpos*, both of which indicate "wrist" (the carpus). Radialis again is derived from the Latin word *radii*, which means "spoke" (used to describe the radius of the forearm).[3,4]

Origin: The tendinous portion of the FCR begins approximately 15 cm proximal to the radial styloid, and the muscular portion ends approximately 8 cm from the radial styloid.[5,6]

Course: The tendon is located on the radial superficial aspect of the forearm. It is ulnar to the radial artery, radial to the median nerve and the tendon of the PL, and superficial to the tendon of the FPL. It enters a fibro-osseous tunnel at the proximal border of the trapezium. In this tunnel, it is bounded radially by the body of the trapezium, palmarly by the trapezial crest and transverse carpal ligament, and ulnarly by a retinacular septum. This septum is continuous with the transverse carpal ligament and separates the tendon from the contents of the carpal tunnel. The tendon is in direct contact with the trapezium and lies in close relation to the distal aspect of the radius, the scaphoid tubercle, the scaphotrapeziotrapezoid (STT) joint, and the carpometacarpal (CMC) joint of the thumb.[5] Nigro has divided the fibro-osseous tunnel for the FCR into four sections. These sections, from proximal to distal, are (1) the forearm aponeurosis that encircles the FCR tendon (palmar carpal ligament), (2) the tunnel formed between the radial insertions of the flexor retinaculum and the scaphoid tubercle, (3) the tunnel formed at the trapezial groove, and (4) the insertion of the FCR tendon at the second metacarpal base.[7]

Insertion: The FCR tendon is inserted at three locations. A small slip inserts into the trapezial crest or tuberosity, 80%

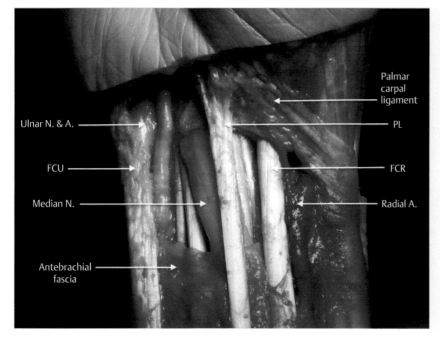

Fig. 28.1 Dissection of the volar distal forearm showing the Flexor Carpi Radialis (FCR) tendon and Palmaris longus (PL) tendons along with the median nerve, the ulnar nerve and the radial artery. The Flexor Carpi Ulnaris (FCU) tendon is also seen.

Ulnar N. & A.

FCU

Median N.

Antebrachial fascia

Palmar carpal ligament

PL

FCR

Radial A.

of the remaining tendon is inserted on the base of the second metacarpal, and 20% inserts on the base of the third metacarpal. The deep palmar arch is located 2 to 3 mm distal to the insertion of the tendon.[5]

Characteristics: The FCR tendon is covered with a synovial sheath that extends from the musculotendinous origin till the metacarpal insertion. This sheath is thin proximally and consists only of paratenon. Four to five cm proximal to the radial styloid, the tendon is circumferentially invested by the transverse fibers of the antebrachial fascia and thickens to about 3 mm at the level of the trapezial crest. The FCR tendon gradually changes from a relatively flat and wide configuration in the forearm to an elliptical shape at the wrist. The fibers of the FCR tendon undergo a torsion of approximately 180° as it progresses from proximal to distal. Half of this torsion occurs in the forearm and half in the sheath of the FCR at wrist level. The rotation of its fibers is constant and is usually 180° in the clockwise direction in the right forearm and anticlockwise in the left forearm.[8] Simovitch et al have suggested the presence of a putative wrist annular pulley for the FCR tendon in 80% of the cadavers in their study. This pulley was present 1.5 cm proximal to the wrist flexion crease and measured approximately 2.1 × 1.5 cm in size.[9] The maximum excursion of the FCR tendon in adults is 4 cm.[10]

Variations: An absence of the FCR has been reported.[11] Other variations of the FCR tendon include slips of attachment to the base of the fourth metacarpal and the tubercle of the scaphoid. The FCR brevis is a small muscle that arises from the palmar surface of the radius between origins of the FPL and the PQ. The tendon of the FCR brevis inserts into base of the second and third metacarpal.[12]

Clinical correlations: Volar wrist ganglions are the second most commonly seen ganglion in the hand and wrist (18–20%). They arise from the radiocarpal joint or the STT joint and are intimately related to the FCR tendon sheath and the radial artery. A relatively uncommon pathology involving the FCR tendon sheath is FCR tendinitis. This may be primary as a result of tendon irritation within the narrow confines of the trapezial tunnel or secondary in association with scaphoid cysts, STT osteoarthritis (OA), thumb CMC joint OA, or scaphoid fractures.[5] Attritional rupture of FCR has been reported in association with STT osteoarthritis.[13]

A split tendon graft can be harvested from the FCR tendon. This is useful in patients who need a short graft but lack the PL. This tendon graft can be harvested by using two to three small transverse incisions.[14] The split FCR tendon graft with the distal insertion preserved is frequently used in ligamentous reconstruction following excision of the trapezium (LRTI procedure)[15] and in scapholunate ligament reconstruction (Brunelli or the three ligament tenodesis procedure).[16,17]

The tendon of the FCR is commonly transferred to the extensor digitorum communis (EDC) in patients with radial nerve palsy. Although the FCU is stronger, the FCR is a better choice for this transfer, having a greater excursion. In addition, in patients who have a low radial nerve palsy (posterior interosseous nerve palsy) and intact radial wrist extensors, preserving the FCU maintains balance between the radial and ulnar deviators of

the wrist. A split transfer of the FCR tendinomuscular unit has also been described to provide independent thumb and finger extension.[18]

28.1.2 Palmaris Longus

Etymology: Palmaris is derived from the Latin word *palma*, which means "pertaining to the palm." Longus is the Latin for "long."[3,4]

Origin: The tendon of the PL begins in the midforearm and has a relatively small musculotendinous portion. A study in a Japanese population estimated that the intramuscular length of the tendon was approximately 0.6 to 1.2 cm.[19]

Course: The PL tendon is initially deep to the antebrachial fascia. In the distal third of the forearm, approximately 5 cm proximal to the distal wrist crease, it passes through an oval opening in the antebrachial fascia to become subcutaneous.[20] The PL tendon is ulnar to the FCR and superficial to the median nerve (▶ Fig. 28.1). At the level of the wrist, the PL tendon is superficial to the flexor retinaculum, which is in continuity with the antebrachial fascia (▶ Fig. 28.2).

Insertion: Distal to the flexor retinaculum, the PL tendon broadens in a fanlike fashion to merge into the palmar aponeurosis (PA; ▶ Fig. 28.2). The PA can be divided into two layers: the superficial one formed by longitudinal fibers (that is in 3 layers),

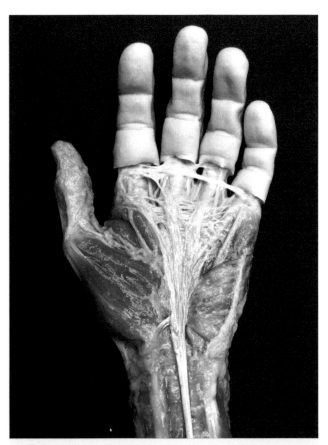

Fig. 28.2 Dissection of the palm and distal forearm shows the palmaris longus tendon and the palmar fascia.

and a deep one, adherent to the skin formed by transverse fibers continuous laterally with the deep fascia of the hand. The PL tendon is in continuity only with the longitudinal fibers of the PA. In addition to the insertion into the PA, fibrous expansions arise from each side of the distal part of the PL tendon that insert into the deep fascia overlying the thenar and hypothenar eminences. The expansions to the thenar eminence were generally thicker.[20]

Characteristics: A study in a Japanese population determined that the mean length and width of the PL tendon were 16.6 ± 1.8 cm and 0.4 ± 0.08 cm, respectively. They also determined that the length of the tendon correlated with the length of the forearm and was approximately 50.7 ± 6.5% of forearm length.[19] This corresponds to earlier reports in Caucasian populations also.[20,22] The mean cross-sectional area of the PL tendon is 3.1 mm^2, mean volume is 529 mm^3, and stiffness is 42.0 ± 4.1 N/mm.[22]

Variations: The PL muscle is one of the most variable muscles in the human body, not only in terms of its absence but also in terms of muscle variations and anomalies. Its absence was first reported in 1559 by Colombo in *De Re Anatomica Libri* and has been the subject of several cadaveric as well as in vivo studies.[23] The highest reported prevalence of absence of the PL tendon (64%) was reported in the Turkish population. The overall prevalence of the absence of the PL tendon in different Caucasian populations is approximately 22%. In contrast, it is quite low in Black (3%), Asian (4.5%), and Native American (7.1%) populations. There is disagreement in the literature regarding the symmetry of absence and whether absence is more common in women. Given the wide variations between the different ethnic groups, we feel that a general figure for the absence of the PL tendon cannot be quoted. It is, therefore, important for surgeons to observe these variations and be familiar with the values of the ethnic groups they treat or study.[23]

Many variations in morphology of the PL tendon have been reported, including tendon multiplicity and anomalous insertions into antebrachial fascia, thenar fascia, carpal bones, or the FCU tendon.[24]

Clinical correlations: The tendon of the PL is the most frequently used source of a tendon graft. A single PL tendon graft can be used to reconstruct a single FDP tendon from its insertion till the palm. If a longer graft is required (till the forearm) or multiple fingers need to be reconstructed, one must consider other grafts such as the plantaris or fascia lata. The PL tendon has also been used for reconstruction of collateral ligaments of the metacarpophalangeal (MCP) and interphalangeal (IP) joints and for correction of the swan neck deformity.

The PL has been used as a motor to provide palmar abduction in patients with low median nerve palsy. The tendon of PL is harvested along with a strip of the PA and transferred to the insertion of the abductor pollicis brevis. This tendon transfer, also known as the Camitz transfer, is especially valuable in low demand patients with severe long-standing carpal tunnel syndrome.[25] The PL has also been used as a motor to restore thumb extension by a transfer to the extensor pollicis longus in patients with radial nerve palsy.[26]

A number of clinical maneuvers have been described in literature to determine the presence of the PL tendon preoperatively. We prefer the use of the resisted wrist flexion test described by Mishra in determining the presence of the PL. In

this test, the examiner passively hyperextends the MCP joints of the fingers to make the PA taut. The patient is then asked to attempt active flexion of the wrist. The tendon of the PL can then be clearly visualized.[27]

28.1.3 Flexor Carpi Ulnaris

Etymology: Flexor is derived from the Latin word *flexus*, meaning "bent" (thus flexor indicates "that which bends," or "bending"). Carpi is derived from Latin word *carpalis* and Greek word *karpos*, both of which indicate "wrist" (the carpus). Ulnaris is derived from the Latin word *ulna*, which means "elbow."[3,4]

Origin: The tendon of the FCU is formed in the distal third of the muscle along the anterolateral border. It is quite thick and unlike the FCR has muscle fibers inserting into it almost till the level of its insertion.

Course: The tendon of the FCU is quite short, and in the distal half of the forearm, the ulnar artery and nerve pass deep and radial to the FCU tendon (▶ Fig. 28.1).

Insertion: The FCU tendon inserts mainly onto the pisiform, with extensions onto the hook of hamate and the base of the fifth metacarpal via the pisohamate and pisometacarpal ligaments. In addition, some fibers insert into the flexor retinaculum and the bases of the third and fourth metacarpals. The pisiform is believed to be a sesamoid bone that lies within the FCU tendon.

Characteristics: The FCU tendon is approximately 47 ± 4.7 mm in length and has a cross-sectional area of 27.4 ± 3.6 mm^2.[28] Unlike the tendons of the FCR and the digital flexors, the FCU does not have a tendon sheath.[29] In addition to its function as a flexor and ulnar deviator of the wrist, the tendon of the FCU plays a role in stabilizing the wrist; in the strong power grip, such as when holding a hammer; and in stabilizing the pisiform. When a subject is asked to abduct the small finger against resistance, the FCU synergistically contracts to stabilize the pisiform, and this in turn stabilizes the origin of the abductor digiti minimi. This can be used to test the function of the FCU by palpating the FCU tendon while asking the subject to abduct the small finger against resistance. The maximum excursion of the FCU tendon in adults is 3.3 cm.[10]

Variations: Many variations of the insertion of the FCU tendon have been described. In addition to the multiple insertions described earlier, it may have extensions to the metacarpals of the small, ring, or long fingers or to the capsule of the CMC joints. A split FCU tendon with the ulnar nerve passing between the split has also been described.[30]

Clinical correlations: There have been reports of patients with FCU tendinopathy. These patients present with pain about 3 to 4 cm proximal to the pisiform and histology shows features of tendinosis (degeneration) and not tendinitis (inflammation).[31] The FCU has been used as a motor in tendon transfers for radial and median nerve palsies. A split FCU transfer with independent innervation based on both heads of the FCU has also been described.[32] The FCU is designed optimally for force generation and less for excursion. Therefore, the FCR may represent a better option for tendon transfer.

The ulnar nerve and artery lie deep and radial to the FCU tendon. The ulnar nerve can be blocked by infiltrating local anesthetic agent deep to the palpable FCU tendon. In order to obtain a complete block of the ulnar nerve, the dorsal branch of the ulnar nerve needs to be blocked by injecting a wheal of anesthetic around the ulnar styloid.

28.1.4 Flexor Digitorum Superficialis/Sublimis

Etymology: Flexor is derived from the Latin word *flexus* meaning "bent" (thus flexor indicates "that which bends," or bending). Digitorum is derived from the Latin word *digitus* or *digitorum*, indicating the digits. Superficialis denotes its superficial location in the forearm. Sublimis is again derived from Latin, meaning "superficial."

Origin: The FDS has two heads of origin—a proximal humeroulnar head and a distal radial head. The median nerve and ulnar artery pass below the muscular arch formed by the two heads of the FDS. The humeroulnar head lies in a deeper plane. It has a complex digastric anatomy with a large flat common tendon that connects a single proximal muscle belly to two or three separate distal muscles that give rise to the tendons to the index, ring, and small fingers. The tendon to the index and small fingers arises completely from the distal muscle bellies, whereas the tendon to the ring finger arises partly from distal muscle belly and partly from the humeroulnar head.[33] The radial head lies in a superficial plane and gives rise to the tendon to the long finger. Although the FDS is often thought of as four independent muscles, only the long finger FDS has truly independent function. The superficialis tendons to the index, ring, and small fingers have a common proximal muscle belly, act as a conjoined unit, and do not have completely independent actions.

Course: The FDS tendons to the ring and long fingers are superficial and central, whereas the tendons to the index and small fingers are deep and located radially and ulnarly, respectively (▶ Fig. 28.3). This arrangement of tendons is maintained in the forearm and in the carpal tunnel. Once the tendons exit from the carpal tunnel, they diverge toward the respective fingers. In the forearm, these tendons are deep to the PL, FCR, PT, and radial artery and are superficial to the FDP, FPL, ulnar artery, and median nerve. In the palm, the tendons of the FDS are deep to the superficial palmar arch and the digital branches of the median and ulnar nerves (▶ Fig. 28.4) and are superficial to the tendons of the FDP, along with the lumbricals and the deep palmar arch.[34]

At the level of the MCP joint, the FDS tendon changes from a relatively oval configuration to a flattened tendon. This divides into two slips over the proximal third of the proximal phalanx to form an interval for the passage of the tendon of the FDP—the "bifurca" (▶ Fig. 28.5). The two slips of the FDS rotate 180° with the radial slip moving in a clockwise direction and the ulnar slip in an anticlockwise direction (▶ Fig. 28.6). The slips of the FDS encircle the FDP tendon as they pass from proximal to distal. They are initially palmar to the FDP tendon, then become lateral, and finally end up dorsal to the FDP tendon (▶ Fig. 28.7). As the two slips approach each other dorsal to the FDP tendon at the level of the neck of the proximal phalanx, they divide again into a radial and an ulnar band. The radial band of the radial slip and the ulnar band of the ulnar slip continue straight ahead (linear bands), whereas the ulnar band of the radial slip and the radial band of the ulnar slip decussate in an **X** pattern behind the FDP tendon (▶ Fig. 28.8) forming the chiasm of Camper.[35] The chiasma can be variable in terms of anatomy and morphology.[36]

Insertion: These crossing bands join with the linear bands to form the triangular insertion of the FDS tendon into the lateral crests on the palmar aspect of the shaft of mid-middle phalanx (▶ Fig. 28.8), lying on either side of the FDP tendon (▶ Fig. 28.7).

Characteristics: The FDS is the prime flexor of the proximal interphalangeal (PIP) joint of the fingers. It also contributes to flexion at the wrist and the MCP joint. When making a fist, it has a slight adduction component and brings the fingers together. The small finger FDS is also believed to have a minor opposing action at the CMC joint.[30] There are also differences in strength and available excursion between the FDS tendons to the four fingers. The long finger FDS is 75% stronger than the ring or the index fingers, while the small finger FDS is 50% weaker than the

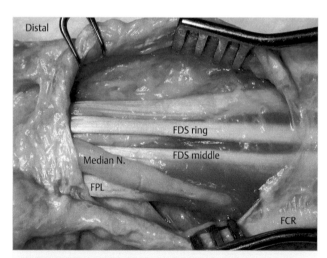

Fig. 28.3 Volar distal forearm dissection showing the Flexor Digitorum Superficialis (FDS) tendons as well as the median nerve. The FDS tendons to the ring and middle fingers are superficial and central, whereas the tendons to the index and small fingers are deep and located radially and ulnarly respectively. Flexor carpi radialis: FCR, flexor digitorum superficialis: FDS, flexor pollicis longus: FPL.

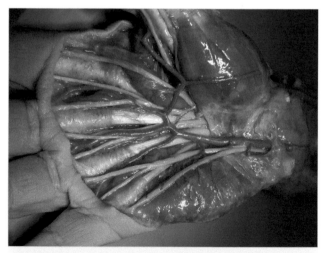

Fig. 28.4 In the palm, the tendons of the FDS are deep to the superficial palmar arch and the digital branches of the median and ulnar nerves, and superficial to the tendons of the FDP along with lumbricals and the deep palmar arch.

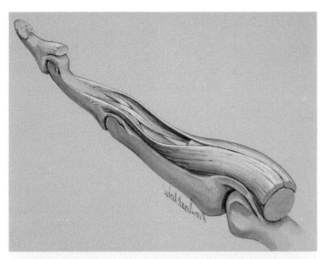

Fig. 28.5 This diagram shows the orientation of the FDS tendon in the digit and its relationship to the FDP tendon. The anatomy and fiber orientation of the "bifurca" and the Camper Chiasma are clearly seen. (Copyright Kleinert Institute, Louisville, KY).

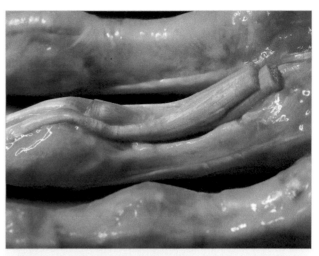

Fig. 28.7 Relationship of the FDS and the FDP. The FDP tendon is passing thru the "bifurca" of the FDS.

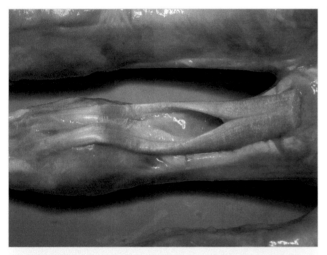

Fig. 28.6 Dissection showing the anatomy of the FDS tendon in the digit. The anatomy and the fiber orientation of the "bifurca" and the Camper's Chiasma are well visualized.

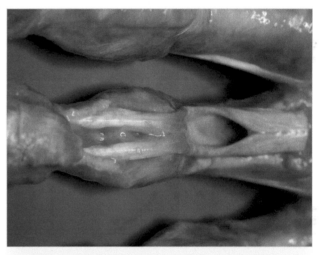

Fig. 28.8 View of the FDS at the level of the proximal phalanx and the PIP joint showing the "bifurca" and the Camper's Chiasma and the insertion of the FDS onto the base of the middle phalanx.

index or ring finger FDS.[33] The maximum excursion of the FDS tendon in adults is 6.4 cm.[10]

Variations: Most variations of the FDS involve the muscle belly. They include accessory muscle slips that connect the muscle to other forearm flexors, absence of the radial head, and the presence of anomalous muscles in the palm that can result in carpal tunnel syndrome.[30] The muscle belly and/or the tendon to the small finger may be absent. The prevalence of absence of FDS to the small finger can vary from 6.5% in Asian populations up to 21% in Caucasian populations.[37]

Clinical correlations: When evaluating an injured hand for the presence of a flexor tendon injury, one must differentiate between an injury to the FDS and the FDP. The FDP can be easily evaluated by checking flexion of the distal interphalangeal joint (DIP), as it is the only flexor of that joint. Testing for injury to the FDS is more complex, because the PIP joint is flexed both by the FDS and the FDP. Therefore, one needs to check the function of the FDS while blocking the action of the FDP. The standard

test for the FDS takes advantage of the fact that the FDP tendons to the long, ring, and small fingers share a common muscle belly and lack independent function. The finger being tested is allowed to flex while the examiner blocks the action of the FDP tendon by preventing flexion of the DIP joint of the other two fingers. The standard test is not reliable for the index finger, because the index finger FDP has an independent muscle belly. In addition, the action of the FDS to the small finger may be dependent on the FDS to the ring finger, and they may need to be tested together.[38] We prefer to use the test described by Mishra to evaluate the FDS.[39] In this test, the subject is asked to press the fingertip pulp of all the fingers together against the proximal part of the palm, such that the DIP joint is kept extended. If the FDS is acting, the DIP joint remains in a position of extension to hypertension while the MCP and PIP joints are fully flexed. If the FDS of any of the fingers is injured or absent, the DIP joint flexes. This test works on the principle that the FDP can flex the PIP joint only after it has flexed the DIP joint.

If the DIP joint is maintained in extension, PIP joint flexion is purely a function of the FDS.

The FDS tendon is often used is a motor for tendon transfers, because it is believed to have an independent function, making it easy to retrain, and its function at the donor finger can be taken over by the FDP. However as previously mentioned, only the FDS tendon to the middle finger is truly independent. The index and small finger FDS tendons are closely linked as they arise from a common proximal muscle. They have independence only of their distal fibers. If one of these tendons is transferred to the dorsal side of the forearm (nonsynergistic transfers), only the distal fibers would transfer, as the proximal muscle belly would need to simultaneously be a flexor and an extensor. In addition, the index finger FDS is necessary for pulp pinch with the thumb and the small finger FDS is quite slender and often absent. For these reasons, the FDS tendons to the long or ring finger are preferred for tendon transfers. The FDS to the long finger is most suited for nonsynergistic transfers. One must also be aware of the morbidity associated with these transfers. The loss of FDS can result in a swan neck deformity in mobile hands from loss of the volar restraint and a PIP joint flexion contracture from tenodesis of the stump of the divided FDS. The loss of FDS of the middle finger will result in inability to perform a chuck grip (pulp-to-pulp pinch between the index finger, middle finger, and thumb), and the loss of the ring finger FDS may result in a decrease in grip strength. The use of the ring finger FDS for a transfer to the dorsum of the forearm or hand may require division of the band of muscle fibers that often connects it to the digastric tendon in the midforearm.[33,40]

28.1.5 Flexor Digitorum Profundus

Etymology: Flexor is derived from the Latin word *flexus,* meaning "bent" (thus flexor indicates "that which bends," or "bending"). Digitorum is derived from the Latin word *digitus* or *digitorum,* indicating the digits. Profundus is derived from the Latin word *profundus,* indicating "deep," and refers to the muscle location in a deeper plane in the forearm.

Origin: The myotendinous junction of the FDP is in the midforearm, and the four FDP tendons arise parallel to each other. The muscle bellies of the long, ring, and small finger FDPs are connected to one another, whereas the index finger FDP is relatively independent.

Course: The four tendons extend distally parallel to each other and deep to the tendons of the FDS in the forearm. After passing through the carpal tunnel, the tendons diverge toward their respective digits. The long and ring finger FDP tendons are linked closely and share tendon fibers in the distal forearm. There may also be interconnected tendinous cross-connections in the carpal tunnel. In the palm, they are deep to the FDS, the superficial palmar arch, and the digital branches of the median and ulnar nerves but superficial to the deep palmar arch (▶ Fig. 28.4). The lumbrical muscles arise from the FDP tendons in the palm. The first and second lumbricals innervated by the median nerve (from the sensory branches) are unipennate and arise from the radial border of the FDP tendons to the index and long fingers, respectively. The third and fourth lumbricals innervated by the ulnar nerve are bipennate and arise from contiguous sides of the long/ring finger FDP and the ring/small finger

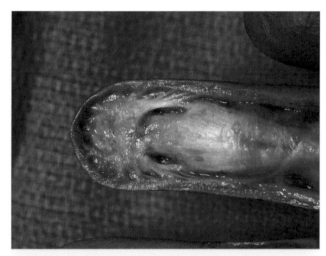

Fig. 28.9 At its insertion, The FDP tendon divides into two and has a broad insertion to the volar aspect of the distal phalanx.

FDP, respectively. At the level of the MCP joint, the FDP tendon passes between the two slips of the FDS to become palmar to the FDS (▶ Fig. 28.6 and ▶ Fig. 28.7).

Insertion: The FDP tendon is divided into two slips and inserted into the palmar surface of the proximal third of the distal phalanx (▶ Fig. 28.9).

Characteristics: The FDP is the largest and strongest of all forearm muscles and about 50% stronger than the FDS. The FDP is mainly a flexor of the finger joints with limited MCP joint and wrist flexion. Electromyographic studies have shown that the FDP performs most of the unloaded flexion movement of the fingers, whereas the FDS comes in when more strength is needed and powers individual finger motion.[41] The maximum excursion of the FCR tendon in adults is 7 cm.[10]

Variations: Variations of the FDP are less frequently observed than variations of the FDS. In addition to accessory muscles and tendinous slips from the FDP to the radius, FPL, and so forth, an anomalous accessory FDP tendon lying ulnar to the FDP to the index finger and a rare congenital anomaly of the FDP causing a flexion contracture of the long and ring fingers have been reported.

Clinical correlations: Avulsion of the FDP tendon commonly involves the ring finger. Many reasons have been offered as to why this injury frequently occurs in the ring finger. The ring finger becomes the longest digit in grip and absorbs more force than other fingers. The FDP insertion of the ring finger is weaker than that of the middle finger. The small finger is protected because it slips away during forcible grasp and the index finger has an independent FDP muscle belly. The ring finger also has limited independent range of motion, because (1) it is closely linked to the long and small finger FDP bellies, (2) it has a bipennate lumbrical, and (3) it has juncturae tendinae on both sides.[42]

28.1.6 Flexor Pollicis Longus

Etymology: Flexor is derived from the Latin word *flexus,* meaning "bent" (thus flexor indicates "that which bends," or "bending"). Pollicis is derived from the Latin word *pollex,* indicating thumb. Longus is again the Latin for "long." The FPL is the longest flexor of the thumb.[3,4]

Origin: The FPL has a long and variable musculotendinous junction that extends from mid forearm to the distal forearm. The unipennate muscle fibers lie on the deep and radial side of the tendon. In 45 to 60% of subjects, an accessory head of the FPL known as Gantzer muscle may join the proximal end of the FPL tendon.[43]

Course: The FPL tendon extends distally in the same plane as the tendons of the FDP and is the most radial flexor tendon (▶Fig. 28.3). It is located radial to the median nerve and the FDP in the carpal tunnel. After passing through the carpal tunnel, it passes deep to the superficial palmar arch and the opponens pollicis and between the superficial and deep heads of the flexor pollicis brevis. It then enters its fibro-osseous sheath and passes between the two sesamoid bones of the thumb.

Insertion: The FPL tendon inserts into the palmar surface of the base of the distal phalanx.

Characteristics: The FPL is the sole flexor of the thumb IP joint. However, the strength of thumb pinch arises mainly from the adductor pollicis and the flexor pollicis brevis that together have one-third more tension capability than the FPL.[44] The maximum excursion of the FPL tendon in adults is 5 cm.[10]

Variations: The most common variation of the FPL tendon is an anomalous connection between the FPL and the index finger FDP tendon in the forearm. This was described by Linburg and Comstock in 1979, and individuals with this anomaly are unable to independently flex the thumb and index finger.[45,46] The incidence of this anomaly can vary from 20 to 37% depending on the population studied. Most cases are asymptomatic, but this anomaly can be problematic in musicians or security staff. The surgical division of this interconnection and any associated thickened tenosynovium is effective treatment. Other rare anomalies of the FPL tendon include absence of the FPL, usually seen in patients with a hypoplastic thumb, and anomalous insertions into the proximal and distal phalanx, the carpal tunnel, and the extensor pollicis longus.[1]

Clinical correlations: The FPL tendon is more difficult to repair and has a potential for a poorer result than seen with other flexor tendons. Many reasons have been proposed for this. The proximal end of the FPL tendon retracts to a greater extent compared with the other tendons, as there are no restraints on retraction. In addition, authors have noted a greater tendency for shortening of the FPL muscle and have had considerable difficulty in pulling the proximal tendon end out to length when FPL repair is attempted after 48 hours.[47] The stress on repaired finger flexor tendons is relieved by using other uninjured fingers, and each finger has only to generate 25% of the total force that the fingers exert together. However, the repaired thumb flexor tendon has to withstand the entire normal power.[48]

In a patient with a thumb laceration and a divided FPL tendon, it is prudent to make an incision in the wrist crease to look for the retracted proximal end instead of blindly groping in the thenar muscles. The FPL tendon can be easily identified below the FCR radial to the FDP. The FPL tendon has an extensive vinculum brevis over the distal third of the proximal phalanx. If the FPL tendon is avulsed or divided within 2.5 cm of its insertion on the distal phalanx, the intact vinculum brevis will keep the FPL tethered at the laceration site and transmit some of the pulling force of the tendon to the distal phalanx. However, this

flexion force is less than normal and can easily be detected by applying resistance.

An attritional rupture of the FPL tendon is classically associated with rheumatoid arthritis and results from attrition from a scaphoid osteophyte. This is also known as Mannerfelt lesion. The rising use of volar locking plates for fixation of distal radius fractures has seen an increase in reports of the attritional ruptures of the FPL tendon. This usually results from placement of the plates beyond the watershed line of the distal radius. At this level, it is difficult to cover the implant adequately with soft tissue or the pronator quadratus muscle.[49]

28.2 Flexor Sheath

The flexor tendon sheath is a unique, closed, mesenteric system that surrounds the digital flexor tendons (FDS, FDP, and FPL). The flexor sheath has two major components, namely the synovial (membranous) component and the retinacular (pulley) component. The synovial layer is thin and begins at the level of the wrist. The retinacular layer is thicker, consisting of a series of fibrous tissue condensations also known as pulleys. It begins at the neck of the metacarpal and lies superficial to the synovial component.[50] The combination of the synovial and retinacular components distal to the neck of the metacarpal results in the formation of a fibro-osseous tunnel for the passage of the flexor tendons. The floor of this fibro-osseous tunnel is formed by the transverse metacarpal ligament; the volar plates of the MCP joint, PIP joint, and DIP joint; and the palmar surfaces of the proximal and middle phalanxes. This fibro-osseous tunnel is also known as the digital flexor sheath and has three important functions. First, it allows for smooth gliding of digital flexor tendons (FDS, FDP, and FPL) in flexion and extension. Second, it provides a pulley that prevents bowstringing of the flexor tendon and improves the mechanical advantage during flexion. Third, it plays a nutritive role by providing a contained bursal environment for synovial fluid.[51]

28.2.1 Synovial (Membranous) Component

The synovial component is a double-walled synovial tube that is sealed at both ends. The inner layer of synovium is in close proximity to the surface of the flexor tendon and is known as the visceral layer, while the outer layer of synovium is related to the overlying retinacular layer and is known as the parietal layer. The visceral and parietal layers form a series of culde-sacs. There are two main cul-de-sacs at either end of the digital flexor sheath as well as a series of cul-de-sacs at either end of each of the pulleys. The proximal cul-de-sac is a double cul-de-sac to accommodate both flexor tendons and begins 10 to 14 mm proximal to end of the metacarpal head. The culde-sacs allow for lengthening and contraction of the synovial component during flexion and extension.[51] The synovial layers were thickest in the space between the pulleys, due to the formation of the cul-de-sacs, and thin and attenuated under the pulleys.

Amis and Jones found that the synovial component did not have a continuous smooth internal surface. It did not attach directly to the edge of the pulleys but rather overlapped it, resulting in the formation of a free floppy synovial edges at the margins of the pulleys. The largest of these overlaps occurred at the distal end of the A2 pulley. The authors hypothesized that sutured or partially cut tendons could trigger on this free edge, and this could be a major contributor to the failure of tendon repairs in zone 2.[52]

The synovial component for all digits ends at the level of the DIP joint. Robb examined the relationship of the termination of the synovial component and the insertion of the FDP and FPL and found that the synovial component extended till the insertion in only 41% of digits.[53] The synovial components of the index, long, and ring fingers begin along with the retinacular component of these fingers (metacarpal neck). However, the thumb and small finger synovial components begin at the level of the wrist.

The thumb synovial component begins 2 cm proximal to the radial styloid and the portion of the synovial sheath covering the FPL tendon from the wrist till the thumb MCP joint is known as the radial bursa. Similarly, the small finger synovial sheath begins at the same level as the radial bursa (2 cm proximal to the wrist crease) and is continuous with the synovial sheath covering the FDS and FDP in the palm and the wrist. This portion of the synovial sheath is known as the ulnar bursa and continues distally to the region of the mid palm for the ring, long, and index fingers. It then continues as the small finger synovial sheath beyond the metacarpal neck.[54] In a study of 367 hands using air insufflation, Scheldrup found communication between the radial and ulnar bursa in 85% of hands. The pattern already described was the most common pattern, being noted in 71.4% of hands. The ulnar bursa communicated with the small finger in 81%, the ring finger in 3.5%, the middle finger in 4%, and the index finger in 5.2% of cases.[55]

The visceral and parietal layers of the synovial component form a closed system filled with synovial fluid. The synovial fluid acts both as a lubricating agent and a nutritional agent, and the synovial layers act as a dialyzing membrane that allows the diffusion of nutrients. This is especially important in the avascular friction surfaces of the tendon and pulleys.[56]

Clinical correlations: The synovial component of the flexor tendon sheath provides an ideal environment for bacterial growth. It is closed and has poor blood supply, and the synovial fluid provides nutrition. Any infection within the synovial sheath rapidly destroys the gliding mechanism and the blood supply leading to necrosis of the tendons. This can lead to formation of adhesions and severe limitation of motion. If left untreated, infection can spread along the tendon sheath to the radial and/or ulnar bursa leading to a horseshoe abscess. The synovial sheath may rupture in the distal forearm and discharge the purulent contents into the space of Parona. The space of Parona is a potential space in the distal forearm superficial to the pronator quadratus and deep to the FDP tendons.[57]

28.2.2 Retinacular (Pulley) Component

The retinacular component consists of a series of thickenings of fibrous tissue that overlies the synovial component. These thickenings are known as pulleys. The retinacular component begins at the neck of the metacarpal and ends at the level of the DIP joint (IP joint for the thumb). It is segmental and not continuous, and each segment is represented by a pulley. The pulleys have been classified into four types based on their appearance: transverse, annular, cruciate, and oblique.[50,51]

Retinacular System of the Fingers

The retinacular component of the fingers includes one transverse pulley, five annular pulleys, and three cruciate pulleys. The transverse pulley is also known as the PA pulley (▶Fig. 28.10). The annular pulleys are numbered from proximal to distal as A1, A2, A3, A4, and A5, (▶Fig 28.11) whereas the cruciate pulleys are numbered from proximal to distal as C1, C2, and C3 (▶Fig. 28.12, and ▶Fig. 28.13). The relationship of the pulleys to the retinacular system of the digit is depicted in ▶Fig. 28.11. The arrangement of the pulleys from proximal to distal for the fingers is PA, A1, A2, C1, A3, C2, A4, C3, and A5, respectively.

Palmar aponeurosis pulley: This pulley is formed by the transverse fibers of the PA. It is located 1 to 3 mm distal to the beginning of the synovial component at the level of the metacarpal neck. It is approximately 10 mm long and anchored on each side by the vertical fibers of Legueu and Juvara that attach to the deep transverse metacarpal ligament (▶Fig. 28.10). This pulley is not as closely applied to tendon as the other pulleys; however, close approximation was noted with increased tension on the PA as in grasping.[50] The average breaking strength of the PA pulley was found to be 16.5 kg. The loss of flexion increases from 5.7%, seen with absence of A1 and A2 pulleys, to 12.6%, seen with absence of PA, A1, and A2 pulleys.[58]

Annular pulleys: The odd-numbered annular pulleys (A1, A3, and A5) are present over the joints (MCP, PIP, and DIP) respectively, whereas the even-numbered annular pulleys (A2 and A4) are located over the shafts of the proximal and middle phalanx, respectively. The A1 pulley begins over the distal third of the volar plate of the MCP joint, with two-thirds of the fibers arising from the volar plate and one-third from the proximal portion of the palmar plate. The average length of the A1 pulley is 8 to 11 mm (▶Fig. 28.14 and ▶Fig. 28.15). The usual configuration for the A1 pulley is a single pulley, although occasionally it may be represented by two or three annular bands. The average breaking strength of the A1 pulley is 31.6 kg. The A2 pulley begins immediately after the A1 pulley, and the separation between them may range from 0.4 to 4.1 mm

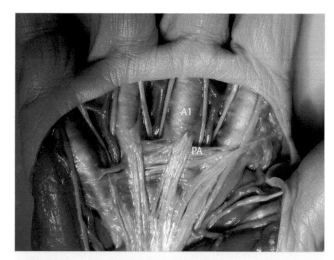

Fig. 28.10 Palmar Aponeurosis (PA) pulley.

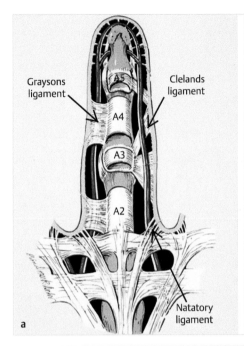

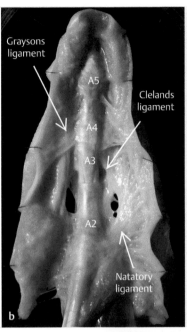

Fig. 28.11 (a, b) Diagram and dissection showing the relationship of the annular pulleys to the retinacular system of the digit. (a. Diagram Copyright Kleinert Institute, Louisville, KY).

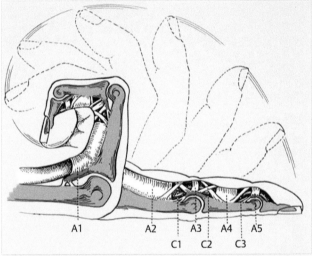

Fig. 28.12 Diagram showing all the pulleys in the digit and their alignment in flexion and extension of the finger. (Copyright Kleinert Institute, Louisville, KY).

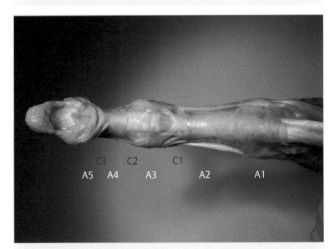

Fig. 28.13 Dissection showing the annular and cruciate pulleys in the digit.

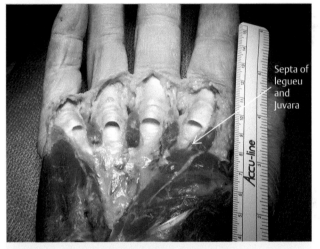

Fig. 28.14 Dissection of the entrance to the pulley system in the digit showing A1 pulley with the tendons removed.

(►Fig. 28.12 and ►Fig. 28.16). The A2 pulley is located over the shaft of the proximal phalanx. The average length of the A2 pulley is 16.8 mm, and it is distinctly thicker at the distal end. The average breaking strength of the A2 pulley is 14 kg. The A3 pulley is located over the PIP joint (►Fig. 28.17). The average length is 2.8 mm, and the average breaking strength is 7.1 kg. The A4 pulley is located over the midportion of the middle phalanx and it is 6.7 mm in length and thickest in the midportion (►Fig. 28.18). The average breaking strength of the A4 pulley is 19.7 kg. The A5 pulley is thin, arises from the volar plate of the DIP joint, and measures 4.1 mm in length.[59,60] The A1 and A2 pulleys are constant, whereas A3 was noted in 87%, A4 in 98%, and A5 in 93% of specimens.[50]

Cruciate pulleys: Two patterns of cruciate pulleys have been identified. They may either be a single oblique loop or Y- shaped (ypsiliform). The three cruciate pulleys (C1, C2, and C3) are located at the distal ends of the A2, A3, and A4 pulleys, respectively (►Fig. 28.12 and ►Fig. 28.17). These cruciate pulleys can become narrower and accommodate the annular pulleys during

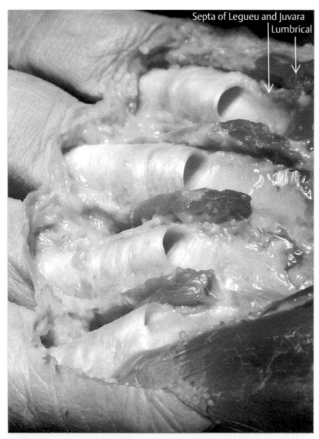

Fig. 28.15 The A1 pulleys and the A2 pulleys. The septa of Legueu and Juvara and the lumbricals are visible.

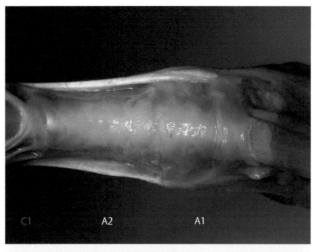

Fig. 28.16 The A1, A2, and C1 pulleys.

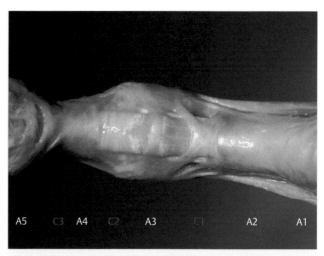

Fig. 28.17 The annular and cruciate pulleys of the digit.

acute flexion. The C3 pulley may not always be a separate structure from the A4 pulley.[50]

Nourishment of the Flexor Tendons

The flexor tendons in the synovial sheath are nourished by the synovial fluid. In addition, the dorsal aspects of the tendons are nourished by blood vessels through the vincula longae (long vincula) and vincula brevia (short vincula) (▶ Fig. 28.18a and b).

Retinacular System of the Thumb

The retinacular component of the thumb includes two annular pulleys and one oblique pulley. The arrangement of the pulleys from proximal to distal for the thumb is A1 (▶ Fig. 28.19), oblique pulley, and A2, respectively (▶ Fig. 28.20). The A1 pulley of the thumb arises partly from the volar plate of the thumb MCP joint and partly from the base of the proximal phalanx. It is 7 to 9 mm long and 0.5 mm thick. The oblique pulley is located over the proximal phalanx and measures 9 to 11 mm in length and 0.5 to 0.75 mm in thickness. The A2 pulley is located over the thumb IP joint and arises from the volar plate. It is relatively thin and measures 8 to 10 mm in length and 0.25 mm in thickness.[54] A study on serial sectioning of the thumb pulleys suggested that the oblique pulley was the most important.[54,61] A recent publication has indicated that there is an additional pulley, the so-called variable annular pulley (Av) between the A1 pulley and the oblique pulley. They suggest that the Av pulley may need to be preserved to prevent bowstringing in patients that undergo A1 pulley release for the treatment of trigger thumb[62] (▶ Fig. 28.20, ▶ Fig. 28.21, ▶ Fig. 28.22, ▶ Fig. 28.23).

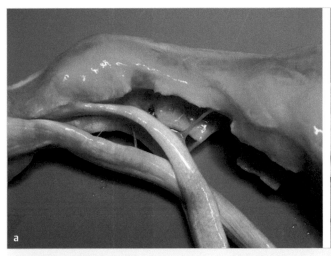

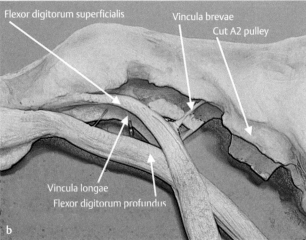

Fig. 28.18 (a, b) The vincula longae and the vincula brevia.

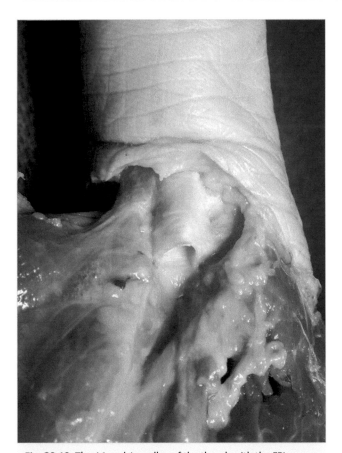

Fig. 28.19 The A1 and Av pulley of the thumb with the FPL tendon removed.

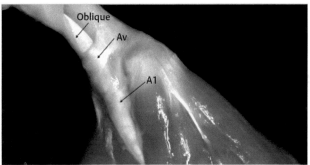

Fig. 28.20 The A1, Av, and Oblique pulley of the thumb.

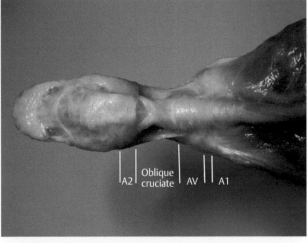

Fig. 28.21 The A1, Av, the Cruciate pulley in place of the classic oblique pulley and A2 pulley. Broad insertion of the FPL on the distal phalanx.

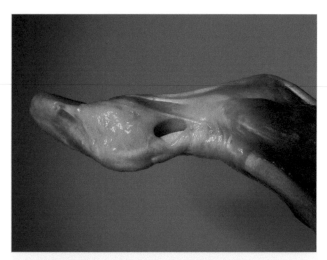

Fig. 28.22 Oblique view of the pulleys of the thumb and FPL tendon. FPL: flexor pollicis longus.

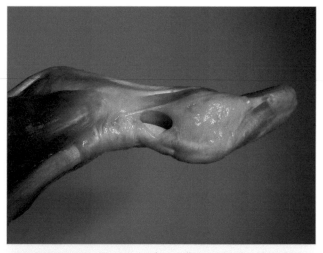

Fig. 28.23 A1, Av, Cruciate, and A2 pulleys of the thumb and FPL. FPL: flexor pollicis longus

References

1. Doyle JR. Forearm. In: Doyle JR, Botte MJ, eds. Surgical Anatomy of the Hand and Upper Extremity. Philadelphia, PA: Lippincott Williams and Wilkins; 2003:407–460

2. Bates SJ, Laurencin CT, Chang J. Flexor tendon anatomy. Medscape reference. 2011. http://emedicine.medscape.com/article/1245236-overview#aw2aab6b3

3. Dorland's Illustrated Medical Dictionary. 32nd ed. Philadelphia, PA: WB Saunders, Elsevier; 2011

4. Stedman's Medical Dictionary. 28th ed. Baltimore, MD: Williams and Wilkins; 2005

5. Bishop AT, Gabel G, Carmichael SW. Flexor carpi radialis tendinitis. Part I: Operative anatomy. J Bone Joint Surg Am 1994;76(7):1009–1014

6. Schmidt HM. Clinical anatomy of the m. flexor carpi radialis tendon sheath. Acta Morphol Neerl Scand 1987;25(1):17–28

7. Nigro RO. Anatomy of the flexor retinaculum of the wrist and the flexor carpi radialis tunnel. Hand Clin 2001;17(1):61–64, vi

8. Lantieri L, Hennebert H, Le Viet D, Guérin-Surville H. A study of the orientation of the fibers of the flexor carpi radialis tendon: anatomy and clinical applications. Surg Radiol Anat 1993;15(2):85–89

9. Simovitch R, Abel M, Arslan O, Frank C. Pulley anatomy for the radial side of the wrist. Clin Anat 2001;14(4):246–247

10. Bunnell S. Surgery of the Hand. 5th ed. Philadelphia, PA: J B Lippincott; 1956

11. Rumball KM, Tonkin MA. Absence of flexor carpi radialis. J Hand Surg [Br] 1996;21(6):778

12. Ho SY, Yeo CJ, Sebastin SJ, Tan TC, Lim AY. The flexor carpi radialisbrevis muscle—an anomaly in forearm musculature: a review article. Hand Surg 2011;16(3):245–249

13. Irwin LR, Outhwaite J, Burge PD. Rupture of the flexor carpi radialis tendon associated with scapho-trapezial osteoarthritis. J Hand Surg [Br] 1992;17(3):343–345

14. Umarji S, Pickford M. Re: a novel technique for harvesting a split flexor carpi radialis (FCR) tendon graft. J Hand Surg Eur Vol 2008;33(6):817–818

15. Eaton RG, Littler JW. Ligament reconstruction for the painful thumb carpometacarpal joint. J Bone Joint Surg Am 1973;55(8):1655–1666

16. Garcia-Elias M, Lluch AL, Stanley JK. Three-ligament tenodesis for the treatment of scapholunate dissociation: indications and surgical technique. J Hand Surg Am 2006;31(1):125–134

17. Brunelli GA, Brunelli GR. [A new surgical technique for carpal instability with scapho-lunar dislocation. (Eleven cases)]. Ann Chir Main Memb Super 1995;14(4-5):207–213

18. Lim AY, Lahiri A, Pereira BP, Kumar VP, Tan LL. Independent function in a split flexor carpi radialis transfer. J Hand Surg Am 2004;29(1):28–31

19. Ito MM, Aoki M, Kida MY, Ishii S, Kumaki K, Tanaka S. Length and width of the tendinous portion of the palmaris longus: a cadaver study of adult Japanese. J Hand Surg Am 2001;26(4):706–710

20. Stecco C, Lancerotto L, Porzionato A, et al. The palmaris longus muscle and its relations with the antebrachial fascia and the palmar aponeurosis. Clin Anat 2009;22(2):221–229

21. Wehbé MA. Tendon graft donor sites. J Hand Surg Am 1992;17(6):1130–1132

22. Carlson GD, Botte MJ, Josephs MS, Newton PO, Davis JL, Woo SL. Morphologic and biomechanical comparison of tendons used as free grafts. J Hand Surg Am 1993;18(1):76–82

23. Sebastin SJ, Puhaindran ME, Lim AY, Lim IJ, Bee WH. The prevalence of absence of the palmaris longus—a study in a Chinese population and a review of the literature. J Hand Surg Am 2005;30B(5):525–527

24. Reiman AF, Daseler EJ, Anson BJ, Beaton LE. The palmaris longus muscle and tendon: a study of 1600 extremities. Anat Rec 1944;89:495–505

25. Sebastin S. Chung KC. Tendon transfers for carpal tunnel syndrome. In: Chung K, ed. Operative Techniques in Hand and Wrist Surgery. 2nd ed. Philadelphia, PA: Elsevier Saunders; 2011:166–173

26. Sebastin S, Chung KC. Tendon transfers for radial nerve palsy. In: Chung KC, ed. Operative Techniques in Hand and Wrist Surgery. Philadelphia, PA: Elsevier Saunders; 2011:200–208

27. Sebastin SJ, Lim AY. Clinical assessment of the palmaris longus—too many newer techniques? J Plast Reconstr Aesthet Surg 2006;59(7):784–786

28. Loren GJ, Lieber RL. Tendon biomechanical properties enhance human wrist muscle specialization. J Biomech 1995;28(7):791–799

29. Shin AY, Deitch MA, Sachar K, Boyer MI. Ulnar-sided wrist pain. Diagnosis and treatment. J Bone Joint Surg 2004;86A:1560–1574

30. Botte MJ. Muscle anatomy. In: Doyle JR, Botte MJ, eds. Surgical Anatomy of the Hand and Upper Extremity. Philadelphia, PA: Lippincott Williams and Wilkins; 2003:111–129

31. Budoff JE, Kraushaar BS, Ayala G. Flexor carpi ulnaris tendinopathy. J Hand Surg Am 2005;30(1):125–129

32. Lim AY, Kumar VP, Sebastin SJ, Kapickis M. Split flexor carpi ulnaris transfer: a new functioning free muscle transfer with independent dual function. Plast Reconstr Surg 2006;117(6):1927–1932

33. Brand PW, Hollister A. Mechanics of individual muscles at individual joints. In: Brand PW, Hollister A, eds. Clinical Mechanics of the Hand. 2nd ed. St. Louis, MO: CV Mosby; 1985:317–319

34. Yu HL, Chase RA, Strauch B. Extrinsic digital flexors. In: Yu HL, Chase RA, Strauch B, eds. Atlas of Hand Anatomy and Clinical Implications. St. Louis, MO: Mosby, Elsevier; 2004:284–299

35. Shrewsbury MM, Kuczynski K. Flexor digitorum superficialis tendon in the fingers of the human hand. Hand 1974;6(2):121–133

36. Gonzalez MH, Nikoleit J, Weinzweig N. The chiasma of the flexor digitorum superficialis tendon. J Hand Surg [Br] 1998;23(2): 234–236

37. Sebastin SJ, Lim AY. Clinical assessment of absence of the palmaris longus and its association with other anatomical anomalies—a Chinese population study. Ann Acad Med Singapore 2006;35(4):249–253

38. Sebastin SJ, Chung KC. Examination of the hand and wrist. In: Chung KC, ed. Hand and Wrist Surgery—Operative Techniques. 2nd ed. Philadelphia, PA: Elsevier; 2012:2–12

39. Mishra S. A new test for demonstrating the action of flexor digitorum superficialis (FDS) tendon. J Plast Reconstr Aesthet Surg 2006;59(12):1342–1344

40. Malaviya GN. Flexor digitorum superficialis—revisited. Indian J Lepr 2005;77(4):305–316

41. Long C II, Conrad PW, Hall EA, Furler SL. Intrinsic-extrinsic muscle control of the hand in power grip and precision handling. An electromyographic study. J Bone Joint Surg Am 1970;52(5):853–867

42. Manske PR, Lesker PA. Avulsion of the ring finger flexor digitorum profundus tendon: an experimental study. Hand 1978;10(1): 52–55

43. Dykes J, Anson BJ. The accessory tendon of the flexor pollicis longus muscle. Anat Rec 1944;90:83–89

44. Fahrer M. The thenar eminence. In: Tubiana R, ed. The Hand. Vol 1. Philadelphia, PA: W B Saunders; 1981

45. Low TH, Faruk Senan NA, Ahmad TS. The Linburg-Comstock anomaly: incidence in Malaysians and effect on pinch strength. J Hand Surg Am 2012;37(5):930–932

46. Linburg RM, Comstock BE. Anomalous tendon slips from the flexor pollicis longus to the flexor digitorum profundus. J Hand Surg Am 1979;4(1):79–83

47. Sirotakova M, Elliot D. Early active mobilization of primary repairs of the flexor pollicis longus tendon. J Hand Surg [Br] 1999;24(6):647–653

48. Nancarrow D. Repair of the flexor pollicis longus tendon. J Hand Surg [Br] 2000;25(4):409–410

49. Matityahu AM, Lapalme SN, Seth A, Marmor MT, Buckley JM, Lattanza LL. How placement affects force and contact pressure between a volar plate of the distal radius and the flexor pollicus longus tendon: a biomechanical investigation. J Hand Surg Am 2012

50. Doyle JR. Anatomy of the finger flexor tendon sheath and pulley system. J Hand Surg Am 1988;13(4):473–484

51. Strauch B, de Moura W. Digital flexor tendon sheath: an anatomic study. J Hand Surg Am 1985;10(6 Pt 1):785–789

52. Amis AA, Jones MM. The interior of the flexor tendon sheath of the finger. The functional significance of its structure. J Bone Joint Surg Br 1988;70(4):583–587

53. Robb JE. The termination of flexor tendon sheaths. Hand 1979;11(1):17–21

54. Doyle JR, Blythe WF. Anatomy of the flexor tendon sheath and pulleys of the thumb. J Hand Surg Am 1977;2(2):149–151

55. Scheldrup EW. Tendon sheath patterns in the hand; an anatomical study based on 367 hand dissections. Surg Gynecol Obstet 1951;93(1):16–22

56. Lundborg G, Myrhage R. The vascularization and structure of the human digital tendon sheath as related to flexor tendon function. An angiographic and histological study. Scand J Plast Reconstr Surg 1977;11(3):195–203

57. Ono S, Sebastin SJ, Chung KC. Overview of hand infections. In: Butler CE, ed. UpToDate. Waltham, MA: UpToDate; 2012

58. Manske PR, Lesker PA. Palmar aponeurosis pulley. J Hand Surg Am 1983;8(3):259–263

59. Manske PR, Lesker PA. Strength of human pulleys. Hand 1977;9(2):147–152

60. Doyle JR. Anatomy of the flexor tendon sheath and pulley system: a current review. J Hand Surg Am 1989;14(2 Pt 2):349–351

61. Zissimos AG, Szabo RM, Yinger KE, Sharkey NA. Biomechanics of the thumb flexor pulley system. J Hand Surg Am 1994;19(3): 475–479

62. Bayat A, Shaaban H, Giakas G, Lees VC. The pulley system of the thumb: anatomic and biomechanical study. J Hand Surg Am 2002;27(4):628–635

29 The Extensor Tendons

David Elliot

29.1 Introduction

If one looks at the development of the extensor mechanism from amphibian to mammal and from monkey to man and also observes the difference between the extensors of our feet and our hands, one realizes that the function of this system in the hand has been continually changing throughout evolution. When mammals crawled onto land, then walked on four feet, the extensors of the wrists and ankles were needed to swing the proximal part of the limb and the body forward over the wrist, after which the extensors of the digits were needed to hyperextend the metacarpophalangeal (MCP) and metatarsophalangeal (MTP) joints as the digital flexors propelled the forward-moving animal off the ground. When apes began to stand on two legs, the relative importance of this function diminished for the front feet, which were now becoming hands, and was increasingly replaced by grasping function as they swung from tree to tree. However, hyperextending MCP joints remained useful for four-limbed running. When we moved out of the trees and the hand became entirely an instrument of prehension, sophisticated by development of the opposing thumb, the MCP joints stiffened and lost much of their hyperextensibility and the extensor system of the hand became largely reduced in importance to a means of setting the flexed digits back to rest and opening the hand sufficiently for the now-dominant flexor system to start the next grasping and/or opposing activity.

While the proximal extensor system in the hand was becoming less important, the one in the finger was evolving into a very complicated system of control which allows us to stack bones, one on top of another, and control their fall forward into flexion, stopping this at any point to allow us to maintain fixed positions of the fingers with variable degrees of flexion of the three joints of the fingers. If you consider each finger as a series of four building bricks sitting on top of each other, it requires a very complicated engineering system to hold four bricks in a position of partial flexion of each brick/brick surface indefinitely, with the bricks in a half falling position, then allow variation of the relative position of the bricks slowly and periodically. This system of control has fallen to the extensor complex in the finger.

It is so complex that few of us fully understand it, and it becomes a headache if injured, unless repaired immediately and before it sets the fingers into various collapsed positions. The anatomy alone, as is elaborated further in this chapter, suggests that this system is complex: the MCP joint has an extensor which works not by direct attachment to the proximal phalanx but rather by lifting a loop around the palmar surface of the base of the proximal phalanx. The proximal interphalangeal (PIP) joint is extended by not one but indeed four muscles: a long extensor that works well with the MCP flexed but not extended, two interossei, and a lumbrical that links the system to the flexor system in a manner whose exact function is debated. These four PIP extensors are linked and interwoven

in a complex manner, with two of the three end parts able to slide up and down the lateral edges of the PIP joint. The distal interphalangeal (DIP) joint has two extensors, each of which has contributions from all four of the muscles that extend the PIP, such that DIP extension is inevitably linked to extension of the PIP. Moreover, Landsmeer's oblique ligament, linking the palmar side of the PIP to the extensor side of the DIP, connects the two joints such that they must move simultaneously and in a linked manner. This complexity has fascinated many of the greatest hand surgeons of the last century, and a great deal has been written about both its anatomy and the failures of this system as a result of pathology or injury.[1-19]

29.2 The Extensors Proximal to the Fingers

29.2.1 Extensor Retinaculum

This structure is discussed first, as it is integral to discussion of all of the wrist and long digital extensors. The extensor retinaculum is a strong fibrous band extending obliquely across the back of the wrist. Its purpose is to prevent the extensor tendons bowstringing away from the skeleton or displacing excessively in a radial or ulnar direction on activation of their muscles proximally (▶Fig. 29.1).[20,21,22,23] It is a strengthened part of the fascia of the forearm (▶Fig. 29.2) that attaches radially to the anterior border of the radius bone (▶Fig. 29.3) and to the triquetral and pisiform bones at its ulnar end (▶Fig. 29.4). Along its course, it attaches to a series of ridges on the dorsum of the radius

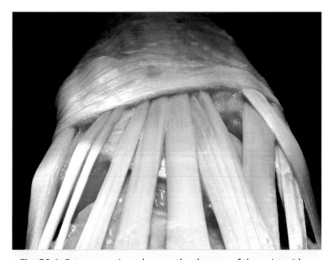

Fig. 29.1 Extensor retinaculum on the dorsum of the wrist with the extensor tendons going distally. This dissection shows 2nd dorsal compartment (ECRL, ECRB), 3rd dorsal compartment (EPL), 4th dorsal compartment (EDC and EI), 5th dorsal compartment (EDM) and 6th dorsal compartment (ECU).

and ulna (▶Fig. 29.5), creating six tunnels through which the extensor tendons pass (▶Fig. 29.6), with the tendons lying between grooves on the dorsal surfaces of the distal parts of the forearm bones and the overlying retinaculum, each tendon being enclosed in a synovial sheath where it passes through its respective tunnel.[4,5,23]

29.2.2 Extensors of the Wrist

These comprise three musculotendinous units, the extensor carpi radialis longus (ECRL), the extensor carpi radialis brevis (ECRB; ▶Fig. 29.7), and the extensor carpi ulnaris (ECU;

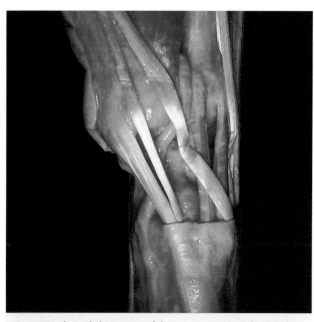

Fig. 29.3 The radial insertion of the extensor retinaculum to the anterior border of the radius. The 1st, 2nd, 3rd, and 4th compartments as well as the radial artery in the anatomical snuffbox is visible.

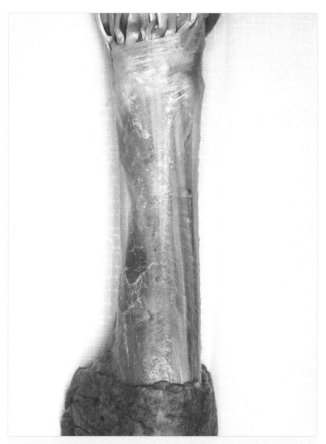

Fig. 29.2 The fascia of the forearm thickens to form the extensor retinaculum.

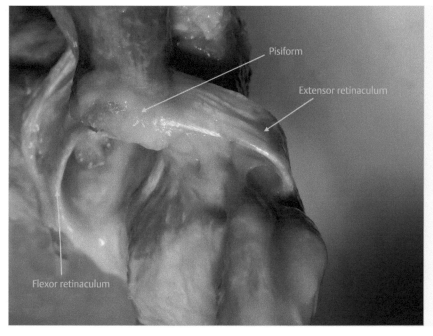

Pisiform

Extensor retinaculum

Flexor retinaculum

Fig. 29.4 On the ulnar side the extensor retinaculum and the flexor retinaculum are both inserted into the pisiform.

▶ Fig. 29.8).[24] Many variants of these muscles are described[22, 25-29] and only the most common variants are given hereafter.[24]

The radial nerve, from nerve roots C6/7 and C7/8, innervates ECRL and ECRB respectively, and the posterior interosseous nerve, from nerve roots C7/8, innervates ECU. The innervation of the radial wrist extensors more proximally by the main radial nerve gives rise to the difference of muscle palsies seen between a proximal injury of the radial nerve, in which all of the wrist and digital extensors are denervated, and injuries more distally in which the radial wrist extensors remain functional and wrist extension remains, albeit with radial deviation.

The ECRL muscle arises mainly from the lower third of the lateral supracondylar ridge of the humerus and from the anterior aspect of the lateral intermuscular septum. The muscle is overlapped proximally, on its radial border, by the brachioradialis muscle as it runs distally along the radial aspect of the

extensor compartment, overlying the proximal radioulnar joint and the proximal third of the radius. The muscle gives rise to its tendon at the junction of the proximal and middle thirds of the

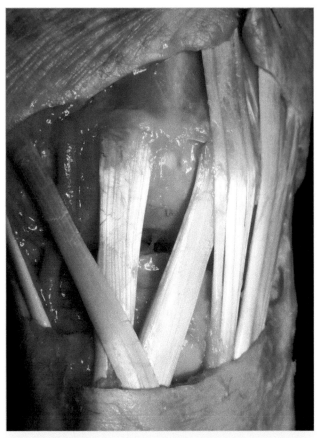

Fig. 29.7 The insertion of the ECRL onto the base of the 2nd metacarpal and the insertion of the ECRB onto the base of the 3rd metacarpal. ECRB: extensor carpi radialis brevis, ECRL: extensor carpi radialis longus.

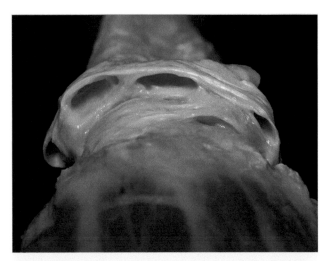

Fig. 29.5 The extensor retinaculum attaches to a series of ridges on the dorsum of the radius forming the compartments through which the various extensor tendons pass from the forearm to the hand.

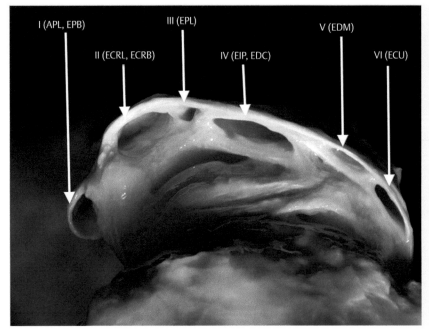

I (APL, EPB)
II (ECRL, ECRB)
III (EPL)
IV (EIP, EDC)
V (EDM)
VI (ECU)

Fig. 29.6 The six compartments of the extensor retinaculum. APL: abductor pollicis longus, ECRB: extensor carpi radialis brevis, ECRL: extensor carpi radialis longus, ECU: extensor carpi ulnaris, EDM: extensor digiti minimi, EIP: extensor indicis proprius, EPB: extensor pollicis brevis, EPL: extensor pollicis longus.

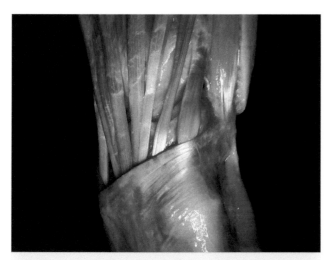

Fig. 29.8 The ulnar side of the wrist showing the 4th, 5th and 6th compartment tendons and the insertion of the ECU.

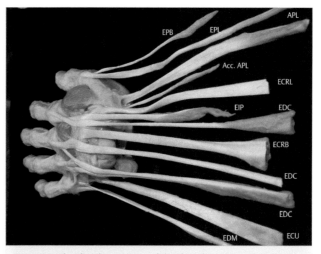

Fig. 29.9 The distal insertions of the dorsal tendons of the hand with the extensor retinaculum removed. APL: abductor pollicis longus, ECRB: extensor carpi radialis brevis, ECRL: extensor carpi radialis longus, ECU: extensor carpi ulnaris, EDC: extensor digitorum communis, EDM: extensor digiti minimi, EIP: extensor indicis proprius, EPB: extensor pollicis brevis, EPL: extensor pollicis longus.

forearm. This flat, wide tendon continues along the ulnar border of the radius, adjacent to the brachioradialis tendon, to pass under the abductor pollicis longus (APL) and extensor pollicis brevis (EPB) tendons. It then passes through the second compartment of the extensor retinaculum, which lies between the overlying retinaculum and a wide groove on the dorsum of the radius, immediately lateral to the first compartment, containing the APL and EPB tendons (see hereafter). As it emerges from the extensor retinaculum, the extensor pollicis longus (EPL) tendon crosses it before the ECRL tendon inserts into the dorsum of the second metacarpal bone (▶Fig. 29.9). The ECRB muscle arises from the common extensor origin attachment to the lateral epicondyle of the humerus, from the radial collateral ligament of the elbow joint, and from the intermuscular septum separating it from the adjacent extensor digitorum communis (EDC) muscle in the proximal forearm extensor compartment. The muscle lies adjacent to the ECRL muscle, on its ulnar side, giving rise to a flat, wide tendon in the middle third of the forearm. This runs adjacent to the ECRL tendon under the APB and EPB muscles, through the second extensor retinacular compartment and under the EPL tendon, to attach to the base of the third metacarpal and the adjacent parts of the second and, sometimes, fourth metacarpal bases. Attachment to the third metacarpal base (▶Fig. 29.7 and ▶Fig. 29.9) is the basis for the "piano-key" sign, in which the extended middle finger is subjected to forced passive flexion to activate the ECRB muscle and cause proximal forearm pain, identifying posterior interosseous nerve compressions in which this nerve lies against a sharp fascial edge of the ECRB muscle in the proximal forearm. The attachments of the ECRB tendon to the second and fourth metacarpals allow for complete removal of the third metacarpal base in ray amputations of the middle finger, to achieve better alignment of the index and ring fingers, without defunctioning of the ECRB.[30] While debate continues as to which of the two units should be used, the fact that there are two radial wrist extensors has allowed for one or other to be used for tendon transfers with no seeming loss of wrist extension or radial deviation. Their very wide and flat contour also makes them a convenient source of free tendon, as an alternative to palmaris longus, when operating on the dorsum of the wrist, hand, and fingers. The ECU muscle arises from the lateral epicondyle of the humerus, as

the most ulnar component of the common extensor origin, and from a septum attaching to the ulnar border of the ulna. This septal attachment extends as far distally as the junction of the middle and distal thirds of the ulna. This septum also gives rise, on its flexor aspect, to the flexor carpi ulnaris (FCU) and flexor digitorum profundus (FDP) muscles. The ECU muscle gives rise to its tendon in the distal third of the extensor compartment of the forearm, with the muscle reaching distally to a variable extent. The tendon then runs distally through the sixth extensor retinacular compartment, immediately ulnar to the ulnar styloid, between the retinaculum and a groove on the dorsoulnar aspect of the ulnar head, to attach to the tubercle on the dorsoulnar side of the base of the fifth, or little finger, metacarpal (▶Fig. 29.8). In addition to acting as wrist extensors, these three musculotendinous units are partly responsible, in conjunction with their flexor equivalents, for radial and ulnar wrist movements.

29.2.3 Extensors of the Thumb

The extensor tendons of the thumb are the APL, the EPB, and the EPL (▶Fig. 29.3), all of which are innervated by the posterior interosseous nerve, from nerve roots C7 and 8.[24] The APL muscle belly lies just distal to the supinator in the extensor compartment in the mid forearm. It arises from the lateral aspect of the posterior part of the ulna in its middle third, the adjacent interosseous membrane, and the middle third of the posterior surface of the radius. The EPB muscle, arising from the posterior surface of the radius and the adjoining interosseous membrane just distal to the APL origins, lies immediately adjacent and distal to the APL muscle belly. The distal part of both the APL and the EPB muscles as well as their tendons lie side by side obliquely across the radial wrist extensors (ECRL and ECRB). Any friction between the tendons in this anatomical location can result in swelling under the tight investing fascia causing pain and crepitus in a condition

347

known as "intersection syndrome". The APL and EPB tendons continue distally to the base of the thumb, passing through the first extensor retinacular compartment in a groove in the lateral border of the radius, immediately dorsal to the radial styloid (▶Fig. 29.10). Frequently, they pass under the extensor retinaculum in separate tunnels, and it is necessary to identify all of these when releasing de Quervain's stenosing tenovaginitis (▶Fig. 29.11).[31] Most commonly, the EPB has a single tendon, or sometimes two, while the APL commonly has several tendons which insert mostly into the base of the first metacarpal but sometimes also into the trapezium and muscles of the thenar eminence (▶Fig. 29.12). The APL largely acts to stabilize the base of the thumb. The EPB tendon continues distally along the dorsal surface of the first metacarpal to

insert most commonly into the base of the proximal phalanx of the thumb (▶Fig. 29.13). However, the insertion of the EPB is variable and this tendon may extend more distally to attach to the base of the distal phalanx. The EPL muscle, much larger than the EPB, arises from the lateral aspect of the posterior part of the ulna in its middle third, just distal to the APL origin, and from the adjacent interosseous membrane. The muscle belly passes obliquely under the long finger extensor muscles proximal to the extensor retinaculum to form the EPL tendon, which enters the third extensor retinacular compartment. This is a separate tunnel formed between the retinaculum and a narrow groove on the dorsolateral surface of the radius (▶Fig. 29.6), lying immediately radial to the fourth extensor compartment, housing the long finger extensors. The EPL tendon curls around the ulnar, then distal, side of the palpable landmark

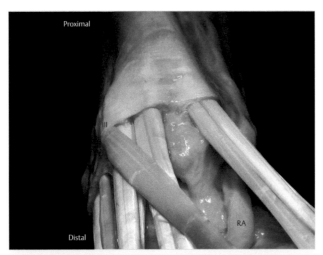

Fig. 29.10 The first (I) dorsal compartment tendons (APL and EPB), the second (II) dorsal compartment (ECRL and ECRB), the 3rd compartment (III) tendon (EPL) . The radial artery (RA) is seen in the anatomical snuff box.

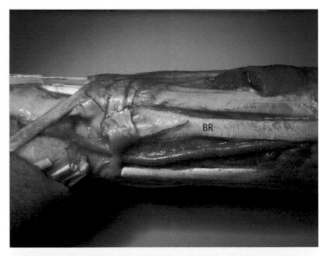

Fig. 29.11 The radial side of the wrist with the 1st dorsal compartment tendons removed. The Brachioradialis (BR) tendon inserting onto the radius forms the floor of the 1st compartment. The EPB is dorsal to the APL and often passes in its own tunnel in the 1st compartment. The radial artery is seen in the anatomical snuff box. APL: abductor pollicis longus, EPB: extensor pollicis brevis.

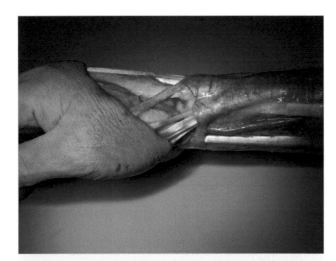

Fig. 29.12 The radial side of the wrist with all the tendons in place. The EPB is the narrowest tendon and is dorsal to the wider APB. The APB often has multiple tendons. The main APB tendon inserts into the base of the I metacarpal. The accessory APL tendons insert onto the base of the 1st metacarpal, trapezium and thenar muscles. The radial artery is passing from the volar forearm along the anatomical snuff box to the dorsum of the wrist. APB: Abductor pollicis brevis, APL: abductor pollicis longus, EPB: extensor pollicis brevis.

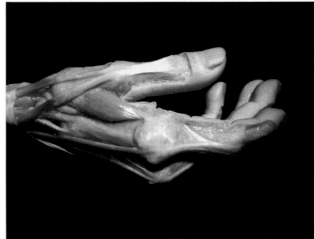

Fig. 29.13 The EPL runs from the 3rd extensor compartment towards the thumb, joining the EPB at the MP joint and inserting with a broad insertion at the base of the distal phalanx of the thumb. EPB: extensor pollicis brevis, EPL: extensor pollicis longus, MP: Metacarpophalangeal.

of Lister's tubercle on the dorsoulnar aspect of the distal radius (►Fig. 29.14), where it is prone to attrition rupture during the weeks after radial wrist injury, possibly as a result of interruption of its blood supply. It then crosses over the distal parts of the radial wrist extensor tendons, running obliquely toward the thumb. At the base of the thumb, it lies at a distance from the EPB tendon, with a space between the two when both muscles are activated giving rise to the "anatomical snuffbox" (►Fig. 29.3). It then passes along the ulnar border of the first metacarpal onto the dorsolateral aspect of the MCP joint, where it lies immediately adjacent to the EPB tendon (►Fig. 29.13), held in position by transverse aponeurotic fibers having the same functions as the sagittal bands in zone 5 of the finger extensor tendons (see later). Because the EPL tendon approaches the thumb from the dorso-ulnar direction, not only is it an extensor of the MCP and interphalangeal (IP) joints of the thumb but it also has an adduction action, which can give rise to confusion in diagnosis when other thumb base muscles are inactivated. Just distal to the MCP joint, on the dorsum of the proximal phalanx, it is joined on the radial and ulnar sides by tendinous extensions of the APB (radial) and the adductor pollicis and first dorsal interosseous muscles (ulnar), respectively, (►Fig. 29.15 and ►Fig. 29.16), before attaching to the base of the distal phalanx.[32] The involvement of these muscles in extension of the IP joint, and the variable insertion of the EPB tendon give rise to a variability of extension of the MCP and IP joints after division of the EPL more proximally than the MCP joint that can be confusing. The distal EPL tendon is a thick structure capable of taking a core suture of the

kind used in flexor tendon repair and does not need the postoperative protective splinting necessary after repairing the distal extensors in zones 1 and 2 in the fingers. In fact, such protection may compromise the vital rapid flexion–extension activity of the thumb IP joint essential to fine pinch function.[33]

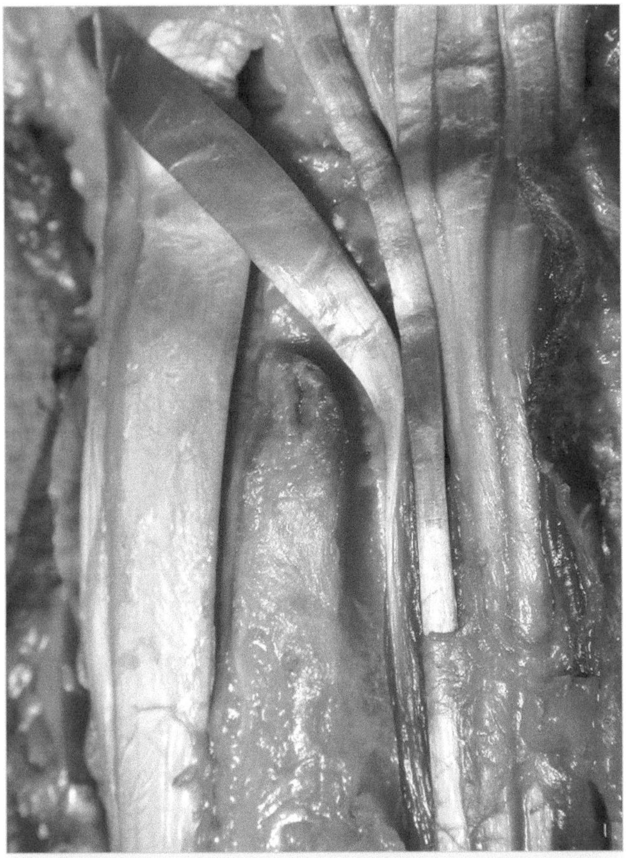

29.2.4 Extensors of the Finger Metacarpophalangeal Joints

It is convenient to consider the extensor system of the MCP joints of the fingers as a single system, although it is also involved in extending the IP joints of the fingers beyond the

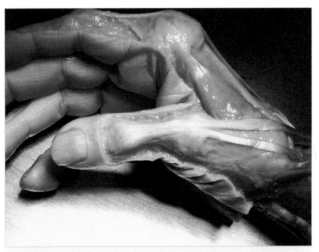

Fig. 29.15 The EPL approaches the thumb from the ulnar direction forming the ulnar border of the anatomical snuff box and thus acts as an adductor of the thumb in addition to being an extensor. At the level of the MP joint and over the dorsum of the proximal phalanx, it is joined on the radial side by the EPB tendon and on the ulnar side by the insertion of the AP and the first dorsal interosseous muscle. AP: abductor pollicis, EPB: extensor pollicis brevis, EPL: extensor pollicis longus, MP: Metacarpophalangeal.

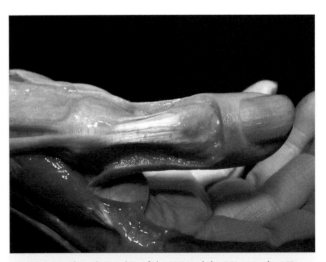

Fig. 29.16 The relationship of the EPB and the EPL over the MP joint and over the proximal phalanx of the thumb. The EPL inserts with a thick and broad insertion that is reinforced by extension of the EPB onto the base of the distal phalanx. EPB: extensor pollicis brevis, EPL: extensor pollicis longus, MP: Metacarpophalangeal.

Fig. 29.14 The Lister's tubercle and its relationship to the 2nd and 3rd compartment tendons.

MCP joints; this is considered later. This system is subdivided into zones 5, 6, 7, 8, and 9 in the Verdan classification (the zones 1, 2, 3, and 4 are in the fingers) for convenience of description of the anatomical variations within its different parts. ▶Fig. 29.17a and b shows the current modification of Verdan's subdivision of extensor tendon injuries by Doyle.[34,35,36] Classifying the different parts allows us to consider each part of this system separately with respect to its particular functional and surgical significance. Without this classification, we could not begin to discuss any of the problems, primary and secondary, simple and complex, that befall each part of the extensor system.

It has been recognized for centuries that the extensors of the fingers are very variable between individuals, with respect to both their muscle component in the forearm and the actual tendon patterns crossing the dorsum of the wrist and hand.[4,5,37–56] Only the most common variants are discussed hereafter.[24]

This system comprises the extensor indicis proprius (EI) to the index finger only; the EDC to all four fingers; and the extensor quinti, or digiti minimi (EDM), to the little finger only (▶Fig. 29.9 and ▶Fig. 29.14). All of these muscles are innervated by the posterior interosseous nerve, from nerve roots C7

and C8. The EDC and EDMin muscles originate from the lateral epicondyle of the humerus in the common extensor origin, while the EI arises from the middle third of the ulna on its radial border and from the adjacent interosseus membrane, immediately distal to the EPL attachment.

All of these muscles give rise to their respective tendons in the distal third of the forearm before passing under the extensor retinaculum. EI passes through the radial side of the fourth compartment of the extensor retinaculum adjacent to the EDC tendons that occupy the bulk of the available space in this compartment. EDMin passes through a separate compartment of the retinaculum, the fifth, which lies against the distal radioulnar joint (▶Fig. 29.6). Zone 9 of Verdan's classification includes the most proximal part of this system: the extensor muscles. The attached tendons running distally to the extensor retinaculum on the dorsum of the wrist constitute zone 8. While the details of the muscle proximal attachments are not usually of particular interest to the surgeon, their innervation by the posterior interosseous nerve and knowledge of the course and ramification of this nerve after its passage through the supinator muscle is of importance, as laceration of the muscles in the mid forearm may cut the terminal branches of the nerve,

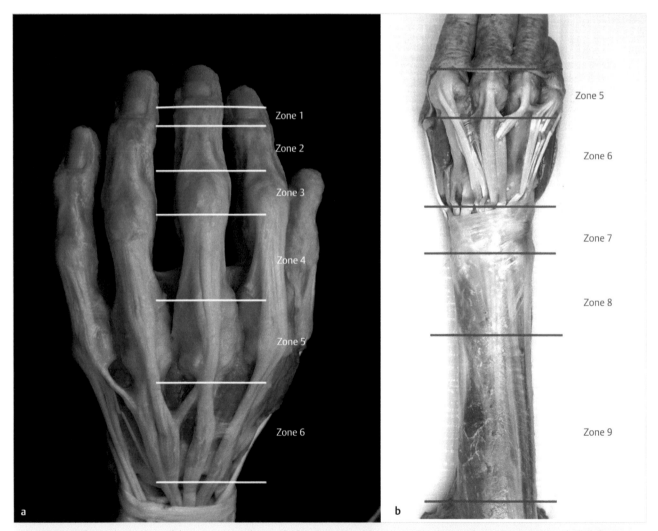

Fig. 29.17 (a, b) Verdan's zones of the extensor tendons in the hand, wrist and forearm with splitting of zone 8 into two, such that the new zone 8 includes only the tendinous part of the long extensors in the forearm and the new zone 9 includes the muscular part of the long extensors in the forearm.[34]

making suture of the muscles a pointless exercise unless the nerve divisions can be reconnected. The main benefit of Doyle's split of Verdan's original zone 8 into two zones is a recognition that the new zone 8 is a tendon injury of tendons of significant size and that strong suture of these is possible. Zone 9 is a muscle injury and thus is less safe to mobilize early unless the trauma surgeon has looked carefully within each muscle for the tendon extension and has carried out strong tendon repairs of these intramuscular extensions.

Zone 7 is that part of the finger extensors, passing through compartments four and five of the extensor retinaculum, the purpose of which is to prevent bowstringing of the finger extensor tendons off the back of the wrist—an ugly, if not particularly functionally disabling, defect. Avoiding this complication after lacerating injury at this level is almost always possible by careful consideration of the level of tendon injury, then appropriate resection of enough of the retinaculum to allow both tendon repair(s) and free gliding of the repair(s) while leaving a strap 1 cm in width of the retinaculum in place. While this requires that the tendon surgery be carried out around and under this strap, bowstringing can usually be avoided. This is possible because of the longitudinal dimension of the extensor retinaculum: this is variable but is always several centimeters, allowing a retaining retinacular strap to be placed where appropriate to the repairs. In the rare circumstance in which the extensor retinaculum of compartment four has been destroyed, it must be replaced by a tendon reconstruction, commonly with palmaris longus, or half of the ECRB or ECRL as a free graft or by turnover of the retinaculum from the more ulnar and/or radial parts of this structure. Before the advent of recent drug treatment of rheumatoid arthritis, the hand surgeons most frequently explored zone 7 to carry out synovectomy. This synovium may also be involved in tuberculosis and gout. In rheumatoid arthritis, tendon ruptures at this level are most commonly of the extensor tendons to the ring and little fingers and are more frequently due to attrition on osteophytes on the dorsum of the distal radioulnar joint than synovial tendon injury. However, the middle finger extensor lies radial to these osteophytes, and rupture of this tendon should alert the surgeon to a synovial origin of the problem. In my experience, rupture by osteophytes from the wrist under the tendons in compartment four is very rare. During this surgery, the extensor retinaculum also needs be preserved, except in case when the wrist movement into extension is minimal or absent. Wrist surgeons are aware of the presence of the terminal branches of the posterior interosseous nerve innervating the wrist, lying deep to the radial tendons in the fourth compartment. Division of this nerve is also used to prevent and treat secondary hypersensitivity on the dorsum of the hand after injury and relocation of the superficial radial nerve and, less commonly, the dorsal branch of the ulnar nerve.[57]

Zone 6 of the finger extensors (▶Fig. 29.18) is that part of their course in which they run across the dorsum of the hand to the MCP joints, at which point they are defined as zone 5. The EI tendon passes to the MCP joint of the index finger on the ulnar side of the EDC tendon to this finger. Over the MCP joint, the two tendons coalesce to become a single long extensor tendon (▶Fig. 29.18). EI is, perhaps, best known to the hand surgeon in its various roles as a tendon transfer. Its loss from the index finger occasionally results in a slight loss of index extension at the MCP joint. Usually, there is no loss of either full extension of this joint or of the ability to point with

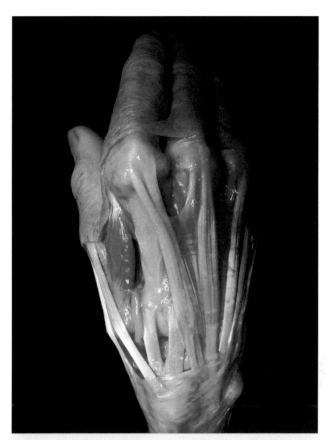

Fig. 29.18 Zones 5 and 6 of the extensor tendons over the MP joint and the dorsum of the hand. The relationship of the EDC to the index and the EI tendon over the MCP joint is clearly seen. EDC: extensor digitorum communis, EI: Extensor indicis, MCP or, MP: Metacarpophalangeal.

the extended index finger alone.[58,59,60] It is suggested that this is because the EDC is named inappropriately: although this muscle starts from the common extensor origin on the lateral epicondyle of the humerus as a single muscle, it quickly splits into four muscles whence the four main tendons arise.[59] Occasionally, the extensor indicis is absent, giving rise to a need to use another motor for tendon transfers. The ECRB makes a suitable alternative after extension, either using the palmaris longus tendon or using half the wide tendon of ECRB itself as its own extension.

The precise pattern of the EDC in zone 6 is inconstant, with the number of tendons running to each finger being very variable. Usually, only one tendon runs to the index finger, but the middle and ring fingers may have two or three EDC tendons. The EDC tendon to the little finger may be an entirely separate tendon. It is frequently absent distally. When absent, it is usually replaced at the metacarpal neck level by a thick juncturae tendinum attaching proximally to the extensor tendon of the ring finger, or its more ulnar tendon if two tendons are present, at the level of the middle part of the little finger metacarpal.

Between the communis tendons are connections called juncturae tendinum that are usually three in number but that are variable both in design and in position between the extensor retinaculum and the MCP joints (▶Fig. 29.19 and ▶Fig. 29.20).[5,22,34,49,52,55,58,61,62,63] Usually the juncturae become thicker and more defined as one moves from radial to ulnar,

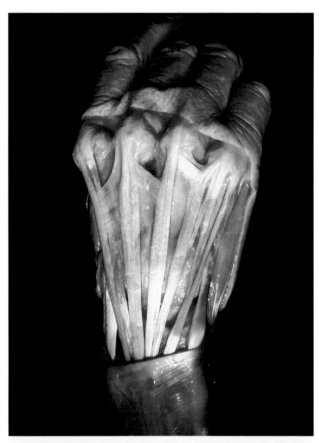

Fig. 29.19 Zone 6 of the extensor tendons showing the juncturae tendinum.

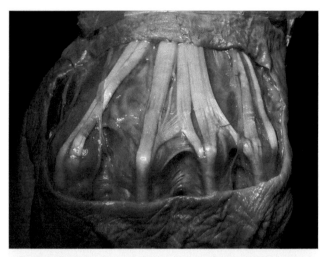

Fig. 29.20 The juncturae between the ring finger EDC and the EDC to the middle and ring fingers. The juncturae slide distally with MP joint flexion. EDC: extensor digitorum communis.

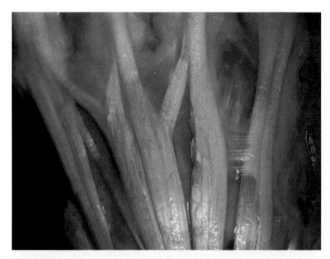

Fig. 29.21 The juncturae from the ring EDC to the middle and small finger EDCs with the digits in extension. EDC: extensor digitorum communis.

with the flimsy junctura between the communis tendons of the index finger and middle finger being nearest to the wrist (▶Fig. 29.21) and that between the ring and little fingers lying close to the MCP joint. The juncturae move distally during finger flexion. The tension in them increases with this movement, as the transverse metacarpal arch widens distally toward the MCP joints. When in their most distal position, the juncturae contribute to stabilizing the extensor tendons over the heads of the metacarpals during full finger flexion. Brand[64] also demonstrated that they have a lateral stabilizing effect on the extended MCP joints. They may give rise to a diagnostic problem when the main tendons of one finger, commonly the middle finger, are divided close to, or over, the MCP joint and the patient can maintain extension of this finger through an intact junctura connecting the distal part of the cut tendon to the intact tendon of the next finger (usually the ring finger). However, extension of the involved finger in this way is usually only partial and/or extension of the MCP joint cannot be entirely achieved actively even if retained once the joint is extended passively. The juncturae are generally divided in realignment or replacement of the MCP joints in rheumatoid disease to prevent ongoing ulnar pull on each joint by the more ulnar extensor tendons after repositioning of the fingers radially. Where the EDC tendon to the little finger is absent and replaced by connection through the juncture to the ring finger extensor, there is a danger of losing EDC function to the little finger if this juncturum tendinum is divided.

The EDMin crosses the dorsum of the hand ulnar to the communis tendon of the little finger to coalesce with this tendon over the MCP joint to become a single long extensor tendon (▶Fig. 29.19). EDMin commonly has two slips, sometimes one, and occasionally more. In the absence of adductor muscle function of the little finger in motor ulnar nerve dysfunction, activity of this muscle is responsible for the abducted position of the little finger.[65]

It is now realized that many of the extensor tendons divided over the MCP joint, and more proximally, are substantial and capable of taking a core suture of the kind used in flexor tendon repair. In some individuals, particularly more distally in zones 5 and 6, the tendons are flatter and require use of horizontal mattress sutures, rather than flexor core sutures. Even when this is necessary, previous fixed postoperative protective splinting regimes after repairing these tendons are unnecessary and early mobilization is possible. Following slightly behind the changes to more aggressive mobilization of acute flexor tendon injuries, mobilization of extensor repairs in zones 5 to 9 has evolved from immobilization to rubber band traction systems of early mobilization to mobilization without rubber bands, in splints blocking full flexion for the short period of time when the repairs are considerably less than full strength.[33, 66,67,68,69,70,71,72]

29.3 Extensors of the Fingers

The extensor system of the fingers (▶Fig. 29.22) consists of two structural components—the tendons themselves, motored by the muscles of the forearm and innervated by the radial nerve (*the extrinsic extensors*) and the muscles within the hand (*the intrinsic extensors*), innervated by the ulnar and median nerves.[1,73] and the *extensor retinacular system*.

In a broader context, the latter are part of the fibrous structures of the hand which divide the hand into compartments enclosing the tendons, nerves, blood vessels, and bones, and act to retain and stabilize the tendons and skin.[74] In respect of the extensor system of the fingers, the retinacular system comprises various fascial structures, mostly running transversely or obliquely to the longitudinal course of the extensor tendons, whose purpose is to retain the tendons by restraining their movements in the sagittal plane. These structures lie mostly across the MCP joint, the

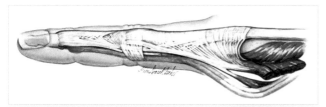

Fig. 29.22 Diagram of the extensor system of the digit. (Copyright Kleinert Institute, Louisville, KY).

proximal phalanx, and the PIP joint and they have particular functional significances at each joint which will be described later in the text. However, they not only act to restrain the sagittal movements of the extensor tendons but also act as means of transmitting variations of tension between the two extensor systems. This allows the interplay between the two, required to achieve the complex movements and relative positioning of the three finger joints which we recognize as the different flexion and extension maneuvers of which a finger is capable.

29.3.1 Extrinsic Extensors of the Fingers and the Retinacular System

The extrinsic extensor tendons act most proximally to assist extension of the wrist. They then extend the fingers at the MCP joints and become a part of the extensor mechanism of the finger, acting in concert with the intrinsic muscles and the retinacular system. Extension of the fingers is synergistic with wrist flexion, and the effective excursion of the extrinsic extensor tendons is increased by flexion of the wrist.[1,11,14,75,76]

Zone 5 is that part of the finger extensors which overlies the four MCP joints of the fingers. The long extensors continue over the MCP joints, being separated from them by small bursae. The long tendons are held centrally on top of the joints, particularly during flexion, by that part of the retinacular system called the *sagittal bands* (▶Fig. 29.23).[5,7,18,77,78,79,80,81] These fibroaponeurotic structures run transversely from the long tendons around the lateral aspect of the joint, external to the joint capsule and collateral ligaments, to attach to the palmar plate ligament on the palmar side of the joint (▶Fig. 29.24 and ▶Fig. 29.25). Although the long extensor tendons have an attachment of their deeper fibers to the MCP joint capsule and thence to the base of the proximal phalanx dorsally, this remains lax except during full hyperextension of the joint and is

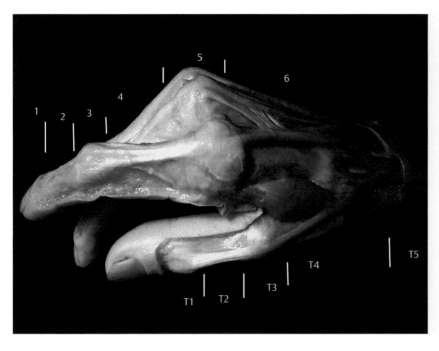

Fig. 29.23 The extensor expansion at the level of the MP joint and proximal phalanx showing the extensor tendon, the sagittal band, the interosseous contribution and the dorsal digital expansion. Verdan's extensor zones in the finger and the thumb are marked.

not the means of extension of this joint.[4,78,82,83,84,85,86,87,88] Rather, the joint is extended by the pull of the long tendon on the palmar plate, through the sagittal bands, akin to lifting a bucket by its handle. During active extension of the joints, the sagittal bands also have a stabilizing effect on the joint, the collateral ligaments being relaxed in this joint position. If a radial sagittal band is either disrupted traumatically[1,5,15,89] or attenuated with disease or age,[90] the long extensor tendon moves onto the ulnar side of the joint on flexing the joint and extension is impossible actively, although it can be maintained if the joint is restored to the extended position passively. Acting on their own, without involvement of the intrinsic muscles, the extrinsic tendons can

only act to extend the IP joints if the MCP joint is held in slight flexion. This is utilized by tendon transfers placing the MCP joints in slight flexion in patients with paralysis of the intrinsic muscles secondary to ulnar nerve dysfunction. Otherwise, they can only hyperextend the MCPs and the IP joints remain flexed, creating the classical claw hand.

The long, or extrinsic, extensor tendon continues over the proximal phalanx. A triangular membrane of transverse and oblique fibers, known as the *dorsal digital expansion* or the *interosseous hood*,[87] with its base proximally and in continuity with the transverse fibers of the sagittal bands, connects the long tendon to the intrinsic muscle tendons laterally and covers the dorsum and sides of the proximal phalanx (▶Fig. 29.22, ▶Fig. 29.23, ▶Fig. 29.24, ▶Fig. 29.26, and ▶Fig. 29.27). The continuous fascial system of the dorsal digital expansion and the sagittal bands is also known as the *MCP extensor hood*. This hood links and relates the various tensions in the two extensor tendon systems. As the long extensor tendon lies over the middle part of the proximal phalanx, its central part receives fibers from the lumbrical and interosseous tendons lateral to it and this central part passes over the dorsum of the PIP joint as the *central slip*, or *proximal conjoint extensor tendon*, to attach to the dorsum of the base of the middle phalanx, thickening as a fibrocartilaginous plate just before attaching to the bone.[91] The extrinsic tendon itself divides at this level such that its lateral fibers join with the adjacent intrinsic tendons on each side of the dorsal digital expansion to form the *lateral bands*, or *conjoint lateral extensor tendons*, which pass

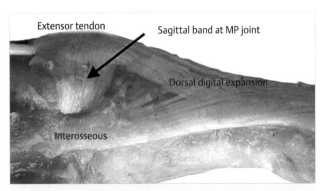

Fig. 29.24 The continuous fascial system of the dorsal digital expansion and the sagittal bands is also known as the MCP extensor hood. Verdan's extensor zones in the digits and in the thumb.

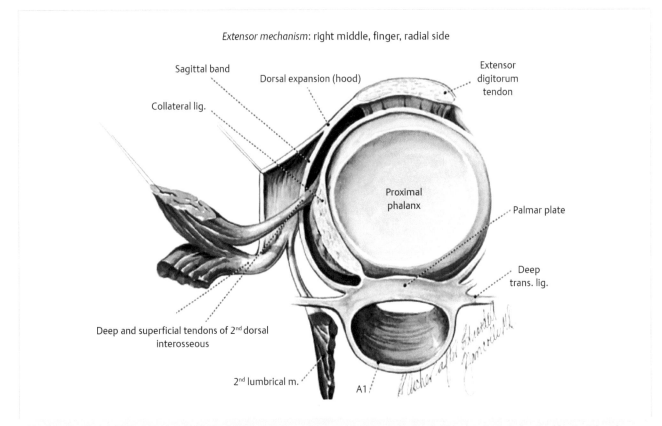

Fig. 29.25 Diagram showing the relationship of the various structures at the MCP joint level. (This drawing was inspired by Dr. Eduardo Zancolli). (Copyright Kleinert Institute, Louisville, KY).

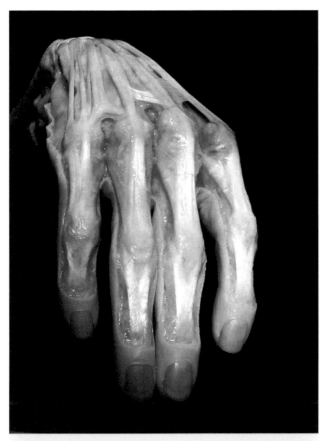

Fig. 29.26 The extensor system over the dorsum of the hand and the digits. The different types of juncturae tendinum are visible. The MCP extensor hood is clearly visible.

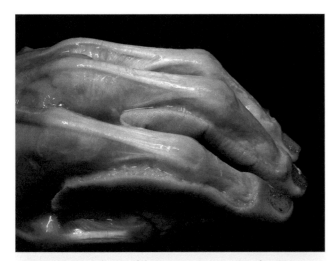

Fig. 29.27 Lateral view of the extensor system over the MP joint, proximal phalanx, PIP joint and middle phalanx. The contribution of the interosseous and lumbricals is clearly seen. MP: metacarpophalangeal, PIP: proximal interphalangeal joints.

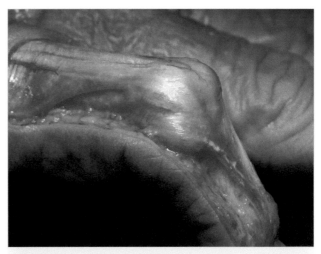

Fig. 29.28 The extensor mechanism over the PIP joint showing the lateral bands and the central slip. The interosseous contribution is also visible. PIP: proximal interphalangeal joints.

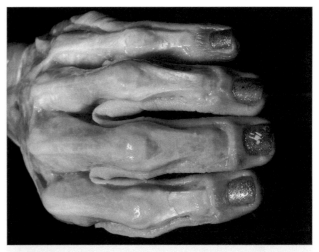

Fig. 29.29 Dorsal view of the extensor mechanism over the digits.

over the dorsolateral aspects of the PIP joint (►Fig. 29.28).[3] The dorsal digital expansion consists of layers of crisscrossing fibers that change their geometrical arrangement as the finger moves from flexion to extension, allowing the lateral bands to displace volarly during flexion and return to the dorsum of the finger on extension (►Fig. 29.28 and ►Fig. 29.29).[5,92,93]

The principal parts of the retinacular system at the PIP joint are made up of two parts, although the various named ligaments are a continuum. Dorsally, the *triangular ligament* lies between the lateral bands just distal to the PIP joint and acts to limit their lateral and palmar movement during joint flexion (►Fig. 29.29 and ►Fig. 29.30).[87,94,95] This dorsal retaining system also includes the *arciform fibers*, running transversely over the actual joint itself, mingling with the fibers of the central slip and acting similarly to the triangular ligament (►Fig. 29.31a, b). Both of these fascial structures are stretched in the Boutonniere deformity and shortened in swan-neck deformity. Laterally, the *transverse ligament of Landsmeer* runs obliquely across the lateral aspect of the PIP joint and functions to fix the extensor tendons in position relative to the skeleton (►Fig. 29.32a, b).[7,87,96] Dorsally, it attaches to the lateral border of the lateral band. At its palmar end, it is attached to the palmar plate of the joint.

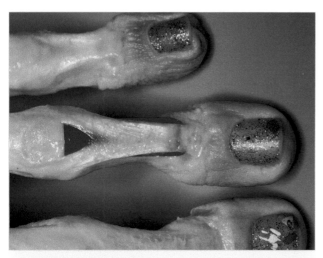

Fig. 29.30 The two lateral bands come together over the middle phalanx to form the distal conjoint extensor tendon that inserts into the distal phalanx.

It lies immediately over, but entirely free from, the collateral ligament of the joint. To its superficial fibers are attached the cutaneous, or Cleland's, ligament.[74,97,98] Distally, the free edge of the ligament is obvious. The principal function of the transverse ligament of Landsmeer is to limit the dorsal movement of the lateral bands during PIP extension.

The lateral bands continue distally over the middle phalanx, remaining distinct initially, although lightly adherent, as they pass over the middle phalanx. Over the middle part of the middle phalanx, they fuse to form the *distal conjoint extensor tendon*. This attaches to the dorsum of the base of the distal phalanx, acting to extend the DIP joint (▶ Fig. 29.33).

Landsmeer's oblique ligaments attach to the lateral aspect of the distal half of the proximal phalanx and to the A2 flexor pulley deep to the lateral bands of the extensors (▶ Fig. 29.34a, b).[7,98,99,100] They pass across the lateral aspect of the PIP joint deep to the transverse ligament of Landsmeer and palmar to the axis of the joint, then continue distally around the middle phalanx to converge with the lateral aspects of the distal conjoint tendon proximal to the DIP joint. The primary function of this ligament, unlike that of the other parts

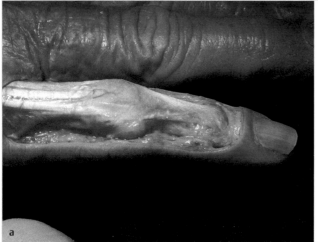

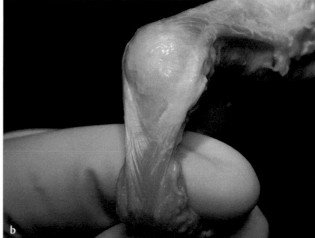

Fig. 29.31 (a) The triangular ligament connects the two lateral bands and prevents them subluxing palmarly. (b) Palmar subluxation of the lateral bands of the extensor mechanism on cutting the triangular ligaments.

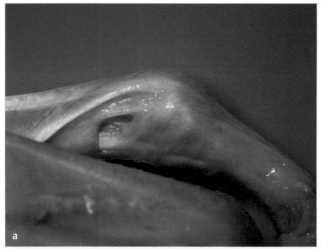

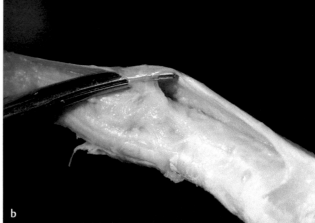

Fig. 29.32 (a, b) Transverse retinacular ligament of Landsmeer.

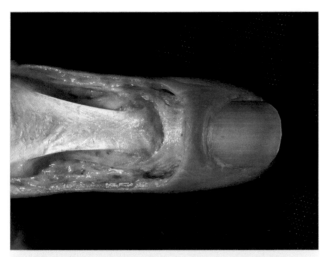

Fig. 29.33 The extensor mechanism over the middle phalanx and the DIP joint. The triangular ligament joins the two lateral bands over the proximal part of the middle phalanx and prevents their palmar subluxation on flexion of the digit. DIP: Distal interphalangeal.

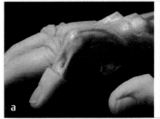
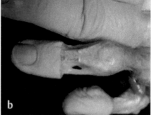

Fig. 29.34 (a, b) Oblique retinacular ligament of Landsmeer.

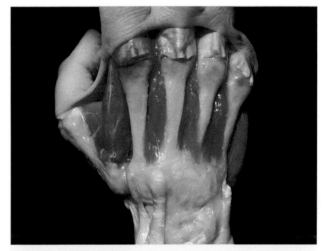

Fig. 29.35 Dorsal interossei.

previously described, is not to retain the extensors over the skeleton but to link the movements of flexion and extension of the IP joints. As the two ligaments pass palmar to the axis of the PIP joint and attach to the extensor tendons of the DIP joint, extension of the PIP joint forces corresponding extension of the DIP joint in a dynamic tenodesis.[1,7,11,17,18,19,101,102,103,104,106] Other authors suggest that this ligament plays a role in maintaining the extensor tendon centrally over the middle phalanx and increasing the lateral stability of the PIP joint.[3,5,76,100,107,108] This part of the retinacular system has variable degrees of development between individuals and individual fingers. The ligaments are normally present on both sides of the finger, but usually the radial ligament is slightly longer and stronger.[83,108]

29.3.2 Intrinsic Extensors of the Fingers

The intrinsic extensor muscles of the fingers comprise the dorsal interossei, the palmar interossei, and the lumbricals. The interossei lie between, and originate from, the metacarpal bones. They are all innervated from nerve roots C8 and T1, through the motor branch of the ulnar nerve.

These muscles are involved not only in the extension of the IP joints of the fingers but also in the flexion and lateral movements of the MCP joints.[108,109,110] It is evident from anatomical studies that these various activities of the intrinsic muscles are achieved in part because the muscles themselves are made up of various and functionally separate parts, with tendons inserting distally to different structures to achieve different motor actions and in part by a complicated interaction between the intrinsic muscles and the extrinsic flexors and extensors, which is conducted through the retinacular system.[14,16,17,81,111,112,113,114,115] Mostly, this is not pertinent to their extension function and is not discussed further here. It is clear that only parts of the intrinsic muscles are involved in finger extension and that the anatomical terminology, which states no more than that these muscles lie between the (metacarpal) bones, is a gross

simplification of the presence of several muscles with different functions being contained in this locality.[17,78,87,95,116,117,118,119]

The Dorsal Interossei

The four bipennate dorsal interossei (▶ Fig. 29.35) take origin from the proximal two-thirds of the lateral surfaces of both adjacent metacarpals of each of the four intermetacarpal spaces. This attachment is more pronounced from the metacarpal bone of the finger into which the muscle will insert. The first dorsal interosseous muscle arises in the first web space and inserts into the radial side of the index finger extensor system. The second and third dorsal interossei arise from the second and third intermetacarpal spaces, respectively, and insert into either side of the middle finger extensor system. The fourth dorsal interosseous arises in the fourth intermetacarpal space and inserts into the ulnar side of the ring finger extensor system. The tendon of each muscle arises just proximal to the MCP joint, then passes distally over the lateral surface of the joint capsule, dorsal to the deep transverse ligament. As it crosses the MCP joint, each dorsal interosseous tendon gives off a short tendon which passes deep to the lateral corner of the proximal part of the dorsal digital expansion, where this attaches to the deep transverse ligament. This tendon attaches to the base of the proximal phalanx and, in the case of the second, third, and fourth dorsal interossei, to the adjacent palmar plate ligament. Muscle action through these attachments serve to abduct the fingers from the resting midline position of the middle finger. The bulk of the dorsal interosseous tendon passes superficial to this junction of the dorsal digital expansion and the deep transverse ligament and coalesces with the other intrinsic tendons on the lateral surface of the proximal part of the proximal phalanx to become the lateral edge of the dorsal digital expansion, then the lateral band. The equivalent functions for the little finger are provided by the abductor digiti minimi muscle and tendon, also innervated from the C8 and T1 nerve roots through the motor branch of the ulnar nerve, which has equivalent distal insertions to the second, third, and fourth dorsal interossei.

The Palmar Interossei

The four palmar interossei (▶Fig. 29.36 and ▶Fig. 29.37), which are smaller, arise from the palmar surface of the metacarpal of the finger into which they will insert. Their innervation is the same as that of the dorsal interossei. The first and second palmar interossei arise on the ulnar sides of the first and second metacarpals, respectively. The third and fourth palmar interossei arise from the radial side of the fourth and fifth metacarpals. As with the dorsal interossei, they insert partially into the bases of the proximal phalanges, in the case of the first palmar interosseous, to act as adductors of the corresponding digits toward the middle finger, and partly, into the lateral edge of the dorsal digital expansion, after passing dorsal to the deep transverse metacarpal ligament.

The Lumbricals

The four lumbrical muscles (▶Fig. 29.37 and ▶Fig. 29.38) take origin from the FDP tendons. With the fingers extended, the origins lie in the proximal part of the palm. When the fingers are flexed, the bulk of the muscles lie within the carpal canal.[120] The first and second lumbricals, arising from the radiopalmar surfaces of the FDP tendons to the index and middle fingers, are innervated from the C8 and T1 nerve roots through the median nerve. They pass to the radial side of the respective fingers. The third and fourth lumbricals are innervated from the same nerve roots but through the motor branch of the ulnar nerve. This pattern of innervation is not absolutely constant. The two ulnar lumbricals are usually bipennate, arising from two adjacent profundus flexor tendons, the third arising from the FDP tendons to the middle and ring fingers and passing to the radial side of the ring finger and the fourth arising from the FDP tendons of the little and ring fingers and passing to the radial side of the little finger. The lumbrical tendons pass on the palmar side of the deep transverse ligament and pass distally to coalesce with those interossei on the radial sides of the fingers to form the radial lateral edge of the dorsal digital expansion, then the radial lateral band. They have no insertion into the bases of the proximal phalanges.

29.4 Involvement of the Extensors in Control of Flexion of the Finger

The extensor mechanism described above glides distally on finger flexion. It does not, however, play a passive role in finger

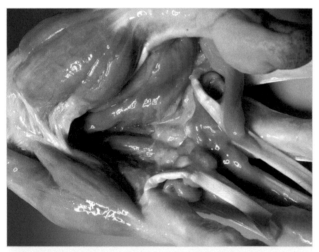

Fig. 29.36 Palmar interossei and lumbricals.

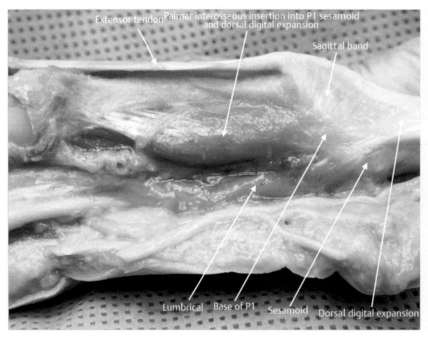

Extensor tendon Palmar interosseous insertion into P1 sesamoid and dorsal digital expansion

Sagittal band

Lumbrical   Base of P1   Sesamoid   Dorsal digital expansion

Fig. 29.37 Longitudinal view at the metacarpal and MP joint level showing the palmar interosseous inserting into the P1, sesamoid and dorsal digital expansion. The lumbrical contribution to the dorsal digital expansion is clearly seen.

flexion, being involved in a number of ways in the process whereby the three joints of the finger flex simultaneously. In this process, the PIP joint initiates flexion, the two proximal joints then flex together, and the distal joint follows a little later. Simultaneous joint flexion is necessary for most efficient prehension in that it places all of the palmar surfaces of the finger onto the object being grasped, maximizing the contact surface and the sensory communication with the object.

The dorsal digital expansion and sagittal bands cover the metacarpal head and the MCP joint during complete extension of the finger but displace approximately 2 cm distally in full flexion to cover the joint and the proximal part of the proximal phalanx. As the fibers of the dorsal expansion begin to move distally, as a result of contraction of the long flexors and initiation of IP flexion, they become aligned with the intrinsic tendons and exert a passive force on the intrinsic muscles such that the viscoelastic pull of these muscles places tension on the dorsal expansion fibers to begin MCP joint flexion.[108,121] If the extrinsic extensor of the finger is activated voluntarily during this process, this process of starting MCP flexion is blocked and the long flexors flex only the IP joints to create *hook grip*. This tightening of the dorsal digital expansion has a secondary effect of stabilizing the distally displaced extensor tendons over this part of the skeleton of the finger. In this, it is aided by the juncturae tendinum moving distally and tightening across the wider transverse metacarpal arch at the MCP level.[19, 61] During gentle flexion of the fingers, it can be seen that the index finger extensors over the MCP move in an ulnar direction, those of the middle remain central and those of the ring and little fingers move in a radial direction. When gripping is strengthened, the extensors of the index, ring, and little fingers move in the opposite directions, indicating the active involvement of the first dorsal interosseous, the fourth dorsal interosseous, and the abductor digiti minimi, respectively, in this tensioning process.

On initiation of IP flexion by activation of the profundus tendon, the PIP joint flexes first, the DIP joint being prevented initially from flexing by the taut oblique retinacular ligament of Landsmeer.[19,61] As the PIP joint flexes, the oblique retinacular ligament relaxes to allow DIP joint flexion, but this can continue

only by relaxation of the extensor system. In itself, the distal migration of the extensor mechanism allows flexion of the MCP and PIP joints but is not quite adequate to allow full flexion of all three joints. During PIP joint flexion, the lateral bands move laterally and in a palmar direction, opening the rhombus enclosed by these two structures over the PIP joint and middle phalanx, which is known as *Winslow's rhombus* after the French anatomist who first described it and this mechanism in Paris in 1732 (▶Fig. 29.38). This provides the relative lengthening of the extensor system necessary to allow the DIP joint to flex, thereby completing digital flexion.[84,94,95,122,123] The mechanism of opening of the rhombus is explained by the attachments of the distal fibers of Landsmeer's transverse retinacular ligament and the dorsal fibers of the Landsmeer's oblique retinacular ligament to the lateral bands. As the PIP joint begins to flex and the extensor lateral bands move distally, these retinacular

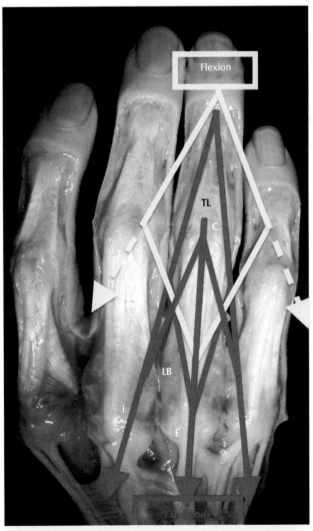

Fig. 29.39 The rhombus of Winslow is formed by the long digital extensor tendon (E), the lateral bands (LB) and the intrinsic contributions (i). Also shown are the central slip insertion to the base of the middle phalanx and the triangular ligaments (TL). In the flexion of the digit (*Yellow*), the rhombus widens by the lateral shifting of the lateral bands and the triangular ligaments tighten to limit this migration. In extension of the digit (*Red*), the rhombus narrows and the oblique ligaments limit their medial migration.

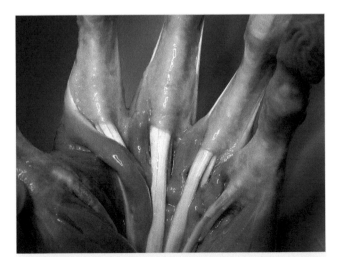

Fig. 29.38 Index finger lumbrical arising from the FDP tendon and inserting into the dorsal digital expansion of the extensor mechanism. FDP: flexor digitorum profundus.

structures tense and oblige the lateral bands to slide laterally and in a palmar direction, opening the rhombus. This effect can be demonstrated by a simple experiment, first carried out by Hauck in 1923[84] in which the two lateral bands are sutured together just proximal to the PIP joint. It is then observed that passive flexion of the finger achieves flexion of the two proximal joints, but not of the distal joint, flexion of only the but not the distal joint, reminding us that this mode of reconstruction of the central slip also requires that an extensor tenotomy be carried out over the middle phalanx if we expect to have a flexing DIP joint postoperatively. Therefore, DIP flexion is inevitably linked to PIP flexion by two passive actions of the retinacular system at the PIP level as a result of PIP joint flexion. These actions are: (1) increasing relaxation of the oblique retinacular ligament of Landsmeer and (2) opening of the rhombus of Winslow.

29.5 Involvement of the Extensors in Control of Extension of the Finger

This, of course, is the primary function of the extensor tendons. The activities of the system are, to some extent, easiest understood by considering a reversal of their role during finger flexion to return the finger to the neutral point of extension.

Activation of the extrinsic extensor muscles pulls the long extensor tendon proximally, moving the sagittal bands and the dorsal digital expansion proximally to cover the metacarpal head. This movement relaxes the dorsal digital expansion, evident from the increased lateral mobility of the long tendon as the MCP joint straightens, releases the joint from its flexion force by this retinacular component linking the extrinsic and intrinsic extensors and allows the more proximal sagittal bands to pull on the palmar plate ligament of the MCP joint and lift it into the straight, or neutral, position. When the MCP joints hyperextend, now involving the extrinsic tendon attachments to the bases of the dorsum of the proximal phalanges, the excursion of the extrinsic tendon is insufficient to also fully extend the IP joints, which flex slightly. The intrinsic extensors are now activated to extend the IP joints.

At the PIP joint level, the pull of the extrinsic and intrinsic extensors on the central slip extend this joint in a complex interplay of both sets of extensor muscles and the lumbrical muscles,[78,84,99,108,124,125,126] while a combination of proximal migration of the lateral bands under these forces and narrowing of Winslow's rhomboid extend the DIP joint in a linked manner.[95] The involvement of the (tightening) oblique retinacular ligament of Landsmeer in DIP extension remains debated, but this ligament does tighten as the PIP extends.

29.6 Conclusion

There is a common perception that the particular skill needed to treat flexor tendon injuries is not necessary for the extensor apparatus; this is not the case for various reasons.[2,11,24,127,128,129,130] The fact that the extensor system has no synovial tunnels, excepting across the wrist, could be considered a design fault.[4,24] It relies on a layer of connective tissue between the tendon and the skin and another between the tendon and the

bone to allow movement. A major problem after any inflammatory pathology, trauma, or operations (as the body does not differentiate between the latter two) is the manner in which these layers accumulate edema in response to the trauma, with the sticky fibrin in the edema then turning to scar tissue and having exactly the same effect as if the interstitial spaces had been filled with a slow-setting glue.[131] These adhesions, and their effect on extensor tendon gliding, are the most common long-term disability of trauma not only to the extensor system but indeed to all other parts of the hand, because of the migration of edema onto the dorsum of the hand and digits. We spend hours of surgical and therapy thought and time trying to keep injured extensors moving while, after extensor tendon suture, balancing this need against the need to protect weak tendon repairs from snapping: this constitutes 90% of our efforts in dealing with the extensor system. This perhaps underlies the comments of past masters: "To suture a tendon, then to splint it for 5 weeks is to make sure of failure" (Couch, 1939)[132] and "My first attempts at repair of tendons in the fingers resulted in immediate success, but as the succeeding days went by motion became less and less, until at the end of a few weeks it was nil" (Bunnell, 1949).[133] This "glue" deposition varies in degree from patient to patient, as well as with the severity of the trauma or pathology, and we all have patients whose hands cannot work, whatever the primary cause, because they cannot flex to allow full gripping as a result of the extensor system's having become stuck to its surrounds.

A further "design fault" is illustrated in (▶Table 29.1)[133], which shows the movement of the extensor tendon needed to move the finger joints through a range of movement of 10° each.[19,94,134] The movements are very small, so even slight restriction of the movement of the extensor tendons significantly affects the movement of the digits.

It is also a reality of surgical practice that the picture presented to us as trainees of a clean cut of the substantial extensor tendon, at whatever place along its length, requiring suture and early mobilization to prevent adhesion to its surrounds is too simplistic. This simple concept does not have any bearing on the far more complex concept of how to restore function. When the extensor tendon is shredded, or completely absent, or overlies a smashed phalanx, or has no overlying skin at all. Not only are the extensor tendons flimsy in the fingers, difficult to suture, and difficult to move early after suture without rupturing the repair[135], but also, taken in the wider perspective of injury to the dorsal aspect of the digits, hand, and forearm, the injury is frequently complex both in its mechanism and in the number of structures injured. Sixty percent of extensor tendon injuries have associated joint, bone, and/or skin complicating injuries, with the end result rarely being determined simply by the state of the extensor tendon.[136]

Table 29.1 The excursions of the long extensor tendons of the hand (Elliot and McGrouther, 1986).[134]

Tendon excursions per ten degrees of joint motion (mm)				
	EI	EDC3	EDC4	EDMIN
Wrist	2.0	2.0	2.0	1.4
MCP	1.5	1.5	1.4	1.1
PIP	0.9	0.8	0.7	0.7
DIP	0.7	0.7	0.6	0.6

References

1. Eaton RG. The extensor mechanism of the fingers. Bull Hosp Joint Dis, 30:39–47,1969
2. Entin MA. Repair of the extensor mechanism of the hand. Surg Clin North Am, 40:275–285,1960
3. Harris C, Rutledge GL. The functional anatomy of the extensor mechanism of the finger. J Bone Jt Surg 54A: 713–726,1972
4. Kaplan EB. Functional and Surgical Anatomy of the Hand. Philadelphia: Lippincott, 1953
5. Kaplan EB. Anatomy, injuries and treatment of the extensor apparatus of the hand and digits. Clin Orthop, 13:24–41,1959
6. Laine VAI, Sairanen E, Vainio K. Finger deformities caused by rheumatoid arthritis. J Bone Jt Surg, 39A: 527–533, 1957
7. Landsmeer JMF. Anatomy of the dorsal aponeurosis of the human finger and its functional significance. Anat Rec, 104:31–44,1949
8. Landsmeer JMF. Anatomical and functional investigation on the articulation of the human fingers. Acta Anat (Basel), 25 (suppl 24):1–69,1955
9. Landsmeer JMF. The coordination of finger joint motions. J Bone Jt Surg, 45A: 1654–1662, 1963.
10. Landsmeer JMF. Atlas of Anatomy of the Hand. New York: Churchill Livingstone, 1976
11. Littler JW. The finger extensor mechanism. Surg Clin N Amer, 47:415–423,1967
12. Littler JW. On the adaptability of man's hand. Hand, 5: 187–191,1973
13. Littler JW. The digital extensor-flexor system. In Reconstructive Plastic Surgery. Volume 6. Converse JM (Ed). Philadelphia: Saunders 3166–3183,1977
14. Littler JW, Burton RI, Eaton RG. The dynamics of digital extension. AAOS Sound Slide Program 467,468,1976
15. Micks JE, Hager D. Role of the controversial parts of the extensor of the finger. J Bone Jt Surg, 55A: 884,1973
16. Micks JE, Reswick JB. Confirmation of differential loading of lateral and central fibers of the extensor tendon. J Hand Surg, 6:462–467,1981
17. Stack HG. Muscle function in the fingers. J Bone Jt Surg, 44B:899–909,1962
18. Tubiana R, Valentin P. The physiology of the extension of the finger. Surg Clin N Amer, 44:907–918,1964.
19. Zancolli E. Anatomy and Mechanics of the Extensor Apparatus of the Fingers. In: Structural and Dynamic Basis of Hand Surgery. (2nd Ed.). Philadelphia: Lippincott: 3–63,1979
20. Juvara E. Contribution á l'étude du ligament annulaire dorsal du carpe et des gaines synoviales des tendons de la face posteriéure et externe du poignet, Arch Sci Méd (Paris), 3:261–299,1898
21. Palmar AK, Skahen JR, Werner FW, Glisson RR. The extensor retinaculum of the wrist: an anatomical and biomechanical study. J. Hand Surg 10B: 11–16,1985
22. Schmidt H-M, Lanz U. Surgical Anatomy of the Hand. New York: Thieme, 223–230,231–239,243–247,2004
23. Taleisnik J, Gelberman RH, Miller BW, Szabo RM. The extensor retinaculum of the wrist. J Hand Surg, 9A: 495–501,1984
24. Davies DV, Coupland RE. Myology. Gray's Anatomy. Edition 4. London: Longmans, 673–681,690–693,1958
25. Albright JA, Linburg RM. Common variations of the radial wrist extensors. J Hand Surg, 3:134–138,1978
26. Gruber W. Ueber den Musculus radialis externus accessories. Arch Anat Physiol, 388–397,1877
27. Kosugi K, Shibata S, Yamashita H. Anatomical study on the variation of extensor muscles of the human forearm. Jikeikai Med, 34:51–69,297–304,1987
28. Wood J. Variations in human mycology. Proc R Soc Lond, 15: 229–244,1866
29. Wood VE. The extensor carpi radialis intermedius tendon. J Hand Surg, 13A: 242–245,1988
30. Lyall HA, Elliot D. Total middle ray amputation. Journal of Hand Surgery, 21B: 675–680,1996
31. de Quervain F. Ueber eine Form von chronischer Tendovaginitis. Korrespondenzblatt fur Schweizer Arzte 25: 389–394,1895
32. McFarlane RM. Observations on the functional anatomy of the intrinsic muscles of the thumb. J Bone Jt Surg, 44A: 1073–1088,1962
33. Khandwala AR, Webb J, Harris SB, Foster AJ, Elliot D. A comparison of dynamic extension splinting and controlled active mobilisation of complete divisions of extensor tendons in zones 5 and 6. J Hand Surg, 25B: 140–146,2000
34. Doyle, JR. Extensor tendons – acute injuries. In: Green's Operative Hand Surgery. Edition 4. Green DP, Hotchkiss RN, Pederson WC (Eds.). New York: Churchill Livingstone, 1950–1987,1999
35. Kleinert HE, Verdan C. Report of the committee on tendon injuries. J Hand Surg, 8:794–798,1983
36. Verdan CE. Primary and Secondary Repair of Flexor and Extensor Tendon Injuries. In Flynn JE (Ed) Hand Surgery. Baltimore: Williams and Wilkins: 20–75,1966.
37. Baumann JA. Valeur, variations et équivalences des muscles extenseurs, interosseux, adducteurs et abducteurs de la main et pied. Acta Anat, 4:10–16,1974
38. Cauldwell EW, Anson BJ, Wright RR. The extensor indicis proprius muscle. Quart Bull North-West Univ Med School, 17:267–269,1943
39. Cusenz BJ, Hallock GG. Multiple anomalous tendons of the fourth dorsal compartment. J Hand Surg 11A: 263–264,1986
40. Dostal GH, Lister GD, Hitchinson D, Mogan JV, Davis PH. Extensor digitorum brevis manuis associated with a dorsal wrist ganglion: a review of five cases. J Hand Surg, 20A: 35–37,1995
41. El-Badawi MGY, Butt MM, Al-Zuhair AGH, Fadel RA. Extensor tendons of the fingers: arrangement and variations. Clin Anat 8: 391–398,1995
42. Gonzalez MH, Gray T, Ortinau E, Weinzweig. The extensor tendons to the little finger: an anatomic study. J Hand Surg, 20A: 844–847,1995
43. Gonzalez MH, Weinzweig N, Kay T, Grindel S. Anatomy of the extensor tendons to the index. J Hand Surg 21A: 988–991,1996
44. Kaplan EB, Spinner M. Important muscular variations of the hand and forearm. In Functional and Surgical Anatomy. Edition 3. Spinner M (Ed.). Philadelphia: Lippincott, 1984

45. Le Double A-F. Traité des variations du système musculaire de l'homme et de leur signification au point de vue de l'anthropologie zoologique. Paris: Schleicher Frères, 1897

46. Leslie DR. The tendons on the dorsum of the hand. Aus NZ J Surg23: 253–256,1954

47. Mestdagh H, Bailleul JP, Vilette B, Bocquet F, Depreux R. Organisation of the extensor complex of the digit. Anat Clin7: 49–53 ,1985

48. Ogura T, Inoue H, Tanabe G. Anatomic and clinical studies of the extensor digitorum brevis manus. J Hand Surg 12A: 100–107,1987

49. Schenck RR. Variations of the extensor tendons of the finger. J Bone Joint Surg46A: 103–110,1964

50. Schroeder von HP, Botte M. The extensor medii proprius and anomalous extensor tendons of the middle finger. J Hand Surg16A: 1141–1145,1991

51. Schroeder von HP, Botte M. Anatomy of the extensor tendons of the fingers. Variations and multiplicity. J Hand Surg, 20A: 27–34,1995

52. Schroeder von HP, Botte M, Gellman H. Anatomy of the juncturae tendinum of the hand. J Hand Surg, 15A: 595–602,1990

53. Tan ST, Smith PJ. Anomalous extensor muscles of the hand: a review. J Hand Surg24A: 449–455,1999

54. Testut L. Les Anomalies Musculaires Chez l'Homme Expliquées par l'Anatomie Comparée, leur Importance en Anthropologie. Paris: Masson, 1884

55. Steichen JB, Petersen DP. Junctura tendinum between extensor digitorum communis and extensor pollicis longus. J Hand Surg9A: 674–676, 1984

56. Verdan C. Les anomalies musculo-tendineuses et leur significance en chirurgie de la main. Rev Chir Orthop 67: 221–230,1981

57. Lluch A. Treatment of Radial Neuromata and Dysesthesia. Techniques in Hand and Upper Extremity Surgery 5: 188–195,2001

58. Kitano K, Tada K, Shibata T, Yoshida T. Independent index extension after indicis proprius transfer: excision of juncturae tendinum. J Hand Surg21A: 992–996,1996

59. Moore JR, Weiland AJ, Valdata L. Independent index extension after extensor indicis transfer. J Hand Surg 12A: 232–236,1987

60. Noorda RJP, Hage JJ, Groot PJM, Bloem JJAM. Index finger extension and strength after indicis proprius transfer. J Hand Surg 19A: 844–849,1994

61. Agee J, Guidera M, The functional significance of the juncturae tendinae in dynamic stabilization of the metacarpophalangeal joints of the fingers. American Society for Surgery of the Hand. Atlanta, 1980

62. Schroeder von HP, Botte M. The functional significance of the long extensors and juncturae tendinum in finger extension. J Hand Surg 18A: 641–647,1993

63. Wehbé MA. Junctura anatomy. J Hand Surg, 17A: 1124–1129 1992

64. Brand PW. Clinical Mechanics of the Hand. St Louis: Mosby, 1985

65. Wartenberg R. A sign of ulnar nerve palsy. JAMA 112: 1688, 1939

66. Allieu Y, Asencio G, Gomis R, Teissier J, Rouzaud JC Suture des tendons extenseurs de la main avec mobilisation assistée. A propos de 120 cas. Rev Chir Orthop, 20 Suppl 1:68–73,1984

67. Allieu Y, Asencio G, Rouzaud JC. Protected passive mobilization after suturing of the extensor tendons of the Hand. In: Tubiana R (Ed) The Hand. Philadelphia: Saunders, Vol 3: 57–163,1988

68. Evans RB. Immediate active short arc motion following extensor tendon repair. Hand Clinics, 11: 483–510,1995

69. Frère G, Moutet F, Sarorius C, Vila A. Controlled postoperative mobilization of sutured extension tendons of the long fingers. Ann Chir Main 3:139–144,1984

70. Levame JH. Rééducation de Traumatisés de la Main. Paris: Archee: 105–109,1965

71. Marin-Braun F, Merle M, Sanz J, Foucher G, Voiry MH, Petry D. Primary repair of extensor tendons with assisted post-operative mobilization. A series of 48 cases. Ann Chir de la Main, 8: 7–21,1989

72. Sylaidis P, Youatt M, Logan A. Early active mobilisation for extensor injuries. J Hand Surg 22B: 594 – 596,1997

73. Rabischong PO. L'innervation proprioceptive des muscles lombricaux de la main chez l'homme. Rev Chir Orthop 48: 234–235,1962

74. Milford L. The retaining ligaments of the digits of the hand. Gross and microscopic study. Philadelphia, Saunders, 1968

75. Littler JW. The hand and wrist. In A Textbook of Orthopedics. Howorth MB (Ed.). Philadelphia: Saunders, p.284. 1952

76. Sarrafian SK, Kazarian LE, Topouzian VK, Sarrafian VK, Siegelman A. Strain variation in the components of the extensor apparatus of the finger during flexion and extension. A biomechanical study. J Bone Jt Surg 52A: 980–990,1970

77. Bunnell S. Surgery of the intrinsic muscles of the hand other than those producing opposition of the thumb. J Bone Jt Surg24A: 1–31,1942

78. Cruveilhier J. Traité d'Anatomie Descriptive. Vol 1. Ed 1. Paris: Baillière. 1837

79. Legueu MMF, Juvara E. Des aponeuroses de la paume de la main. Bull Soc Anat (Paris), 393–400,1892

80. Poirier P, Charpy A. Traité d'Anatomie Humaine. Paris: Masson and Cie, 1899

81. Tubiana R, Valentin P. The anatomy of the extension of the finger. Surg Clin N Amer44: 897–906,1964

82. Braithwaite F, Channell GD, Moore FT, Whillis J. The anatomy and function of the extensor complex. Brit J Plast Surg 2: 175–187,1949

83. Engelhart E, Schmidt H-M. Zur klinischen Anatomie der Dorsalaponeurose der Finger beim Menschen. Verh Anat Ges81: 311–313,1987

84. Hauck G. Die Ruptur der Dorsalapooneurose am ersten Interphalangealgelenk, zugleich ein Beitrag zur Anatomie und Physiologie der Dorsalaponeurose. Arch Klin Chir123: 197–232,1923

85. Horner WE. Lessons in Practical Anatomy for the Use of Dissectors. Philadelphia: Carey and Lea. 1827

86. Kaplan EB. Functional significance of the insertions of the extensor communis in man. Anat Rec92: 293–303,1945.

87. Montant R, Baumann A. Recherches anatomiques sur le système tendineux des doigts de la main. Ann Anat Pathol 14: 311–336,1937

88. Seifert E. Zur Kenntnis der Dorsalaponeurose der Finger. Arch Orthop Unfallchir16: 557–562,1919

89. Carroll C, More JR, Weiland AJ. Posttraumatic ulnar subluxation of the extensor tendons: a reconstructive technique. J Hand Surg 12A: 227–231,1987

90. Love GJ, MacLean JGB. Ulnar subluxation of the extensor tendons in elderly osteoarthritic females: a neglected diagnosis. J Hand Surg 32E: 45–49,2007

91. Slattery PG. The dorsal plate of the proximal interphalangeal joint. J Hand Surg15B: 68–73,1990

92. Schultz RJ, Furlong J. Observations on the fiber pattern of the extensor mechanism of the finger at the level of the proximal interphalangeal joint. Bull Hosp Jt Dis39: 100–101,1978

93. Schultz RJ, Furlong J, Storace A. Detailed anatomy of the extensor mechanism at the proximal aspect of the finger. J Hand Surg6: 493–498,1981

94. Bunnell S. Surgery of the Hand. Philadelphia, Lippincott; 1944

95. Winslow JB. Exposition Anatomique de la Structure du Corps Humain. Paris: Desprez and Desessartz, 1732.

96. Testut L. Traité d'Anatomie Humaine. 3rd Ed. Vol 1. Paris: Doin, 1896

97. Cleland J. On the cutaneous ligaments of the phalanges. J Anat Physiol12: 526–527,1878

98. Weitbrecht J. Syndesmologia sive historia ligamentorum corporis humani quam secundum observationes anatomicas concinnavit et figuris ad objecta recentia adumbratis illustravit. Petersburg: Typographia Academiae Scientiarum, Petropoli; 1742. A description of the ligaments of the human body, arranged in accordance with anatomical dissections and illustrated with figures drawn from fresh subjects. (Translated by Kaplan EB. Philadelphia: Saunders; 1969.)

99. Haines RW. The extensor apparatus of the finger. J Anat85: 251–259,1951

100. Shrewsbury MM, Johnson RK. A systematic study of the oblique retinacular ligament of the human finger: its structure and function. J Hand Surg2: 194–199, 1977

101. Hahn P, Krimmer H, Hradetzky A, Lanz U. Quantitative analysis of the linkage between the interphalangeal joints of the index finger. J Hand Surg20B: 696–699,1995

102. Kleinman WB, Petersen DP. Oblique retinacular ligament reconstruction for chronic mallet deformity. J Hand Surg9A: 399–404,1984

103. Steinheil I. Beiträge zur Anatomie und Funktion der Fingersehnen. Med Inaug Diss, Tübingen, 1959

104. Stack HG. A study of muscle function in the fingers. Ann Roy Coll Surg Engl33: 307–322,1963

105. Thompson JS, Littler JW, Upton J. The spiral oblique retinacular ligament. J Hand Surg 3: 482–487,1978

106. Wilhelm A. Zur Anatomie und Chirurgie des Strecksehnenapparates der Hand unter Berücksichtigung neuerer Operationsmethoden. Hefte Unfallheilk101: 1–18,1969

107. Bendz P. The functional significance of the oblique retinacular ligament of Landsmeer. A review and new proposals. J Hand Surg10B: 25–29,1985

108. El-Gammal TA, Steyers CM, Blair WF, Maynard JA. Anatomy of the oblique retinacular ligament of the index finger. J Hand Surg18A: 717–721,1993

109. Long C, Brown ME. Electromyographic kinesiology of the hand. Muscles moving the long finger. J Bone Jt Surg46A: 1683–1706,1964

110. Stack HG. The anatomy of the muscles and tendons of the hand. P.95 In the Second Hand Club. Stack HG, Bolton H (Eds.). Brentwood: Westbury Press, 1975

111. Goldner JA. Deformities of the hand incidental to pathological changes of the extensor and intrinsic muscle mechanisms. J Bone Jt Surg35A: 115–131,1953

112. Ketchum LD, Thompson D, Pocock G, Wallingford D. A clinical study of forces generated by the intrinsic muscles of the index finger and the extrinsic flexor and extensor muscles of the hand. J Hand Surg 3: 571–578,1978

113. Smith RJ. Balance and kinetics of the finger under normal and pathological conditions. Clin Orthop104: 92–111,1974

114. Snow JW, Switzer H. Method of studying the relationships between the finger joints and the flexor and extensor mechanism. Plast Reconstr Surg 55: 242–243,1975

115. Spoor CW, Landsmeer JM. Analysis of the zigzag movement of the human finger under influence of the extensor digitorum tendon and the deep flexor tendon. J Biomech9: 561–566,1976

116. Albinus BS. Historia muscolorum hominis. Leyden: folio; 1734

117. Bichat MFX. Traité d'Anatomie Descriptive. Paris: Goben and Cie; 1801–1803

118. Bouvier M. Note sur une paralysie partielle des muscles de la main. Bull Acad Nat Med18: 125–139,1851–52

119. Salisbury CR. The interosseous muscles of the hand. J Anat71: 395–403,1936

120. Yii NW, Elliot D. A study of the dynamic relationship of the lumbrical muscles and the carpal tunnel. J Hand Surg19B: 439–443,1994

121. Chase R. Muscle tendon kinetics. Am J Surg 109: 277–282, 1965

122. Henle J. Handbuch der Muskellehre des Menchen. Braunschweig: Vieweg; 1871

123. Schöenig von G. Ueber den Abriss der Strecksehne von der Phalanx des Nagelgliedes. Arch Klin Chir35: 237,1887

124. Blackhouse KM, Catton WT. An experimental study of the functions of the lumbrical muscles in the human hand. J Anat 88: 133–141,1954

125. Duchenne GB. Physiologie des mouvements démontrée à l'aide de l'expérimentation électrique et de l'observation clinique, et applicable à l'étude des paralysies et des deformations. Paris: Baillière, 1867

126. Long C. Intrinsic-extrinsic muscle control of the fingers. J Bone Jt Surg 50A: 973–984,1968

127. Elliott RA. Injuries to the extensor mechanism of the hand. Orthop Clin North Amer1: 335–354,1970

128. Flatt AE. The Care of Minor Injuries of the Hand. St Louis: Mosby, 1979

129. Kelly AP. Primary tendon repairs. A study of 789 consecutive tendon severances. J Bone Jt Surg41A: 581–598,1959.

130. Tubiana R. Surgical repair of the extensor apparatus of the fingers. Surg Clin North Am 48: 1015–1031,1968

131. Kulkarni M, Harris SB, Elliot D. The significance of extensor tendon tethering and dorsal joint capsule tightening

after injury to the hand. Journal of Hand Surgery 31B: 52–60,2006

132. Couch JH: The principles of tendon suture in the hand. Can Med Assoc. 41(1):27–30,1939.

133. Bunnell S: Surgery of the Hand. 2nd Ed., Philadelphia, Lippincott, 1949

134. Elliot D, McGrouther DA. The Excursions of the long extensor tendons of the hand. J Hand Surg 11B: 77–80,1986

135. Kilgore ES, Graham WP. The hand. Surgical and Nonsurgical Management. Philadelphia: Lea and Febiger, 1977

136. Newport ML, Blair WF, Steyers CM. Long-term results of extensor tendon repair. Journal of Hand Surgery. 15A: 961–966,1990

30 The Interossei

Indranil Chakrabarti

30.1 Anatomy and Biomechanics

The interossei are muscles that occupy the space between the metacarpals of the hand. They comprise two groups: one slightly palmar to the mid coronal plane and one slightly dorsal. They are numbered 1 to 4, starting with the most radial and progressing ulnarward (▶ Fig. 30.1).

They fill the space *between* the bones, hence named interossei. There are usually four dorsal and three palmar interossei (▶ Fig. 30.2 and ▶ Fig. 30.3), but variations do occur, and it is not unusual to find a fourth palmar interosseus.[1]

This also gives rise to a degree of confusion when looking at the muscles in situ, because it is sometimes difficult to tell which muscle is palmar and which is dorsal. The latter are

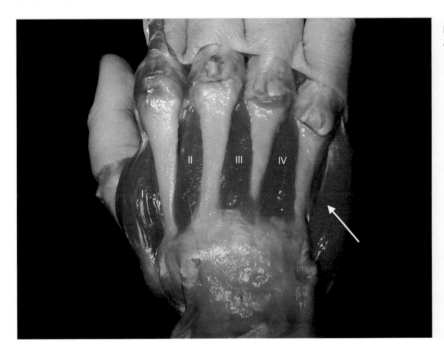

Fig. 30.1 The dorsal interossei (I–IV) and the abductor digiti minimi (*arrow*).

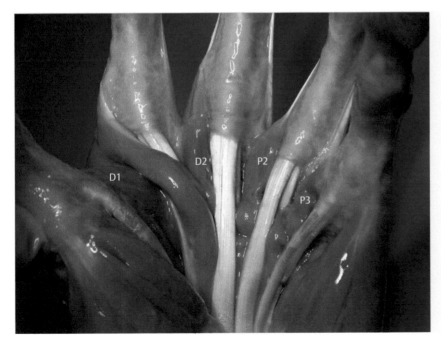

Fig. 30.2 The first two dorsal interossei (D1 and D2) and the last two palmar interossei (P2 and P3).

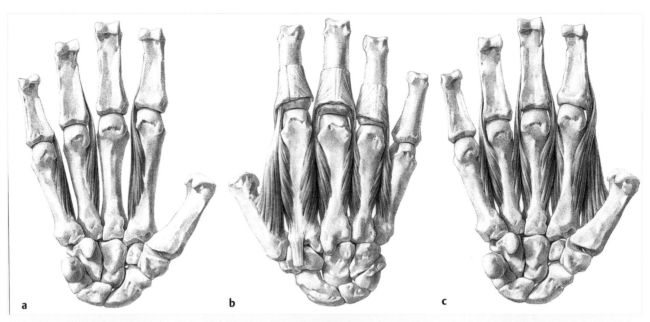

Fig. 30.3 (a) The three palmar interossei from the anterior aspect. (b) The dorsal interossei from the posterior aspect. (c) The dorsal interossei from the anterior aspect. (From Schmidt H-M, Lanz U. Surgical Anatomy of the Hand. Stuttgart, Germany: Thieme; 2004.)

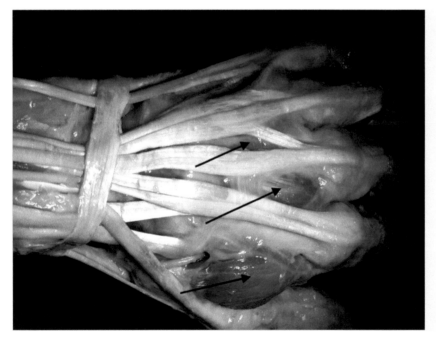

Fig. 30.4 The dorsal interossei bulging though (*arrows*).

prominent on the dorsum of the hand (▶Fig. 30.4) underneath the extensor tendons, and it is the first dorsal interosseus that one notices immediately, with the others bulging underneath the deep fascia below. It is for this reason that "guttering" is so easily evident in the presence of a chronic ulnar nerve lesion: the "ulnar-minus hand."

The palmar interossei are *unipennate* muscles, while the dorsal interossei are *bipennate*, each one being attached almost throughout its length to the metacarpal and having a very short tendon in relation to its total length. The mean length of the dorsal interossei is 1.3 cm and that of the palmar interossei is 1.7 cm, with the former occupying about 37% of the total volume of the intrinsic muscles of the hand and the latter 16%.[2]

The excursion of each muscle/tendon unit is limited, but the proportionate power exerted is very high indeed, because when it contracts, each muscle exerts its effect using a short lever arm; the fulcrum of its action is effectively the middle of the metacarpal head, with the line of pull being about a centimeter away, at the level of the metacarpophalangeal joint. The strength required to hold a piece of paper between two fingers, for example, is proportionately very high.

The dorsal interossei abduct the fingers and the palmar interossei adduct them. This is easily remembered by employing the acronyms DAB, for "dorsal abduct," and PAD, for "palmar adduct." Since the abductor digiti minimi abducts the little finger, it functions in the same way and would be referred to as the

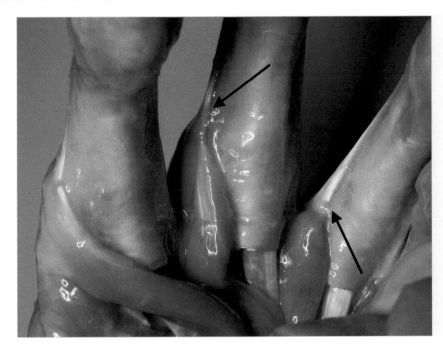

Fig. 30.5 The interossei join the lumbricals to form the conjoint tendons (*black arrows*).

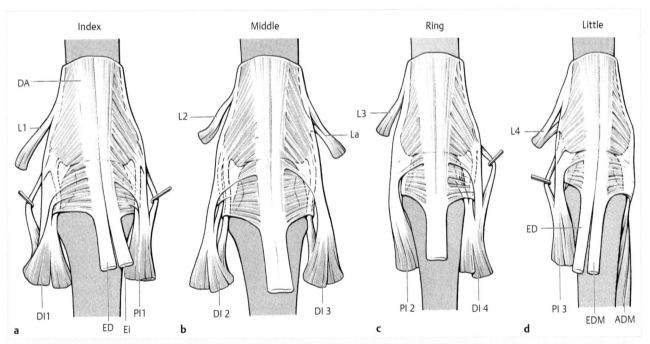

Fig. 30.6 Insertions of the dorsal and palmar interossei and the lumbricals in the fingers. **a.** Index finger; **b.** Middle finger; **c.** Ring finger; **d.** Little finger. (From Schmidt H-M, Lanz U. Surgical Anatomy of the Hand. Stuttgart, Germany: Thieme; 2004.)

fifth dorsal interosseus were it not for the fact that it does not lie between two bones.

The interossei combine with the lumbricals at the level of the metacarpophalangeal joint to form a conjoint tendon (▶Fig. 30.5 and ▶Fig. 30.6).

This is joined distally, after it has merged with the extensor expansion just before the proximal interphalangeal joint, by *Landsmeer's oblique retinacular ligament*, a structure that begins its course more volarly and takes its origin from the phalanx itself and the fibrous flexor sheath, continuing onward to

merge with the lateral slips as they converge and form the terminal extensor tendon (▶Fig. 30.7).

The lumbricals, interossei, and oblique retinacular ligament of Landsmeer run parallel at the level of the proximal phalanx[3]; the conjoint tendon thereby *extends* the proximal interphalangeal joint while, at the same time, *flexing* the metacarpophalangeal joint (▶Fig. 30.8).

It is worth noting that the first palmar interosseus is on the ulnar side of the index, whereas the first lumbrical is on the radial side; therefore, the index does not have an ulnar conjoint

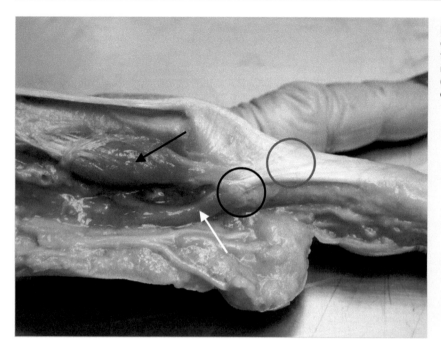

Fig. 30.7 The interosseus (*black arrow*) combines with the lumbrical (*white arrow*) to form the conjoint tendon (*black circle*), which merges with the dorsal extensor expansion (*red circle*). More distally, this blends with the oblique retinacular ligament of Landsmeer.

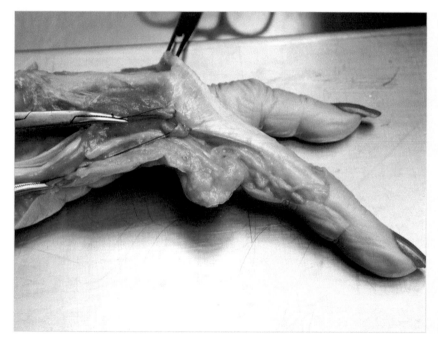

Fig. 30.8 The conjoint tendon flexes the metacarpophalangeal joint and extends the proximal interphalangeal joint.

tendon. One needs to consider this when contemplating a crossed intrinsic transfer for a patient who has ulnar deviation of the fingers in conditions such as rheumatoid arthritis.

It is easy to mistake the adductor pollicis for the first dorsal interosseus. The former lies deep to the latter and has two "heads," or sites of origin: one (the deep head) from the thumb metacarpal and the other (the transverse head) from the middle metacarpal. They insert at the base of the proximal phalanx of the thumb. Mardel and Underwood[4] considered adductor pollicis to be the real first palmar interosseus muscle, and functionally, it is. The first dorsal interosseus also has two heads: one

from the thumb metacarpal and one from the index. It inserts into the base of the index proximal phalanx on its radial side (▶ Fig. 30.9 and ▶ Fig. 30.10).

The anthropoid apes also have interossei similar to humans, with gorillas, gibbons, and orangutans having the same number. However, chimpanzees appear to have extra three interossei, which may be considered palmar but are in fact *intermediate*, lying between the dorsal and palmar layers, and can be thought of as *short flexors*.[5] In many ways this resembles the short flexors of the human foot and may reflect the fact that the chimpanzees often use their upper limbs to walk on and to propel themselves.

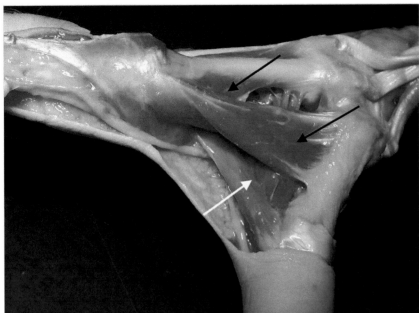

Fig. 30.9 Two heads of the first dorsal interosseus (*black arrows*) and the adductor pollicis (*white arrow*), which may be considered the true first palmar interosseus.

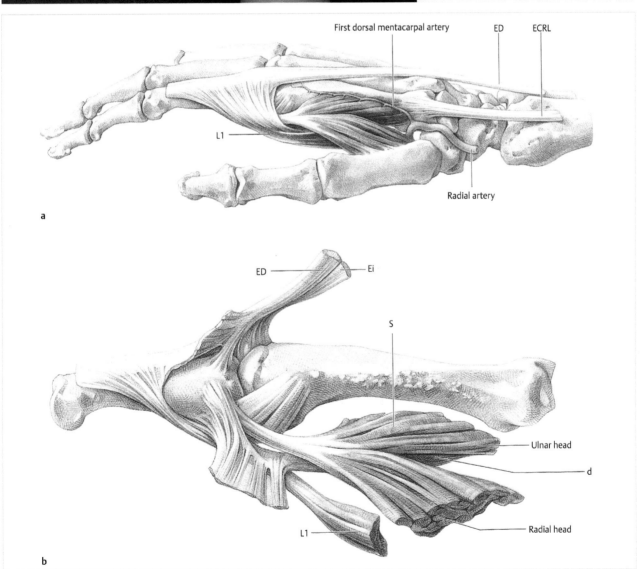

Fig. 30.10 Anatomy of the first dorsal interosseous. (a) muscles in place; (b) detailed origins and relations of structures. (From Schmidt H-M, Lanz U. Surgical Anatomy of the Hand, Thieme, Stuttgart, 2004.)

The interossei are supplied by the deep branch of the ulnar nerve after it has passed through Guyon's canal into the palm.

30.2 Function

So why do we need to abduct (and, indeed, *adduct)* our fingers? Surely it is enough to be able to flex and extend them individually or en masse, thereby allowing the hand to carry out most of the functions of daily living? In order to understand this, one needs to consider how we use our fingers to grip. Although numerous types of grip have been described by various authors, Sollerman's description of eight types of grips is particularly useful: diagonal volar, transverse volar and spherical volar (which provide power) and extension grip, lateral pinch, five-finger pinch, pulp pinch, and tripod pinch (which are useful for "fine" tasks).

Transverse volar, diagonal volar, and extension grips all require *adduction* of the fingers in order to provide strength, while spherical volar grip requires *abduction* (▶ Fig. 30.11).

Tripod pinch, lateral pinch, five-finger pinch, and pulp pinch require a functioning first dorsal interosseous (▶ Fig. 30.12).

It is interesting, therefore, to see that all eight grips involve the interossei. They may be small, but they are important.

Where would we be without abduction? One need only ask a musician. Would it be possible for a pianist, flautist, violinist, or guitarist (or practically any musician) to play if he or she were unable to abduct and adduct the fingers?

Liszt and Rachmaninov,[7,8] who were both virtuoso pianists and composers, and Paganini (a violinist and composer) were all able to abduct their fingers more than most people. This is because they almost certainly had Marfan's syndrome. Rachmaninov, for example, could "span a twelfth," which allowed

him a level of performance that few could match. His compositions (and those of Liszt) are well known for being difficult to play for this very reason.

One should, of course, consider all sorts of activities and skills. Artists and craftsmen all over the world, in all walks of life, rely on functioning interossei.

This train of thought inevitably leads to the following question: Can a surgeon operate without active abduction and adduction of the fingers? Would he or she be able to use a pair of dissecting scissors, a needle-holder, an arthroscope, or a probe?

These are thought-provoking questions that inevitably arise while studying the anatomy of these muscles.

This chapter has dealt, so far, with the interossei alone. Clearly this is a slightly artificial conceit, since these muscles act alongside the other muscles and tendons in the hand (especially the lumbricals, as the "*intrinsics*") in a complex and intimate way. It isn't until one sees a patient with an ulnar nerve lesion that one appreciates how important they are. Because the strong, unopposed extensors of the metacarpophalangeal joints cause hyperextension, the "ulnar claw" develops, grip is weakened, and significant functional deficit ensues. Patients complain of an inability to perform basic day-to-day tasks ("I can't do up my buttons or tie my shoelaces"; "I can't pick up coins") and life becomes difficult.

It is crucial that one take these features into account when operating on the hand. If plating of a metacarpal fracture is undertaken, the interossei are inevitably interfered with. They may be stripped off the bone and a bulky plate may be applied. This causes adhesions which prevent the smooth gliding of the muscle–tendon unit and also compromises its biomechanical properties, resulting in stiffness of the metacarpophalangeal and proximal interphalangeal joints.

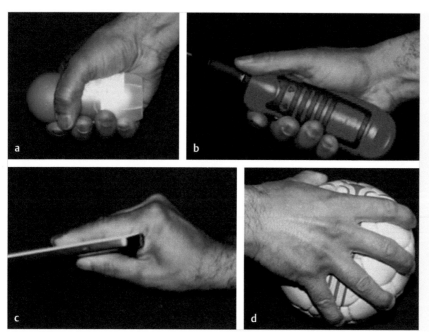

Fig. 30.11 Power grips: transverse volar, (**a**) diagonal volar, (**b**) and extension grip (**c**) require *adduction*, while spherical volar grip (**d**) requires *abduction*.

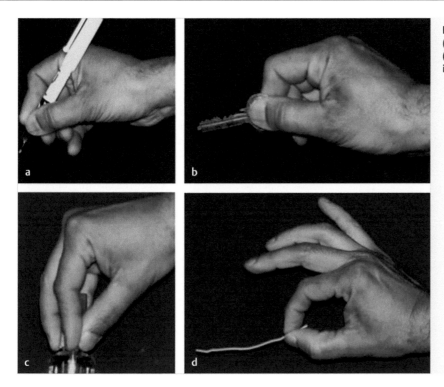

Fig. 30.12 Tripod pinch, (**a**) lateral pinch, (**b**) five-finger pinch, (**c**) and pulp pinch (**d**) all require a function first dorsal interosseus (*arrow*).

30.3 Summary

The interossei, both dorsal and palmar, are extremely important muscles. Structurally they resemble other muscles that are attached to long bones (e.g., the vasti of the femur and triceps brachii) in being attached throughout their length to the bone of origin. As a result, they have relatively short tendons with little excursion and a great deal of power in relation to their size. Where they differ is in their relationship to other muscles: they work in conjunction, principally, with the lumbricals. Bio-mechanically they are indeed supremely efficient and allow the hand to perform tasks that require strength, precision, or both simultaneously.

Functionally, they are vital.

References

1. McMinn RMH, Hutchings RT. A Colour Atlas of Human Anatomy. Wolfe Medical Publications; London 1977
2. Linscheid RL, An K, Gross RM. Quantitative analysis of the intrinsic muscles of the hand. Clin Anat 1991;4:265–284
3. Landsmeer JM. The anatomy of the dorsal aponeurosis of the human finger and its functional significance. Anat Rec 1949;104(1):31–44
4. Mardel S, Underwood M. Adductor pollicis. The missing interosseous. Surg Radiol Anat 1991;13(1):49–52
5. Hepburn D. The comparative anatomy of the muscles and nerves of the superior and inferior extremities of the anthropoid apes, part 1. J Anat Physiol 1892;26(Pt 2):149–186
6. Sollerman C, Ejeskär A. Sollerman hand function test. A standardised method and its use in tetraplegic patients. Scand J Plast Reconstr Surg Hand Surg 1995;29(2):167–176
7. Basnayake V. Enthusiasms: a tropical wreath for Liszt. Br Med J (Clin Res Ed) 1986;293(6562):1626–1627
8. Young DAB. Rachmaninov and Marfan's syndrome. Br Med J (Clin Res Ed) 1986;293(6562):1624–1626

31 Lumbricals

Jaehon M. Kim and Chaitanya S. Mudgal

31.1 Introduction

The lumbricals have the unique feature of being the only muscle in the body which originates from its own antagonistic muscle. The lumbricals originate from flexor digitorum profundus (FDP) and insert onto the radial lateral band at the level of proximal phalanx.[1] The primary function of the lumbricals is to extend the interphalangeal joints, but there exists a complex interplay of tension between flexor and extensors. In reality, both origin and insertion of lumbricals are highly variable, and the detailed report of anatomy and function in literature is sparse. The purpose of this chapter is to summarize what we know about lumbricals in existing literature along with illustrative cases of pathomechanics.

31.2 Detailed Anatomy

31.2.1 Origin

A detailed account of lumbrical anatomy was carefully demonstrated in a cadaveric study by Eladomikadachi et al.[2] There are four cylindrical lumbricals in each hand, based on their insertion site (index to small finger). The origins of each muscle are diverse and do not correspond to their respective tendon. The first lumbrical is the most consistent with its origin at the radial aspect of index finger FDP at the level of proximal half of the metacarpal bone. The second lumbrical receives contributions from neighboring tendons over 20% of the time.[2] The most variability is seen with third and fourth lumbricals, where over 50% derived origins from other fingers (▶ Fig. 31.1a, b). The third and fourth lumbricals commonly share fibers from adjacent FDP and occasionally derive their entire fibers from the neighboring tendons. This, in part, may explain the less independent extension of ring and small fingers compared with index and long fingers, especially with extension.

31.2.2 Insertion

The distal lumbrical insertions always attach to the radial side of the lateral band at the level of proximal phalanx. A shared insertion to the oblique or transverse fibers of the extensor apparatus is common and is seen in up to 60% of lumbrical muscles.[2] Minor contributions to the volar plate and proximal phalanx are also present. The highest frequency of variations is observed once again in the ulnar fingers. The fibrous hood of the dorsal apparatus, which is a broad interconnection of various tendons and ligaments, crosses majority of the joints in the fingers (▶ Fig. 31.2). The central portion corresponds to the extensor digitorum communis (EDC), tethered centrally by the

sagittal bands on either side. The tendons of interossei and lumbrical run volar to the axis of the metacarpophalangeal (MCP) joint, and once they become the lateral band, they swoop dorsally around the proximal phalanx forming the conjoint lateral band (▶ Fig. 31.2). The attachments of lumbricals are distal and dorsal to the interossei. The subsequent crossing of PIP and DIP joints occurs dorsal to the flexion–extension axis of these joints, and volar shift of the conjoint lateral band is prevented by the triangular ligament at the level of middle phalanx (▶ Fig. 31.3). To prevent dorsal dislocation, transverse retinacular ligaments (▶ Fig. 31.4) anchor the lateral bands to the pulley of the flexor tendons on either side of the PIP joint. The terminal tendon, which combines the EDC and two lateral bands, attaches to a bony ridge at the base of the distal phalanx.

31.2.3 Mechanics

Based on anatomic dimensions carefully measured by Jacobson et al, lumbricals have the longest fiber length, measuring 40 to 50 mm among the intrinsic muscles. In fact, the fiber length of lumbricals is similar to that of extrinsic muscles of the hand which originate from the forearm.[3] Due to almost full extension of muscle fibers relative to the entire muscle length, the lumbricals are designed for high excursions. This construct allows for ability to maintain constant contractile force during various position of the FDP.[3] In contrast, the physiologic cross-sectional area of lumbricals (similar to other intrinsic muscles) is small (0.06–0.11 cm^2) which reduces the capability for force production.[3]

31.3 Nerve Supply

The median nerve is responsible for innervation of the two radial lumbricals and occasionally the third lumbrical. The first lumbrical is always innervated by the radial digital nerve of the index finger (▶ Fig. 31.5).[4] The second lumbrical is innervated by the common digital nerve to the index and middle fingers (▶ Fig. 31.5). In 25% cases, the third lumbricals are innervated by the median nerve.[5] At the level of proximal third metacarpal bone, the nerve enters the muscle on its radial–palmar aspect.

The third and fourth lumbricals are innervated by the deep (motor) branch of the ulnar nerve. The ulnar nerve emerges from Guyon's canal and divides into superficial sensory and deep motor branches. The superficial sensory branch has a linear course splitting into the digital sensory nerves for ring and small fingers (▶ Fig. 31.6). The deep motor branch passes deep to the flexor digiti minimi brevis and pierces the opponens

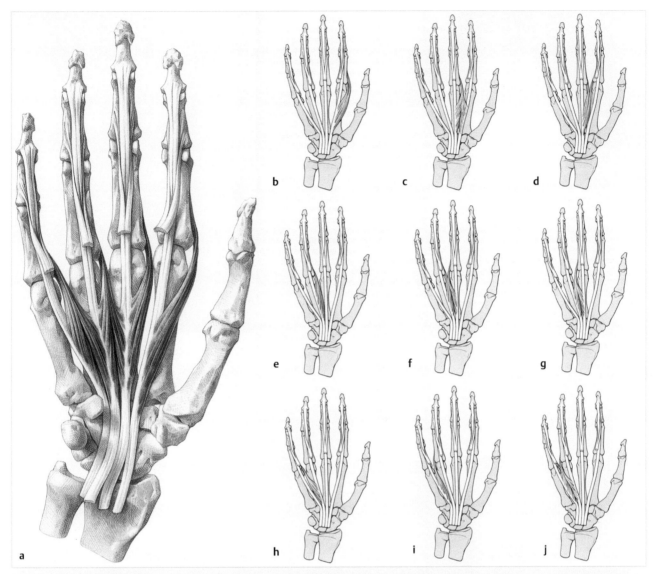

Fig. 31.1 There is a high frequency of variability in the origins of fourth lumbrical. Multiple combinations of fiber origins were observed, including additional derivation from the ulnar aspect of ring flexor digitorum profundus (FDP), few fiber contributions from the adjacent lumbrical, and entire origin from the ring FDP. (**a**) Standard description of lumbrical origin and insertion. (**b–j**) Variations. (From Schmidt H-M, Lanz U. Surgical Anatomy of the Hand. Stuttgart, Germany: Thieme; 2004.)

digiti minimi. The deep motor branch of the ulnar nerve curves radially at the level of proximal third metacarpal. Small longitudinal branches radial to the third and fourth metacarpal bone innervate the lumbricals (▶ Fig. 31.6). A cadaveric study by Hughes et al[6] failed to identify anatomic variation where the nerve extended to innervate the first and second lumbricals in 10 hand specimens.

31.4 Function

Forces generated by the lumbricals are transmitted through the lateral bands, and various anatomic features allow the

lumbricals to perform a complex array of functions. Primarily, the lumbricals are one of the independent extensors of proximal interphalangeal (PIP) and distal interphalangeal (DIP) joints (▶ Fig. 31.7). The origin and insertion onto its antagonistic tendon allow the contraction of the lumbrical to relax its corresponding FDP. During flexion of the interphalangeal joints, the FDP contracts and lengthens the lumbricals. With full extension of the fingers, the lumbricals contract and the FDPs relax.

Secondly, the lateral band demonstrates its own function independent of the EDC. Even after the EDC has competed its excursion, the lumbricals acting through the lateral band can further extend the middle and distal phalanx.[7] When the MCP and PIP joints are passively hyperextended (increasing tension

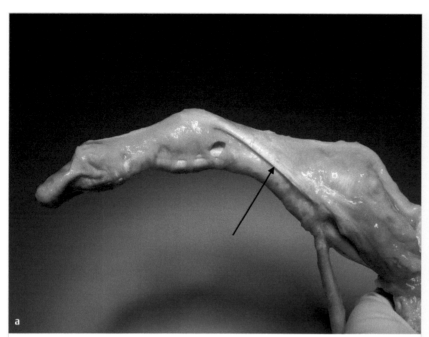

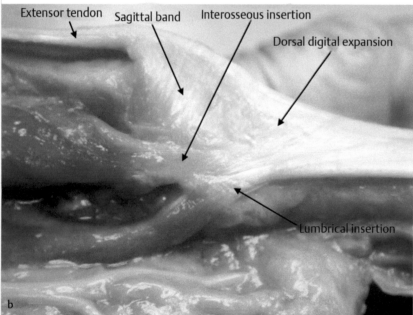

Extensor tendon   Sagittal band   Interosseous insertion

Dorsal digital expansion

Lumbrical insertion

Fig. 31.2 (a,b) The fibrous sheath of the dorsal apparatus interconnects three major tendons: two lateral bands and the extensor apparatus, which consists of extensor digitorum communis and the central slip. Both interosseous and lumbricals contribute to the lateral band (*thin arrow*). The distal insertion of lumbricals attaches distal and dorsal to the interosseous.

on the FDP), the distal phalanx can be actively flexed and extended with full independence. On the contrary, if the MCP and PIP joints are forcefully flexed, permitting complete relaxation of the dorsal apparatus (via the lumbricals), the FDP is subsequently without tension; it is then impossible for the distal phalanx to actively extend. For optimal function, the lumbricals require a taut anchor, which is achieved by the tension of the respective FDP (▶ Fig. 31.8).

FDP and flexor digitorum sublimis (FDS) are considered to be the primary flexors of MCP joint. The lumbricals also may function as a flexor of MCP joint without the aid of these two extrinsic muscles. Although this conception has been debated, cadaveric biomechanical studies have supported it when lumbricals have been tested in isolation.[8] The amount of generated force during flexion is unclear. Despite the radial insertion of lumbricals, the overall alignment is relatively parallel to the

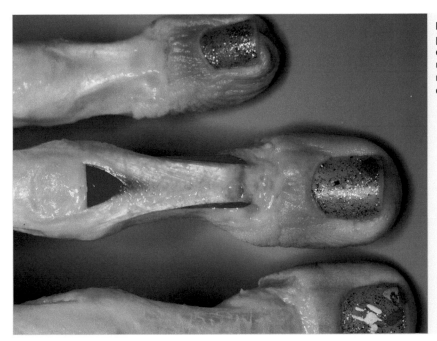

Fig. 31.3 The triangular ligament distal to proximal interphalangeal joint prevents volar displacement of the lateral bands. Attenuation of this ligament may lead to volar migration of lateral bands and Boutonniere deformity in chronic settings.

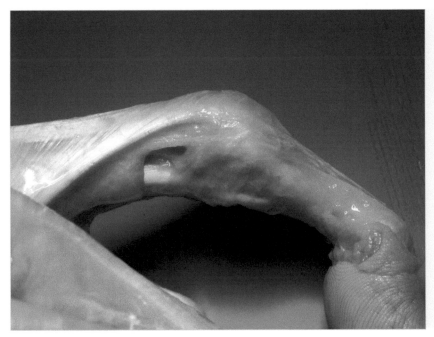

Fig. 31.4 The transverse retinacular ligament originates from the flexor tendon sheath at the volar aspect of proximal interphalangeal (PIP) joint and attaches to the lateral band. It functions to prevent dorsal shift, which would lead to hyperextension of PIP joint and flexion of distal interphalangeal joint, known as the "swan-neck" deformity.

long axis of the finger. Hence, there is minimal contribution to the abduction of the index and long fingers and the adduction of the ring and small fingers. Volar and dorsal interossei play more influential roles during lateral digital motion.

31.5 Pathologic Manifestations

The pathologies of intrinsic muscles (i.e., ischemic contractures) are difficult to treat and are generally irreversible by surgical means. Most important are the kinetics and the interplay of lumbricals to the overall function of the hand. Since the lumbricals originate and attach to flexors and extensors, it is impossible to discuss lumbrical dysfunction in isolation. The implications for treatment and rehabilitation strongly depend on understanding this concept. We have selected two examples of flexor and extensor pathologies that are affected through the lumbricals.

31.5.1 Extensor Lacerations

Mechanical open severance of the central slip at the PIP joint or closed rupture leads to imbalance of force favoring the

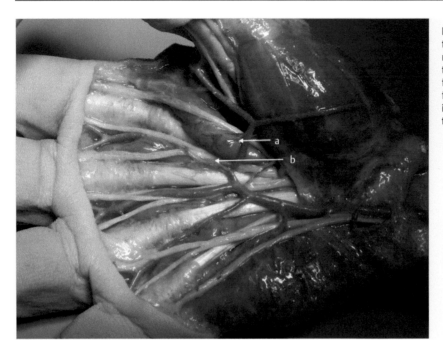

Fig. 31.5 The median nerve exits the carpal tunnel and branches into common digital nerves and the motor branch. The nerve to the first lumbrical receives its contribution from the radial digital nerve to the index finger (**a**), while the second lumbrical is innervated by the common digital nerve to the second web space (**b**).

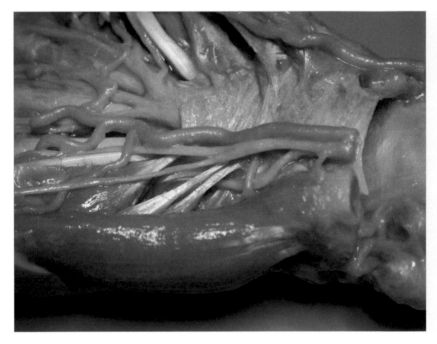

Fig. 31.6 The deep motor branch of the ulnar nerve curves radially at the level of proximal metacarpals. Small longitudinal branches innervate the third and fourth lumbricals.

unopposed flexors. The flexion of PIP joint causes proximal migration of lumbrical origin along with the contracted flexors. Over the course of several weeks, triangular ligament stretches and the lateral bands migrate palmarly. The tension on the lumbricals and lateral bands forcibly extends the DIP joint. The position of finger with flexion of PIP joint and hyperextension of DIP joint is known as "Boutonniere" deformity, meaning "buttonhole."[7] The central slip should be acutely repaired surgically, or in select cases, closed ruptures, if seen early, may be treated by splinting of the PIP joint in extension.

31.5.2 Lumbrical Plus

The force transmission from FDP to extensor apparatus via lumbrical is tightly balanced. Scarred or ischemic contracture of the lumbrical or lengthened FDP due to tendon grafting with suboptimal tension in the graft will favorably direct the tension toward the extensor apparatus during flexion. A voluntary contraction of the FDP will, therefore, paradoxically extend the interphalangeal joints. This is known as the "lumbrical plus" finger. The occurrence of lumbrical plus finger is rare, because

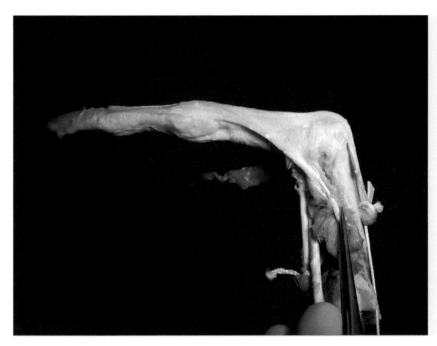

Fig. 31.7 The lumbricals serve as independent extensors of proximal interphalangeal and distal interphalangeal joints. Even with the MCP joint held flexed, the interphalangeal joints are capable of full active extension. The forceps is providing the tension on the lumbrical to hold the finger in extension.

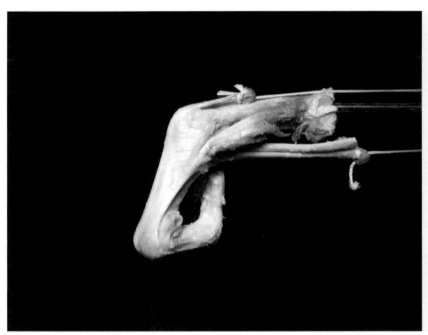

Fig. 31.8 In order for lumbricals to function, it requires a taut anchor. The tension of the flexor digitorum profundus is lost during maximal flexion, and the lumbricals lose adequate tensioning. This phenomenon can be maintained by holding the metacarpophalangeal and proximal interphalangeal joints in flexion. The lumbrical appears loose. In this position, it is impossible to actively extend the distal interphalangeal joint.

the origin of each lumbrical does not always correspond directly with its corresponding FDP. The lumbricals may have to be released or resected to correct this problem.

References

1. Smith RJ. Balance and kinetics of the fingers under normal and pathological conditions. Clin Orthop Relat Res 1974; (104):92–111
2. Eladoumikdachi F, Valkov PL, Thomas J, Netscher DT. Anatomy of the intrinsic hand muscles revisited: part II. Lumbricals. Plast Reconstr Surg 2002;110(5):1225–1231
3. Jacobson MD, Raab R, Fazeli BM, Abrams RA, Botte MJ, Lieber RL. Architectural design of the human intrinsic hand muscles. J Hand Surg Am 1992;17(5):804–809
4. Lauritzen RS, Szabo RM, Lauritzen DB. Innervation of the lumbrical muscles. J Hand Surg [Br] 1996;21(1):57–58
5. Sunderland S, Ray LJ. Metrical and non-metrical features of the muscular branches of the median nerve. J Comp Neurol 1946;85(2):191–203
6. Hughes LA, Clarke HM. Normal arborization of the deep branch of the ulnar nerve into the interossei and lumbricals. J Hand Surg Am 1995;20(1):10–14
7. KAPLAN EBMD. 3 Anatomy, injuries and treatment of the extensor apparatus of the hand and the digits. Clin Orthop 1959; (1959):24–41
8. Ranney DA, Wells RP, Dowling J. Lumbrical function: interaction of lumbrical contraction with the elasticity of the extrinsic finger muscles and its effect on metacarpophalangeal equilibrium. J Hand Surg Am 1987;12(4):566–575

32 Compartments of the Hand

Ethan W. Blackburn

32.1 Introduction

A thorough knowledge of the discrete myofascial compartments of the hand is critical when a surgeon is confronted with a severely injured hand with possible compartment syndrome. The causes of compartment syndrome of hand are numerous, ranging from restrictive dressings to industrial accidents.[1] Surgeons must have a high level of clinical suspicion even after seemingly innocuous injuries such as injection injury or careless intraoperative positioning. Failure to diagnose compartment syndrome of the hand can lead to intrinsic muscle necrosis, followed by fibrosis and loss of function. Litigation often stems from missed compartment syndrome with an average malpractice award of 280,000.[2] Understanding the anatomy and variability of the hand compartments is required for prompt and effective treatment of this potentially devastating problem.

Studies have supported the presence of distinct myofascial compartments of the hand, and much of the contemporary teaching for treating compartment syndrome is founded on this.[3] It should be noted that some research supports little to no tough fascial tissue surrounding these compartments.[4] While anatomical studies are controversial, clinical studies documenting the results of neglected compartment syndrome support prompt and aggressive treatment.[5] Until further research is available, we recommend aggressive treatment with surgical decompression when clinical suspicion is high. As Ortiz and Berger pointed out, fasciotomy wounds may present a cosmetic challenge, but this is far outweighed by the potential dysfunction of an undiagnosed hand compartment syndrome.[6]

Hand compartments are enclosed spaces by connective tissue or bone. Typically, the hand has been divided into six spaces (▶Fig. 32.1 and ▶Fig. 32.2): the thenar, hypothenar, adductor, interosseous, carpal tunnel, and digit. It should be noted that some surgeons refer to each volar and dorsal interosseous muscle as a separate space.

32.1.1 Thenar Compartment

The thenar compartment contains the flexor pollicis brevis, abductor pollicus brevis, and the opponens pollicus. These muscles are innervated primarily by the recurrent branch of the median nerve with variable contributions of the deep branch of the ulnar nerve.[7] The thenar fascia extends from the palmar surface of the thumb metacarpal, surrounds the muscles, and inserts back onto the thumb metacarpal.[1] In 52% of cadaveric hands, a second discrete compartment is found within the thenar group.[8] The flexor pollicis brevis was found to be an isolated compartment in 38% of hands, while the abductor pollicis brevis as confined space was found in only 10% of cadaveric specimens.

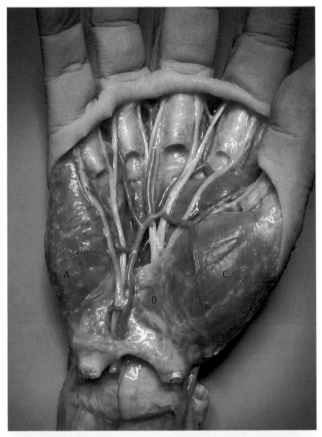

Fig. 32.2 Volar view of the hand with skin, subcutaneous tissues, palmar aponeurosis, and flexor tendons removed. The hypothenar compartment (A), carpal tunnel (B), and thenar compartment (C) are visualized. The median nerve has been transected proximal to the carpal tunnel, and the palmar cutaneous branch of the median nerve was removed with subcutaneous tissues.

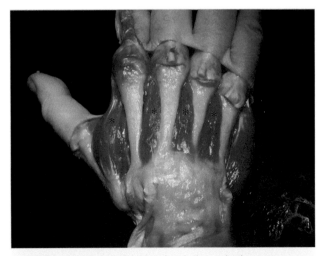

Fig. 32.1 Dorsal view of the hand with skin and subcutaneous tissues and finger extensors removed. From left the right, the first through fourth dorsal interossei (*), and the abductor digiti minimi (A) are visualized.

32.1.2 Adductor Compartment

The adductor pollicis is the largest and most powerful thenar muscle.[7] Its transverse head spans between the thumb and third metacarpal while its oblique head commonly originates from the third and fourth metacarpal (▶Fig. 32.3). The deep branch of the ulnar nerve with the deep palmar arch and associated veins pierce a space formed between the two heads. DiFelice et al reported the adductor was a separate space in 71% of hands while 19% of the time it was combined with the first dorsal interosseous.[8] These authors found the adductor pollicus and the first dorsal interosseous space continuous with the midpalmar space in 5% of specimens. Isolated chronic compartment syndrome of the first dorsal interosseous has been reported.[9–11]

32.1.3 Interossei

The dorsal interossei are finger abductors away from the axis of the third ray, while the volar interossei adduct the fingers.[7] Both muscle groups are metacarpophalangeal joint flexors and proximal interphalangeal joint extenders. The three volar interossei are bipennate muscles that arise from the second, fourth, and fifth metacarpal, pass volar to the deep transverse metacarpal ligament, and insert onto the dorsal apparatus. The radial head of the first dorsal interossei arises from the ulnar aspect of the first metacarpal, while the ulnar head arises from the radial aspect of the second metacarpal. These tendons have a primarily bony insertion onto the base of the second proximal phalanx. The radial artery and vena comitans pass through a gap between the two origins of this muscle. The second, third, and fourth dorsal interossei originate from their adjacent metacarpals and pass volar to the deep transverse metacarpal. They insert into proximal phalanx and dorsal apparatus. The second dorsal interossei inserts onto the radial aspect of the middle finger, the third on the ulnar aspect of the middle finger, and the fourth on the ulnar aspect of the ring finger. These muscles flex the metacarpophalangeal joints and extend the proximal interphalangeal joints. The second and third dorsal interossei are responsible for the radial and ulnar deviation of the middle

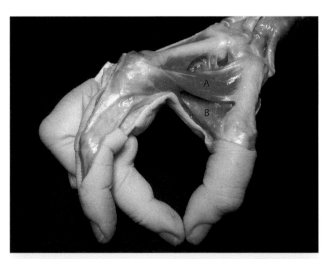

Fig. 32.3 Dorsal radial view of the hand with skin, subcutaneous tissues, and extensor tendons removed. The first dorsal interosseous (A) and adductor pollicus (B) are visualized.

finger, and the first and forth abduct the index and ring fingers relative to the third ray, respectively.

The interosseous compartments have been the subjects of considerable debate in several studies. Halpern and Mochizuki examined the interossei by removing the dorsal skin, injecting Renografin dye followed by radiographic evaluation and dissection.[3] The authors discovered that the dye injected into the dorsal interossei did not extravasate into the volar interossei and thus concluded that these muscles resided in separate compartments. More recent studies have reexamined these results with several modifications to the study design. Guyton et al left the skin intact and used continuous pressure monitoring with real-time computed tomography to visualize the injected contrast in the second dorsal interosseous.[4] These authors demonstrated that the barrier between volar and dorsal interossei became incompetent at only 15 mm Hg. Contrast was visualized spreading to adjacent interossei at pressures less than 35 mm Hg.

DiFelice et al demonstrated significant variability in the interosseous spaces.[8] The first dorsal interosseous was a separate space in 76% of hands, and it was combined with the adductor pollicus in 19% hands, with this space continuous with the midpalmar space 5% of the time. The second, third, and fourth interosseous groups were separate compartments in 48, 29, and 57% of hands, respectively. The second interosseous group was in separate volar and dorsal compartments in 48% of specimens. The third and fourth dorsal and volar interossei were separate compartments 67 and 38% of the time, respectively. All interossei spaces opened into the midpalmar space or the carpal canal 4 to 5% of the time.

32.1.4 Hypothenar Compartment

The hypothenar muscles include the abductor digiti minimi, opponens digiti minimi, and flexor digiti minimi. The abductor digiti minimi arises from the pisiform and pisohamate ligament and inserts onto the ulnar aspect of the small finger proximal phalanx, the palmar plate, and a sesamoid if present.[7] It is an abductor of the small finger and a flexor of the metacarpophalangeal joint. The flexor digiti minimi is variably present, but when it is distinct it takes origin from the ulnar hook of the hamate and flexor retinaculum. It is primarily a flexor of the fifth metacarpophalangeal joint. The opponens digit minimi is found deep to the other two hypothenar muscles and comprises two heads that originate from the hook of the hamate and flexor retinaculum and converge onto the ulnar shaft of the fifth metacarpal. The deep branch of the ulnar artery and nerve pass through a hiatus between the two heads of the opponens digiti minimi. The muscle adducts and slightly flexes the fifth metacarpal aiding to deepen the palm.

DiFelice et al observed a single hypothenar myofascial space in 24% of hands, with at least two distinct spaces in the remaining 76% hands.[8] The abductor digiti minimi was a distinct space in 43% of hands, while the opponens digiti minimi and the flexor digiti minimi were separate spaces 43 and 38% of the time, respectively.

32.1.5 Carpal Tunnel

The carpal tunnel is the space bound by the transverse carpal ligament palmarly, the volar extrinsic wrist ligaments dorsally, the scaphoid and trapezium radially, and the hamate and pisiform ulnarly. Eight finger flexors, the flexor pollicus longus and the median nerve travel from the forearm to the hand through the carpal tunnel. Acute carpal tunnel syndrome may be precipitated by distal radius fracture, carpal fracture, or less commonly, by inflammatory conditions or coagulopathy.[12–15] It is characterized by rapid onset of pain with progressive neurologic dysfunction in the median nerve distribution. This must be differentiated from median nerve contusion that presents as median nerve dysfunction immediately following injury that is nonprogressive.[16] Median nerve contusion may be monitored with rest and elevation, while acute carpal tunnel syndrome warrants urgent surgical decompression.[15]

32.1.6 Finger

The fingers do not contain discrete compartments, but when massive swelling occurs, neurologic and vascular compromise must be monitored. Schnall et al measured tissue pressures in 14 patients with flexor tenosynovitis.[17] Eight fingers measured pressures greater than 30 mm Hg. The authors irrigated the tendon sheath and left a midlateral incision open to relieve pressure while allowing active mobilization.

32.2 Compartment Monitoring

Compartment pressure should be used when physical examination is inconclusive. Various methods have been used successfully for measuring and monitoring compartment pressures.[18–21] We prefer the Stryker Intra-compartmental Pressure Monitor (Stryker, Kalamazoo, MI) because the setup is quick, the device is straightforward to use, and it is accurate.[18] The device does not allow for continuous pressure monitoring. It is our opinion that a patient with a clinical exam worrisome enough to warrant continuous monitoring should be considered for surgical release.

32.3 Compartment Release

The compartments of the hand can be accessed through multiple incisions (▶Fig. 32.4, ▶Fig. 32.5, and ▶Fig. 32.6). A longitudinal dorsal incision between the index and long, and a second incision between the ring and small metacarpals is used to access dorsal and volar interossei. Careful dissection is performed to ensure complete release along the entire length of the metacarpals. The thenar compartment is accessed from an incision along the radial aspect of the thenar eminence. The hypothenar incision is over the ulnar aspect of the hypothenar eminence. Care must be taken during release of the thenar and hypothenar spaces to avoid injury to the motor branches of the

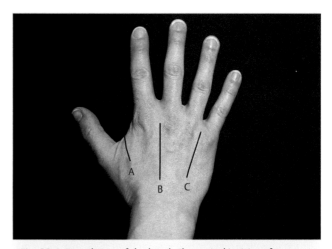

Fig. 32.4 Dorsal view of the hand. The typical incisions for release of the adductor compartment and first dorsal interosseous (A), the second and third dorsal interossei (B), and the fourth interosseous (C) are demonstrated. Incisions should be positioned to avoid exposure and desiccation of the extensor tendons, as the wounds are typically left to heal by secondary intention.

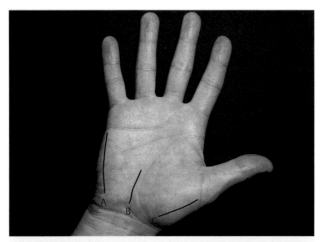

Fig. 32.5 Volar view of the hand. The typical incisions for release of the hypothenar compartment (A), carpal tunnel (B), and thenar compartment (C) are demonstrated.

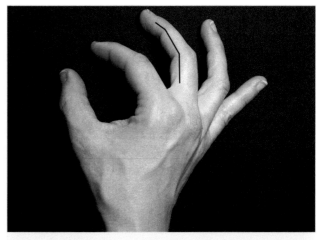

Fig. 32.6 Dorsal radial view of the hand with the fingers splayed. The midlateral incision for the finger is demonstrated.

median and ulnar nerves, respectively. The adductor compartment is addressed through a longitudinal incision centered over the first web space dorsally.

A standard open carpal tunnel release is adequate in cases of acute carpal tunnel syndrome. If the carpal tunnel release is performed in conjunction with a volar approach to the radius through the flexor carpi radialis sheath, a separate carpal tunnel incision is recommended. This protects the palmar cutaneous branch of the median nerve as it crosses the wrist crease.

32.4 Conclusion

The myofascial compartments of the hand are highly variable. Neglected compartment syndrome of the hand can lead to significant dysfunction. A high level of clinical suspicion for compartment syndrome must be maintained when the surgeon encounters a tense, swollen hand. The condition is diagnosed clinically, and compartment pressure monitoring may be used when physical examination is inconclusive. When diagnosed in a timely fashion, the expedient release of the hand myofascial spaces with careful attention to the variable anatomy previously discussed will avoid complications of muscle necrosis and contracture and likely decrease patient morbidity.

References

1. Seiler JG III, Olvey SP. Compartment syndromes of the hand and forearm. J Am Soc Surg Hand 2003;3(4):184–198
2. Gulli B, Templeman D. Compartment syndrome of the lower extremity. Orthop Clin North Am 1994;25(4):677–684
3. Halpern AA, Mochizuki RM. Compartment syndrome of the interosseous muscles of the hand. Orthop Rev 1980; (9):121–127
4. Guyton GP, Shearman CM, Saltzman CL. Compartmental divisions of the hand revisited. Rethinking the validity of cadaver infusion experiments. J Bone Joint Surg Br 2001;83(2):241–244
5. Ouellette EA, Kelly R. Compartment syndromes of the hand. J Bone Joint Surg Am 1996;78(10):1515–1522
6. Ortiz JA Jr, Berger RA. Compartment syndrome of the hand and wrist. Hand Clin 1998;14(3):405–418
7. Schmidt H-M, Lanz U. Surgical Anatomy of the Hand. Thieme; Stuttgart 2004.
8. DiFelice A Jr, Seiler JG III, Whitesides TE Jr. The compartments of the hand: an anatomic study. J Hand Surg Am 1998;23(4): 682–686
9. Abdul Hamid A. First dorsal interosseous compartment syndrome. J Hand Surg: J Brit Soc Surg Hand 1987;12(2):269–272
10. Styf J, Forssblad P, Lundborg G. Chronic compartment syndrome in the first dorsal interosseous muscle. J Hand Surg Am 1987;12 (5 Pt 1):757–762
11. Phillips JH, Mackinnon SE, Murray JF, McMurtry RY. Exercise-induced chronic compartment syndrome of the first dorsal interosseous muscle of the hand: a case report. J Hand Surg Am 1986;11(1):124–127
12. Chiu KY, Ng WF, Wong WB, Choi CH, Chow SP. Acute carpal tunnel syndrome caused by pseudogout. J Hand Surg Am 1992;17(2):299–302
13. Olerud C, Lönnquist L. Acute carpal tunnel syndrome caused by fracture of the scaphoid and the 5th metacarpal bones. Injury 1984;16(3):198–199
14. Ford DJ, Ali MS. Acute carpal tunnel syndrome. Complications of delayed decompression. J Bone Joint Surg Br 1986;68(5):758–759
15. Schnetzler KA. Acute carpal tunnel syndrome. J Am Acad Orthop Surg 2008;16(5):276–282
16. McDonald AP III, Lourie GM. Complex surgical conditions of the hand: avoiding the pitfalls. Clin Orthop Relat Res 2005; (433):65–71
17. Schnall SB, Vu-Rose T, Holtom PD, Doyle B, Stevanovic M. Tissue pressures in pyogenic flexor tenosynovitis of the finger. Compartment syndrome and its management. J Bone Joint Surg Br 1996;78(5):793–795
18. Boody AR, Wongworawat MD. Accuracy in the measurement of compartment pressures: a comparison of three commonly used devices. J Bone Joint Surg Am 2005;87(11): 2415–2422
19. Shuler MS, Reisman WM, Whitesides TE Jr, et al. Near-infrared spectroscopy in lower extremity trauma. J Bone Joint Surg Am 2009;91(6):1360–1368
20. Mubarak SJ, Owen CA, Hargens AR, Garetto LP, Akeson WH. Acute compartment syndromes: diagnosis and treatment with the aid of the wick catheter. J Bone Joint Surg Am 1978;60(8): 1091–1095
21. Rorabeck CH, Castle GS, Hardie R, Logan J. Compartmental pressure measurements: an experimental investigation using the slit catheter. J Trauma 1981;21(6):446–449

33 Hand Spaces

Amit Gupta and Ghazi M. Rayan

33.1 Introduction

Hand spaces can be affected by injury, inflammatory process, or infection.[1] A thorough knowledge of the anatomy of these spaces is essential for proper understanding of pathophysiology and surgical management of conditions involving these spaces.

There are two varieties of hand spaces: (1) *potential anatomical spaces* that are bordered within muscle planes or by fascial bands and (2) *true anatomical spaces* that are lined by synovial membrane.

Based on their anatomical location, hand spaces can be classified into the following types:

I. Perionychium and pulp space
II. Superficial potential spaces
    1. Digital spaces
       • Dorsal
       • Palmar
    2. Dorsal hand spaces
       • Subcutaneous
       • Subaponeurotic
    3. Palmar hand spaces
    4. Interdigital web spaces
III. Synovial spaces
    1. Extensor tendon sheath
    2. Flexor tendon sheath
    3. Radial and ulnar bursae
IV. Deep potential spaces
    1. Space of Parona.
    2. Thenar space.
    3. Mid palmar space.
    4. Lumbrical spaces.
    5. Hypothenar space.

33.2 Perionychium/Pulp Space

The nail plate is made of solid keratin and has a root and body. The nail root is contained in the nail socket. The proximal cornified thin skin layer that covers the nail plate is the eponychium, which extends a variable distance onto its surface. The lateral skin fold is called the paronychium, whereas the distal skin beneath the nail margin is the hyponychium.

Kanavel described the anatomy of the distal pulp as a "closed sac of connective tissue framework isolated and different from the rest of the finger."[1] Multiple fibrous bands (▶ Fig. 33.1, ▶ Fig. 33.2, and ▶ Fig. 33.3) extend from the periosteum of the distal phalanx to the dermis, dividing the pulp into numerous compartments that are potential spaces for spread of infection from the nail bed.[2]

Subungual or paronychial infection may occur de novo or spread from a pulp space. The tight septa can cause considerable swelling and pain from pressure caused by purulence

or bleeding. Infection is contained in the pulp for a while, but if not relieved either by spontaneous drainage or surgically, it can spread to the bone, causing osteomyelitis of the distal phalanx, to the distal interphalangeal joint, causing septic arthritis, or to the flexor tendon sheath, causing septic flexor tenosynovitis.

33.3 Superficial Spaces

33.3.1 Subcutaneous Dorsal and Palmar Digital Spaces

The dorsal skin of the digit is loose and attached to the deeper structures at the metacarpophalangeal (MCP), proximal, and distal interphalangeal joints by *dorsal paratendinous cutaneous system* that arises from the central and terminal tendons, respectively, and insert directly into the dermis deep to the dorsal skin crease of the finger joints[3] (▶ Fig. 33.4). These fibers are probably a continuation of *Cleland's ligaments* and were originally described by Cleland.[3]

Thus the dorsal subcutaneous areas over the middle and proximal phalanges are potential spaces that can be filled with fluid, blood, pus, or granulation tissue. The space over the proximal phalanx has direct connection to the loose subcutaneous space on the dorsum of the hand, as the paratendinous cutaneous system over the MCP joint is less robust and the skin on the dorsum of the MCP joint is much more mobile.

The primary function of the cutaneous ligaments is to provide stability to the skin by tethering it to the deeper fascial or bony structures. The *Cleland's ligaments* attach in the vicinity of the lateral borders of these joints and lie dorsal to the digital neurovascular bundles. The *Grayson's ligaments* are slender fibrous strips that extend from the flexor tendon sheath to the palmar skin of the digits and lie volar to the neurovascular bundle[3] (▶ Fig. 33.5). The dorsal digital cutaneous creases form areas of skin tether to the deeper fascial structures (▶ Fig. 33.4). Between the adjacent digital creases are potential subcutaneous spaces that can harbor infection.

At the palmar digital skin creases, the skin is attached to the deeper structures (▶ Fig. 33.6). The area in between the palmar digital creases form a potential space for fluid collection.

33.3.2 Superficial Dorsal Hand Spaces

The superficial dorsal spaces include the *dorsal subcutaneous* and the *dorsal subaponeurotic space*[1] (▶ Fig. 33.7 and ▶ Fig. 33.8).

The dorsal subcutaneous space lies between the loose dorsal skin of the hand and the deeper extensor tendons and the dorsal aponeurosis.[1,4] Distally it communicates with the space over the proximal phalanx, as the paratendinous cutaneous fibers are less robust over the dorsum of the MCP joints. The wrist skin creases define the limit of this space proximally. This large

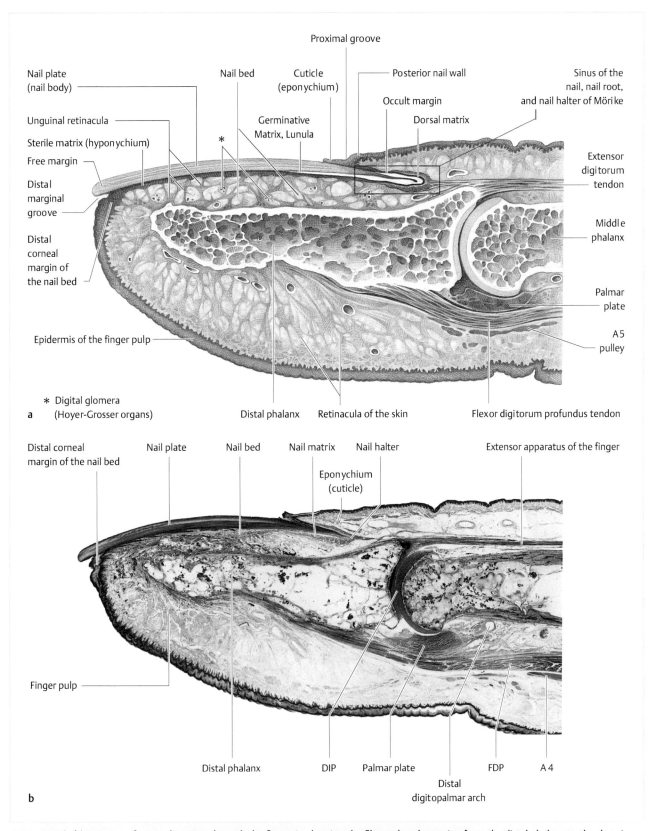

Fig. 33.1 (a,b) Diagram of sagittal section through the fingertip showing the fibrous bands running from the distal phalanx to the dermis. (From Schmidt H-M, Lanz U. Surgical Anatomy of the Hand. Stuttgart, Germany: Thieme; 2004.)

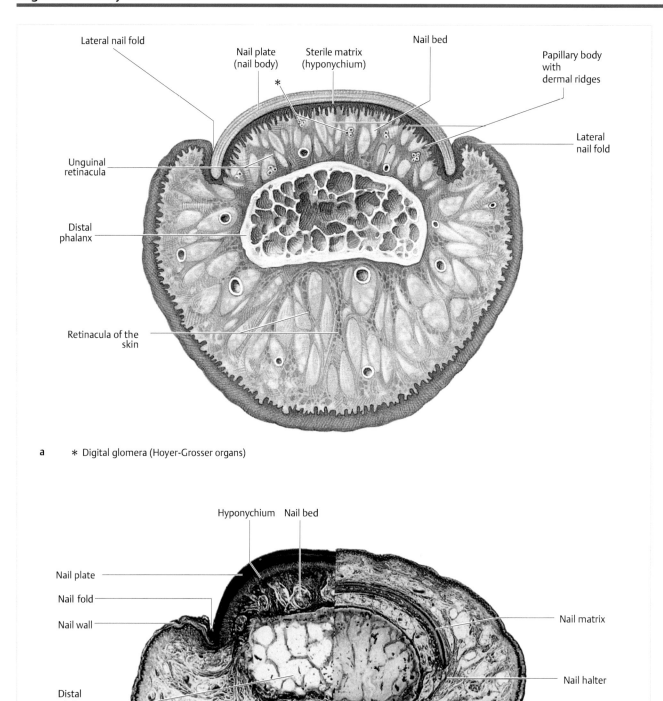

a   * Digital glomera (Hoyer-Grosser organs)

Fig. 33.2 (a,b) Diagram of axial section of the pulp and nail along with the distal phalanx showing the detailed anatomy of the fingertip. (From Schmidt H-M, Lanz U. Surgical Anatomy of the Hand. Stuttgart, Germany: Thieme; 2004.)

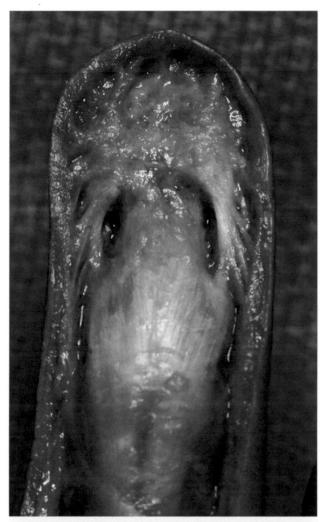

Fig. 33.3 Dissection of the fingertip showing the insertion of the FDP tendon and the fibrous septae running from the distal phalanx to the pulp skin and the spaces they create. Also seen are the interosseous ligaments of Flint.

space on the dorsum of the hand and fingers can be potentially increased by poor finger position after injury whereby the MCP joint is hyperextended and the proximal interphalangeal (PIP) joint is flexed (▶Fig. 33.9). Placing the hand in the intrinsic plus or "safe position" with the wrist slightly extended, the MCP joints flexed, and PIP joints extended pulls the dorsal skin tight and reduces the size of this space and decreases edema fluid accumulation in this space.

The deeper dorsal subaponeurotic space lies between the aponeurotic network of the extensor tendons and their connections superficially and the periosteum over the metacarpals (▶Fig. 33.7 and ▶Fig. 33.8) and the fascia covering the interosseous muscles.[1,4] On the radial and ulnar sides, the aponeurotic sheath merges with the fascia covering the dorsal interosseous muscles and the periosteum of the thumb and the small finger compartments as well as the capsules of these MCP joints, forming what Kanavel termed a "truncated cone." The thin fascia between the extensor tendons—*intertendinous fascia of*

Anson—extends to the space between the thumb and index metacarpals, connecting the extensor tendons of these two digits[5] (▶Fig. 33.10). Therefore, this aponeurosis spans the first dorsal interosseus muscle and fascia as well as the adductor pollicis muscle and forms a curved edge on the dorsum of the first web space. Thus, the dorsal subaponeurotic space extends to the thumb metacarpal on the radial side.

33.3.3 Palmar Subcutaneous Space

The palmar fascial complex and its extensions tether the dermis, especially in central portion of the palm. The palmar skin is very adherent to the deeper structures at the palmar creases (▶Fig. 33.6). However, there are many areas of the palmar skin, especially in the thenar and hypothenar areas and over the first web space, that are loosely attached to the underlying structures and contain some adipose tissue (▶Fig. 33.11). These areas form potential subcutaneous spaces for infection. The subcutaneous infection remains localized, because the fascial bands like those at palmar creases tether the skin and limit these spaces. The palmar subcutaneous space over the first web space readily communicates with the dorsal subcutaneous space (▶Fig. 33.12).

33.3.4 Interdigital Web Spaces

The three interdigital web spaces between the fingers are made up of loose connective tissue and some adipose tissue. They have no clear boundaries.[1] They are located between heads of metacarpals, the capsuloligamentous structures of the MCP joints, and the overlying extensor mechanisms. The interpalmar plate ligaments (IPPL) lie farther proximally deep and in line with each of the three web spaces (▶Fig. 33.13). The palmar boundaries of these spaces are the natatory ligaments and the skin and dorsal is the skin that is inclined toward the palm (▶Fig. 33.14). The thumb index web space freely communicates with the dorsal subcutaneous space and the palmar thenar subcutaneous space.

Infection of the interdigital web space may extend dorsally and palmarly, resulting in an "hourglass" or "collar-button" abscess.

33.4 Synovial Spaces

33.4.1 Extensor Tendon Sheaths

The synovial sheaths surround the extensor tendons deep to the extensor retinaculum in the wrist area (▶Fig. 33.15). These synovial sheaths extend proximal and distal to the retinaculum and help the tendons glide under the retinaculum.[1,5] The most common cause of synovitis in this region is inflammatory tenosynovitis associated with rheumatoid arthritis, although acute and chronic infection can also affect this area.

33.4.2 Flexor Tendon Sheaths

As they enter the fingers from the palm, the flexor tendons pass through fibro-osseous tunnels that guide, modulate, control, and nourish the tendons (▶Fig. 33.16). The curved palmar surfaces of

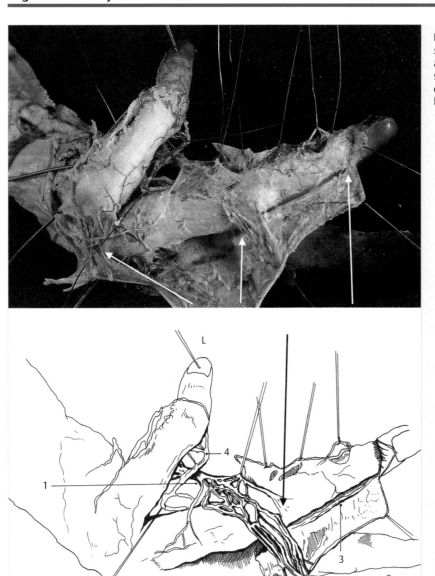

Fig. 33.4 *Dorsal paratendinous cutaneous system* arising from the extensor tendons and attaching to the dermis at the PIP joint skin crease. (From Zancolli EA, Cozzi EP. Atlas of Surgical Anatomy of the Hand. New York, NY: Churchill Livingstone; 1992.)

the phalanges, the palmar plate of the MCP, and the interphalangeal (IP) joints form the dorsal floor of the tunnel. The synovial sheath is anchored to the bones with thick and strong pulleys. Doyle and Blythe[6] introduced a system of nomenclature for the palmar pulleys that is commonly used (▶ Fig. 33.17). Manske and Lesker[7] included the transverse fibers of the palmar aponeurosis as an extra pulley that was later clarified to be the transverse ligament of the palmar aponeurosis (TLPA; ▶ Fig. 33.18).

The pulley system is a closed system surrounding the flexor tendons. The sheaths extend from the level of the neck of the metacarpals to the flexor digitorum profundus tendon insertion in the distal phalanx. The sheath contains synovial fluid that is produced by the epithelial cells of the synovial layer.

This closed space is a suitable growth medium for bacteria, as it is avascular and the synovial fluid provides ready nourishment. In this closed system, if infection is introduced either through penetrating wound or from extension of a felon into the flexor sheath, the bacteria can multiply and cause increased pressure in a closed system, thus rendering the tendons avascular and susceptible to rupture or adhesions.

33.4.3 Radial and Ulnar Bursae

The flexor sheath of the flexor pollicis longus (FPL) tendon extends further proximally to almost 1 to 2 cm proximal to the proximal edge of the transverse carpal ligament and forms the radial bursa[1] (▶ Fig. 33.19 and ▶ Fig. 33.20). Thus, infection in the FPL tendon synovial sheath can spread proximal to the carpal tunnel into the forearm.

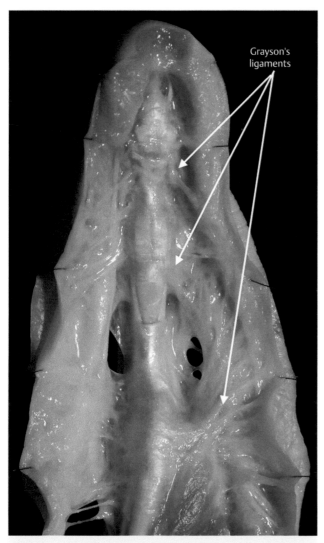

Fig. 33.5 Dissection of the digit showing Grayson's ligaments.

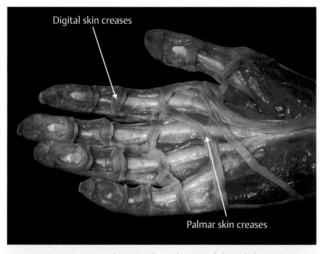

Fig. 33.6 Dissection showing the palmar and digital skin creases. The subcutaneus spaces between the creases are potential areas for fluid collection.

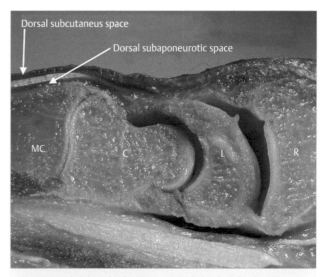

Fig. 33.7 The dorsal subcutaneous and the dorsal subaponeurotic spaces in the back of the hand.

In addition, the flexor sheath of the flexor digitorum profundus to the small finger also extends proximal to the transverse carpal ligament and widens just distal to the transverse carpal ligament.[5] The flexor tendons of the index, long, and ring fingers invaginate the ulnar bursa (▶Fig. 33.19).

In a large proportion of cases (85%), the radial and ulnar bursae communicate with each other[5] (▶Fig. 33.20). Therefore, distal infection of the small finger tendon sheath can spread to the forearm through the proximal extension of the sheath. Similarly, infection from the flexor tendon sheath of the thumb can spread to the forearm. Theoretically, small finger synovial infection may spread to the thumb synovial space and vice a versa through communication between the radial and ulnar bursae, giving rise to "horse-shoe" abscess.

33.5 Deep Potential Spaces

33.5.1 Space of Parona

Francesco Parona,[8] in 1876, described the space that carries his name. Also called the "retroflexor space," it is a potential space deep to the flexor tendons in the distal forearm overlying the fascia that covers the pronator quadratus muscle (▶Fig. 33.19). Parona's space contains the deep fatty tissue of the distal forearm (▶Fig. 33.21 and ▶Fig. 33.22). The radial and ulnar bursa do not communicate with the space of Parona but infection may spread to the space due to rupture of either bursa.

33.5.2 Thenar Space

The thenar space is an ill-defined triangular space situated in the thenar region. Proximally, it extends to the distal border of the flexor retinaculum. Distally, it extends to the proximal transverse palmar crease.

It is bounded on the palmar aspect by the palmar aponeurosis and dorsally by the oblique fascia over the adductor pollicis muscle[9] (▶Fig. 33.23). Medially it extends to the origin of the adductor

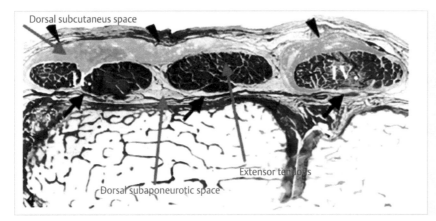

Fig. 33.8 Cross sectional specimen showing the dorsal subcutaneous and the dorsal subaponeurotic spaces. (From Thurmuller P, Schubert M, Bade H. Functional gliding space of the dorsal side of the human hand. The Anatomical Record 2002 267; 242-251. With permission.)

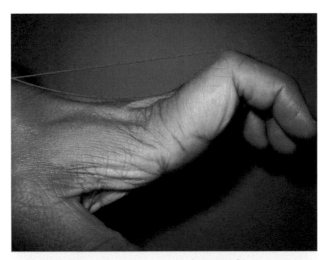

Fig. 33.9 MP joint hyperextension and PIP joint flexion increases the potential space on the dorsum of the hand.

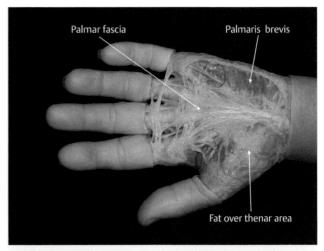

Fig. 33.11 Detailed dissection showing the palmar fascia and the potential subcutaneous spaces in the first web, thenar and hypothenar areas.

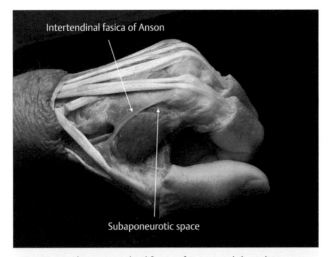

Fig. 33.10 The intertendinal fascia of Anson and the subaponeurotic space in the first web space.

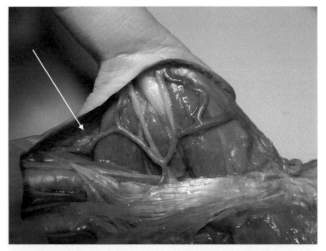

Fig. 33.12 The potential first web subcutaneous space that makes for easy communication between the palmar and dorsal subcutaneous spaces.

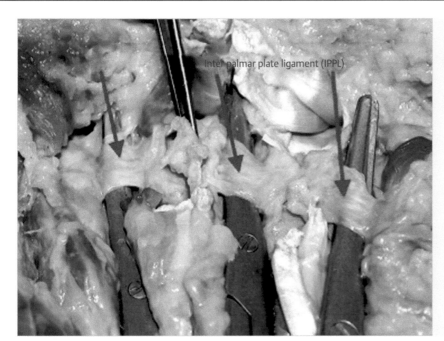

Fig. 33.13 The Inter Palmar Plate Ligaments (IPPL) form proximal boundaries of the interdigital web spaces. (Photo Courtesy of Dr. Ghazi M. Rayan.)

Inter palmar plate ligament (IPPL)

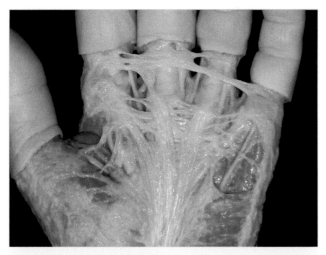

Fig. 33.14 The natatory ligaments form the palmar boundary of the interdigital web spaces.

pollicis muscle in the middle finger metacarpal shaft, and laterally it extends to the insertion of the adductor pollicis muscle and the adductor fascia to the thumb proximal phalanx[5] (▶ Fig. 33.24).

The thenar space has communication with the forearm space, the subcutaneous web of the thumb through the fascial sheath of the first lumbrical muscle, and it may also communicate with the second lumbrical canal.

The thenar space contains the FPL tendon with its sheath, the flexor tendons of the index with their sheath, the first lumbrical muscle in the distal part, the palmar digital vessels and nerves of the thumb, and the radial nerves and vessels of the index ray.

The thenar space may become infected by spread of infection from the thumb or index finger. This results in marked swelling in the thenar region.

33.5.3 Midpalmar Space

The midpalmar space is completely covered by the central aponeurosis[10] (▶ Fig. 33.18, ▶ Fig. 33.23, and ▶ Fig. 33.24). It is a triangular space with apex proximal between the thenar and hypothenar fascia. Distally it extends to the distal palmar crease and the TLPA, which gives attachments to the septa of Legueu and Juvara (▶ Fig. 33.18). This space occupies an area deep to the midpalm and communicates with the forearm space.

Dorsally, it is bounded by the periosteum covering the index, middle, and ring metacarpals and the fascia covering the interossei of the second, third, and fourth spaces. Medial and lateral boundaries of the space are ill defined but correspond to the septa of Legueu and Juvara at the index and small fingers.

The midpalmar space contains the flexor tendons of the long, ring, and small fingers; the second, third, and fourth neurovascular canals, including the lumbrical muscles; and the common digital nerves and vessels of the small, ring, middle, and the ulnar side of the index fingers, as well as the formation of superficial palmar arch by these vessels. Midpalmar space infection develops by direct penetrating injury. Flexor tenosynovitis of the small finger tracks through this space without involving it. This space infection can cause distension and swelling that flattens the concavity of the palm and may extend to the web spaces.

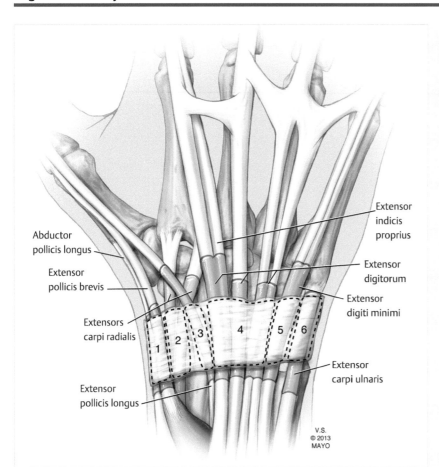

Fig. 33.15 Diagram of the synovial sheaths around the extensor tendons deep to the extensor retinaculum in the dorsum of the wrist. (From Mayo Clinic.)

Abductor pollicis longus

Extensor pollicis brevis

Extensors carpi radialis

Extensor pollicis longus

Extensor indicis proprius

Extensor digitorum

Extensor digiti minimi

Extensor carpi ulnaris

V.S.
© 2013
MAYO

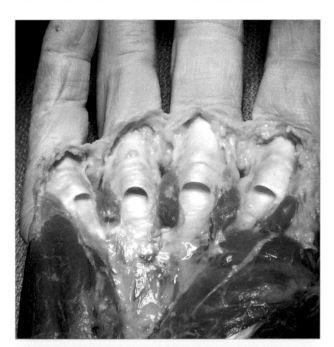

Fig. 33.16 Palmar dissection showing the entrance to the fibro-osseous tunnel of the finger flexors.

The distal midpalmar space contains multiple channels formed by the septa of Legueu and Juvara that attach to the central palmar aponeurosis through the TLPA.[11] There are eight septa that form seven channels: four flexor tendon and three neurovascular canals (▶Fig. 33.25, ▶Fig. 33.26, ▶Fig. 33.27, ▶Fig. 33.28, ▶Fig. 33.29, ▶Fig. 33.30, ▶Fig. 33.31, and ▶Fig. 33.32).

Legueu and Juvara were two French anatomists who described these septa in 1892. Their original description was very succinct, being in the form of a brief communication. Bilderback and Rayan[12] described in detail the anatomy of these septa and their attachments (▶Fig. 33.25, ▶Fig. 33.28, ▶Fig. 33.29, ▶Fig. 33.30, ▶Fig. 33.31, and ▶Fig. 33.32).

33.5.4 Lumbrical Spaces

The lumbrical muscles pass with the common digital neurovascular structures from the proximal palm to the finger through the three neurovascular canals formed by the vertical septa of Legueu and Juvara (▶Fig. 33.25 and ▶Fig. 33.27). In doing so, they form a communication channel from the midpalmar space to the digital web space and infection can track along these channels. Midpalmar space infection can also be drained by incisions extending into the interdigital web spaces.

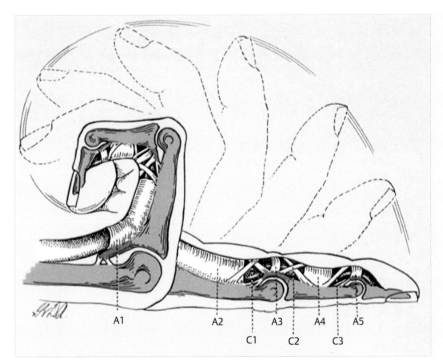

Fig. 33.17 The palmar flexor pulley system. (Kleinert Institute, Louisville, KY.)

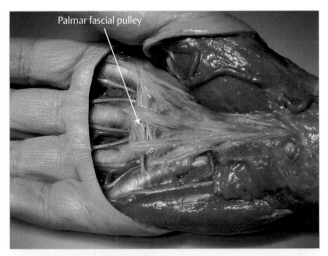

Fig. 33.18 Palmar fascial pulley or the Transverse Ligament of the Palmar Aponeurosis (TLPA).

33.5.5 Hypothenar Space

This space is of minor importance. It is located over the hypothenar muscles. It is bordered dorsally by the periosteum of the fifth metacarpal and the fascia of the deep hypothenar muscles. The palmar and ulnar boundaries are the palmar fascia and the fascia over the superficial hypothenar muscles.[10] The radial boundary is the radial border of the hypothenar muscles.

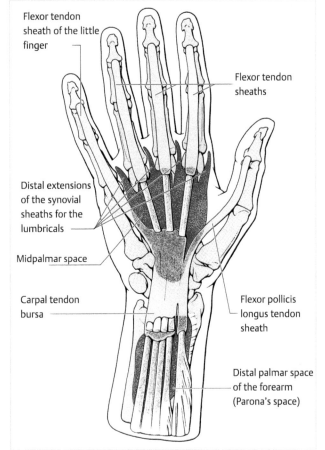

Fig. 33.19 Diagram showing the digital flexor sheaths, the radial and ulnar bursae. (From Schmidt H-M, Lanz U. Surgical Anatomy of the Hand. Stuttgart, Germany: Thieme; 2004.)

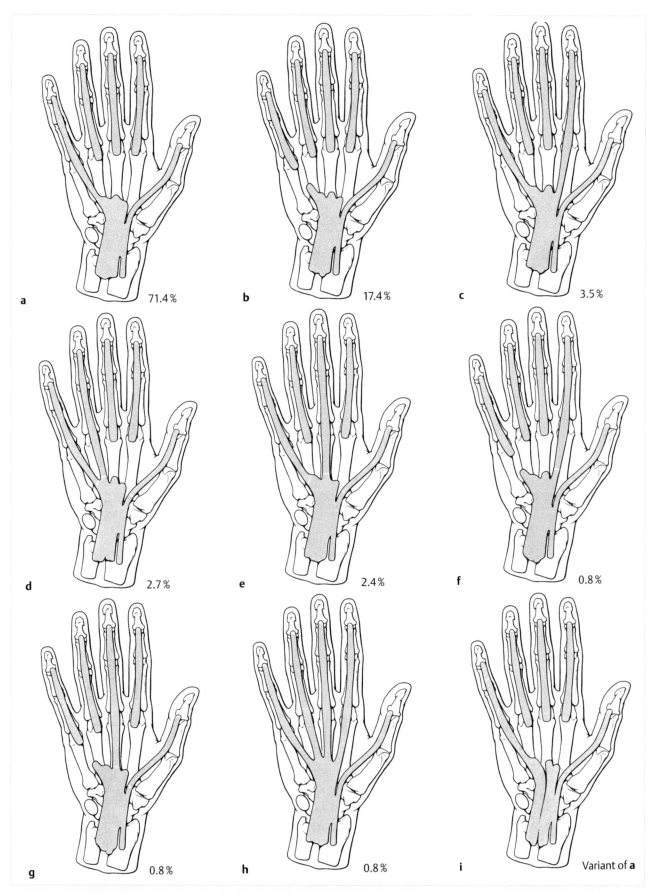

Fig. 33.20 (a–i) Diagram showing the variations of the radial and ulnar bursae. (From Schmidt H-M, Lanz U. Surgical Anatomy of the Hand. Stuttgart, Germany: Thieme; 2004.)

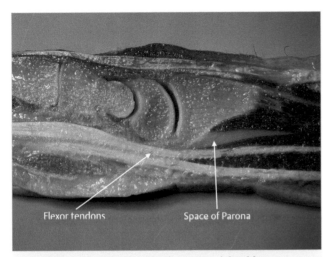

Fig. 33.21 Coronal section thru the wrist and distal forearm showing the fat pad in the space of Parona.

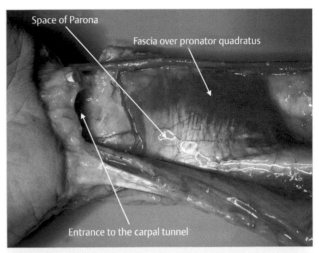

Fig. 33.22 The potential space of Parona and the fascia over the pronator quadratus.

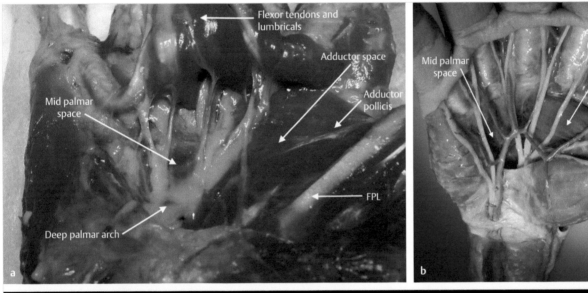

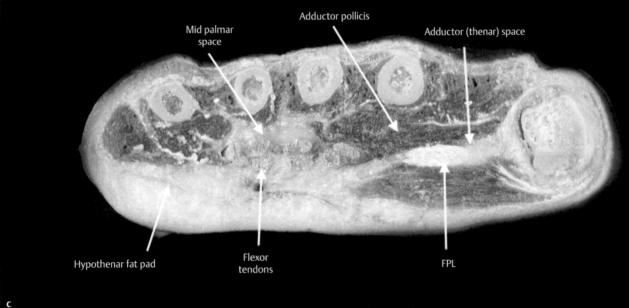

Fig. 33.23 (a) Dissection of the palm (b) Dissection of the palm with the flexor tendons removed and the arteries injected and (c) cross section through the palm showing the thenar (adductor) space and the mid palmar space.

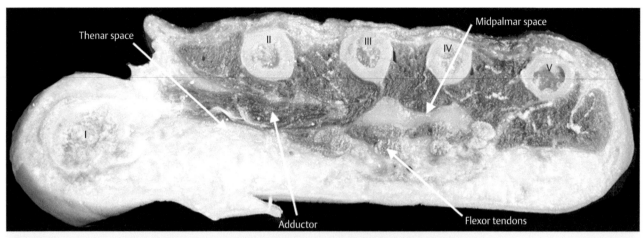

Fig. 33.24 Cross section through the palm showing the anatomy of the Thenar and the Midpalmar Spaces.

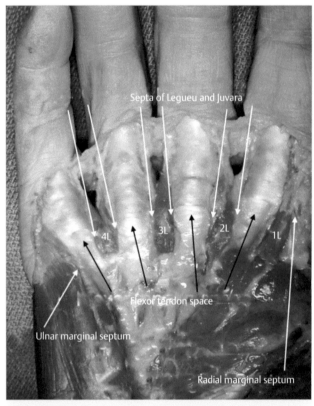

Fig. 33.25 Dissection of the palm with the flexor tendons removed showing the flexor sheaths, the lumbrical muscles, the septa of Legueu and Juvara, the radial and ulnar marginal septae.

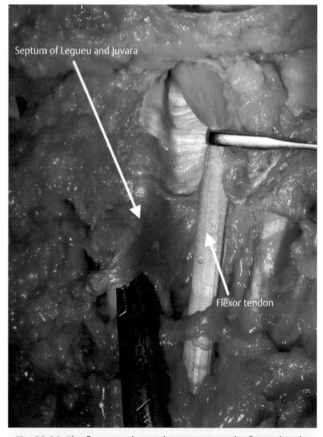

Fig. 33.26 The flexor tendon at the entrance to the flexor sheath showing the septum of Legueu and Juvara.

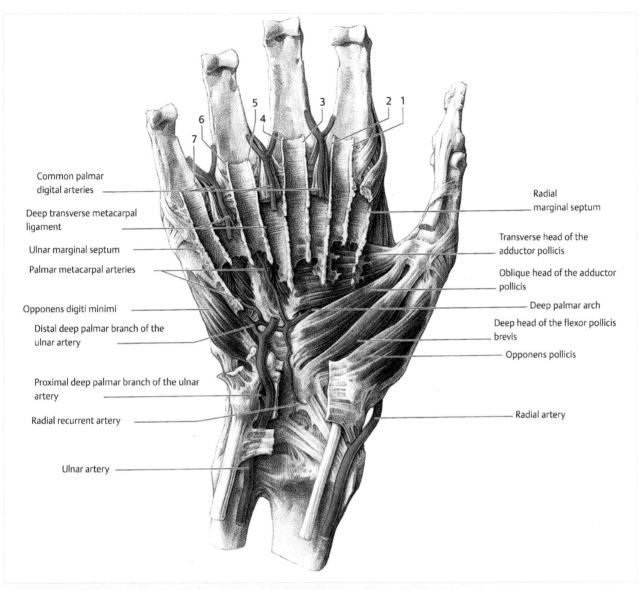

Common palmar digital arteries

Deep transverse metacarpal ligament

Ulnar marginal septum

Palmar metacarpal arteries

Opponens digiti minimi

Distal deep palmar branch of the ulnar artery

Proximal deep palmar branch of the ulnar artery

Radial recurrent artery

Ulnar artery

Radial marginal septum

Transverse head of the adductor pollicis

Oblique head of the adductor pollicis

Deep palmar arch

Deep head of the flexor pollicis brevis

Opponens pollicis

Radial artery

Fig. 33.27 Diagram of palmar anatomy with the flexor tendons removed. The flexor sheaths as well as septa of Legueu and Juvara are seen. (From Schmidt H-M, Lanz U. Surgical Anatomy of the Hand. Stuttgart, Germany: Thieme; 2004.)

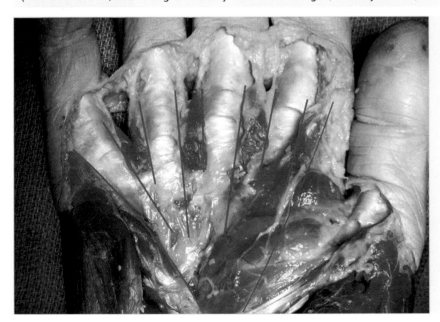

Fig. 33.28 Deep dissection of the palm at the entrance to the fibrous flexor sheaths. The 9 septa and 8 canals are marked.

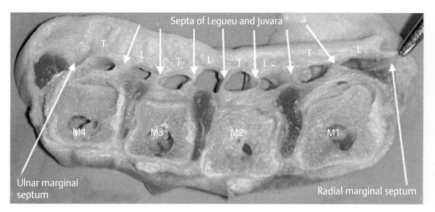

Fig. 33.29 Axial section thru the palm showing the tendon spaces (T) and the septa of Legueu and Juvara. (Photo courtesy of Dr. Ghazi M. Rayan.)

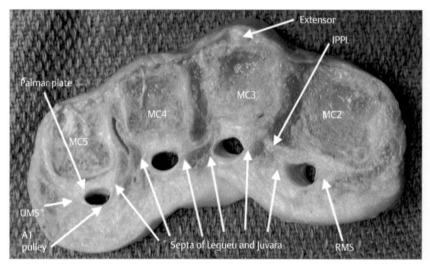

Fig. 33.30 Axial section thru the metacarpal heads showing the IPPLs and the Septa of Legueu and Juvara. (Photo courtesy of Dr. Ghazi M. Rayan.)

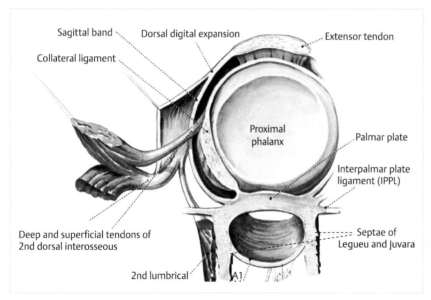

Fig. 33.31 Diagrammatic representation of the anatomy at the MP joint level showing the base of the proximal phalanx, the palmar plate, The IPPL and Septa of Legueu and Juvara. (Kleinert Institute, Louisville, KY.)

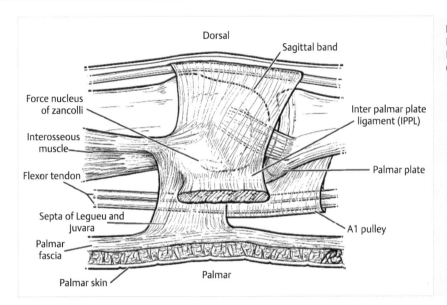

Fig. 33.32 Diagram of the anatomy at the MP joint level showing the palmar plate, the IPPL, and the septa of Legueu and Juvara. (Courtesy of Dr Ghazi M. Rayan.)

References

1. Patel DB, Emmanuel NB, Stevanovic MV, et al. Hand infections: anatomy, types and spread of infection, imaging findings, and treatment options. Radiographics 2014;34(7):1968–1986

2. Zook EG. Anatomy and physiology of the perionychium. Hand Clin 1990;6(1):1–7

3. Zancolli EA, Cozzi EP. Atlas of Surgical Anatomy of the Hand. New York, NY: Churchill Livingstone; 1992

4. Thurmüller P, Schubert M, Bade H, Notermans HP, Knifka J, Koebke J. Functional gliding spaces of the dorsal side of the human hand. Anat Rec 2002;267(3):242–251

5. Schmidt H-M, Lanz U. Surgical Anatomy of the Hand. Stuttgart, Germany: Thieme; 2004

6. Doyle JR, Blythe W. The finger flexor sheath and pulleys: anatomy and reconstruction. Amer. Acad. Orthop. Surg. (AAOS) Symposium on tendon surgery in the hand. St. Louis, MO: CV Mosby; 1975: 81–87

7. Manske PR, Lesker PA. Palmar aponeurosis pulley. J Hand Surg Am 1983;8(3):259–263

8. Malenfant J, Walters A, Kralovic S, et al. Francesco Parona (1842-1908) and his contributions to our understanding of surgery through anatomy. Clin Anat 2013;26(5):547–550

9. Spinner M. Kaplan's Functional and Surgical Anatomy of the Hand. 3rd ed. Philadelphia, PA: J.B. Lippincott Company; 1984

10. DiFelice A Jr, Seiler JG III, Whitesides TE Jr. The compartments of the hand: an anatomic study. J Hand Surg Am 1998;23(4): 682–686

11. Bojsen-Moller F, Schmidt L. The palmar aponeurosis and the central spaces of the hand. J Anat 1974;117(Pt 1):55–68

12. Bilderback KK, Rayan GM. The septa of Legueu and Juvara: an anatomic study. J Hand Surg Am 2004;29(3):494–499

34 The Carpometacarpal Joints

Amy L. Ladd

34.1 Introduction

The structural anatomy reflects the functional demands of the carpometacarpal (CMC) joints: they create an architectural foundation for the digits to position, manipulate, and respond to surfaces and objects that the human hand encounters. The proximal transverse arch of the CMC joints comprises the distal carpal row and the proximal five metacarpals, completed by the transverse carpal ligament; it stabilizes the hand and disperses forces, similar to a masonry arch. J. William Littler likened this to a fixed arch, while the activity at the metacarpal heads creates an adaptive arch (▶Fig. 34.1). Similarly, a fixed longitudinal unit of the second and third metacarpals and the distal carpal row permits the thumb and fingers to create gross and powerful action or, conversely, the intricate fine movement unique to the human hand.[1] The third CMC (CMC-3) joint serves as the keystone and is the rigid, neutral axis of the hand and forearm.

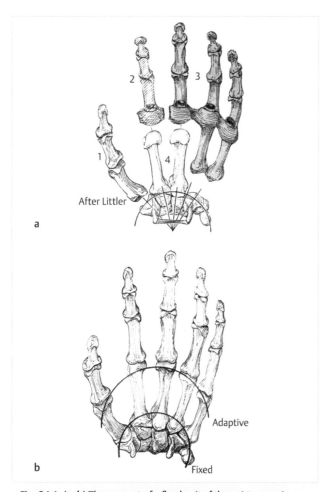

Fig. 34.1 (a, b) The concept of a fixed unit of the wrist comprises a longitudinal arch of the second and third metacarpal, along with the distal carpal row. The rigid transverse carpal arch of the carpometacarpal joints stabilizes the adaptive arch of the metacarpal heads, and the transverse carpal ligament completes the arch. (After Littler, from Hentz and Chase.)[1]

Emanating in either direction, the CMC articulations become increasingly mobile. The muscles and tendons within the palmar arch enable their dynamic capabilities, acting upon the distal segments to create the range of palmar excursion from a flat hand to the rotation and flexion of palmar cupping. At either end the especially mobile thumb CMC (CMC-1) and the small finger CMC (CMC-5) permit the opening and prehension that affords a powerful grip, extending the vector of the forearm to create a strong powerful lever arm, unique to human function.[2] The resourceful thumb also creates a precision pinch; the balance between stability and mobility arguably comes at a price with its vulnerability for osteoarthritis. The proprioception and sensibility within the ligaments, muscles, and the glabrous, tactile skin communicate with the brain to carry out object manipulation.[3]

The block like joints have variable curvature and interdigitations (▶Fig. 34.2), stronger dorsal than palmar carpometacarpal ligaments, and intermetacarpal ligaments (▶Fig. 34.3). Five primary ligaments stabilize CMC-1 with a dorsal and volar intermetacarpal ligament attaching to the second metacarpal.[4,5] The CMC-2 through CMC-5 joints possess 9 dorsal ligaments and 11 palmar ligaments, an interosseous ligament, and an intraarticular ligament between CMC-3 and CMC-4. Intermetacarpal ligaments exist between each of the metacarpals.[6,7]

Following Hilton's law,[8] the joints are innervated regionally by each of the terminal branches of the median, radial, and ulnar nerves, with CMC-1[9] and likely CMC-5 having the most cross-innervation. Similarly, the terminal carpal and digital branches of the radial and ulnar artery and anterior interosseous artery provide their blood supply. The synovium is typically continuous with occasional disruption between the hamate and fourth and fifth metacarpal.[10]

34.2 Thumb Carpometacarpal Joint

In concert with the human brain, the thumb coordinates elite, precise function with the fingers. Its demands create a paradox between mobility and stability: uniquely poised to grasp a shot put or pen a beautiful script. To oppose its neighbors with stable pinch and grasp, it recessed over millions of years from a three-phalanx digit to the current two phalanges and metacarpal upon a mobile saddle joint.[2,11–13] With the trapezium's terminal post at the radial carpal arch establishing the thumb's offset position, its coordinates lie tangential to the plane of the thorax and fingers, respectively (▶Fig. 34.4).[14–17] Composite opposition to hold a pen requires positioning and stabilizing muscles across the CMC joint, imparting abduction, flexion, translation, and pronation; additional contributors are the metacarpophalangeal (MCP) and interphalangeal joints.[18] Human prehension requires an opposable strong thumb, the small finger's hypothenar complex,[19] and wrist positioning in the "dart-thrower's motion"[20,21] with thumb and forearm in line, extending the lever arm and imparting mechanical advantage to throw a fast ball or swing a golf club.[2,3]

The trapezium's metacarpal surface is gently comma-shaped (left) or C-shaped (right) with the ulnar–radial axis as a vertical

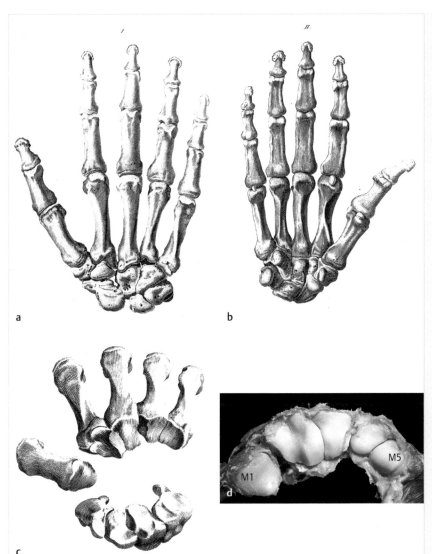

Fig. 34.2 An early 18th-century engraving demonstrates the osteology of the hand: (a) the dorsal and (b) volar views and (c) the opened view of the carpometacarpal joints. (d) The transverse arch is visualized, demonstrating the metacarpal articulations and dorsal and volar intermetacarpal ligaments with the carpal bones removed. M1, first metacarpal; M5, fifth metacarpal. (a–c with permission, AL Ladd.)

reference to this shape (▶Fig. 34.5). The loose configuration relies upon ligament and muscular stability. The concavo-convex saddle trapezial surface creates "reciprocal reception" (gray) with the metacarpal to permit wide circumduction (▶Fig. 34.6). The larger ulnar surface and eccentric contact provides a "rollback" or "screw-home" mechanism, similar to a knee.[18,22] Although largely considered a "saddle" joint, its eccentric morphology permits slide, glide, rotation, and translation circumduction, which includes features reminiscent of a ball-and-socket joint; arguably, the combined motion is somewhere between the two.[23] The trapezium's prominences and multiple articulations with the first and second metacarpal, trapezoid, and scaphoid secure its anchoring position as the radial abutment of the transverse arch and its relationship with the proximal carpal row (▶Fig. 34.7).

The CMC joint's investing ligaments are stout dorsally and thin volarly, both as measured in thickness and cellular content.[24–26] The structural difference has been verified from outside-in gross dissection, inside-out arthroscopically, and radiographic position on a total of 47 cadavers as follows

(▶Fig. 34.4, ▶Fig. 34.8, ▶Fig. 34.9, and ▶Fig. 34.10). The *dorsal deltoid complex* emanates from the dorsal tubercle and distally fans across the dorsum of the metacarpal (▶Fig. 34.8). The stout collagen is organized and cellular and possesses proprioceptive mechanoreceptors known as Ruffini endings near ligamentous attachments.[4,8,9] Conversely, the *volar ligaments* are thin, capsular structures, variable in location, with thenar muscles intimal to their presence (▶Fig. 34.9) that variably take origin upon the trapezium. Absence of organization and proprioceptive nerve endings support the concept that muscular activity contributes to volar stability. Muscle is rich in proprioceptive muscle spindles, and their presence in thenar muscles has been demonstrated with conditioning experiments in both central and peripheral evoked potential testing.[27,28] These findings support thenar strengthening in functional CMC rehabilitation with favorable MCP flexed positioning, preventing hyperextension.[29,30] The anterior oblique "beak" ligament (AOL) has been implicated for its importance in the presence and creation of arthritis, and reconstructing it surgically is important.[31–34] Although current evidence for the AOL's being an attenuated, thin structure challenges its historic

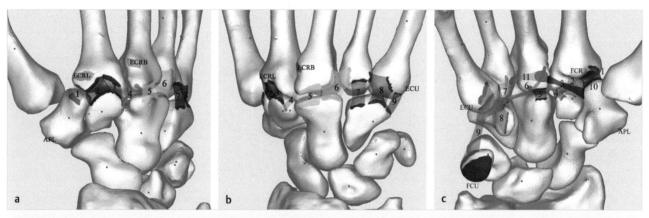

Fig. 34.3 The dorsal carpometacarpal (CMC) and intermetacarpal ligaments are shown; the block like joint configuration and these stout ligaments confer stability. The most rigid is the third CMC (CMC-3) joint, with increasing mobility toward the small finger and thumb. (**a**) A dorsal view of a three-dimensional (3D) model of a right wrist. The *solid colored areas* show ligament attachment locations, and the *transparent colored areas* show the paths of the ligaments. 1, dorsal second metacarpal radial base–trapezium ligament; 2, dorsal second metacarpal radial base–trapezoid ligament; 3, dorsal second metacarpal ulnar base–trapezoid ligament; 4, dorsal third metacarpal radial base–trapezoid ligament; 5, dorsal third metacarpal radial base–capitate ligament; 6, dorsal third metacarpal ulnar base–capitate–fourth metacarpal radial base ligament; 7, dorsal fourth metacarpal ulnar base–hamate ligament; 8, dorsal fourth metacarpal ulnar base–hamate–fifth metacarpal radial base ligament. APL, abductor pollicis longus; ECRB, extensor carpi radialis brevis; ECRL, extensor carpi radialis longus. (**b**) A dorsal view of a 3D model of a right wrist. The *solid colored areas* show ligament attachment locations, and the *transparent colored areas* show the paths of the ligaments. 1, dorsal second metacarpal radial base–trapezium ligament; 2, dorsal second metacarpal radial base–trapezoid ligament; 3, dorsal second metacarpal ulnar base–trapezoid ligament; 4, dorsal third metacarpal radial base–trapezoid ligament; 5, dorsal third metacarpal radial base–capitate ligament; 6, dorsal third metacarpal ulnar base–capitate–fourth metacarpal radial base ligament; 7, dorsal fourth metacarpal ulnar base–hamate ligament; 8, dorsal fourth metacarpal ulnar base–hamate–fifth metacarpal radial base ligament; 9, dorsal fifth metacarpal ulnar base–hamate ligament. ECRB, extensor carpi radialis brevis; ECRL, extensor carpi radialis longus; ECU, extensor carpi ulnaris. (**c**) A palmar view of a 3D model of a right wrist. The *solid colored areas* show ligament attachment locations, and the *transparent colored areas* show the paths of the ligaments. 1, palmar second metacarpal–trapezium ligament; 2, palmar second metacarpal–trapezoid ligament; 3, palmar third metacarpal radial base–trapezium ligament; 4, palmar third metacarpal radial base–trapezoid ligament; 5, palmar third metacarpal–capitate ligament; 6, palmar third metacarpal ulnar base–hamate ligament; 7, palmar fourth metacarpal ulnar base–hook of hamate ligament; 8, palmar fifth metacarpal–hook of hamate ligament; 9, the third metacarpal, fourth metacarpal, fifth metacarpal, hamate–pisiform ligament; 10, second metacarpal–trapezium interosseous ligament; 11, palmar third metacarpal–fourth metacarpal–fifth metacarpal ligament. APL, abductor pollicis longus; ECU, extensor carpi ulnaris; FCR, flexor carpi radialis; FCU, flexor carpi ulnaris. (Reproduced with permission from Nanno M, Buford WL Jr, et al. Three-dimensional analysis of the ligamentous attachments of the second through fifth carpometacarpal joints. Clin Anat 2007;20(5):530–544.)

importance, the emphasis on both restoring the palmar stability and strengthening with surgical reconstruction, along with postoperative rehabilitation to maximize functional return, complements both current and historical emphasis on thenar muscular coupling as integral to palmar support.

The *ulnar complex* creates a checkrein effect: the ulnar collateral ligament or, more appropriately, the volar trapeziometacarpal ligament and the dorsal trapeziometacarpal ligament span from their more central locations proximally to a conjoined attachment directly ulnarly.[4,5,18,] The stout ulnar complex may be critical to volar concentration of forces (▶ Fig. 34.10).

34.3 Second Carpometacarpal Joint

The second metacarpal articulates primarily with the trapezoid, with a small facet articulating with each of the trapezium and the capitate (▶ Fig. 34.2 and ▶ Fig. 34.7d). The radial aspect of the index finger provides a stable platform for the thumb's lateral pinch, and the index ray is relatively rigid compared with the mobile thumb. The small articulating facet of the second metacarpal on the trapezial surface is positioned dorsally and oriented coronally (volarly). This relationship provides enough pronation, abduction, and flexion to provide a small amount of rotation[35,36] that is

critical for both three-jaw grasp and pinch.[2] The CMC-2, in concert with thumb CMC-1, exhibits evolutionary distinction from hominins and extant great apes that make it uniquely human.[2]

34.4 Third Carpometacarpal Joint

The third metacarpal serves as a keystone to its adjacent metacarpals and has the richest ligamentous attachments of the finger CMC joints. CMC-3 provides stability to the carpus and, along with its primary articulation of the capitate, provides the neutral axis to the forearm. An intra-articular ligament between the third and fourth metacarpal, dividing two articular facets between the two bones, and an intra-articular ligament between the capitate and hamate are typically found,[6] lending additional stability to this critical joint (▶ Fig. 34.11).

34.5 Fourth Carpometacarpal Joint

The fourth metacarpal articulates with the third and fifth metacarpals, and the hamate constitutes its primary carpal surface with typically one or two dorsal and volar small facets articulating with the capitate[37] (▶Fig. 34.11). CMC-4 possesses the most variability of the finger basilar joints in shape and articulation—in a study of 142 cadaveric wrists, Viegas and colleagues found the majority of specimens to have a flat metacarpal surface (85.9%), with conical shape

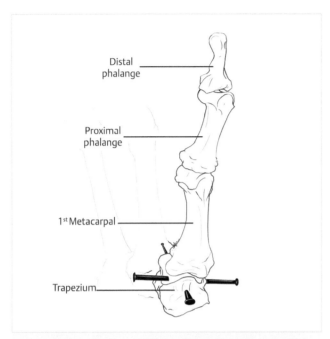

Fig. 34.4 The motion arcs of the metacarpal upon the trapezium are flexion-extension and abduction-adduction. Pronation-supination represents composite rotation and translation of this triaxial joint based on morphology and muscular activity (Fick, Cooney, Zancolli, Haines). The thumb position in relation to the fingers represents a completion of the carpal arch, which places the carpometacarpal joint obliquely volar to the adjacent fingers and proximally oriented on its radial aspect. The arcs of motion thus are out of phase with the fingers. Image redrawn from computed tomography surface rendering of a normal right hand. (Image used with permission from S Hegmann.)

(14.1%) less common.[37] The centrifugal increase in mobility away from CMC-3 adds to the cupping capability, with CMC-4 and CMC-5 providing the ulnar prehension critical for grasp.[2] The fourth metacarpal is the most slender of the metacarpals[38] and the interval between the third and fourth metacarpal cited as the most frequent location of axial dislocation[39]: the variability and vulnerability of this joint is perhaps related to its importance to evolutionary adaptation of human grasp.[2,37]

34.6 Fifth Carpometacarpal Joint

The fifth metacarpal articulates with the fourth metacarpal, and with it shares the support of the hamate (Fig. 34.2). It is relatively flat, but along with the fourth metacarpal, it provides a gentle concave reciprocating surface for the slightly convex surface of the hamate. In addition, in the volar–dorsal plane it has a gentle convex configuration, thus having a biconcave-convex feature, or gentle saddle shape less developed than but similar to the thumb CMC (▶Fig. 34.12). This affords mobility second only to CMC-1, provided by the strong hypothenar complex. It possesses both dorsal and volar CMC ligaments[37] and also possesses spanning ligaments to the hook of the hamate, pisiform, and fourth metacarpal (▶Fig. 34.13). CMC-4 and CMC-5 together complete ulnar prehension critical for human grasp.[2,3]

34.7 Summary

The strong and stable CMC joints of the hand provide the platform for subtle independence of intricate fine motor activity of the fingers, or conversely, powerful manipulation and thrust of objects as the terminal unit that the long lever the arm, affords. The most stable is CMC-3, with increasing mobility occurring in a centrifugal pattern toward the thumb and small finger, thus providing their critical role in manipulative capabilities.

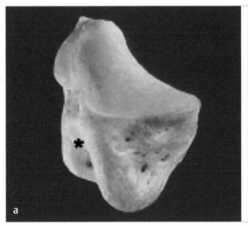
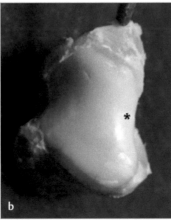

Fig. 34.5 (a) The trapezium devoid of articular cartilage. This is a right trapezium with the metacarpal articular surface facing upward. The ulnar side is toward the top, and the flexor carpi radialis groove is marked with an *asterisk*. (From the Bassett Anatomy collection, Stanford University, with permission.) (b) The metacarpal surface is gently comma-shaped (*left*) or C-shaped (*right*, as indicated here) as positioned in viewing one's own thumb from above, with the radial side closest to the body. The *asterisk* corresponds to the gentle concavity on the dorsal side. The pin emanates from the ulnar position at the trapezoid articulation; the shape is in reference to the ulnar–volar axis. (With permission from AL Ladd.)

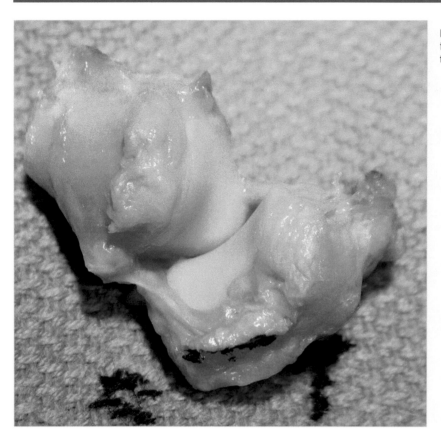

Fig. 34.6 The reciprocal articulating surfaces of a right first metacarpal upon the trapezium. (With permission from AL Ladd.)

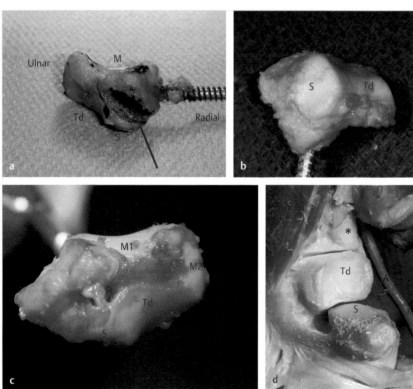

Fig. 34.7 The osteology of the trapezium; articular cartilage intact. (**a**) The flexor carpi radialis (FCR) groove runs volar and in an oblique direction (*arrow*); since the FCR runs relatively longitudinally in the palm, this orientation indicates the offset and oblique position of the trapezium relative to the rest of the fingers. (**b**) The scaphoid (S) and trapezoid (Td) facets of the trapezium are visualized. (**c**) As viewed from the dorsal side, the S, Td, second metacarpal (M2), and first metacarpal (M1) articular facets of the trapezial are seen. (**d**) The M2–Td articulation viewed from the volar side, with articulation trapezial facets visualized; the trapezium is removed. Note the dorsally positioned trapezial facet of the M2 (*), which illustrates the volar position of the body of trapezium relative to the remainder of the transverse fixed arch. A, dorsal branch radial artery; M1, articular facet of first metacarpal; S, scaphoid; Td, trapezoid. (Images a–c courtesy AL Ladd.)

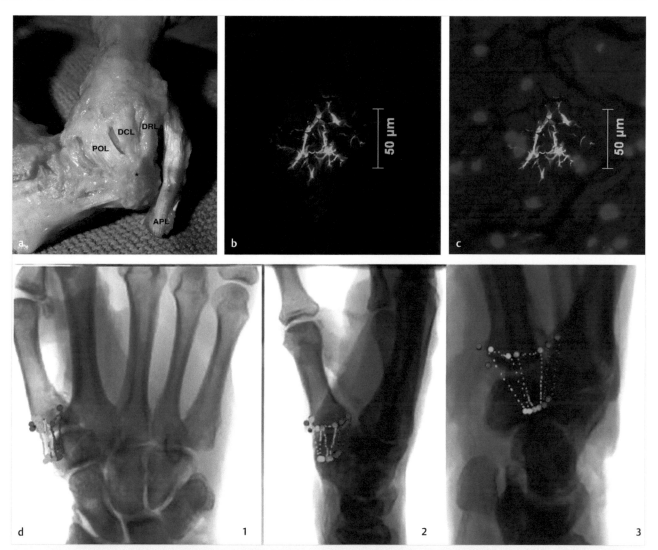

Fig. 34.8 The dorsal ligamentous anatomy presented from gross dissections, immunohistochemical staining, and radiographic marking. (a) The stout dorsal ligaments form a deltoid complex emanating from the dorsal tubercle (*), representing the dorsal radial ligament (DRL), dorsal central ligament (DCL), and posterior oblique ligament (POL) in a left hand. (b, c) Dorsal ligament immunofluorescent PGP9. 5 and 4′,6-diamidino-2-phenylindole (DAPI) staining demonstrating a Ruffini ending (b) and nucleated collagen (c). These were essentially absent in all volar ligaments examined. (d) The radiographic representation of the dorsal ligaments with anteroposterior, lateral, and Robert's views.[1–3] DRL (*green*), DCL (*orange*), POL (*magenta*), and APL (*red*). (Image d courtesy AL Ladd.)

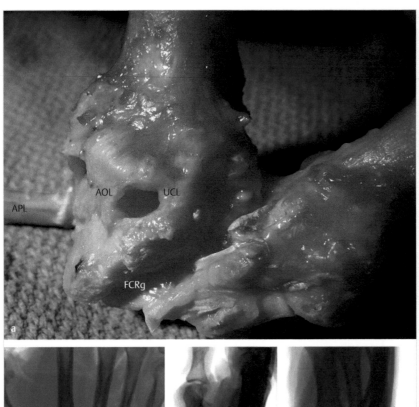

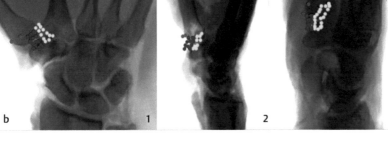

Fig. 34.9 The volar ligamentous anatomy from gross dissections and radiographic marking. (**a**) The volar ligaments in passive extension: anterior oblique ligament (AOL) and ulnar collateral ligament (UCL). The window between the thin ligaments is commonly found intimal to the thenar muscles. (**b**) The radiographic representation of the volar ligaments with anteroposterior, lateral, and Robert's views[1,2,3]. AOL (*blue*), UCL (*yellow*), APL (*red*). FCRg, the obliquely oriented flexor carpi radialis groove. (Images a and b courtesy AL Ladd, E Hagert.)

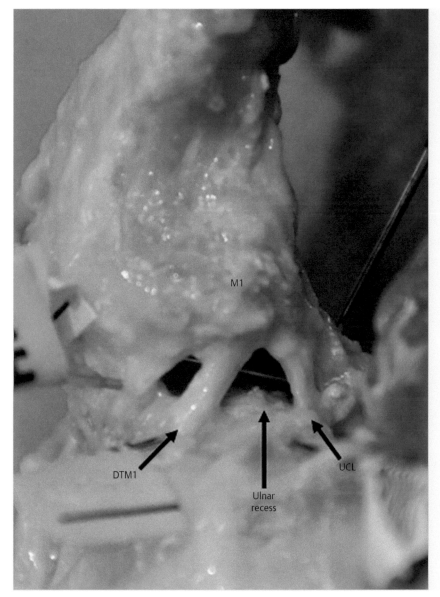

Fig. 34.10 The ulnar checkrein complex: the ulnar collateral ligament, or more appropriately, the volar trapeziometacarpal ligament and the dorsal trapeziometacarpal ligament span from their more central locations proximally to a conjoined attachment directly ulnarly on the first metacarpal (M1).[4,5,18] (Image courtesy AL Ladd.)

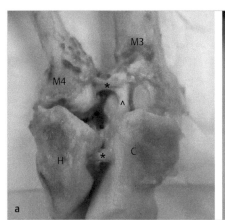
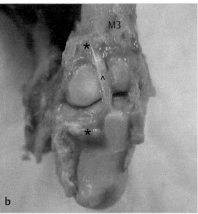

Fig. 34.11 (**a**) Dorsal view and (**b**) lateral view: the intra-articular ligament (^) runs between the third (M3) and the fourth (M4) metacarpal and the capitate (C) and the hamate (H). The interosseous ligament (*) runs between the third and the fourth metacarpal and between the capitate and the hamate. (Images courtesy of S Viegas, with permission.)

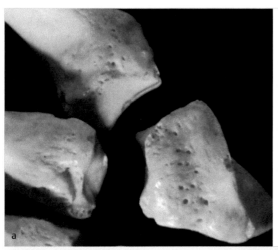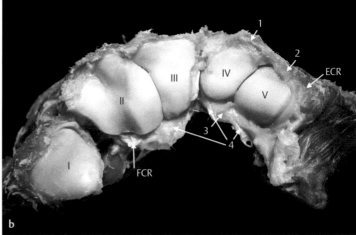

Fig. 34.12 (a) CMC-4 and CMC-5 together create a loose saddle configuration, emulating the thumb's versatility in motion. (b) Anatomical dissection showing the bases of metacarpals with the carpus removed. 1, dorsal fourth metacarpal ulnar base–hamate–fifth metacarpal radial base ligament; 2, dorsal fifth metacarpal ulnar base–hamate ligament; 3, palmar fifth metacarpal–hook of hamate ligament; 4, the third meta-carpal, fourth metacarpal, fifth metacarpal, hamate–pisiformis ligament, 5, hook of hamate–pisiformis ligament; FCR, flexor carpi radialis; FCU, flexor carpi ulnaris; ECU, extensor carpi ulnaris.

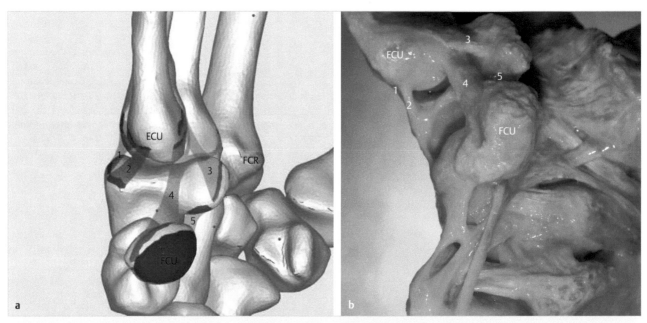

Fig. 34.13 (a) An ulnar view of a three-dimensional model of the right wrist. The *solid colored areas* show ligament attachment locations, and the *transparent colored areas* show the paths of the ligaments. (b) Anatomical dissection showing the fifth metacarpal base, hamate and pisiform. 1, dorsal fourth metacarpal ulnar base–hamate–fifth metacarpal radial base ligament; 2, dorsal fifth metacarpal ulnar base–hamate ligament; 3, palmar fifth metacarpal–hook of hamate ligament; 4, the third metacarpal, fourth metacarpal, fifth metacarpal, hamate–pisiformis ligament; 5, hook of hamate–pisiformis ligament. ECU, extensor carpi ulnaris; FCR, flexor carpi radialis; FCU, flexor carpi ulnaris. (a: Reproduced with permission from Nanno M, Buford WL Jr, et al. Three-dimensional analysis of the ligamentous attachments of the second through fifth carpometacarpal joints. Clin Anat 2007;20(5):530–544.)

References

1. Hentz VR, Chase RA. Hand Surgery: A Clinical Atlas. Philadelphia, PA: WB Saunders Company; 2001

2. Marzke MW, Wullstein KL, Viegas SF. Evolution of the power ("squeeze") grip and its morphological correlates in hominids. Am J Phys Anthropol 1992;89(3):283–298

3. Wilson FR. The Hand: How Its Use Shapes the Brain, Language, and Human Culture. New York, NY: Pantheon Books;1998

4. Ladd AL, Lee J, Hagert E. Macroscopic and microscopic analysis of the thumb carpometacarpal ligaments: a cadaveric study of ligament anatomy and histology. J Bone Joint Surg Am 2012;94(16):1468–1477

5. Bettinger PC, Linscheid RL, Berger RA, Cooney WP III, An KN. An anatomic study of the stabilizing ligaments of the trapezium and trapeziometacarpal joint. J Hand Surg Am 1999;24(4):786–798

6. Nakamura K, Patterson RM, Viegas SF. The ligament and skeletal anatomy of the second through fifth carpometacarpal joints and adjacent structures. J Hand Surg Am 2001;26(6):1016–1029

7. Nanno M, Buford WL Jr, Patterson RM, Andersen CR, Viegas SF. Three-dimensional analysis of the ligamentous attachments of the second through fifth carpometacarpal joints. Clin Anat 2007;20(5):530–544

8. Hilton J. On Rest and Pain: A Course of Lectures on the Influence of Mechanical and Physiological Rest in the Treatment of Accidents and Surgical Diseases, and the Diagnostic Value of Pain, delivered at the Royal College of Surgeons of England in the years 1860, 1861, and 1862. London, England: Bell and Daldy; 1863

9. Lorea DP, Berthe JV, De Mey A, Coessens BC, Rooze M, Foucher G. The nerve supply of the trapeziometacarpal joint. J Hand Surg [Br] 2002;27(3):232–237

10. Gray H. Anatomy of the Human Body. 20th ed. W.H. Lewis. 1918, Philadelphia: Lea & Febiger.

11. Bell C. The Hand—Its Mechanism and Vital Endowments as Evincing Design. 2nd ed. London, England: William Pickering; 1833

12. Napier JR. The form and function of the carpo-metacarpal joint of the thumb. J Anat 1955;89(3):362–369

13. Marzke MW. Evolutionary development of the human thumb. Hand Clin 1992;8(1):1–8

14. Fick A. Die Gelenke mit sattelformigen Filichen. Zeitschrift fur rationelle Medicin; 1854:314–321

15. Haines RW. The mechanism of rotation at the first carpo-metacarpal joint. J Anat 1944;78(Pt 1-2):44–46

16. Cooney WP III, Lucca MJ, Chao EY, Linscheid RL. The kinesiology of the thumb trapeziometacarpal joint. J Bone Joint Surg Am 1981;63(9):1371–1381

17. Zancolli EA, Ziadenberg C, Zancolli E Jr. Biomechanics of the trapeziometacarpal joint. Clin Orthop Relat Res 1987; (220):14–26

18. Bojsen-Moller F. Osteoligamentous guidance of the movements of the human thumb. Am J Anat 1976;147(1):71–80

19. Ladd AL. Upper-limb evolution and development: skeletons in the closet. Congenital anomalies and evolution's template. J Bone Joint Surg Am 2009;91(Suppl 4):19–25

20. Palmer AK, Werner FW, Murphy D, Glisson R. Functional wrist motion: a biomechanical study. J Hand Surg Am 1985;10(1):39–46

21. Crisco JJ, Coburn JC, Moore DC, Akelman E, Weiss AP, Wolfe SW. In vivo radiocarpal kinematics and the dart thrower's motion. J Bone Joint Surg Am 2005;87(12):2729–2740

22. Edmunds JO. Traumatic dislocations and instability of the trapeziometacarpal joint of the thumb. Hand Clin 2006;22(3):365–392

23. Ladd AL, Weiss APC, Crisco JJ, Hagert E, Wolf JM, Glickel SZ. The thumb CMC joint: anatomy, hormones, and biomechanics. 2012 AAOS. Instr Course Lect, in press

24. Hagert E, Lee J, Ladd AL. Innervation patterns of thumb trapeziometacarpal joint ligaments. J Hand Surg Am 2012;37(4):706–714.e1

25. Lee J, Ladd A, Hagert E. Immunofluorescent triple-staining technique to identify sensory nerve endings in human thumb ligaments. Cells Tissues Organs 2012;195(5):456–464

26. Zhang A, van Nortwick S, Hagert E, Yao J, Ladd AL. Thumb CMC ligaments inside and out: a comparative study of arthroscopic and gross anatomy. J Wrist Surg, in press

27. Spitzer A, Claus D. The influence of the shape of mechanical stimuli on muscle stretch reflexes and SEP. Electroencephalogr Clin Neurophysiol 1992;85(5):331–336

28. Segura MJ, Gandolfo CN, Sica RE. Percutaneous cervical stimulation: effects on intraspinal structures. Electroencephalogr Clin Neurophysiol 1991;81(4):299–303

29. Neumann DA, Bielefeld T. The carpometacarpal joint of the thumb: stability, deformity, and therapeutic intervention. J Orthop Sports Phys Ther 2003;33(7):386–399

30. Poole JU, Pellegrini VD Jr. Arthritis of the thumb basal joint complex. J Hand Ther 2000;13(2):91–107

31. Pellegrini VD Jr. The ABJS 2005 Nicolas Andry Award: osteoarthritis and injury at the base of the human thumb: survival of the fittest? Clin Orthop Relat Res 2005;438(438):266–276

32. Pellegrini VD Jr. Osteoarthritis of the trapeziometacarpal joint: the pathophysiology of articular cartilage degeneration. I. Anatomy and pathology of the aging joint. J Hand Surg Am 1991;16(6):967–974

33. Eaton RG, Littler JW. A study of the basal joint of the thumb. Treatment of its disabilities by fusion. J Bone Joint Surg Am 1969;51(4):661–668

34. Eaton RG, Littler JW. Ligament reconstruction for the painful thumb carpometacarpal joint. J Bone Joint Surg Am 1973;55(8):1655–1666

35. Tocheri MW, Marzke MW, Liu D, et al. Functional capabilities of modern and fossil hominid hands: three-dimensional analysis of trapezia. Am J Phys Anthropol 2003;122(2):101–112

36. Lewis OJ. Functional Morphology of the Evolving Hand and Foot. Oxford, England: Oxford University Press; 1989

37. Viegas SF, Crossley M, Marzke M, Wullstein K. The fourth carpometacarpal joint. J Hand Surg Am 1991;16(3):525–533

38. Bergman RA, Thompson SA, Afifi AKFA. Compendium of Human Anatomic Variation: Catalog, Atlas and World Literature. Baltimore, MD, and Munich, Germany: Urban & Schwarzenberg; 1988

39. Garcia-Elias M, Dobyns JH, Cooney WP III, Linscheid RL. Traumatic axial dislocations of the carpus. J Hand Surg Am 1989;14(3):446–457

35 The Metacarpophalangeal Joints

Joanne Labriola and Jeffrey A. Greenberg

35.1 Surface Anatomy of Metacarpophalangeal Joint

The metacarpophalangeal joints are located 1 to 2 cm proximal to the interdigital skin fold. The palmar flexion creases define their location.[1,2] The metacarpophalangeal joint of the index finger is aligned with the proximal palmar flexion crease, the metacarpophalangeal joint of the middle finger is aligned between the distal and proximal palmar flexion creases, and the metacarpophalangeal joints of the ring and small fingers are aligned with the distal palmar flexion crease. The thumb metacarpophalangeal joint is at the level of the first web space, and the palmar flexion crease of the thumb defines the location of its metacarpophalangeal joint.

35.1.1 Skin and Integument

The skin on the dorsal aspect of the metacarpophalangeal joints is mobile, while the skin on the palmar aspect of the metacarpophalangeal joints is firmly fixed to the palmar fascia. The adherence of the palmar skin via the vertical septae that run from the skin to the palmar fascia facilitates gripping. The palmar fascia includes the pretendinous bands, superficial transverse metacarpal ligament (also called the transverse ligament of the palmar aponeurosis), and vertical septa.[3–5] The pretendinous bands run superficially and longitudinally in line with the flexor tendons and insert into the skin at the level of the metacarpophalangeal joint. The superficial transverse metacarpal ligament is perpendicular and deep to the pretendinous bands. The vertical septa are the deepest structures and are adjacent to the metacarpal necks. The vertical septa, including the septa of Legueu and Juvara, connect the superficial and deep metacarpal ligaments.[3] The

vertical septa form seven longitudinal compartments in the palm and divide the flexor tendons and A1 pulleys from the neurovascular bundles and lumbricals. The palmar fascia of the thumb includes the thenar muscle fascia, the poorly defined pretendinous band, the proximal commissural ligament, and the distal commissural ligament.[6] The proximal commissural ligament is the radial continuation of the superficial transverse metacarpal ligament. The distal commissural ligament is the radial continuation of the natatory ligament of the digital web spaces.

35.1.2 Osteology

The metacarpophalangeal joint is composed of the metacarpal head and the base of the proximal phalanx (▶Fig. 35.1a–d). The radius of curvature of the metacarpal head is smaller than the radius of curvature of the base of the proximal phalanx.[7] The metacarpal head is larger in the sagittal plane than in the transverse plane (▶Fig. 35.2). The opposite is true for the base of the proximal phalanx. The base of the proximal phalanx is larger in the transverse plane than in the sagittal plane.

The metacarpal head is convex, irregular, and asymmetrical (▶Fig. 35.2). It is narrow dorsally and widens volarly (▶Fig. 35.2), allowing progressively more contact with the base of the proximal phalanx with increasing flexion (▶Fig. 35.3).[2] The metacarpal head and the arc of its articular surface are offset volarly relative to the metacarpal shaft (▶Fig. 35.1d and ▶Fig. 35.4). The radial condyle is larger than the ulnar condyle especially in the second and third metacarpal heads (▶Fig. 35.4a).[8] The asymmetry of the condyles of the metacarpal head may contribute to ulnar drift of the metacarpophalangeal joints in inflammatory arthritis. The base of the proximal phalanx is concave, shallow, and oval (▶Fig. 35.3).

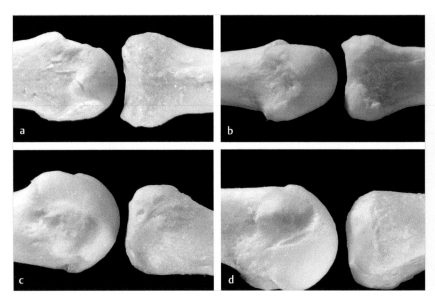

Fig. 35.1 (a) Dorsal view; (b) volar view; (c) radial view and (d) ulnar view of the metacarpal head and base of the proximal phalanx making the metacarpophalangeal joint.

The metacarpal head has dorsal lateral tubercles for the attachment of the collateral ligaments[5] (▶ Fig. 35.5). It also has grooves on its lateral surface that are oriented from palmar proximal to dorsal distal (▶ Fig. 35.5). The tendons of the interosseous muscles lie in these grooves. The base of the proximal phalanx has a dorsal and palmar ridge for the attachment of the metacarpophalangeal joint capsule and, rarely, the direct insertion of the extensor tendon.[5] The palmar ridge extends laterally to form tubercles for the attachment of the collateral ligaments. The base of the proximal phalanx also has dorsal lateral abductor and adductor tubercles. In addition, there is a palmar depression located centrally for the passage of the flexor tendons (▶ Fig. 35.3).

The metacarpophalangeal joint is an ellipsoid joint that allows biaxial motions, including flexion, extension, abduction, adduction, and rotation.[5] The intra-articular space is greater in the sagittal than in the transverse plane, and the synovium has enlarged dorsal and palmar pouches. The metacarpophalangeal joint volume is largest in extension. With flexion, the metacarpophalangeal joint volume decreases and joint constraint increases. The shape of the metacarpal head produces a cam effect: flexion transforms into translation and elongation of collaterals.[1] The collateral ligaments are loose in extension but tighten in flexion and further increase the constraint of the joint. The primary stabilizers of the metacarpophalangeal joint are the collateral ligaments, volar plate, and capsule.[5] The flexor tendons, extensor tendons, and intrinsics add to the dynamic stability of the joint.

35.1.3 Capsule, Collateral Ligaments, and Volar Plate

The capsule surrounds the metacarpophalangeal joint, attaching to the base of the proximal phalanx and the metacarpal neck. It is relatively lax. The metacarpophalangeal joint is supported dorsally by the sagittal bands and the loose insertion of the common extensor tendon (▶ Fig. 35.6). Volarly, the joint is supported by the volar plate (▶ Fig. 35.7 and

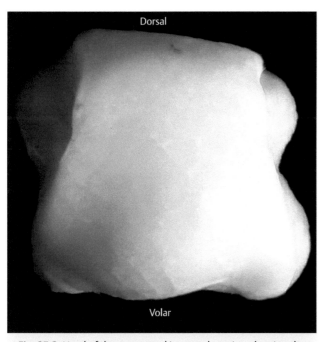

Fig. 35.2 Head of the metacarpal in an end-on view showing the narrow dorsal part and wider volar part.

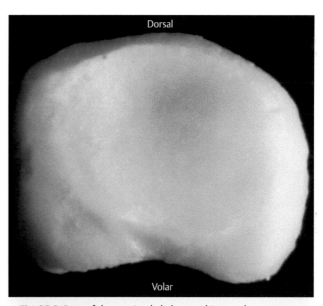

Fig. 35.3 Base of the proximal phalanx making up the metacarpophalangeal joint.

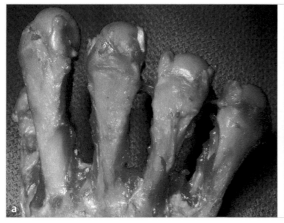
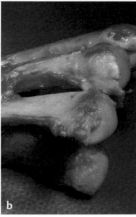

Fig. 35.4 The geometry of the metacarpal heads is demonstrated in the dorsal (**a**) and lateral (**b**) views of the hand. The metacarpal head and the arc of its articular surface are offset volarly relative to the metacarpal shaft. The asymmetric shape of the metacarpal head produces a cam effect as the proximal phalanx moves into flexion, tightening the collateral ligaments.

▶ Fig. 35.8) that is continuous with the deep transverse metacarpal ligament (or the inter palmar plate ligament) (▶ Fig. 35.9) and laterally by the collateral ligaments, sagittal bands, and intrinsic tendons.[2]

The collateral ligaments arise from the dorsal lateral tubercles of the metacarpal head (▶ Fig. 35.5) and insert on the lateral tubercles on the base of the proximal phalanx[5] (▶ Fig. 35.10). The accessory collateral ligaments run from the palmar grooves of the dorsal lateral tubercles of the metacarpal head to the lateral edge of the volar plate (▶ Fig. 35.11). The accessory collaterals then penetrate the deep transverse metacarpal ligament and joint with the fibrous flexor tendon sheath.[5] The collateral ligaments are dorsal to the center of rotation of the metacarpophalangeal joints.[9] They are loose in extension but tighten in flexion (▶ Fig. 35.12). The accessory collaterals are volar to the center of rotation.[9] These ligaments are loose in flexion but tighten in extension.

The collateral ligaments of the metacarpophalangeal joint are asymmetric.[8] The ulnar collateral ligaments are more parallel to the long axis of the finger in the sagittal plane. The radial collateral ligaments are more oblique and attach closer to the joint margins. The angulation of the radial collateral ligament is greatest in the index finger and decreases progressively from the radial to the ulnar side of the hand.[10] The obliquity of the radial collateral ligament of the index finger resists the pronation force on the index finger generated by the first dorsal interosseous muscle. The radial collateral ligament also resists the volar translational forces of the flexors and intrinsic muscles. Biomechanically, the asymmetry of the collateral ligaments leads to supination and ulnar deviation with metacarpophalangeal joint flexion.[1,8,10]

The volar plate of the metacarpophalangeal joint is fibrocartilaginous distally and membranous proximally (▶ Fig. 35.7 and ▶ Fig. 35.8). The distal portion is thicker laterally and is attached to the lateral tubercles at the base of the proximal phalanx.[5] The proximal portion inserts on the metacarpal neck. Laterally, the volar plate attaches to the deep transverse metacarpal ligament.

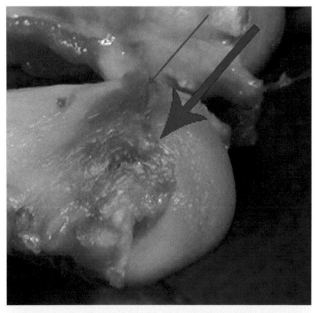

Fig. 35.5 An enlarged view of the lateral aspect of the metacarpal head depicts the dorsolateral tubercle (*blue arrow*). The collateral ligament inserts proximal to the articular surface of the joint on this tubercle. The palmar to dorsal groove for the interosseous is marked by a *red arrow*.

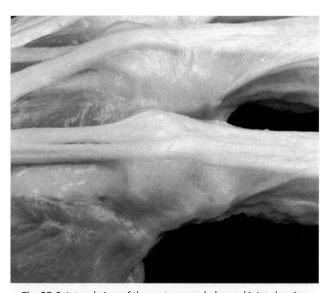

Fig. 35.6 Lateral view of the metacarpophalangeal joint showing the extensor tendon and sagittal band and the collateral ligament traversing distal and volar to insert on the base of the proximal phalanx.

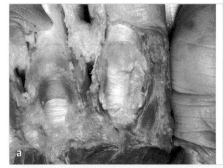
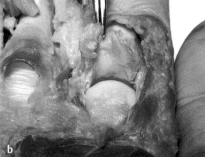
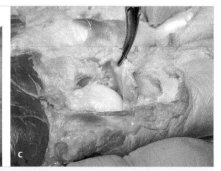

Fig. 35.7 The volar plate provides the main volar support for the metacarpophalangeal joint (**a**) and blends in with the intermetacarpal ligaments on its radial and ulnar sides. The middle finger shows the intact transverse fibers of the volar plate deep to the A1 pulley. In the photo of the index finger, the distal fibrocartilaginous portion of the volar plate remains attached to the base of the proximal phalanx, but the proximal membranous portion of the volar plate has been released from the metacarpal neck and is held by the forceps (**b, c**).

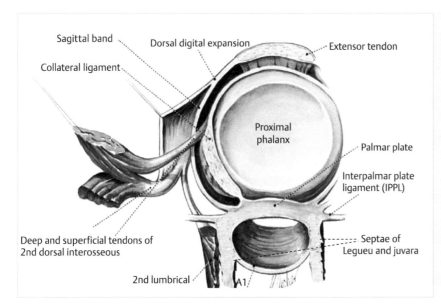

Fig. 35.8 Drawing of the base of the proximal phalanx and the surrounding soft tissues with the metacarpal removed showing the extensor mechanism, the volar plate, and the A1 pulley along with the relationship of the lumbrical and interossei. (From Kleinert Institute, Louisville, KY.)

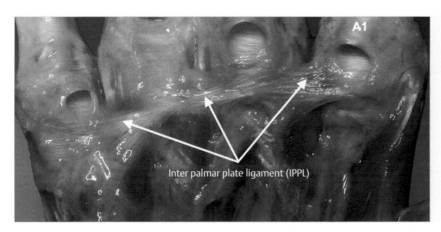

Fig. 35.9 The Inter Palmar Plate Ligament (IPPL) or the Deep Transverse Metacarpal Ligament is a thick and strong structure spanning the palm connecting the palmar plates.

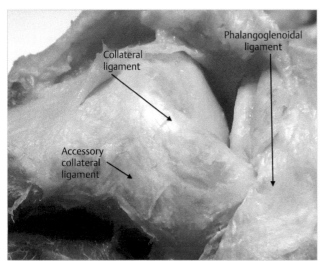

Fig. 35.10 The lateral view of the metacarpophalangeal joint shows the collateral ligament with its dorsolateral metacarpal origin extending distally and volarly to its proximal phalangeal insertion. It also shows the accessory collateral ligament and the phalangoglenoidal ligament.

The volar plate is collapsible and rarely forms checkreins, making metacarpophalangeal joint contractures less common than proximal phalanx contractures.[1]

35.1.4 Deep Transverse Metacarpal Ligament (Inter Palmar Plate Ligament) and the Metacarpal Transverse Arch

The deep transverse metacarpal ligament (▶Fig. 35.9) connects the volar plates of adjacent metacarpophalangeal joints of the index finger through the small finger. This ligament should be called inter palmar plate ligament (IPPL) as the ligaments are attached mainly to the palmar plates and not to the metacarpals. Additionally, the IPPL is a series of three structures attached to the palmar plates. It is continuous with the sagittal bands, the accessory collateral ligaments, the A1 pulleys and flexor sheath (▶Fig. 35.8), the radial collateral ligament of the index finger, and the ulnar collateral ligament of the small finger.[4] In addition, the first dorsal interosseous muscle attaches to the deep transverse metacarpal ligament (or the IPPL) radially and to the abductor digiti minimi and flexor digiti minimi ulnarly.[11] These muscular

411

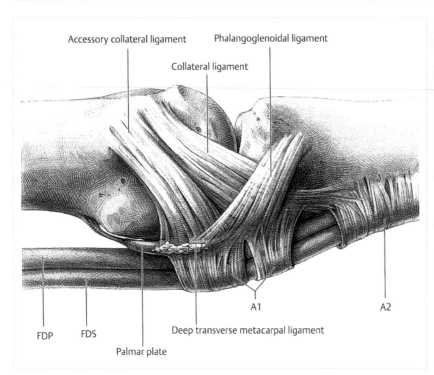

Accessory collateral ligament   Phalangoglenoidal ligament

Collateral ligament

A1   A2

FDP   FDS   Deep transverse metacarpal ligament

Palmar plate

Fig. 35.11 Drawing showing the lateral view of the metacarpophalangeal joint with the collateral ligaments, the accessory collateral ligaments, and the phalangeoglenoid ligament and relationship with the volar plate and flexor sheath. (From Schmidt H-M, Lanz U. Surgical Anatomy of the Hand. Stuttgart, Germany: Thieme; 2004.)

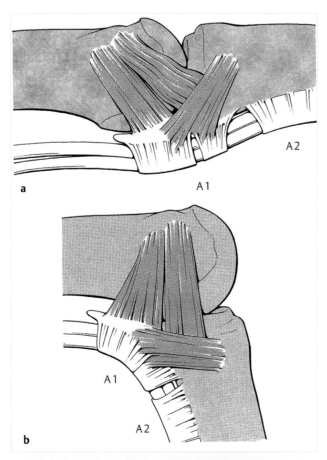

a   A1   A2

b   A1   A2

Fig. 35.12 (a, b) Drawing showing the laxity of the collateral ligament in extension and tightening in flexion of the metacarpophalangeal joint. (From Schmidt H-M, Lanz U. Surgical Anatomy of the Hand. Stuttgart , Germany: Thieme; 2004.)

attachments may provide stability and mobility to the interconnected metacarpophalangeal joints of the fingers.

The deep transverse metacarpal ligament (or the IPPL) is the fundamental structure maintaining the metacarpal transverse arch (▶Fig. 35.4).[12] The metacarpal transverse arch refers to the normal convex relationship between the metacarpal heads and convex contour of the palm. The transverse metacarpal arch influences the normal cascade of the fingers. It allows mobility ulnarly for power grip and cylindrical grasp. It provides stability radially for precision patterns such as tip and chuck pinch. During power grip, the metacarpal transverse arch widens as the fourth and fifth metacarpals descend volarly, and the second and third metacarpals remain fixed.[13] Widening of the metacarpal transverse arch leads to increased ulnar deviation at the metacarpophalangeal joints.[12] During opposition of the fifth metacarpal, this arch narrows as the ulnar metacarpals descend, supinate, and adduct.

35.1.5 Extensor Apparatus

The metacarpophalangeal joints are located within extensor tendon zone V of the eight zones proposed by Verdan for classification of extensor lacerations.[14] In zone V, the extensor apparatus is a tendinous hood composed primarily of the extrinsic extensor tendons and the sagittal bands. The extensor digitorum communis (EDC) tendons lie centrally over the dorsal aspect of the metacarpophalangeal joints (▶Fig. 35.13). The index finger and the small finger have accessory extrinsic extensors—the extensor indicis proprius and the extensor digiti minimi, respectively. These accessory extrinsic extensor tendons are located ulnar to the EDC tendons and also contribute to the extensor hood. The sagittal bands originate on both sides of the metacarpophalangeal joint and attach to

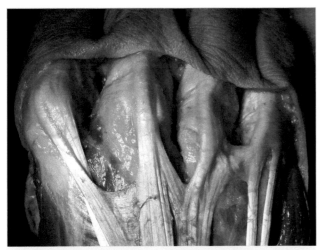

Fig. 35.13 The extensor digitorum communis (EDC) tendons lie centrally over the dorsal aspect of the metacarpophalangeal joints. The extensor indicis proprius and the extensor digiti minimi are ulnar to the EDC tendons. These extrinsic extensor tendons contribute to the extensor hood of the metacarpophalangeal joint.

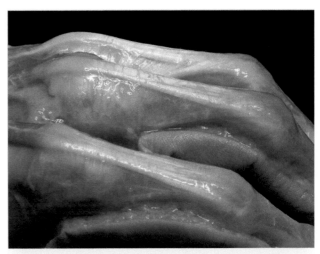

Fig. 35.14 Lateral view of the metacarpophalangeal joint. The sagittal band attaches dorsally to the extrinsic extensor tendon and palmarly to the volar plate. The sagittal bands contribute to and centralize the extensor hood of the metacarpophalangeal joint. The continuation of the lateral bands toward the proximal interphalangeal joint is also visualized.

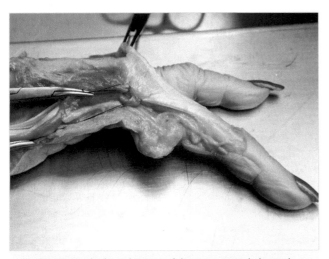

Fig. 35.15 On the lateral aspect of the metacarpophalangeal joint, both the interosseous muscle and the lumbrical (*black sutures*) contribute to the formation of the lateral band.

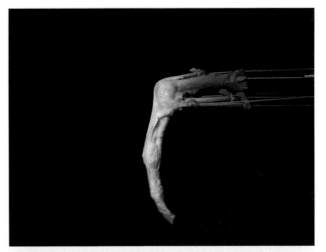

Fig. 35.16 Traction on the intrinsic tendons. The intrinsic tendons are volar to the center of rotation of the metacarpophalangeal joints and, by virtue of their insertion and formation of the lateral bands, are dorsal to the axis of rotation of the proximal interphalangeal joint. Traction on these tendons produces metacarpophalangeal flexion and interphalangeal extension.

the extrinsic extensors and the volar plate[15] (▶Fig. 35.8 and ▶Fig. 35.14). The sagittal bands centralize the EDC tendons, limit their excursion, and prevent extensor tendon bowstringing.[4,5,15] Short articular fibers loosely tether the extensor hood to the dorsal capsule and the base of the proximal phalanx.

The extrinsic extensor tendons extend the metacarpophalangeal joint indirectly by tensioning the sagittal bands. A small percentage of patients may also have a direct bony attachment of the deep fibers of the extensor tendon to the capsule and base of the proximal phalanx. Distal to the metacarpophalangeal joint, the extrinsic extensor tendon trifurcates into a central slip and two lateral bands.[4] The intrinsic tendons, including the lumbricals and interossei, run laterally to the metacarpophalangeal joint and contribute to the lateral bands (▶Fig. 35.15). The intrinsic tendons are volar to the center of rotation of the metacarpophalangeal

joints and act as flexors of this joint (▶Fig. 35.16). A percentage of each dorsal interossei tendon runs between the metacarpophalangeal joint capsule and sagittal bands. This portion of the dorsal interosseous tendon inserts on the abductor or adductor tubercle on the base of the proximal phalanx.[5]

35.1.6 Flexor Tendons and Pulleys

The metacarpophalangeal joint corresponds to the most proximal aspect of flexor tendon zone II of the five zones proposed by Verdan for classification of flexor tendon lacerations.[14] The A1 pulley overlies the metacarpophalangeal joint volarly and arises from the volar plate (▶Fig. 35.7, ▶Fig. 35.8 and

▶Fig. 35.9). It also receives fibers from the accessory collateral ligament.[4] The flexor tendon sheath and A1 pulley are lined with a parietal synovial membrane.[5] A digital bursa separates the parietal synovium on the flexor tendon sheath from the visceral synovium on the flexor tendons within the sheath. In the small finger, the digital bursa is continuous with the ulnar bursa of the palm. Within the flexor tendon sheath at the A1 pulley, the flexor digitorum superficialis lies volar to the flexor digitorum profundus. At this level, the flexor digitorum superficialis begins to flatten and bifurcate. More distally, it rotates laterally and dorsally around the flexor digitorum profundus.

35.2 Neurovascular Anatomy

One volar articular nerve and two dorsal articular nerves innervate the metacarpophalangeal joint.[16] The volar articular nerve is a deep branch of the ulnar nerve. It innervates the palmar and lateral capsule, metacarpal head, flexor tendon sheath, and collateral ligaments. The dorsal articular nerves are branches of the dorsal common digital nerve. They innervate the dorsal capsule, sagittal bands, and dorsal metacarpal head. Nerve density is greater volarly and follows the vascular distribution of the metacarpophalangeal joint.

The metacarpophalangeal joints have a rich blood supply (▶Fig. 35.17) from two anastomotic vascular circles located (1) proximally at the metacarpal neck near the capsular insertion and (2) distally at the base of the proximal phalanx.[17] Four arteries contribute to the anastomotic circles: (1) the palmar metacarpal artery that arises from the deep palmar arch, (2) the proximal lateral dorsal articular branches that arise from the radial artery or deep palmar arch, (3) the common palmar digital artery that arises from the superficial palmar arch, and (4) the proper palmar digital arteries.[17] Both anastomotic vascular circles supply the volar plate, collateral ligaments, and dorsal capsule. Both anastomotic vascular circles supply the volar plate, collateral ligaments, and dorsal capsule.

35.3 Thumb Metacarpophalangeal Joint Surface Anatomy

35.3.1 Osteology

The metacarpophalangeal joint is composed of the metacarpal head and the base of the proximal phalanx. The metacarpal head of the thumb is less convex and spheroid than the fingers and is more expanded volarly. Its articular surface extends volarly as the palmar–lateral articular processes to articulate with the sesamoids. Its radial condyle is larger in the sagittal plane than its ulnar condyle, allowing increasing pronation in conjunction with increasing flexion of the metacarpophalangeal joint.[2] The base of the proximal phalanx of the thumb is shorter, thicker, and wider than those of the fingers.[5] Its articular surface is oval, shallow, and flat. The metacarpophalangeal joint of the thumb is more concentric than the metacarpophalangeal joint of the fingers and is nearly equally stable throughout its arc of flexion and extension.

The metacarpal head has dorsal lateral tubercles for the attachment of the collateral ligaments.[5] It also has a palmar

intercondylar depression for the passage of the flexor pollicis longus. The base of the proximal phalanx has steep dorsal and palmar ridges for the attachment of the metacarpophalangeal joint capsule and a dorsal crest of the insertion of the extensor pollicis brevis. The palmar ridge extends laterally to form tubercles for the attachment of the collateral ligaments. In addition, there is a palmar depression located centrally for the passage of the flexor pollicis longus.

The metacarpophalangeal joint is an ellipsoid joint that allows biaxial motions, including flexion, extension, abduction, adduction, and rotation.[5] As the metacarpal head and base of the proximal phalanx are flat, the metacarpophalangeal joint of the thumb allows much less abduction, adduction, and rotation than the metacarpophalangeal joint of the fingers. Therefore, it primarily functions as a ginglymus (hinge) joint with a primary arc of flexion and extension.

35.3.2 Capsule and Collateral Ligaments

The capsule surrounds the metacarpophalangeal joint, attaching to the base of the proximal phalanx and the metacarpal neck. The metacarpophalangeal joint of the thumb (▶Fig. 35.18) is supported on all sides: (1) dorsally by the extensor hood, (2) volarly by the volar plate and sesamoids, and (3) laterally by the collateral ligaments, sagittal bands, thenar aponeurosis, and adductor aponeurosis.[2] The thenar aponeurosis and adductor aponeurosis blend with the extensor hood dorsally and the volar plate and sesamoids volarly (▶Fig. 35.19).

The collateral ligaments arise from the dorsal lateral tubercles of the metacarpal head and insert on the lateral tubercles on the base of the proximal phalanx.[5] The center of the origin and insertion of the ulnar and radial collateral ligaments have been precisely defined for reconstructive purposes. The center of the origin of the ulnar collateral ligament is 7 mm from the articular surface, 3 mm from the dorsal border, and 8 mm from the volar border of the metacarpal head.[18] The center of insertion of the ulnar collateral ligament is 3 mm from the articular surface, 3 mm from the volar border, and 8 mm from the dorsal border of the base of the proximal phalanx.[18] The center of the origin of the radial collateral ligament is 1 to 2 mm dorsal to the central axis of the lateral condyle of the metacarpal head.[19] The center of insertion of the radial collateral ligament is 3 to 5 mm from the articular surface and is on the palmar half of the lateral tubercle of the base of the proximal phalanx.[19] The accessory collateral ligaments run from the dorsal lateral head of the metacarpal to the lateral edge of the volar plate. The collateral ligaments stabilize the metacarpophalangeal joint against radial and ulnar deviation as well as against dorsal and ulnar translation. The thenar and adductor aponeurosis add to the dynamic stability of the metacarpophalangeal joint.

35.3.3 Volar Plate and Sesamoids

The volar plate of the thumb metacarpophalangeal joint is trapezoidal; the ulnar aspect of the volar plate is longer and thicker than the radial aspect of the volar plate. Unlike the metacarpophalangeal joints of the fingers, the metacarpophalangeal joint of the thumb has well-defined check ligaments. Similar to the

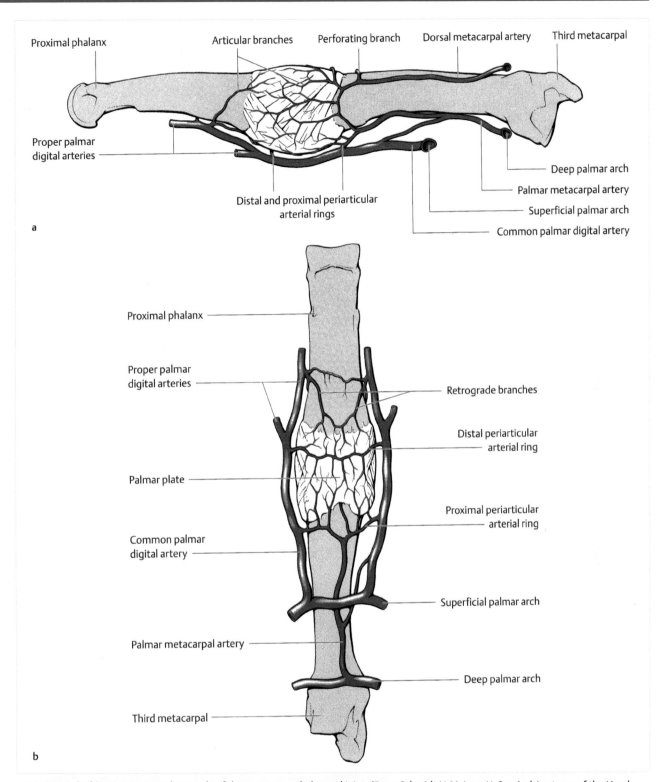

Fig. 35.17 (**a, b**) Extensive vascular supply of the metacarpophalangeal joint. (From Schmidt H-M, Lanz U. Surgical Anatomy of the Hand. Stuttgart, Germany: Thieme; 2004.)

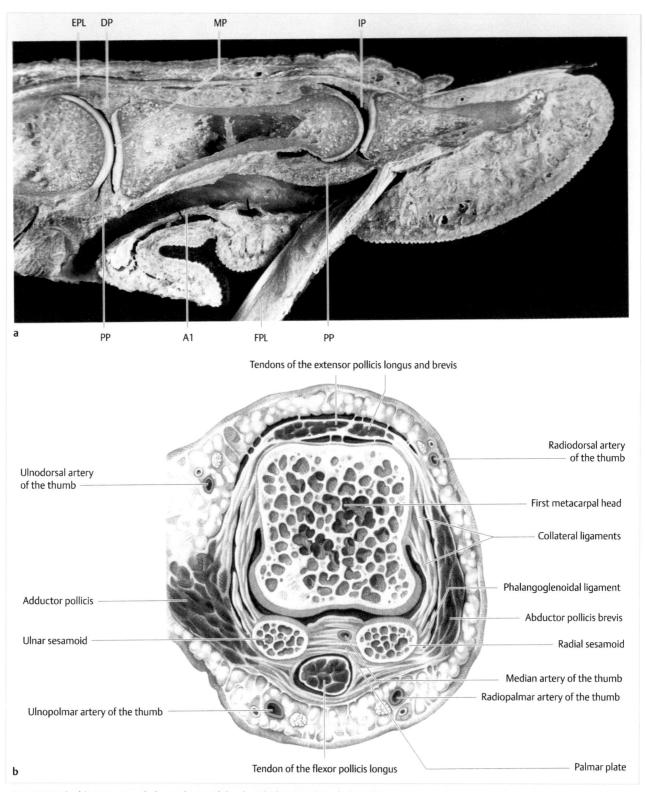

Fig. 35.18 (a, b) Metacarpophalangeal joint of the thumb showing the relation of the structures. (From Schmidt H-M, Lanz U. Surgical Anatomy of the Hand. Stuttgart, Germany: Thieme; 2004.)

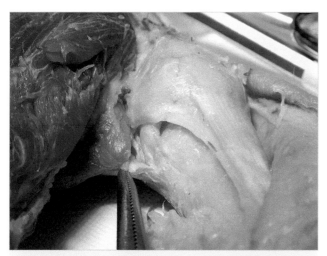

Fig. 35.19 Ulnar view of the metacarpophalangeal joint of the thumb. The adductor aponeurosis (within the forceps) blends with the extensor hood dorsally and the volar plate and sesamoids volarly. The strong ulnar collateral ligament can be seen running deep to the aponeurosis.

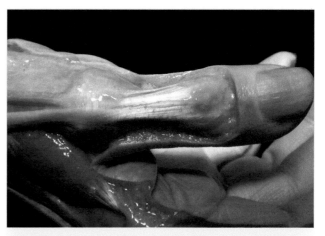

Fig. 35.20 Dorsal view of the thumb with the extensor hood of the metacarpophalangeal joint seen on the left. The extensor hood comprises the extrinsic extensor tendons and the sagittal bands and has contributions from the abductor pollicis brevis, flexor pollicis brevis, and adductor pollicis.

volar plate, the ulnar check ligament is longer and stronger than the radial check ligament.[1]

Two sesamoid bones are embedded in the volar plate. The radial sesamoid is larger and is an insertion site for the abductor pollicis brevis and the flexor pollicis brevis. The ulnar sesamoid serves as an insertion site for the adductor pollicis. Due to their sesamoid attachments, the abductor pollicis brevis, flexor pollicis brevis, and adductor pollicis provide additional volar support to the metacarpophalangeal joint.

35.3.4 Extensor Apparatus

The metacarpophalangeal joint of the thumb is located within Verdan's extensor tendon zone III. In zone III, the extensor apparatus is a tendinous hood composed of the extrinsic extensor tendons and the sagittal bands as well as contributions from the abductor pollicis brevis, flexor pollicis brevis, and adductor pollicis (▶ Fig. 35.20). The extensor pollicis longus tendon lies centrally over the dorsal aspect of the metacarpophalangeal joint of the thumb. The extensor pollicis brevis is located radial to the extensor pollicis longus tendon and contributes to the extensor hood. In addition, the extensor pollicis brevis attaches directly to the dorsal ridge at the base of the proximal phalanx. The sagittal bands originate on both sides of the metacarpophalangeal joint and attach to the extensor pollicis longus dorsally and to the volar plate and sesamoids volarly.[20] The sagittal bands stabilize the centralized extensor tendons, limit their excursion, and prevent extensor tendon bowstringing.[4,5] The broad thenar aponeurosis reinforces the sagittal band radially, and the narrow adductor aponeurosis reinforces the sagittal band ulnarly.[20]

Tension on the extensor pollicis longus indirectly extends the metacarpophalangeal joint by pulling on the sagittal bands. In addition, the extensor pollicis brevis extends the metacarpophalangeal joint through a direct insertion on the base of the proximal phalanx. The extensor pollicis longus, thenar aponeurosis, and adductor aponeurosis continue distally and contribute to interphalangeal joint extension.[5]

35.3.5 Flexor Tendons and Pulleys

The metacarpophalangeal joint is located in the proximal aspect of Verdan's flexor tendon zone II. The A1 pulley overlies the metacarpophalangeal joint volarly and arises from the volar plate. It also receives fibers from the accessory collateral ligament.[4] The flexor tendon sheath and A1 pulley are lined with a parietal synovial membrane.[5] A digital bursa separates the parietal synovium on the flexor tendon sheath from the visceral synovium on the flexor pollicis longus within the sheath. In the thumb, the digital bursa is continuous with the radial bursa of the palm. The flexor pollicis longus passes through a groove between the two sesamoids and also through the interval between the abductor pollicis brevis and flexor pollicis brevis radially and the adductor pollicis ulnarly.

35.4 Neurovascular Anatomy

Innervation of the metacarpophalangeal joint of the thumb is similar to the innervation of the metacarpophalangeal joints of the fingers. One volar articular nerve and two dorsal articular nerves innervate the metacarpophalangeal joint of the thumb.[16] The volar articular nerve is a deep branch of the ulnar nerve. It innervates the palmar and lateral capsule, metacarpal head, flexor tendon sheath, and collateral ligaments. The dorsal articular nerves are branches of the dorsal common digital nerve. They innervate the dorsal capsule, sagittal bands, and dorsal metacarpal head. Nerve density is greater volarly and follows the vascular distribution of the metacarpophalangeal joint.

The metacarpophalangeal joint of the thumb has a rich blood supply from vascular anastomoses located (1) volarly at the metacarpophalangeal joint and (2) dorsally and volarly just distal to the metacarpophalangeal joint. The three arteries that contribute to the blood supply of the thumb are (1) the princeps pollicis artery, (2) the radial artery, and (3) the first palmar metacarpal artery (also called the first commissural artery or the first intermetacarpal artery).[21] These three vessels form the radial digital artery, the ulnar digital artery, the dorsal radial artery, and the dorsal ulnar artery of the thumb. The princeps pollicis artery is the dominant artery to the thumb and most commonly forms the radial digital artery, the ulnar digital artery, and the dorsal ulnar artery. Anastomoses exist between the radial and ulnar arteries and the dorsal and palmar vascular systems.

References

1. Hunt TR, Wiesel SW. Operative Techniques in Hand, Wrist, and Forearm Surgery. Philadelphia, PA: Lippincott Williams & Wilkins; 2011

2. Wolfe S, Pederson W, Kozin SH. Green's Operative Hand Surgery. 6th ed. Churchill Livingstone; 2010

3. Bilderback KK, Rayan GM. The septa of Legueu and Juvara: an anatomic study. J Hand Surg Am 2004;29(3):494–499

4. Leversedge FJ, Goldfarb CA, Boyer MI. A Pocketbook Manual of Hand and Upper Extremity Anatomy Primus Manus. Philadelphia, PA: Lippincott Williams & Wilkins; 2010

5. Yu H, Chase RA, Strauch B. Atlas of Hand Anatomy and Clinical Implications. St. Louis, Mosby; 2004

6. Figus A, Britto JA, Ragoowansi RH, Elliot D. A clinical analysis of Dupuytren's disease of the thumb. J Hand Surg Eur Vol 2008;33(3):272–279

7. Dumont C, Ziehn C, Kubein-Meesenburg D, Fanghänel J, Stürmer KM, Nägerl H. Quantified contours of curvature in female index, middle, ring, and small metacarpophalangeal joints. J Hand Surg Am 2009;34(2):317–325

8. Smith RJ, Kaplan EB. Rheumatoid deformities at the metacarpophalangeal joints of the fingers: a correlative study of anatomy and pathology. J Bone and Joint Surg 1967;49A:31–37

9. Kataoka T, Moritomo H, Miyake J, Murase T, Yoshikawa H, Sugamoto K. Changes in shape and length of the collateral and accessory collateral ligaments of the metacarpophalangeal joint during flexion. J Bone Joint Surg Am 2011;93(14):1318–1325

10. Linscheid RL. Historical perspective of finger joint motion: the hand-me-downs of our predecessors. The Richard J. Smith Memorial Lecture. J Hand Surg Am 2002;27(1):1–25

11. al-Qattan MM, Robertson GA. An anatomical study of the deep transverse metacarpal ligament. J Anat 1993;182(Pt 3):443–446

12. Zancolli E. Pathomechanics and correction of the arthritic ulnar drift before and after cartilage destruction. In: Structural and Dynamic Bases of Hand Surgery. 2nd ed. Philadelphia, PA: J.B. Lippincott Company; 1979

13. Palande DD. Correction of intrinsic-minus hands associated with reversal of the transverse metacarpal arch. J Bone Joint Surg Am 1983;65(4):514–521

14. Verdan CE. Primary and secondary repair of flexor and extensor tendon injuries. In: Hand Surgery. Baltimore, MD: Williams & Wilkins; 1975

15. Young CM, Rayan GM. The sagittal band: anatomic and biomechanical study. J Hand Surg Am 2000;25(6):1107–1113

16. Chen YG, McClinton MA, DaSilva MF, Shaw Wilgis EF. Innervation of the metacarpophalangeal and interphalangeal joints: a microanatomic and histologic study of the nerve endings. J Hand Surg Am 2000;25(1):128–133

17. Bonnel F, Teissier J, Allieu Y, Rabischong P, Mansat M. Arterial supply of ligaments of the metacarpophalangeal joints. J Hand Surg Am 1982;7(5):445–449

18. Bean CHG, Tencer AF, Trumble TE. The effect of thumb metacarpophalangeal ulnar collateral ligament attachment site on joint range of motion: an in vitro study. J Hand Surg Am 1999;24(2):283–287

19. Edelstein DM, Kardashian G, Lee SK. Radial collateral ligament injuries of the thumb. J Hand Surg Am 2008;33(5):760–770

20. Jaibaji M, Rayan GM, Chung KW. Functional anatomy of the thumb sagittal band. J Hand Surg Am 2008;33(6):879–884

21. Ramírez AR, Gonzalez SM. Arteries of the thumb: description of anatomical variations and review of the literature. Plast Reconstr Surg 2012;129(3):468e–476e

36 The Interphalangeal Joint

Hilton P. Gottschalk and Randy S. Bindra

36.1 Introduction

The proximal interphalangeal (PIP) and distal interphalangeal (DIP) joints are critical hinges that lend dexterity to the fingers to perform fine manipulative tasks while affording stability to the hand to allow a powerful grip. While the bony anatomy of the joint is the major determinant of the joint stability and mobility, all structures enveloping the bony scaffold, including joint capsule, ligaments, surrounding tendons, and skin, also contribute to joint integrity and function.

36.2 Proximal Interphalangeal Joint

Of the interphalangeal joints, the PIP joint is most critical to function due to its large arc of motion and its long lever arm. Like elsewhere in the hand, form and function are closely related.[1] Although it has been described as a simple hinge joint,[2,3] the PIP joint is considerably more complex.[1] The PIP joint is responsible for 85% of total encompassment as we grasp an object, which allows us to adapt to surface irregularities. This adaptability allows us to perform an amazing array of functions.

36.2.1 Bony Anatomy

The PIP joint is located midway between the metacarpophalangeal (MCP) joint and the tip of the finger, forming the anatomical and functional center of the digit.[1,4] The central location is not a coincidence but rather is designed to allow congruous finger movement. Like many things in nature, the relative lengths of the phalanges and metacarpals in the hand follow the Fibonacci series (▶Fig. 36.1). This is a mathematical series in which each number is the sum of the previous two numbers and was first described by Fibonacci.[1,4] Thus, the length of the proximal phalanx equals the sum of the lengths of the middle and distal phalanges. Similarly, the length of the metacarpal is equal to the sum of the lengths of the middle and proximal phalanges (See also Chapter 2).

The PIP joint can be best described as a "sloppy hinge" that allows motion in three dimensions. The sagittal plane motion (flexion/extension) is the main movement.[1,2] Not only do the fingers have to flex into the palm, but they also have to stay closely approximated despite their individual lengths.

Proximal Phalangeal Head

The proximal phalangeal head is bicondylar, separated by an intercondylar notch that articulates with a projection, or trochlea, from the middle phalanx (▶Fig. 36.2a, b). This articulation provides some inherent stability in medial, lateral, and rotational directions when the joint is flexed or extended.[3,5,6] The three-dimensional shape of the proximal phalangeal head/neck allows for a rotational component to motion at the PIP joint such that the tips of the fingers converge toward each other with flexion of the joint. Following three components contribute to this phenomenon:

1. The proximal phalangeal heads are roughly trapezoidal in shape, with the volar margin being greater than the dorsal margin (▶Fig. 36.3). In addition, the dorsal and volar margins are tilted such that the index, middle, and small fingers tilt slightly toward the ring finger.[1,2,7]
2. The radius of curvature of each condyle is slightly different.
3. In the coronal plane, the distal margin of the head of the proximal phalanx tilts away from the second web space.[1]

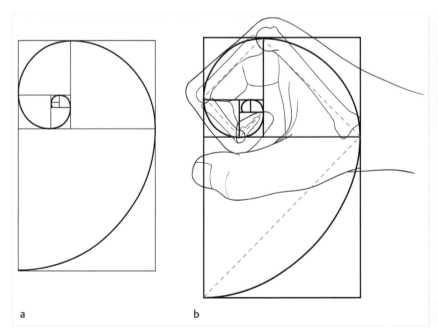

a   b

Fig. 36.1 (a) Line drawing of a Fibonacci spiral approximating a golden spiral. Square sizes are 1,1,2,3,5,8,13,21, and 34. (b) The Fibonacci spiral and tiles are superimposed on a clenched fist. Illustrating the length of proximal phalanx is the sum of the lengths of the middle and distal phalanges.

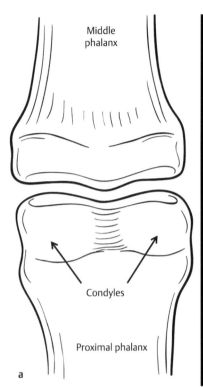

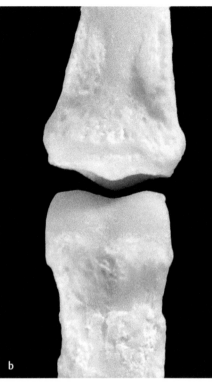

Fig. 36.2 (a, b) Volar view of the proximal phalangeal joint.

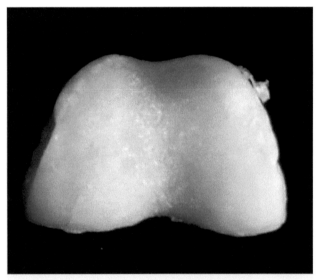

Fig. 36.3 End–on view of the head of the proximal phalanx showing the wider volar portion and the narrower dorsal part.

Essentially, the index finger supinates at the PIP joint in flexion while the ring and small fingers slightly pronate.

Additional features of the proximal phalangeal head include (▶ Fig. 36.4a, b, and c):

1. A dorsally placed pit on the lateral side where the "proper" collateral ligament originates.
2. A flattened area just volar to the pit which serves as an extension of the attachment site for the proper collateral ligament and allows for the ligament complex to glide during flexion and extension.
3. Extension of the intercondylar groove to the volar aspect of the phalanx to accommodate the volar lip of the middle phalanx and allow a 110° arc of motion.

Base of Middle Phalanx

The base of the middle phalanx has two concavities separated by an intercondylar ridge (▶ Fig. 36.5). The fit is not perfectly congruous to the head of the proximal phalanx, to allow for a small amount of rotation. Additional features of the base of the middle phalanx include the following (▶ Fig. 36.6):

1. A base wider than the dorsal margin, with a lateral tubercle on each side where portions of the collateral ligament attach.[1,2]
2. An additional thickening in the dorsal lip for insertion of the central slip of the extensor tendon.
3. The palmar aspect of the middle phalanx contains a roughened area close to the joint surface for attachment of the palmar plate, as well as two small tubercles for capsular attachment.

36.2.2 Stabilizing Restraints

There are three main restraints to the PIP joint: the proper collateral ligament, accessory collateral ligament, and the volar plate. Interestingly, the dorsal aspect of the joint is devoid of major stabilizing structures and only has a thin-walled capsule that allows for some "give" in finger extension with a synovial pouch lying deep to the extensor mechanism.

Proper Collateral Ligament

The proper collateral ligament is the major restraint to varus and valgus angulation of the PIP joint.[6] The proper collateral ligament (PCL) possesses the following properties:

1. It originates from the pit of the proximal phalangeal head and fans out to attach to the thickened lateral margin of the middle phalanx (▶ Fig. 36.7).

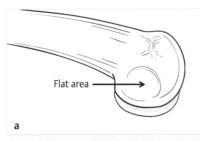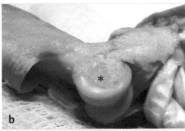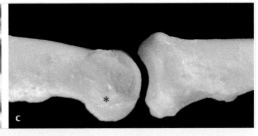

Fig. 36.4 **(a)** The lateral aspect of the proximal phalanx **(b).** Cadaver specimen **(c)** Dried bone specimen with (*) marking flat area.

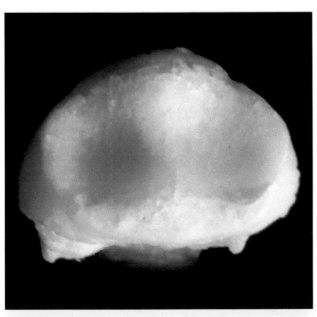

Fig. 36.5 End on view of the base of the middle phalanx showing the bicondylar shape, the volar intercondylar ridge, and the insertion area of the central slip dorsally.

2. It is thicker than the accessory collateral ligament and can cover up to one-third of the lateral width of the PIP joint.
3. At its insertion onto the lateral tubercle of the middle phalanx, the fibers blend with the periosteum into a portion of the metaphysis (▶ Fig. 36.8).
4. The PCL is tight in flexion secondary to the trapezoid cross-sectional shape of the proximal phalanx. The PCL stretches across the condyles and is the major lateral stabilizer at 60° flexion.[1,6]
5. The volar edge blends with the thinner accessory collateral ligament.

Accessory Collateral Ligament

The accessory collateral ligament (ACL) takes origin form the same area as the PCL but fans out in a more volar direction (▶ Fig. 36.9). It has a different structure and design from those of the PCL:
1. The ACL is thinner than the PCL.
2. It has a substantially broader insertion into the tubercles at the base of the middle phalanx, the lateral margins

of the volar plate, and the dorsal fibers of the flexor sheath.[1]
3. The ACL is tight in extension as it rides over the condyles of the proximal phalanx.
4. As it attaches to the sides of the volar plate, it acts as a sling to suspend the volar plate.

Volar Plate

The volar plate is a thick fibrocartilaginous structure covering the volar portion of the PIP joint and is the prime stabilizer on the volar aspect essential for preventing hyperextension. On its palmar aspect, it forms the floor of the flexor tendon sheath, while its dorsal surface lies intra-articular and is lined with synovium.[1,5]

Key anatomic details have been described by Gad[8] and others[1,9] and include the following:
1. It originates deep to the A2 pulley, and its proximal attachments resemble a "swallow's tail," as the lateral attachments extend onto the proximal phalanx beyond the volar lip (▶ Fig. 36.10). The proximal origin of the first cruciate (C1) pulley is confluent with the proximal aspect of the volar plate.[1]
2. The "check" ligaments are the reflected fibers of the flexor sheath/lateral margin and are formed by the confluence of three fascial structures: reflected fibers from dorsal portion of flexor sheath, reflection of the accessory collateral ligament, and lateral margin of the volar plate. The term *checkrein* when used of ligaments describes pathologic thickening of the check ligaments that restrict full extension of the PIP joint.[9]
3. The proximal portion of the volar plate is thin, and there is a space between the condyles and the volar plate to allow passage of transverse arterial feeders from the digital arteries.
4. The volar plate is thickest distally and inserts into the rough area at the base of the middle phalanx. Its fibers do not insert into the volar tubercle of the median ridge, because this is covered with articular cartilage and lies within the PIP joint (▶ Fig. 36.11). It has thin fibers centrally that blend with the volar periosteum of the middle phalanx. This unique feature allows the volar plate to fall away from the joint in flexion.[1]
5. At the lateral margins, the volar plate becomes thicker and confluent with the accessory collateral ligament insertion into the palmar tubercles. This point of attachment has been termed the "critical corner."[1,5]

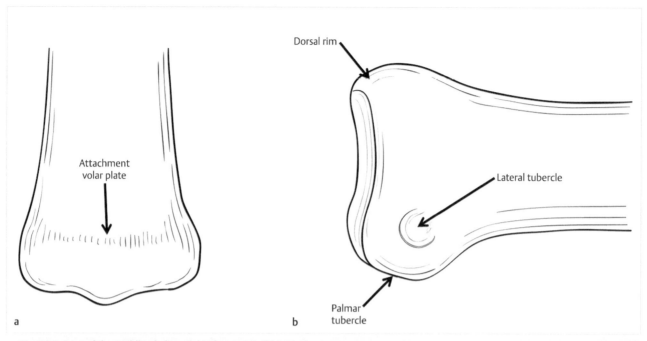

Fig. 36.6 Base of the middle phalanx. (**a**) Volar aspect. (**b**) Lateral aspect.

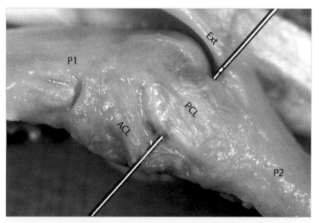

Fig. 36.7 Lateral view of the proximal interphalangeal (PIP) joint. Central slip of extensor tendon (Ext) inserts onto the dorsal rim of the middle phalanx base. The proper collateral ligament (PCL) originates from proximal phalangeal (P1) head and attaches to thickened lateral margin of middle phalanx (P2). A needle is placed at the volar edge of the proper collateral ligament as it blends with the thinner accessory collateral ligament (ACL).

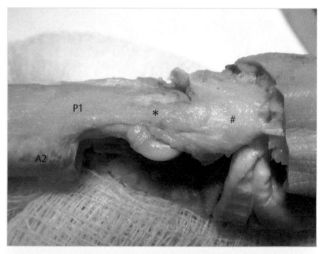

Fig. 36.8 Lateral view of the proximal interphalangeal (PIP) joint with accessory collateral ligament and volar plate removed. Notice the origin of the proper collateral ligament (*) and its attachment (#) as it blends with the periosteum into the meta-physeal portion of the middle phalanx. P1, proximal phalanx; A2, A2 pulley.

The PIP joint has secondary stabilizing structures that consist of the flexor tendons, extensor tendon, lateral bands, neurovascular structures, bony anatomy, and skin. When the joint is axially loaded through tension by the long flexor and extensor tendons, the relatively congruent articulating surfaces come into contact and provide lateral stability.[1] Although the latter do not contribute to digital stability in the normal hand, they can cause considerable compromise to the range of motion when pathologic.

36.2.3 Vascular and Neurologic Structures

The two proper digital arteries give rise to transverse digital arteries that run beneath the check ligaments. The two transverse digital arteries merge in the midline, sending arterial branches to the vinculae, synovium, and joint capsule. The vincular vessel passes through the floor of the flexor sheath

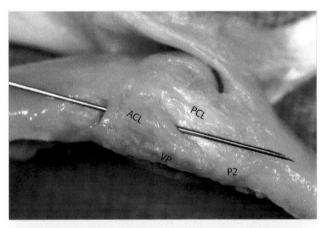

Fig. 36.9 Lateral view of the proximal interphalangeal (PIP) joint. A needle is placed under the accessory collateral ligament (ACL). The accessory collateral ligament is thinner than the proper collateral ligament (PCL) and fans out in a more volar direction and has attachments to the volar plate (VP) and base of the middle phalanx (P2).

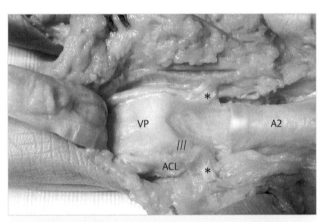

Fig. 36.10 Volar view of the proximal interphalangeal joint. The volar plate (VP) originates deep to the A2 pulley (A2) with proximal attachments resembling a "swallow's tail." Fibers of the cruciate pulley have been split (*). The checkrein ligament (///) comprises the reflected fibers of the flexor sheath, reflection of the accessory collateral ligament (ACL), and lateral margin of the volar plate.

(▶ Fig. 36.12) to provide the major vascular supply to the tendon vincular system.[1,5,9]

The PIP joint is innervated by a constant articular branch arising from the palmar digital nerve at the level of the mid-proximal phalanx.[10,11] The nerve bifurcates near the capsule and enters the joint in the midlateral plane at the junction of the volar plate and lateral capsule. The dorsal sensory nerves do not contribute to articular innervation.[10] A recent study looking at mechanoreceptors in the human finger found that type I nerve endings (Ruffini endings) were distributed more densely in the volar plate at the proximal region of the PIP joint.[12] These nerve endings are stretch receptors and sense the tension in the collagen fibrils, especially those of the volar plate. Type II mechanoreceptors (Pacinian endings respond to pressure and vibratory stimuli) were distributed densely in

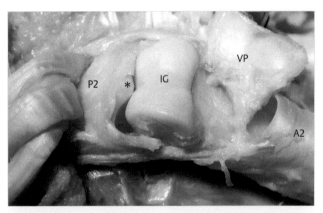

Fig. 36.11 Volar view of the proximal interphalangeal joint with the volar plate (VP) transected, demonstrating increased thickness distally as it inserts at the base of the middle phalanx (P2). Note that the median ridge (*) is devoid of attachment and is covered with cartilage. Also, note the extension of the intercondylar groove (IG) to the volar aspect of the proximal phalanx.

the proximal regions on both the radial and ulnar sides of the volar plate. These regions where the C1 pulley and radial and ulnar accessory collateral ligaments coalesce have been termed the radial assemblage nucleus and ulnar assemblage nucleus, respectively.[12]

36.2.4 Surface Anatomy

The skin creases on the palmar aspect are consistently proximal to their associated PIP joint, ranging from 1.6 to 2.6 mm.[13]

36.3 The Distal Interphalangeal Joint

The DIP joint does not seem to get as much press as its neighbor the PIP joint. Part of the reason is that it is responsible for only 15% of total motion arc as we grasp an object. Illustrating this fact, fusion of the DIP joint is better tolerated than fusion of the PIP joint.[1] However, the importance of the DIP joint lies in its ability to place the terminal pulp of the finger in an optimal position for tactile sensation and precision movements.[14]

There are many similarities between the DIP joint and the PIP joint, as well as some unique features, as discussed hereafter.

36.3.1 Bony Anatomy

1. The bony anatomy includes two condyles separated by an intercondylar groove on the middle phalanx head. The lateral aspects of the condyles provide attachments for the proper and accessory collateral ligaments. The condyles themselves are asymmetric, which allows for deviation of the distal phalanx toward the middle digit.
2. The shape of the middle phalanx head allows for passive hyperextension but limits the range of flexion of the DIP joint.

3. The base of the distal phalanx has a prominent dorsal lip for attachment of the terminal portion of the extensor tendon (▶Fig. 36.13). In skeletally immature patients, the extensor tendon inserts onto the epiphysis, whereas the flexor digitorum profundus (FDP) inserts on the shaft distal to the epiphysis.[14]

4. The distal phalanx has prominent lateral tubercles for attachment of the collateral ligaments.

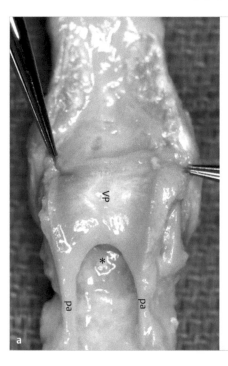
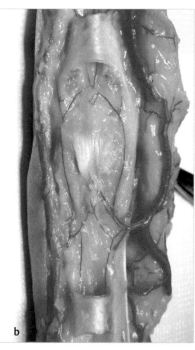

Fig. 36.12 (a, b) Volar view of the volar plate (VP) demonstrating the proximal attachments (pa) resembling a "swallow's tail." There is a space (*) between the condyles and the vol-ar plate to allow passage of arterial feeders that contribute to the vincular system. There are contributions from both digital arteries. This transverse digital artery runs deep to the check rein ligament of the volar plate, connecting one digital artery to the other and is called Edward's arcade. The interconnections are present at the MP joint, PIP joint and DIP joint level.

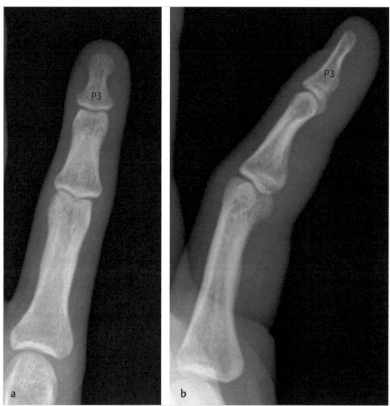

Fig. 36.13 (a) Posteroanterior and (b) lateral radiographs showing the proximal interphalangeal and distal interphalangeal joints. The base of the distal phalanx (P3) has a dorsal rim (*) for attachment of the terminal portion of the extensor tendon.

36.3.2 Synovial Membrane

Two pouches exist (one dorsal and one palmar) lined with synovium. These are potential spaces that contain synovial fluid. During full flexion, the fluid is transferred from the dorsal pouch to the palmar pouch as the triangular ligament forces the fluid palmarly.[14]

36.3.3 Stabilizing Restraints

Similar to the PIP joint, the capsule is thin and flexible dorsally and palmarly but becomes thicker on the lateral aspects as it incorporates with the volar plate. The proper collateral ligaments are cord like structures running from the sides of the head of the middle phalanx to the lateral tubercles of the distal phalanx. The accessory collateral ligaments are fan like and extend to the volar plate.

The DIP joint has a volar plate with a thickened proximal portion attached to the neck of the middle phalanx. There are no well-developed check ligaments on the sides of the volar plate such as are seen in the PIP joint, allowing for hyperextension of the joint.

36.3.4 Vascular and Neurologic Structures

The short vinculum belonging to the FDP tendon splits the volar plate and receives its arterial supply from the distal arterial arch, linking the two palmar digital arteries. Some direct branches from the digital arteries have been documented entering other aspects of the joint.[14]

The DIP joint receives innervation from small articular branches. Chikenji et al[15] examined the distribution of nerve endings in the human DIP joint. In 12 cadavers, they reported a higher density of type II mechanoreceptors (Pacinian-like endings) in the proximal region of the radial and ulnar assemblage nuclei. This correlated to the area of the C3 pulley and accessory ligaments. This suggests that these structures may act as a sensory generator transmitting traction forces through the finger pulley system.[15]

36.3.5 Surface Anatomy

The level of the DIP joint is approximately 3 mm distal to the knuckle on the dorsal surface. When the finger is straightened, the joint interval lies distal to the volar, main flexion crease.[14]

36.4 Biomechanics of Digital Motion

The finger is a chain of joints bridged by long tendons.[16] The chain can flex to wrap around an object or become taut at any angle so as to apply force through the tip. While basic stability of the joints is imparted by the collateral ligaments and the volar plate, dynamic stabilization is a more complex process. Flexion and extension of the interphalangeal joints are not simply the outcome of exclusive actions of the flexors and extensors, respectively, as this would not explain the ability to maintain the finger stability in between full flexion and extension. There is an intricate balancing act between the forces of the extensor mechanism through the long extensor and the intrinsics and the two flexor tendons. The complex interplay between these forces has been demonstrated by electromyography studies.[17,18] The following actions occur during finger flexion:

1. The FDP tendon is active during flexion of the DIP joint.
2. The FDS tendon is active when the wrist is flexed and during firm grasp.
3. The extensor digitorum communis is active during the entire range of finger flexion.
4. The intrinsics are active during simultaneous MCP flexion and PIP extension.[17]

In addition, there is coupling of the DIP and PIP joints by two systems: (1) the spiral oblique ligament and (2) the extensor mechanism.[3] The spiral oblique retinacular ligament (SORL) is a small fibrous band that arises from the flexor sheath proximal to the PIP joint and attaches to the terminal tendon (▶Fig. 36.14).[3,14] The SORL is tensioned by DIP flexion and PIP extension. To offset the tension caused by the FDP tendon (which flexes the DIP joint), the FDS tendon fires to flex the PIP joint.

The extensor mechanism is the second system that couples DIP and PIP flexion through the interplay between the lateral bands and the central slip. As the DIP joint flexes, this creates increased tension in the lateral bands while instantaneously causing a relative laxity of the central slip. The lateral bands resist further DIP joint flexion, while the lax central slips allow PIP flexion. But as the PIP flexes, tension is restored in the central slip, which unloads the lateral bands and permits further DIP joint flexion. Further PIP flexion will allow the lateral bands to slip volarward, which further decreases the extensor moment at the PIP joint. This couple coordinates flexion between the two joints.[3]

The extensor mechanism is powered by the digital extensors and the intrinsics. To create coordinated extension at the PIP and DIP joints, the extensor mechanism trifurcates into a central slip that powers the PIP joint and two lateral bands that bypass the PIP joint to extend the DIP joint. For the finger to achieve full

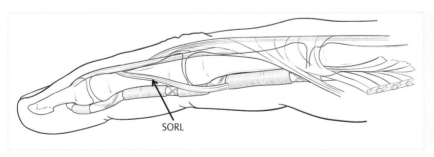

Fig. 36.14 The spiral oblique retinacular ligament is a small fibrous band that arises from the flexor sheath proximal to the proximal interphalangeal joint and attaches to the terminal tendon.

SORL

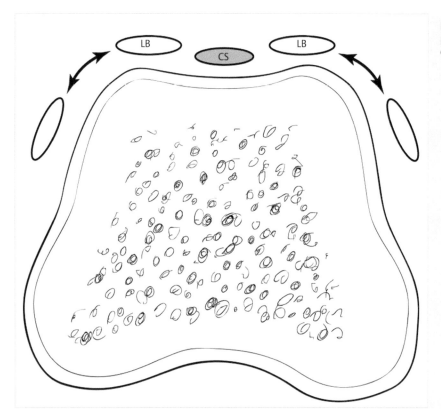

Fig. 36.15 Sloping cross-section of proximal phalangeal head allows dorsopalmar gliding of the lateral bands.

extension at both joints, the central slip and the lateral bands must have the same effective length to tighten simultaneously.[19] With finger flexion, however, the lateral bands would have to lengthen even further to allow flexion of both the PIP and DIP joints. This relative lengthening is achieved by dorsopalmar gliding of the lateral bands, facilitated by the smooth contour of the proximal phalanx condyles and the trapezoidal cross-section of the proximal phalanx head, which is wider on the palmar aspect (▶Fig. 36.15). Digital extension is initiated at the PIP joint with contraction of the central slip. Proximal shift of the extensor mechanism results in tightening of the lateral bands that shift dorsally as they slide onto the narrower dorsal portion of the proximal phalanx head. The two tight lateral bands pull the DIP joint into extension. Hyperextension at the joints is resisted by volar plates and the resting tone in the flexor tendons.

36.5 Summary

In the interphalangeal joints, form closely follows function. Bony geometry provides a scaffold stabilized by the collateral ligaments and volar plate. Movement is provided by a complex interaction between the flexor and extensor tendons. The large arc of motion of the PIP joint and the complex stabilizing structures can result in significant functional loss from small structural changes caused by trauma or pathology.

References

1. Leibovic SJ, Bowers WH. Anatomy of the proximal interphalangeal joint. Hand Clin 1994;10(2):169–178

2. Kuczynski K. The proximal interphalangeal joint. Anatomy and causes of stiffness in the fingers. J Bone Joint Surg Br 1968;50(3): 656–663

3. Gonzalez MH, Mohan V, ElHassan B, Amirouche F. Biomechanics of the digit. J Am Soc Surg Hand 2005;5:48–60

4. Littler JW, Thompson JS. Surgical and functional anatomy. In: Bowers WH. The Interphalangeal Joints. New York, NY: Churchill Livingstone; 1987

5. Leversedge FJ, Goldfarb CA, Boyer MI. A Pocketbook Manual of Hand and Upper Extremity Anatomy: Primus Manus. Philadelphia, PA: Lippincott Williams & Wilkins; 2010

6. Kiefhaber TR, Stern PJ, Grood ES. Lateral stability of the proximal interphalangeal joint. J Hand Surg Am 1986;11(5):661–669

7. Kuczynski K. Less-known aspects of the proximal interphalangeal joints of the human hand. Hand 1975;7(1):31–33

8. Gad P. The anatomy of the volar part of the capsules of the finger joints. J Bone Joint Surg Br 1967;49(2):362–367

9. Watson HK, Light TR, Johnson TR. Checkrein resection for flexion contracture of the middle joint. J Hand Surg Am 1979;4(1):67–71

10. Schultz RJ, Krishnamurthy S, Johnston AD. A gross anatomic and histologic study of the innervation of the proximal interphalangeal joint. J Hand Surg Am 1984;9(5):669–674

11. Chen YG, McClinton MA, DaSilva MF, Shaw Wilgis EF. Innervation of the metacarpophalangeal and interphalangeal joints: a microanatomic and histologic study of the nerve endings. J Hand Surg Am 2000;25(1):128–133

12. Chikenji T, Suzuki D, Fujimiya M, Moriya T, Tsubota S. Distribution of nerve endings in the human proximal interphalangeal joint and surrounding structures. J Hand Surg Am 2010;35(8):286–1293

13. Bugbee WD, Botte MJ. Surface anatomy of the hand. The relationships between palmar skin creases and osseous anatomy. Clin Orthop Relat Res 1993; (296):122–126

14. Gigis PI, Kuczynski K. The distal interphalangeal joints of human fingers. J Hand Surg Am 1982;7(2):176–182

15. Chikenji T, Berger RA, Fujimiya M, Suzuki D, Tsubota S, An KN. Distribution of nerve endings in human distal interphalangeal joint and surrounding structures. J Hand Surg Am 2011;36(3):406–412

16. Landsmeer JM. Functional morphology, functional mechanism, and biomechanics related to surgery of the hand. J Hand Surg Am 1989;14(2 Pt 2):347–348

17. Long C II, Conrad PW, Hall EA, Furler SL. Intrinsic-extrinsic muscle control of the hand in power grip and precision handling. An electromyographic study. J Bone Joint Surg Am 1970;52(5):853–867

18. Long C II. Intrinsic-extrinsic muscle control of the fingers. Electromyographic studies. J Bone Joint Surg Am 1968;50(5):973–984

19. Harris C Jr, Rutledge GL Jr. The functional anatomy of the extensor mechanism of the finger. J Bone Joint Surg Am 1972;54(4):713–726

37 The Nail and Finger Pulp

Nada N. Berry, Reuben A. Bueno, and Elvin Zook

37.1 Introduction

The nail with its perionychium is a unique structure found only on the dorsal distal fingertips of primates. Other animals have adapted these appendages to serve different purposes (claws and hooves). Its flat appearance serves to assist in sensory perception through counter-pressure and accurate manipulation of small objects. It protects the sensitive fingertip and aids in thermoregulation. Loss of a nail leads to aesthetic deformity as well as loss of function.

37.2 Embryology

The Wnt signaling pathway is responsible for regulating dorsal/palmar digital orientation. Specifically, inactivation of the dorsally located Wnt7a pathway leads to ventralization of the dorsal surface, producing digits without nails and finger pads on both sides. Correspondingly in the ventral surface of the limb, gene engrailed-1 (En-1) blocks the Wnt pathway resulting in normal development of pulp structures.[1]

At 10 weeks of gestation, thickened epidermis called sole plate starts to expand and burrow proximally over the underlying dermis, creating the nail grove and laying down the nail-producing matrix. Within the superficial matrix, the cells differentiate into hard keratin, creating the nail plate. At 14 weeks, the plate starts to grow distally along the matrix. As the nail grows, more keratin is deposited, adding to the thickness of the nail while keeping the firm attachment to the underlying tissue. The advancement of the firm plate through the soft tissue creates the nail folds. The nail reaches the tip of the fingers by 32 weeks and in case of the toes by 36 weeks of gestation.[2]

37.3 Anatomy

37.3.1 Surface Anatomy

Eponychium is the most proximal portion of the dorsal fingertip (▶ Fig. 37.1). It allows attachment of tissues to the nail itself. Cuticle or nail veil provides a water tight seal to the underlying space. In cases where cuticle is disrupted and there is frequent water exposure, such as in dishwashers, chronic bacterial and fungal infections are common.

Hyponychium is the junction of the nail to the most distal fleshy fingertip. It contains a keratinous plug that also seals off the underlying space. There are numerous leukocytes within the tissue of the hyponychium averting subungual infections.

Paronychium is the soft tissue that surrounds the lateral edges of the nail. The cells are arranged in an overlapping manor, i.e., as shingles on the roof. Even minor trauma in this area can introduce bacteria underneath the nail, leading to infection or paronychia. These are commonly treated with removal of a portion of or the entire nail under local anesthesia.[3–5]

37.2.2 Longitudinal and Cross-sections of the Fingertip

The hard cornified structure overlying the dorsum of the fingertip is termed the *nail plate* (▶ Fig. 37.2a). Underlying tissue that contributes to the thickness of the nail, called the nail, overlies the periosteum of the distal phalanx and originates distal to the terminal extensor tendon insertion. The two sections of the nail bed are germinal and sterile matrices. The nail fold contains dorsal roof and the ventral floor of the germinal matrix. The dorsal roof contributes to the smoothness and the shine of the nail (▶ Fig. 37.2b). In instances of revision amputations, this portion of the matrix should be removed as well to avoid nail cysts.

When an injured nail bed results in persistent deformity, it may be reconstructed from a nail bed of another digit, usually a toe. It is important to note that sterile matrix can be reconstructed by splitting the sterile matrix of the donor digit, similar to the split thickness skin graft. By doing so, the donor deformity is minimal. On the contrary, reconstruction of the germinal matrix requires full-thickness harvest from the donor digit, producing donor morbidity.[6]

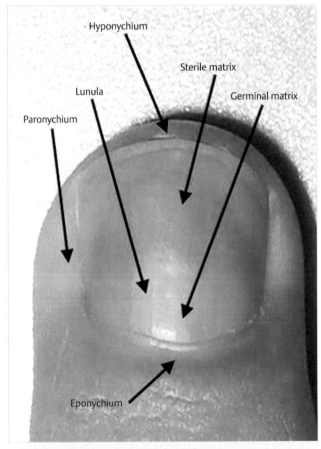

Fig. 37.1 Surface anatomy of the fingertip.

Specialized and viable keratin-producing cells with intact nuclei are located within the germinal matrix. As the nail is pushed distally during growth, the cell nuclei degenerate (▶Fig. 37.2c). These cells without nuclei are located within the sterile matrix. They add keratin to the undersurface of the nail plate, making it thicker and provide firm adherence of the plate

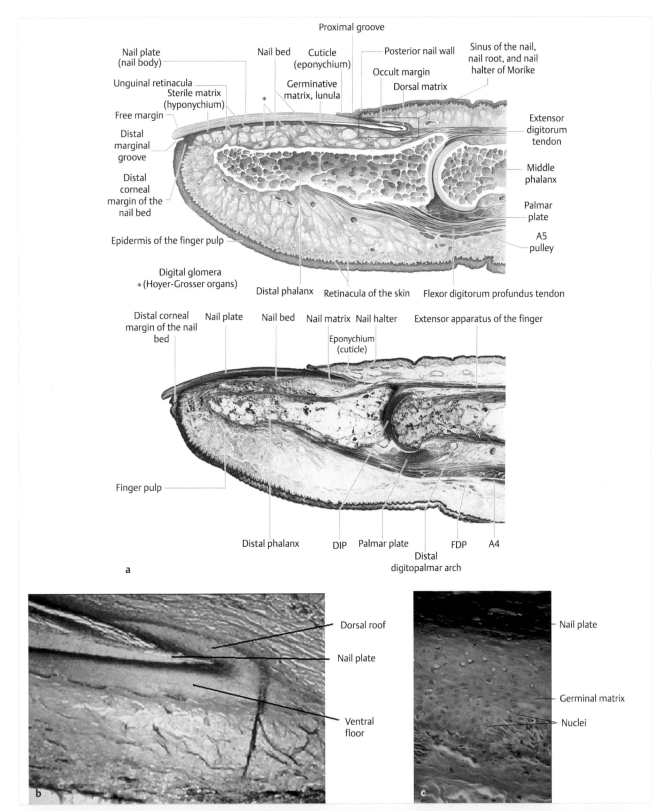

Fig. 37.2 (a) Longitudinal section of the fingertip. (b) Histological section of the sinus of the nail, nail root and nail halter of Morike, (c) As the cells with nuclei divide within the germinal matrix, they are pushed dorsally and distally. As this occurs, the cells flatten and elongate and the nuclei disintegrate. The addition of keratin layers forms a solid rigid sheath of the nail plate. (37.2a from: Schmidt H-M, Lanz U. Surgical Anatomy of the Hand. Stuttgart, Germany: Thieme; 2004).

to the nail bed. Delineation between the two matrices is indicated with a lunula. Lunula is an arc of pale tissue just distal to the eponychium.

Areolar tissue of the volar pad provides softness of the finger pulp. There are multiple fibrous collagen bands within the pulp (▶ Fig. 37.3). Their purpose is not to create the compartments but rather to adhere the skin to the underlying periosteum. These septa need to be released during drainage of a pulp abscess (felon). This area also contains copious sensory appendages that aid in touch perception.

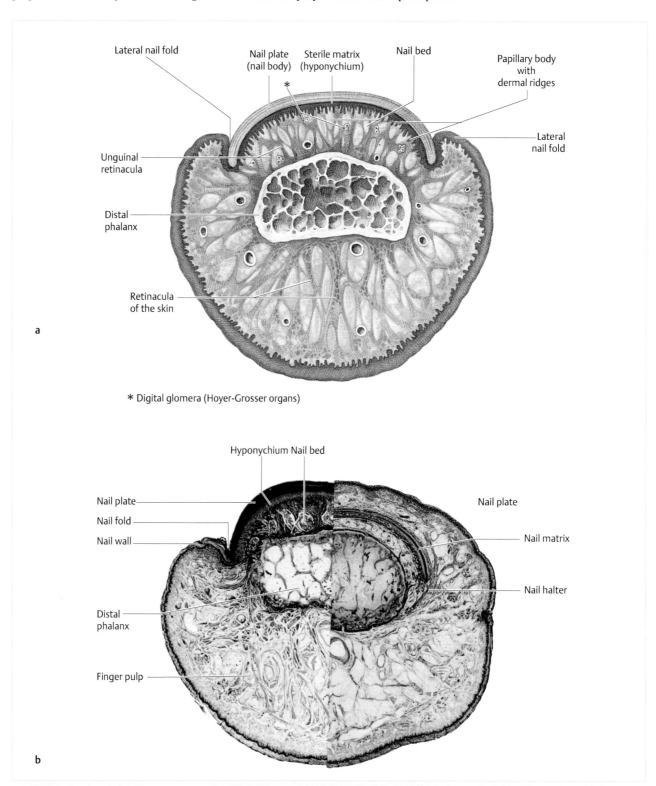

a

* Digital glomera (Hoyer-Grosser organs)

b

Fig. 37.3 (a,b) Cross-section of the fingertip showing the nail structures. (From: Schmidt H-M, Lanz U. Surgical Anatomy of the Hand. Stuttgart, Germany: Thieme; 2004).

There is a thickening of the epithelium on the dorsum of the nail resembling a halter that hold the nail in place. This area is connected to the phalangoglenoid ligament and to the proper phalangeal or interosseous ligament, also called the ligament of Flint (▶Fig 37.3, ▶Fig 37.4, and ▶Fig. 37.5).

37.2.3 Blood Supply to the Fingertip

Digital arteries sendoff branches just proximal to the distal interphalangeal (DIP) joint (▶Fig. 37.6). Terminal branches further divide to supply the nail bed and the volar pulp. The nail bed is supplied by two arches, one at the level of the lunula and the second at the fingertip (▶Fig. 37.7 a–c). Capillaries are very dense within the germinal matrix.

In addition to the volar system, two dorsal branches arise from the digital arteries to supply the dorsal fingertip (▶Fig. 37.7 and ▶Fig. 37.8). Small branches traverse across the eponychium and mid substance of the nail bed.

There is intense vascular supply of the pulp. The two digital arteries cross the digital nerves dorsally and become more midline. There are three specific branching patterns of the arteries in the pulp: the I pattern, the inverted U pattern, and the H pattern (▶Fig. 37.9a–f).

Venous return is composed of the superficial system just deep to the skin of the volar pad and of the deep system, which corresponds to the venae comitans of the digital arteries (▶Fig. 37. 10). The small veins coalesce at the nail fold and continue to course proximally through the network over the dorsal finger (▶Fig. 37.10b). Small transverse and oblique veins

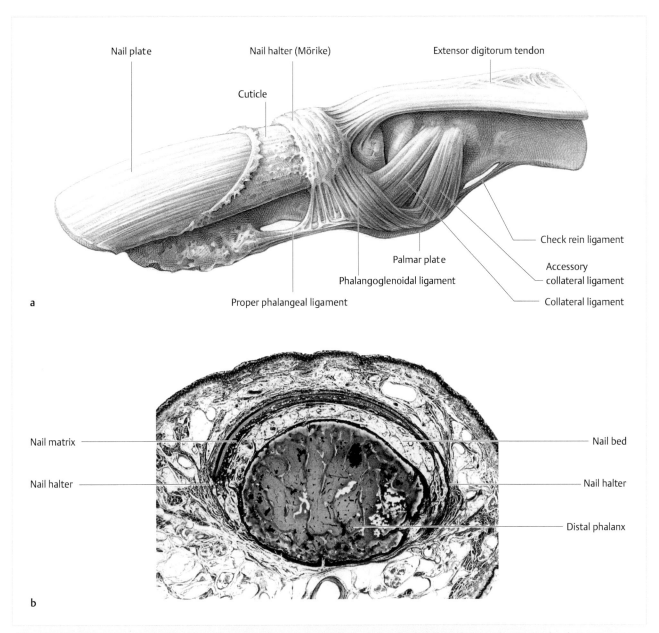

Fig. 37.4 (a,b) Ligaments supporting the nail matrix and cross-section through the distal phalanx showing the proximal nail structures. (From: Schmidt H-M, Lanz U. Surgical Anatomy of the Hand. Stuttgart, Germany: Thieme; 2004).

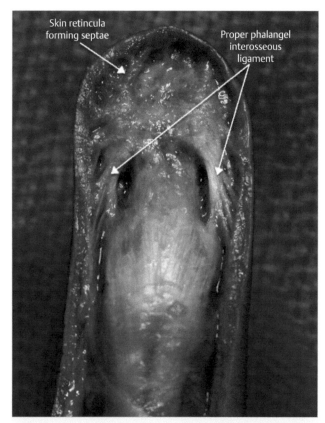

Fig. 37.5 Longitudinal dissection of the pulp of the finger showing the supporting skin retinaculae forming septae. Also seen are the Proper Phalangeal Interosseous ligaments on either side.

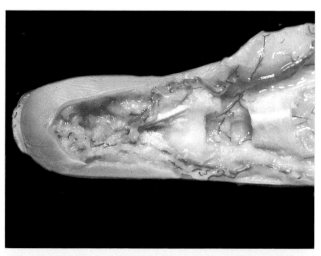

Fig. 37.6 Digital arteries send branches to the distal interphalangeal (DIP) joint. Distal to the DIP, terminal branches divide to supply the nail bed and the pulp.

connect the sides of the finger. Superficial palmar veins at 3–5 and 7–9 o'clock may be suitable for replantation at the level of the eponychium.[7,8]

Venous valves can be encountered within the smallest veins of the fingertip pulp (▶ Fig. 37.11). However, most of them are located where the veins merge together, starting at the nail fold.[9]

37.2.4 Nerve Supply

Digital nerves divide into three terminal branches 0.5 to 1.0 cm from the DIP crease. The first branch extends toward the nail fold, he econd to the nail bed at the level of the lunula, and the final to the hyponychium (▶ Fig. 37.12).

Glomus body (Hoyer-Grosser organ), a specialized organ, aids in thermoregulation and blood flow in the digits and can be identified within the fingertip as well as the ears, nose, and toes (▶ Fig. 37.2a, ▶ Fig. 37.3a, and ▶ Fig. 37.13). The majority of these structures (75–90%) are located in the digits. Benign proliferation of these cells can lead to painful, pin point, and cold sensitivity usually presenting in the subungual space. Bluish appearance of the nail bed can help identify the glomus tumor. Otherwise, magnetic imaging is useful in identification of symptomatic but not easily visible lesions, as well as those as small as 2 mm. Subungual or periungual incision (▶ Fig. 37.14) and meticulous curettage are the treatment of choice.[10,11]

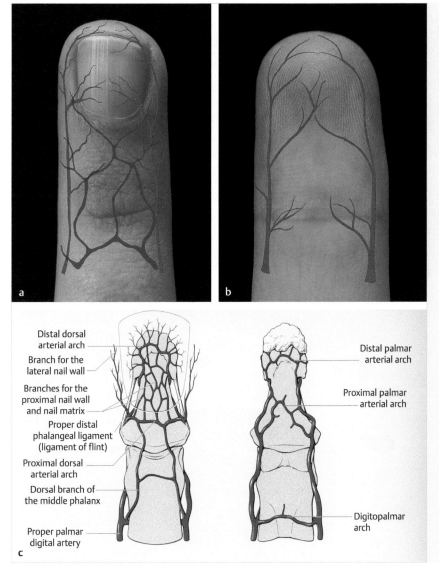

Fig 37.7 (a–c) The nail bed is supplied by two arterial arches—the proximal and distal dorsal arterial arches. In between, there are multitude of blood vessels dividing and reanastomosing. Branches from the distal arch also supply the pulp. The palmar digital arteries also form arches—a digitopalmar arch at the level of the DIP joint and a proximal palmar arch and a distal palmar arch at the distal phalanx level. Arterial branches from the palmar arteries pass deep to the interosseous ligament of Flint to anastomose with the dorsal system. Venous drainage from the perinychium is provided by vessels in the dorsal skin of the finger proximal to the nail wall. (Fig 37.7 b and c from: Schmidt H-M, Lanz, U: Surgical Anatomy of the Hand. Thieme, Stuttgart 2004).

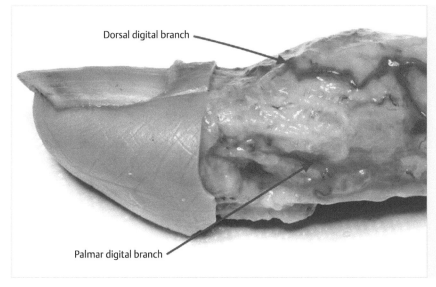

Fig. 37.8 Dorsal and palmar arteries supplying the nail bed and the finger pulp.

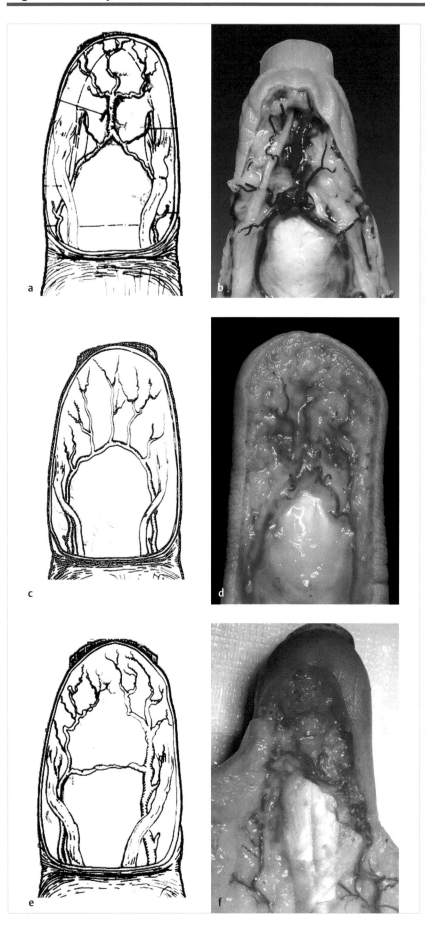

Fig. 37.9 (a–f) Branching patterns of the terminal digital arteries. (a, b) I pattern, (c, d) inverted U pattern, (e, f) and H pattern.

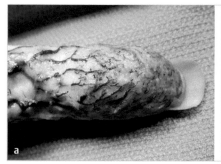
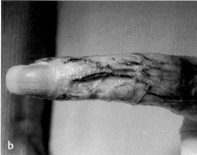

Fig. 37.10 (a, b) Superficial veins of the pulp and dorsal veins.

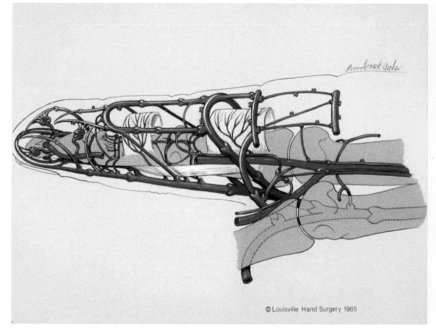

Fig. 37.11 The veins of the pulp and finger draining through volar and dorsal veins to the web vein. The veins have valves at junctions. (From Kleinert Institute, Louisville, KY.)

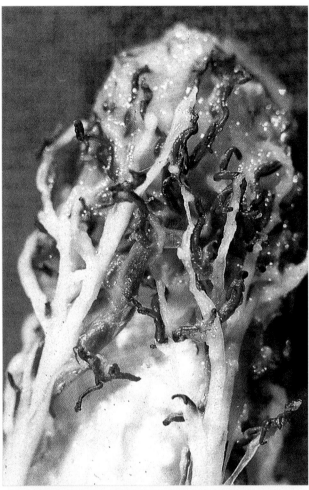

Fig. 37.12 Arteries and nerve branches arborize in the pulp of the digit. (Reproduced with permission from Zancolli EA and Cozzi EP. Atlas of Surgical Anatomy of the Hand. New York, NY: Churchill Livingstone; 1992.)

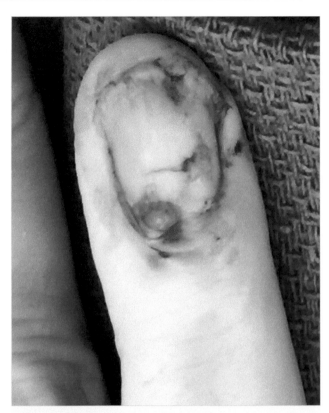

Fig. 37.14 Excision of subungual glomus tumor.

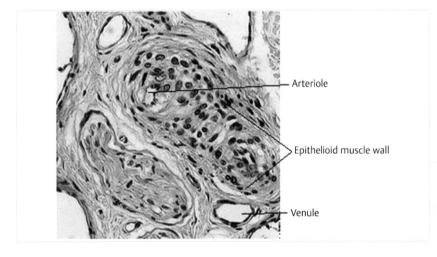

Arteriole

Epithelioid muscle wall

Venule

Fig. 37.13 Glomus body with afferent arteriole, venule, and epithelioid muscle cells. Strongly associated with the sympathetic nerves, this organ aids in thermoregulation through blood flow control.

References

1. Al-Qattan MM. WNT pathways and upper limb anomalies. J Hand Surg Eur Vol 2011;36(1):9–22
2. Oberg KC, Feenstra JM, Manske PR, Tonkin MA. Developmental biology and classification of congenital anomalies of the hand and upper extremity. J Hand Surg Am 2010;35(12):2066–2076
3. Zook EG, Van Beek AL, Russell RC, Beatty ME. Anatomy and physiology of the perionychium: a review of the literature and anatomic study. J Hand Surg Am 1980;5(6):528–536
4. Zook EG. Anatomy and physiology of the perionychium. Hand Clin 1990;6(1):1–7
5. Zook EG. Anatomy and physiology of the perionychium. Hand Clin 2002;18(4):553–559, v
6. Lille S, Brown RE, Zook EE, Russell RC. Free nonvascularized composite nail grafts: an institutional experience. Plast Reconstr Surg 2000;105(7):2412–2415
7. Moss SH, Schwartz KS, von Drasek-Ascher G, Ogden LL II, Wheeler CS, Lister GD. Digital venous anatomy. J Hand Surg Am 1985;10(4):473–482
8. Cheng L, Chen K, Chai YM, Wen G, Wang CY. Fingertip replantation at the eponychial level with venous anastomosis: an anatomic study and clinical application. J Hand Surg Eur Vol 2013;38(9):959–963
9. Venkatramani H, Sabapathy SR. Fingertip replantation: Technical considerations and outcome analysis of 24 consecutive fingertip replantations. Indian J Plast Surg 2011;44(2):237–245
10. Lee IJ, Park DH, Park MC, Pae NS. Subungual glomus tumours of the hand: diagnosis and outcome of the transungual approach. J Hand Surg Eur Vol 2009;34(5):685–688
11. Netscher DT, Aburto J, Koepplinger M. Subungual glomus tumor. J Hand Surg Am 2012;37(4):821–823, quiz 824

Section V

Epilegomena

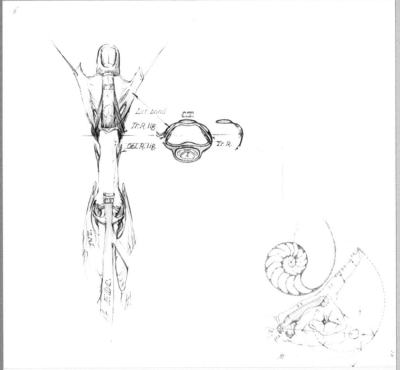

Drawings by Dr William Littler. Courtesy: Dr. Steven Glickel and the American Society for Surgery of the Hand. Courtesy SAGE Publications.

38 Imaging and Anatomy

Herbert P. von Schroeder and Ali Naraghi

38.1 Introduction

Advancing technology has made medical imaging indispensable for assessing, evaluating, and diagnosing specific conditions and injuries of the wrist and upper extremity. The diagnostic value and utility of imaging techniques are improved by choosing the type of studies that are best suited for particular tissue types, anatomical regions, and conditions. This chapter will focus on relevant wrist and upper extremity anatomy and cover how plain radiography, computerized tomography (CT), magnetic resonance imaging (MRI), and ultrasound (US) aid in defining the anatomy and the conditions of the regions.

38.2 Imaging Approach to Wrist Pathology

Imaging of the hand and wrist poses special challenges. The anatomy is complex; many of the structures involved are small. There may be an overlap in radiological findings of symptomatic and asymptomatic individuals, and many of the pathological conditions have a dynamic basis, whereas imaging is typically performed in a static manner. These challenges are best exemplified in imaging of ligamentous injuries of the wrist, where the pathological lesions often involve intricate structures that measure 1 to 2 mm in thickness and may not result in significant malalignment on static images.

Despite advances in imaging techniques, plain radiographs remain an indispensable initial investigation, which often helps narrow the differential diagnosis and guide further investigation. In many cases, no further imaging is warranted following plain radiographs. At least two orthogonal views are necessary, as radiographs only provide a two-dimensional representation of three-dimensional structures, but in practice additional views are usually obtained. The advantages of radiographs include easy access, reproducibility, high spatial resolution for osseous abnormalities, relative lack of artifact from postoperative hardware, and the ability to perform stress views. In addition, plain radiographs allow for easy side-to-side comparison in equivocal cases.

CT provides exquisite osseous detail with a high spatial resolution, but contrast resolution and soft tissue detail has been lacking for imaging wrist structures. Therefore, it is most commonly used to assess occult, complex, or intra-articular fractures, the degree and pattern of joint space loss, the extent and characteristics of osseous lesions, and imaging of postoperative hardware complications. Three-dimensional images reconstructed from the axial images are often helpful by providing an overview of the abnormality, although they typically do not increase diagnostic accuracy or confidence. CT arthrography, with instillation of intra-articular iodinate contrast material, has emerged as an adjunct technique in evaluation of ligamentous and chondral injuries, taking advantage of the high spatial resolution of CT to image the small complex structure.

MRI in many ways is well suited to imaging assessment of the wrist, offering excellent soft-tissue resolution, multiplanar capabilities, and the ability to perform a global assessment of the wrist, and is extensively used in detecting osseous, tendinous, and ligamentous injuries. However, issues related to signal-to-noise ratio and spatial resolution have somewhat limited its accuracy in comparison with arthroscopy in evaluating abnormalities of intrinsic and extrinsic ligaments and articular cartilage, and as a result MR arthrography is often used to identify injuries to these structures. Three-Tesla (3T) MRI systems and advances in coil technology have significantly increased the signal-to-noise ratio, in turn allowing for thinner slice acquisitions and improved spatial resolution. Isotropic data acquisition and high-quality multiplanar reformats of the wrist are now a reality. Despite this, imaging of ligamentous injuries of the wrist is still challenging. Seven-Tesla (7T) MRI is likely to push these boundaries further and has already demonstrated improvements in imaging of the articular cartilage with demonstration of the hyaline cartilage at the interphalangeal joints.[1]

Ultrasound is also widely used for assessing soft-tissue structures. Advantages of ultrasound include a high spatial resolution especially with transducers > 15 MHz, easy side-to-side comparison, assessment of vascularity within soft-tissue masses, and the synovium as well as the ability to perform dynamic assessment. As a result, ultrasound has emerged as the optimal imaging technique for diagnosing tendon injuries.[2]

Advanced imaging techniques are also being used to evaluate the neurovascular structures in the upper extremity. CT angiography of the upper limb has replaced conventional angiography in many centers. MR angiography has improved substantially over the past few years with images of high temporal resolution as well as images of high spatial resolution, clearly depicting the vascular anatomy even in the digital arteries. There has been an interest in imaging of the nerves of the upper extremity using MRI, not only to detect structural changes such as swelling and edema but also to detect functional changes by using diffusion-weighted MRI.

The choice of the imaging modality used will ultimately be guided by the clinical differential diagnosis, the findings on the initial plain radiographs, and the local clinical and radiological expertise. In the majority of cases, this decision is straightforward, but in complex situations a tailored approach is often necessary.

38.3 Anatomical Considerations

The complex anatomy of the wrist consists, in general terms, of two joints, which are appreciated on routine radiographs but better appreciated on sagittal and coronal imaging of the carpus (▶Fig. 38.1). The relatively round capitate of the distal row is well contained in the socket formed by the scaphoid and lunate of the proximal row.

Flexion and extension of the wrist occurs at both the radiocarpal and the midcarpal joints (▶Fig. 38.2). But these motions, as well as radial and ulnar deviation, are oversimplified when considered in only two dimensions, as they do not address the multiple degrees of freedom that occur between and within the carpal rows. Wrist motion is dictated and restricted by the anatomical shapes of the bones and by the position, tension and integrity of the inter- and intracarpal

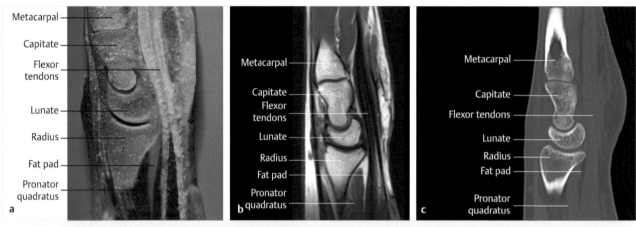

Fig. 38.1 (a) Sagittal section of the wrist and (b) corresponding proton density magnetic resonance imaging and (c) sagittal CT reformat showing articulation of the capitate and lunate and the lunate in the distal radius.

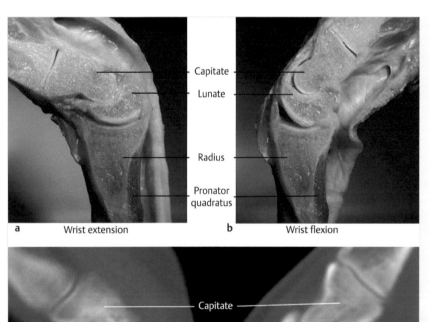

Fig. 38.2 Sagittal section of the wrist in (a) extension and (b) flexion. The wrist capsule and ligaments act as tension bands on the convex side in each respective position. Sagittal CT reformats of the wrist in extension (c) and flexion (d) obtained during a dynamic examination of the wrist demonstrate the degree of motion at the radiocarpal and midcarpal joints.

ligaments and the joint capsule that are crucial to carpal stability. Advances in CT technology, with faster gantry rotation, smaller detectors, and extended coverage now allow for isotropic volumetric acquisitions to be performed through the whole wrist in a fraction of a second. The isotropic datasets (voxels of same dimension in all planes) allow for high-quality reformats and three-dimensional images. In addition, the high temporal and spatial resolution can be utilized to perform true dynamic assessment of wrist biomechanics. Similar experimental work is being undertaken using MRI, and these techniques should enhance our understanding of normal as well as pathological wrist biomechanics.[3] Although fluoroscopy has long been used for dynamic assessment of wrist motion, the advantage of cross-sectional techniques such as CT and MRI for kinematic assessment is the lack of superimposition of multiple bones and the ability to assess the motion of each individual bone.

The TFCC and the distal radius form a shallow socket for the proximal carpal row (▶Fig. 38.3) which is defined not only by the shapes of the radius and TFCC but also by the capsule and the extrinsic ligaments between these structures and the proximal row (see hereafter).

The proximal row is commonly referred to as the intercalated segment in reference to its interposed position between the distal carpal row and the radius/TFCC. The proximal row, consisting of the scaphoid, lunate, and triquetrum, itself forms a socket for the capitate and hamate of the distal row (▶Fig. 38.4). The structural integrity of bones or their ligaments of the proximal row is important to this relationship, and any laxity or disruption results in instability patterns and eventual arthritis. Bone anatomy of the carpus is ideally assessed by CT and three-dimensional (3D) imaging, which is useful for visualization of pathology such as fracture nonunions and osteophytes. Imaging the ligaments of the proximal row remains a challenge given the small size and structure of the ligaments themselves. Conventional MRI has a limited sensitivity for tears of the scapholunate (SL) (60%) and lunotriquetral (LT) (30%) ligaments. Even at 3T there is a modest improvement in accuracy of detecting SL and LT tears.[4] MRI arthrography results in increased sensitivity and specificity, and MRI in radial and ulnar deviation also appears to improve detail but may be limited by coil geometry.[5] CT arthrography appears to be the most accurate imaging technique for diagnosing SL (sensitivity 95%, specificity 96%) and LT (sensitivity 90%, specificity 100%) tear,

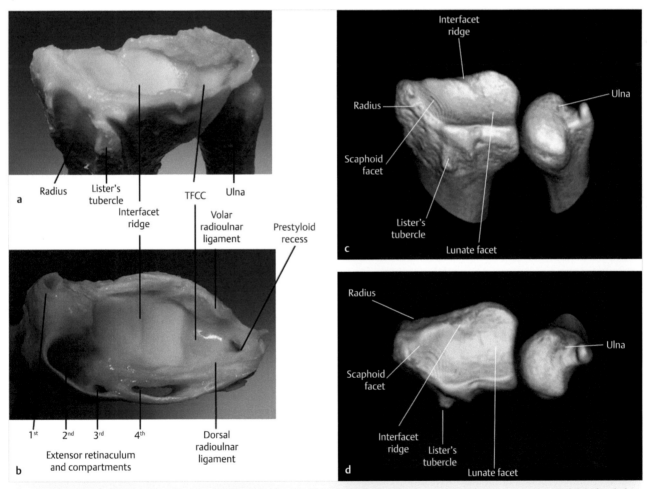

Fig. 38.3 Anatomical dissections of a right distal radius, ulna, and triangular fibrocartilage complex with the carpus removed. (a) The shallow socket for the proximal row is viewed from a posterior view and (b) from a distal viewpoint. Three-dimensional shaded surface display CT images (c, d) through the radiocarpal joint with the carpus segmented out demonstrate the shallow socket of the distal radial articular surface.

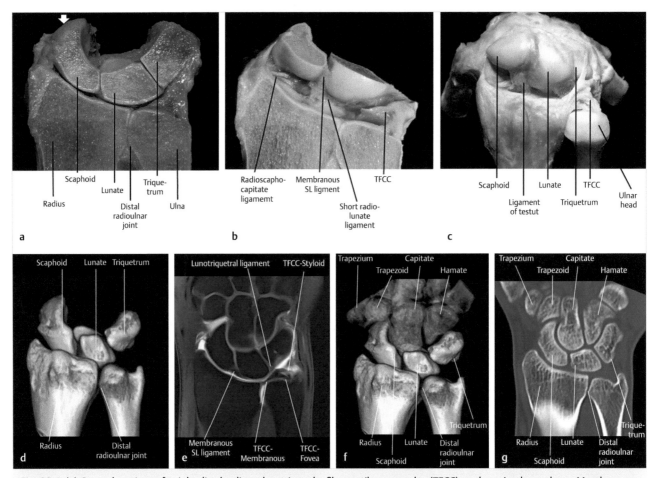

Fig. 38.4 (a) Coronal sections of a right distal radius, ulna, triangular fibrocartilage complex (TFCC), and proximal carpal row. Membranous sections of the scapholunate (SL) and lunotriquetral (LT) ligaments are shown. The articulation with the trapezium and trapezoid is at the arrowhead. (b) With the proximal row in flexion, the volar wrist capsule and ligaments are viewed. (c) Nonsectioned specimen showing intact intracarpal SL and LT ligaments. (d) Three-dimensional computed tomography (3D CT) images through the wrist with the distal carpal row segmented out demonstrate the socket made by the distal articular surfaces of the scaphoid and lunate. (e) Coronal T1 fat-suppressed magnetic resonance arthrogram of the wrist shows the articular surfaces of the radiocarpal and midcarpal joints, including the contribution of the TFCC to the articular surface. The SL and LT ligaments are also clearly visualized. (f) Same 3D CT image as seen in (d), with insertion of the distal carpal row, demonstrates the anatomy of the midcarpal joint. (g) Coronal reformat of the wrist demonstrates the osseous anatomy of the radiocarpal and midcarpal joints.

but this technique lacks sensitivity for assessment of other soft-tissue structures. This technique also has the highest inter observer reliability.[6]

The proximal carpal row forms a socket (▶Fig. 38.4 and ▶Fig. 38.5) for the distal row. The socket is deepened by the wrist capsule and ligaments that cross the midcarpal joint, but despite the constraints, the midcarpal joint is inherently lax. The major extrinsic ligaments on the dorsum of the wrist are the radiotriquetral (RT or radiocarpal) and the dorsal intercarpal (DIC) ligaments (▶Fig. 38.6). The RT ligament originates on the dorsum of the radius as far radial as Lister's tubercle and inserts in the tuberosity on the dorsum of the triquetrum. This anchor point on the triquetrum is an important bony landmark and is also the origin of the DIC ligament, which crosses the wrist to insert into the dorsum of the trapezium and scaphoid. The RT and DIC ligaments lengthen in opposing directions during radial and ulnar deviation of the wrist.[7] The ligaments can be preserved during surgical approaches to the wrist. The DIC crosses the waist of the capitate and not the central portion of the midcarpal joint. The joint is contained only by the capsule in this region, allowing for motion but also leaving potential instability of the region.

The volar intercarpal ligaments (▶Fig. 38.7) are more numerous and complex than their dorsal counterparts. The radioscaphocapitate ligament originates at the radial styloid, crosses the scaphoid waist, and inserts into the volar aspect of the capitate. Between the long and short radiolunate ligaments is the intra-articular ligament of Testut (radioscapholunate ligament), which contains blood vessels to the SL region. Ulnolunate and LT ligaments form the volar aspect of the TFCC and stabilize the proximal row. The ligaments on the radial and ulnar aspect of the wrist converge and insert on the capitate to form an inverted **V**. As seen dorsally, there are no ligaments to cross the central portion of the midcarpal joint on the volar side. Until recently, there has been little attention paid to imaging of extrinsic ligaments in the radiology literature in comparison with assessment of intrinsic ligaments.[8,9] However, isotropic MRI acquisitions with slice thicknesses of 0.5 to 0.6 mm can clearly identify the extrinsic ligaments in all three planes especially when combined with MR arthrography. Ultrasound has also been used to evaluate the extrinsic carpal ligaments.[10] However, the accuracy of imaging in identifying tears of extrinsic ligaments has not been adequately assessed.

Volarly, the carpal ligaments coalesce with the wrist capsule to form the base of the carpal tunnel (▶Fig. 38.8). The carpal tunnel contains the median nerve and nine flexor tendons to the digits. The carpal tunnel can be assessed by ultrasound[11] and by MRI if soft tissue pathology is suspected.[12] The fibrous transverse carpal ligament (flexor retinaculum) comprises the roof of the tunnel that supports to structural concavity of the carpus; the ligament can be quantitated by US.[13] On its ulnar side, the transverse carpal ligament splits to form the superficial

and deep walls of Guyon's canal, containing the ulnar nerve and artery (▶Fig. 38.8b).

The two major blood vessels to the hand (the radial and ulnar arteries), and their anastomotic arches and distal vessels can be assessed by conventional arteriography as well as by CT angiography and MR angiography (▶Fig. 38.9a–d). An appreciation of the anatomy is important for assessing ischemia of the hand, replanting amputated and traumatized regions of the hand, and planning vascular bone or soft tissue transfers.

Dorsally, the extensor tendons are contained in their respective six compartments (numbered from radial to ulnar direction) by the extensor retinaculum (▶Fig. 38.10). The retinaculum is a continuation of the antebrachial fascia. It has an oblique orientation and encloses the tendons onto the distal radius for the first three compartments, or to the carpus for compartments four to six. The first compartment contains the multiple tendon slips of the abductor pollicis longus (APL) and the extensor pollicis brevis (EPB). These tendons may be separated by an intracompartmental septum; the tendons insert into the base of the metacarpal and the base of the proximal phalanx of the thumb, respectively. The intracompartmental septum is best evaluated by ultrasound. The EPB is the ulnar border of the anatomical snuffbox. The second compartment contains the tendons of the extensor carpi radialis longus (ECRL) and brevis (ECRB). The ECRL is radial to the ECRB; they insert into the second and third metacarpals, respectively. The second and third compartments are separated at Lister's tubercle on the dorsum of the radius. The third compartment contains the extensor pollicis longus (EPL) tendon, which uses Lister's tubercle as a fulcrum; the tendon crosses the tendons of the second compartment, defines the ulnar border of the anatomical snuffbox, and inserts in the distal phalanx of the thumb. The first three compartments have the periosteum of the distal radius as their floor. This makes the tendons vulnerable to tendonitis, rupture following radius fracture, or irritation from orthopaedic hardware. The third compartment or the interval created between the third and fourth compartments is commonly used as a surgical approach to the distal radius or to the wrist.

The extensor retinaculum is primarily at the level of the carpus at the fourth compartment. More proximally, the compartment contains the posterior interosseus artery and nerve at its floor. The compartment also contains the extensor digitorum communis (EDC) tendons, the extensor indicis proprius (EIP) tendon, and the relatively common anomalous tendons[14,15] to the fingers. Distally the EDC tendons are interconnected by

Fig. 38.5 (a) The midcarpal socket formed centrally by the lunate and scaphoid and the surrounding wrist capsule and ligaments. The dissection is viewed from the distal aspect with the distal carpal row having been excised. (b) Corresponding three-dimensional computed tomography image with segmentation of the distal carpal row shows the midcarpal socket.

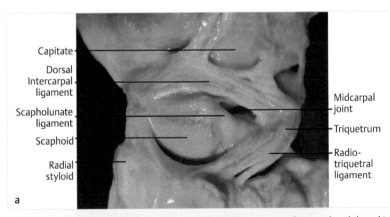

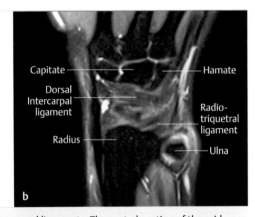

Fig. 38.6 (a) Dorsal aspect of the right wrist with extrinsic radiocarpal and dorsal intercarpal ligaments. The central portion of the midcarpal joint does not have direct ligament constraints. (b) Isotropic coronal SPACE magnetic resonance imaging acquisition through the dorsal aspect of the wrist shows a striated appearance to the dorsal intercarpal and radiotriquetral ligaments.

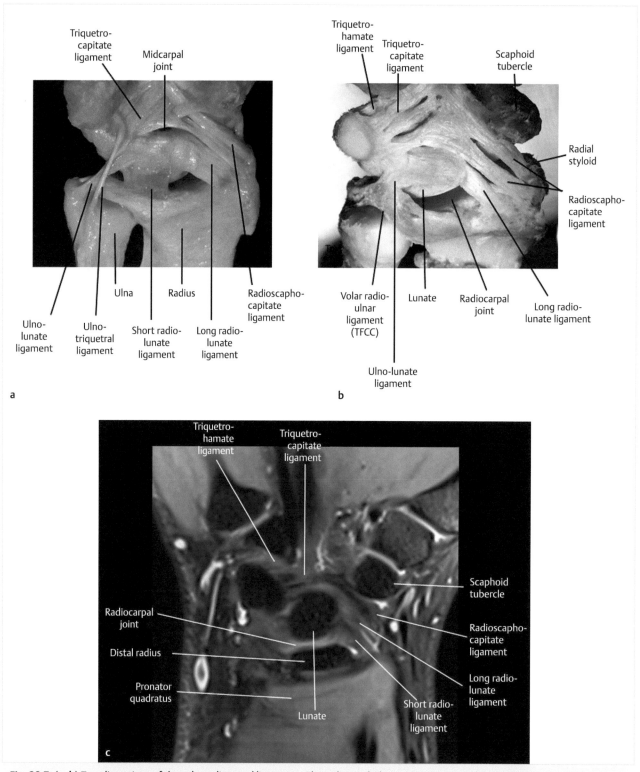

Fig. 38.7 (a, b) Two dissections of the volar radiocarpal ligaments. The radioscapholunate (RSC) crosses the waist of the scaphoid and provides a fulcrum for scaphoid flexion. Note the space between the long and short radiolunate ligaments, which is occupied by the vascular RSC ligament of Testut. The distal ligaments from the proximal to the distal row form and inverted **V** but provide only minimal constraint for the center of the midcarpal joint. (c) Isotropic coronal SPACE magnetic resonance imaging acquisition through the volar aspect of the wrist shows the inverted **V** configuration of the volar extrinsic ligaments with relative central deficiency.

three distinguishable types of juncturae tendinum[16] and continue into the extensor hoods on the dorsum of each of the fingers, which also receives contribution from the intrinsic muscles of the hand.[17]

The fifth extensor compartment contains the extensor digiti minimi (EDM) tendon to the small finger. The compartment is directly over the distal radioulnar joint (DRUJ) (▶ Fig. 38.10) and can be used as a surgical approach to the joint and to the

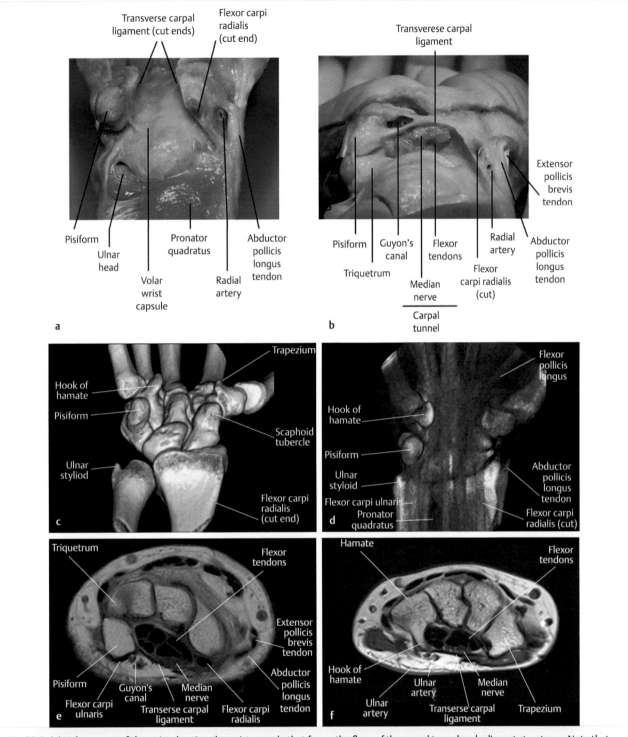

Fig. 38.8 (a) Volar aspect of the wrist showing the wrist capsule that forms the floor of the carpal tunnel and adjacent structures. Note that the flexor carpi radialis (FCR) tendon is adjacent to the carpal tunnel. At this level, the radial artery begins its dorsal direction into the anatomic snuffbox at this level. (b) The contents of the carpal tunnel include the median nerve and nine tendons to the digits. Guyon's canal is structurally separate from the carpal tunnel and contains the ulnar nerve and artery. (c) Coronal three-dimensional computed tomography (3D CT) image showing the bony boundaries of the carpal tunnel. (d) 3D CT image through the volar aspect of the wrist showing the same osseous boundaries of the carpal tunnel as in (d) but with the tendons of the volar wrist also demonstrated. Axial magnetic resonance imaging through the proximal (e) and distal (f) carpal tunnel showing the contents of the carpal tunnel and the transverse carpal tunnel. FCR and FCU are seen outside of the carpal tunnel. The ulnar nerve and artery are also seen within Guyon's canal on the slice through the proximal carpal tunnel.

dorsal aspect of the TFCC. The extensor retinaculum continues over the sixth compartment, containing the extensor carpi ulnaris (ECU) tendon, and finally inserts at the ulnar border of the wrist.

The proximal scaphoid, together with the lunate form a socket for the capitate, but the distal portion of the scaphoid is adjacent to the capitate to stabilize the carpal rows. Distally the scaphoid articulates with the trapezium and trapezoid

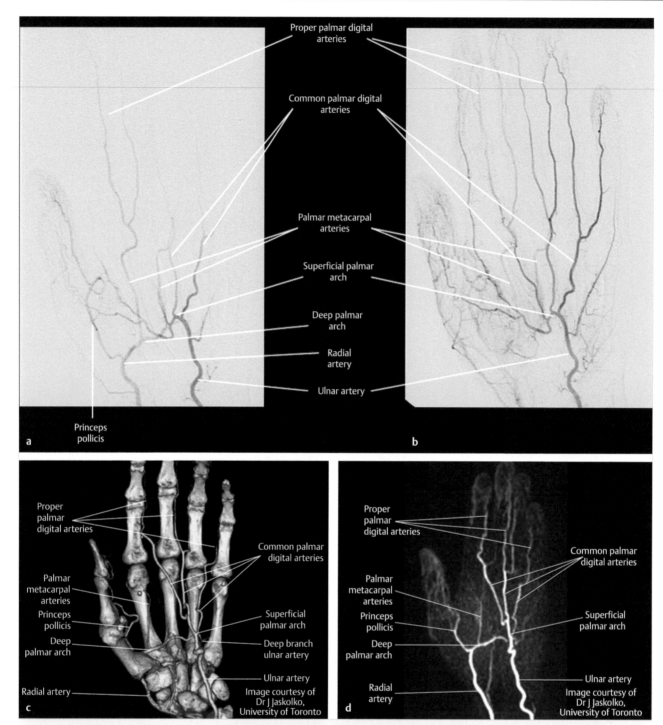

Fig. 38.9 (**a, b**) Images from a conventional arteriogram of the hand demonstrating deep and superficial arches on the early image (**a**) and the common metacarpal, common palmar digital, and proper palmar digital arteries on the later image (**b**). Computed tomography (CT) angiogram (**c**) and magnetic resonance imaging angiogram (**d**) in another patient also demonstrates the arterial anatomy. The relationship of the arteries to the osseous structures is particularly well seen on the CT arteriogram (**c**).

(►Fig. 38.11). Dorsally the scaphoid has a ridge that extends obliquely around the bone (►Fig. 38.11b). The ridge is the site of the capsular attachment through which branches of the radial artery provide the vascular supply to the majority of the bone. The ridge develops osteophytes (►Fig. 38.11c) with age and carpal collapse that may impinge on the dorsal rim of the radius.

Dorsally, the strongest portion of the SL ligament attaches to the ulnar aspect of the scaphoid ridge (►Fig. 38.12a) to the dorsoradial edge of the lunate. The other key structural part of the SL ligament is the volar portion which receives the ligament of Testut. The SL ligament itself is C-shaped in cross-section, with the stout dorsal and volar portions at opposite sides and the membranous portion of the ligament between them. The dorsal and volar bands of the SL ligament are best visualized on MR arthrography, in either the coronal or the axial planes (►Fig. 38.12b).

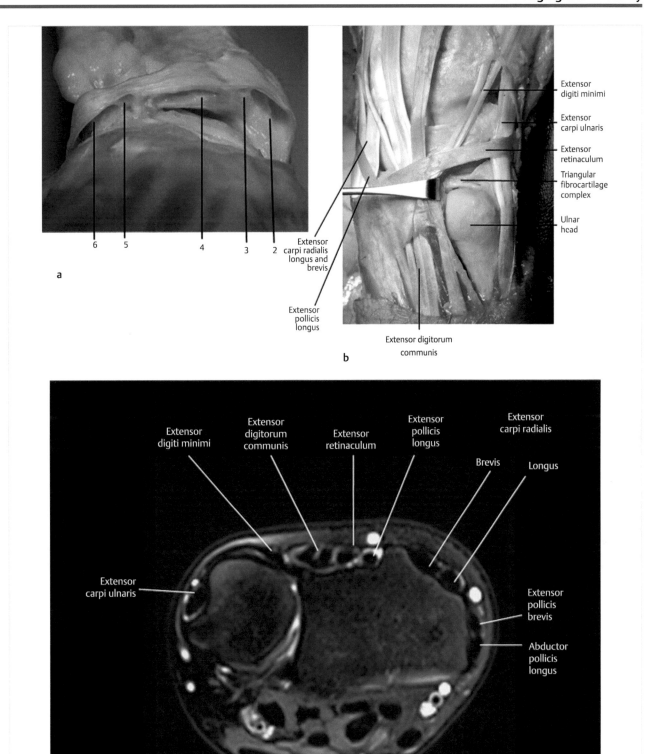

Fig. 38.10 (a) The extensor retinaculum, with tendons removed, is viewed from a distal perspective to show the respective compartments, which are separated by fibrous septa. (b) The extensor tendons within their compartments are used as surgical landmarks to the distal radius. Note that the fifth compartment containing the extensor digiti minimi tendon is directly dorsal to the distal radioulnar joint. (c) Axial magnetic resonance imaging through the distal radius (at Lister's tubercle) and ulna showing the extensor tendons of the six dorsal compartments.

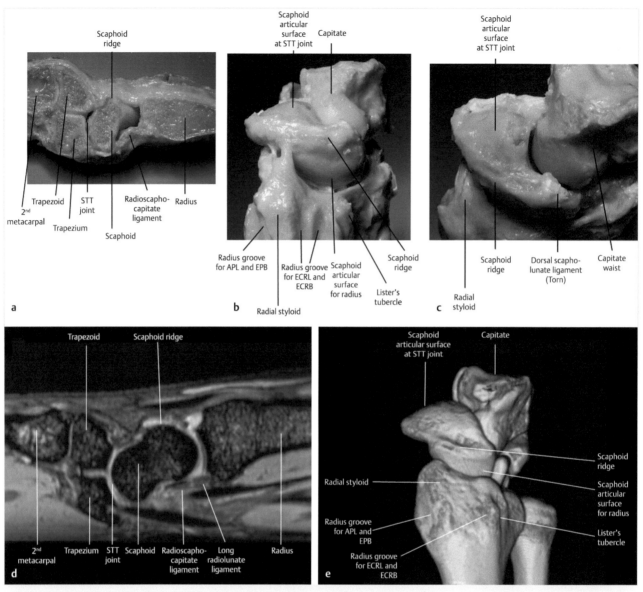

Fig. 38.11 (a) Parasagittal section of the distal half of the scaphoid showing its articulation with the trapezium and the trapezoid. Dorsally the scaphoid ridge attaches to the wrist capsule and contains the major blood supply to the bone. Proximally the scaphoid articulates within its facet of the distal radius. (b) The scaphoid ridge continues obliquely across the bone and separates the proximal articulation with the radius and the distal articulation with the trapezium and the trapezoid. The proximal half of the scaphoid provides part of the socket for the capitate (c), but distally the scaphoid crosses to the distal row and thereby acts to mechanically stabilize the carpus. The ulnar end of the scaphoid ridge is the anchor point for the dorsal scapholunate ligament. (d) Sagittal gradient echo magnetic resonance imaging through the radial aspect of the wrist, demonstrating the articulation of the scaphoid with the radius proximally and with the trapezoid and trapezium distally. (e) Three-dimensional computed tomography scan of the radius with the trapezium and trapezoid segmented out demonstrating the proximal and distal articular surfaces of the scaphoid and the scaphoid ridge.

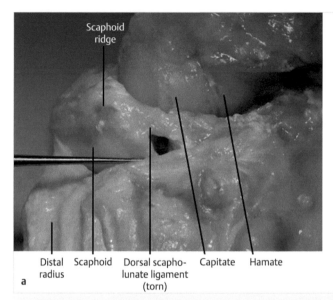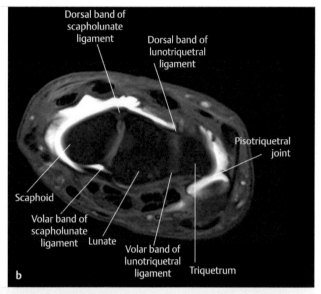

Fig. 38.12 (a) The strongest portion of the scapholunate (SL) ligament, responsible for the integrity of the SL socket for the capitate is seen dorsally between the scaphoid ridge and the dorsal rim of the lunate. Volarly, the ligament has a similar counterpart. (b) Axial T1 fat-suppressed magnetic resonance arthrogram of the wrist following radiocarpal injection demonstrates the intact dorsal and volar bands of the SL and lunotriquetral ligaments. The thick dorsal band of the SL ligament is particularly well visualized.

Volarly, the radioscaphocapitate ligament crosses the waist and supports the scaphoid (▶Fig. 38.13). The flexor carpi radialis (FCR) tendon passes ulnar to the scaphoid tubercle and continues within a groove on the trapezium to its insertion at the base of the second metacarpal. One corner of the transverse carpal ligament attaches in the adjacent region of the trapezium. The ligament also attaches to the scaphoid tubercle and crosses the carpal tunnel to insert into the hook of the hamate and pisiform.

On the ulnar aspect of the wrist, the distal ulna articulates with the TFCC; the TFCC forms a shallow socket for the lunate and triquetrum (▶Fig. 38.14), which in turn articulate with the distal carpal row. The TFCC is major stabilizer of the DRUJ and, together with the capsule of the joint, contains the ulnar head in the shallow sigmoid notch of the radius (▶Fig. 38.14b). The central portion of the TFCC is cartilaginous (▶Fig. 38.14c) and prone to degenerative changes with age (▶Fig. 38.14d), particularly in individuals who have positive ulnar variance. Although the various components of the TFCC, particularly the cartilage, can be easily assessed with routine MRI, the accuracy for detection of TFCC tears has been variable, with reported sensitivities and specificities of 44 to 100% and 52 to 100%, respectively.[18,19] The reported variation is partly dependent on the magnetic field strength, whether routine MRI or MR arthrography is used

and whether the tears are through the cartilaginous disc or through the ulnar side of the TFCC.[20] In general the accuracy is higher at 3T, with MR arthrography and in evaluation of radial sided tears. In particular, the clinically significant ulnar-sided tears and particularly partial undersurface tears have been notoriously difficult to detect, even with MR arthrography with reported sensitivities as low as 17%.[21] The ligamentum subcruentum can result in high signal intensity between the foveal and ulnar styloid attachments of the TFCC, mimicking a tear.[21] The volar and dorsal radioulnar ligaments are the main stabilizers of the DRUJ, whereas the ECU sheath and the volar ulnocapitate, ulnolunate, and ulnotriquetral ligaments stabilize this aspect of the carpus. The dorsal radiotriquetral ligament, although not a part of the TFCC structure, coalesces with the ECU subsheath to insert into prominence on the dorsum of the triquetrum.

The dorsal and volar radioulnar ligaments, which are the key structural portions of the TFCC, insert in and around the fovea of the distal ulna at the base of the ulnar styloid (▶Fig. 38.15). Trauma to the ligaments or to the insertion site of the ligaments will result in DRUJ instability and is one cause for arthritis of the articular surface at the ulnar head (▶Fig. 38.15b). Standard radiography, CT, and MRI can be insensitive for detection of DRUJ instability. In clinically equivocal cases, limited CT

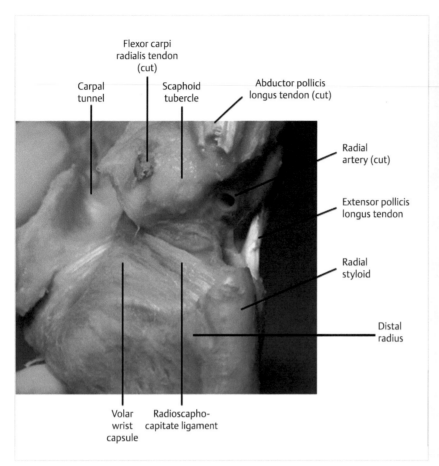

Carpal tunnel

Flexor carpi radialis tendon (cut)

Scaphoid tubercle

Abductor pollicis longus tendon (cut)

Radial artery (cut)

Extensor pollicis longus tendon

Radial styloid

Distal radius

Volar wrist capsule

Radioscapho-capitate ligament

Fig. 38.13 The radioscaphocapitate ligament crosses the waist of the scaphoid and acts as a fulcrum over which the scaphoid flexes and extends. In radial deviation of the wrist, the distal scaphoid is pushed into flexion. The flexor carpi ulnaris courses adjacent to the scaphoid tubercle and across a groove in the trapezium bordered by a ridge. The transverse carpal ligament is anchored adjacent to this and to the scaphoid tubercle.

examination through the DRUJ in pronation, neutral position, and supination has been utilized and a variety of measurements have been proposed for assessment of relationship of the ulnar head to the sigmoid notch to detect subtle subluxation.[23]

The radioulnar ligaments of the TFCC have a complex structure with deep and superficial components (►Fig. 38.16) that may not be appreciated during arthroscopy or imaging, but which can contribute to pain, instability, or clicking. The structure of the TFCC is further complicated by the volar ulno-carpal ligaments. Dorsally, the base of the ECU sheath of the sixth extensor compartment is an integral part of the TFCC (►Fig. 38.17). Subluxation of the ECU tendon at the distal ulna requires a dynamic assessment and this is best performed by ultrasound.

Viewed from the ulnar side, the wrist has a *mini* anatomical snuff box bounded by the ECU and flexor carpi ulnaris (FCU) tendons (►Fig. 38.18). The ECU continues to insert into the base of the fifth metacarpal, whereas the FCU inserts into the pisiform. The mini snuff box contains the distal ulna and ulnar styloid and the bony prominence on the ulnar aspect of the triquetrum that is enveloped by the continuation of the extensor retinaculum. The ulnar artery and nerve lie volar and slightly radial to the FCU tendon (►Fig. 38.19), before coursing to the radial side of the

pisiform at Guyon's canal. The mini snuff box is used for injections or as an arthroscopic portal on the ulnar side of the ECU; however, the dorsal sensory branch also courses through this region (►Fig. 38.20)[24] and is prone to injury, as are the sensory branches of the radial nerve on the radial aspect of the wrist.

The elbow joint consists of three articulations: (1) the capitellum of the humerus articulates with the radial head, (2) the trochlea of the humerus articulates with the ulna, and (3) the radial head articulates with the semilunar notch of the ulna at the proximal radioulnar joint (►Fig. 38.21, ►Fig. 38.22, and ►Fig. 38.23). Stability of the elbow is achieved through articular congruity and the ligaments. The ulnar (medial) collateral ligament (Fig. 38.21) consists of an anterior, posterior, and oblique portion. The anterior and posterior aspects each originate on the humerus and insert into the coronoid process and olecranon of the ulna, respectively. The ligament is subject to laxity and injury with throwing sports. The radial (lateral) ligament originates from the humerus and inserts into the supinator crest of the ulna and into the annular ligament. The annular ligament encircles the head of the radius and maintains it within the semilunar notch. At the elbow, the brachial artery bifurcates into radial and ulnar arteries and also provides recurrent vessels around the joint

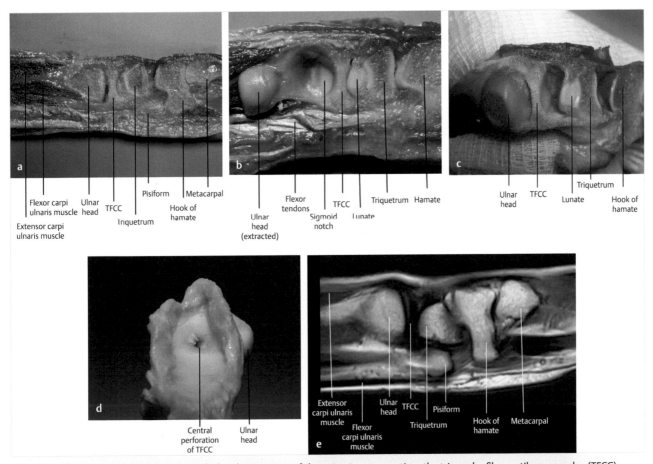

Fig. 38.14 (a) Parasagittal section through the ulnar portion of the wrist. In cross-section, the triangular fibrocartilage complex (TFCC) has an hourglass structure as it forms shallow sockets for the ulnar head and for the triquetrum and lunate of the proximal row. These two bones articulate with the hamate, shown here with its hook. The hamate articulates with the fourth and fifth metacarpals. (b) The socket for the ulnar head is formed not only by the TFCC but also by the sigmoid notch of the distal radius, shown in this anatomical section with the ulnar head flipped out of the distal radioulnar joint. Direct articulation of the TFCC with the lunate is shown. (c) The central portion of the TFCC is cartilaginous and is susceptible to degenerative tears with age and trauma, as seen in (d) from a superior aspect with the carpus removed. (e) Sagittal proton density magnetic resonance imaging through the ulnar aspect of the wrist showing the relationships just described.

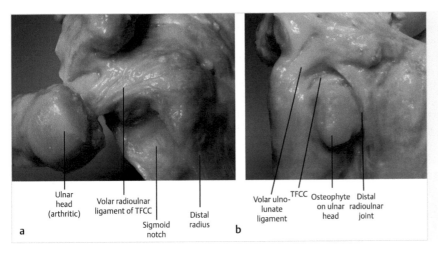

Fig. 38.15 (a) The ligaments of the triangular fibrocartilage complex (TFCC) are the major stabilizers of the distal radioulnar joint, as shown in this anatomical section, with the ulna cut to bring it out of the joint with distal ligaments intact. (b) Osteophytes around the ulnar head from arthritic changes related to chronic TFCC instability.

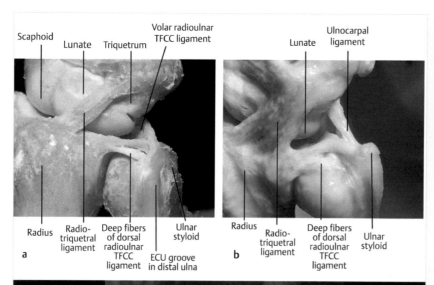

Scaphoid | Lunate | Triquetrum | Volar radioulnar TFCC ligament

Radius | Radio-triquetral ligament | Deep fibers of dorsal radioulnar TFCC ligament | Ulnar styloid | ECU groove in distal ulna

a

Lunate | Ulnocarpal ligament

Radius | Radio-triquetral ligament | Deep fibers of dorsal radioulnar TFCC ligament | Ulnar styloid

b

Fig. 38.16 (**a** and **b**) The dorsal radioulnar ligament of the triangular fibrocartilage complex inserts in layers the base of the ulnar styloid. The ligament and its volar counterpart are the main stabilizers of the distal radioulnar joint. The volar ulnocarpal ligaments contribute to carpal stabilization, as does the dorsal radiotriquetral ligament (**c**) Sagittal T2 fat-suppressed magnetic resonance arthrogram of the wrist illustrating the distal radioulnar ligaments and the ulnotriquetral ligament.

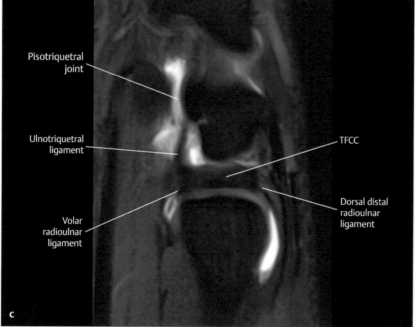

Pisotriquetral joint

Ulnotriquetral ligament

Volar radioulnar ligament

TFCC

Dorsal distal radioulnar ligament

c

(▸ Fig. 38.23, ▸ Fig 38.24). The interosseous arteries, on respective sides of the interosseous membrane, originate off of the ulnar artery. The shoulder is a highly mobile joint and is stabilized by the joint capsule and the rotator cuff. The musculature of the cuff initiates much of the movement of the shoulder. The limited subacromial space between the acromium and the humerus is the site of impingement particularly of the supraspinatus tendon which can progress to degenerative changes. Imaging has an important role in the management of shoulder conditions. Routine radiographs alone may be all that is required for assessing trauma and osteoarthritis of the shoulder. For soft tissue abnormalities, such as rotator cuff impingement or tears, US and MRI are particularly useful (▸ Fig. 38.25, ▸ Fig. 38.26, and ▸ Fig. 38.27). MR or CT arthrography are used for instability, and CT alone is ideal for defining bony detail (▸ Fig. 38.27c). The brachial artery is readily assessed by routine angiography or CT (▸ Fig. 38.28) or by US when performing regional anesthesia.

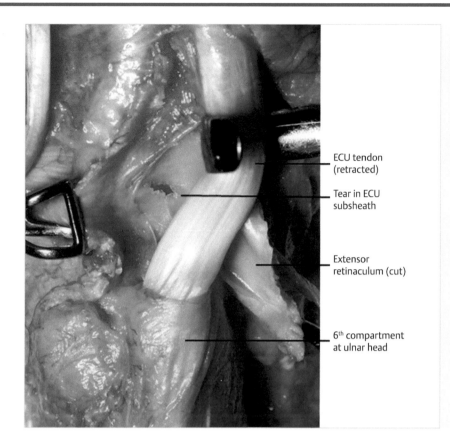

ECU tendon (retracted)

Tear in ECU subsheath

Extensor retinaculum (cut)

6th compartment at ulnar head

Fig. 38.17 The base of the sheath of the extensor carpi ulnaris tendon is an integral part of the triangular fibrocartilage complex and is shown in this dissection with a tear. The extensor retinaculum of the sixth compartment has been cut to mobilize the tendon. The main stability of the tendon is achieved by its fibro-osseus tunnel more proximally between the ulnar head and the ulnar styloid.

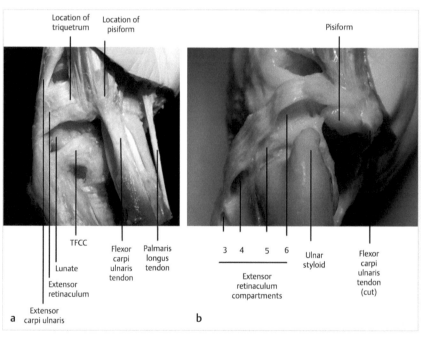

Location of triquetrum

Location of pisiform

Pisiform

TFCC

Flexor carpi ulnaris tendon

Palmaris longus tendon

Lunate

Extensor retinaculum

3   4   5   6

Extensor retinaculum compartments

Ulnar styloid

Flexor carpi ulnaris tendon (cut)

a Extensor carpi ulnaris

b

Fig. 38.18 (a) The ulnar aspect of the wrist is bounded by the flexor and extensor carpi ulnaris tendons to border the *mini* sniff box. The region contains the triangular fibrocartilage complex, lunate and triquetrum, and ulnar styloid **(b)**. The extensor retinaculum crosses over the bony prominence on the ulnar aspect of the triquetrum.

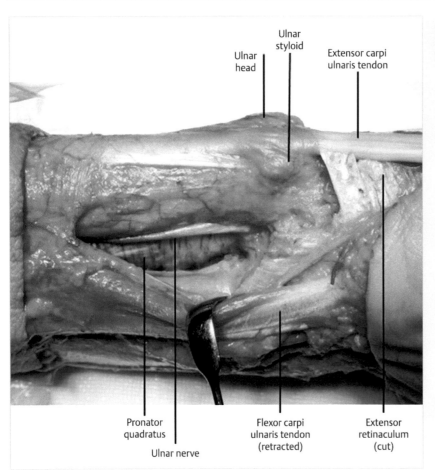

Fig. 38.19 Ulnar side of the wrist with the flexor carpi ulnaris tendon retracted to show the position of the ulnar nerve and artery.

Ulnar styloid

Ulnar head

Extensor carpi ulnaris tendon

Pronator quadratus

Ulnar nerve

Flexor carpi ulnaris tendon (retracted)

Extensor retinaculum (cut)

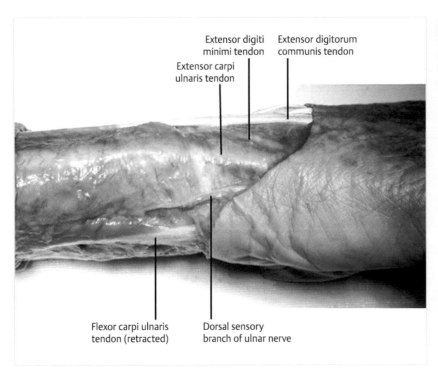

Fig. 38.20 Ulnar side of the wrist showing the dorsal sensory branch of the ulnar nerve crossing the region to provide sensation on the ulnodorsal aspect of the hand and ring and small fingers.

Extensor digiti minimi tendon

Extensor digitorum communis tendon

Extensor carpi ulnaris tendon

Flexor carpi ulnaris tendon (retracted)

Dorsal sensory branch of ulnar nerve

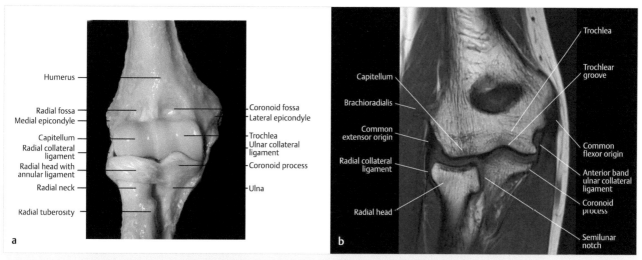

Fig. 38.21 Anterior view of a dissected elbow (**a**) and corresponding magnetic resonance imaging (**b**) with bony and soft tissue detail, including the elbow ligaments.

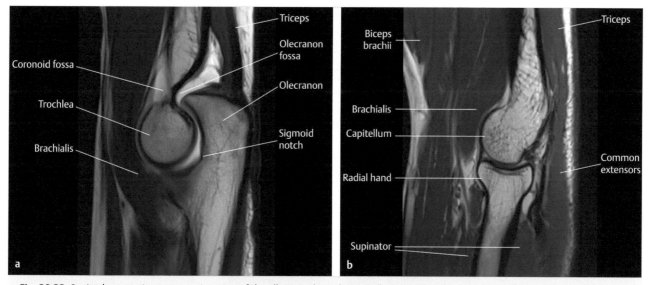

Fig. 38.22 Sagittal magnetic resonance imaging of the elbow at the radiocapitellar joint (**a**) and at the ulnotrochlear aspect of the joint (**b**).

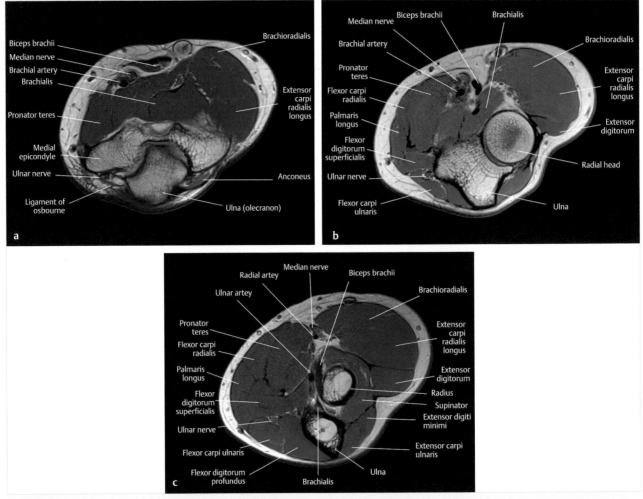

Fig. 38.23 Cross-sectional magnetic resonance imaging (MRI) of the elbow at the proximal aspect of the joint (**a**) as the ulna extends into the olecranon fossa of the distal humerus. At this level, the ulnar nerve is posterior to the medial epicondyle of the humerus, whereas the median nerve and radial artery are medial to the biceps tendon. (**b**) Cross-sectional MRI at the proximal radioulnar joint showing the flexor musculature on the medial aspect of the forearm. (**c**) Proximal forearm with biceps tendon inserting into the radius.

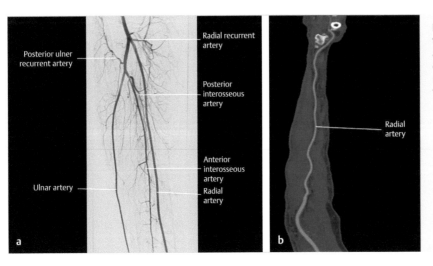

Fig. 38.24 (**a**) Conventional arteriogram of the forearm demonstrating normal arterial anatomy. (**b**) Computed tomography angiogram of the forearm with curved multiplanar reformat reconstructed along the length of the radial artery.

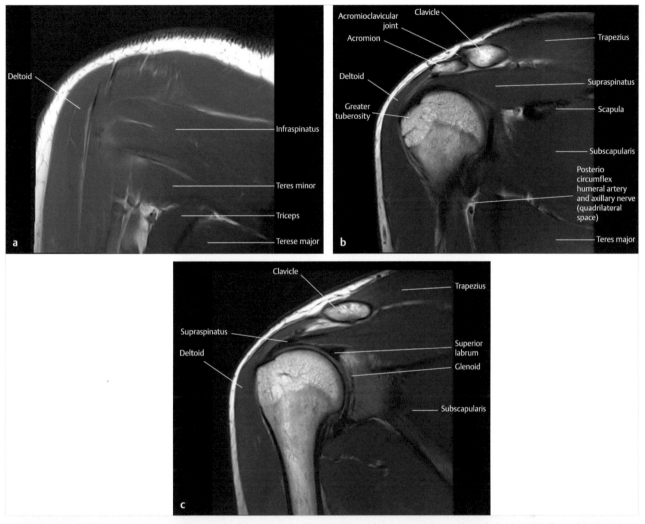

Fig. 38.25 Magnetic resonance coronal imaging of the posterior shoulder musculature (**a**) at the acromioclavicular joint (**b**) and at the glenohumeral joint (**c**).

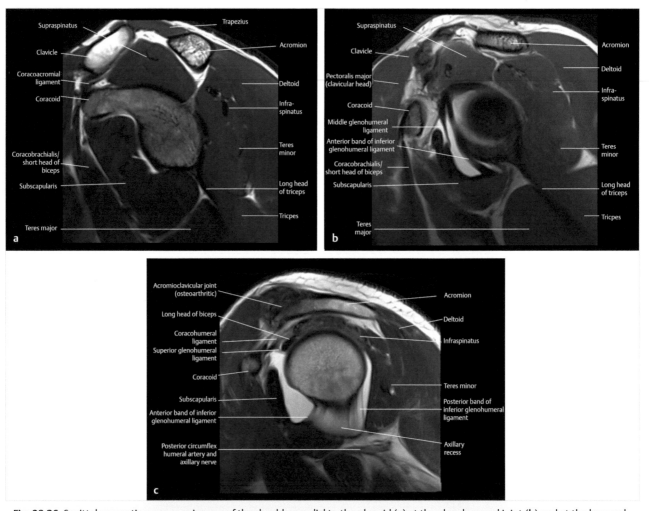

Fig. 38.26 Sagittal magnetic resonance images of the shoulder medial to the glenoid (**a**) at the glenohumeral joint (**b**) and at the humeral head (**c**). Arthritic changes are seen at the acromioclavicular joint.

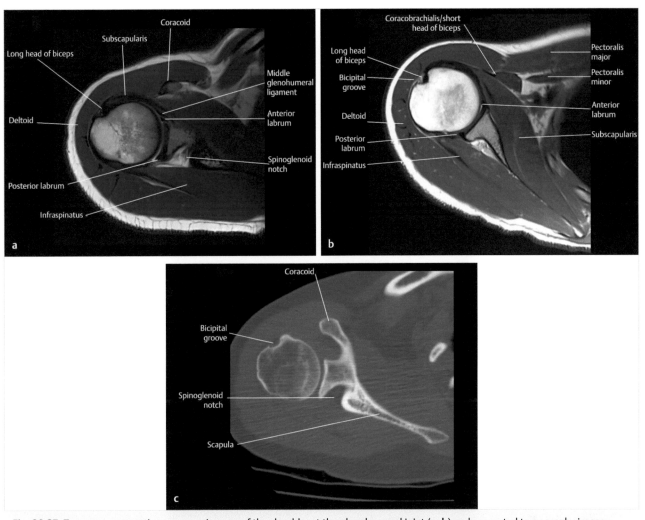

Fig. 38.27 Transverse magnetic resonance images of the shoulder at the glenohumeral joint (**a, b**) and computed tomography image showing bony anatomy (**c**).

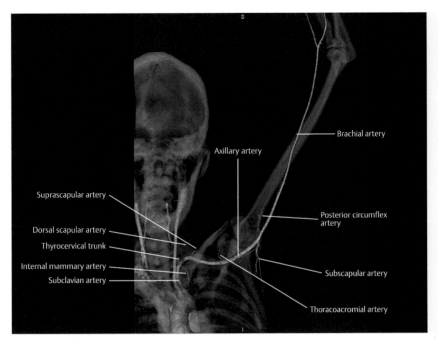

Fig. 38.28 Three-dimensional computed tomography angiogram of the left upper arm demonstrating the normal vascular anatomy from the thorax and neck into the axilla and arm.

References

1. Friedrich K, Komorowski A, Trattnig S. 7T imaging of the wrist. Seminars in Musculoskeletal Radiology 2012;16: 88–92
2. Puippe G.D., Lindenblatt N., Gnannt R., Giovanoli P., Andreisek G., Calcagni M. Prospective morphologic and dynamic assessment of deep flexor tendon healing in zone II by high-frequency ultrasound: preliminary experience. Am J Roentgenol. 2011; 197,6:W1110–W1117
3. Leng S., Zhao K., Qu M., An K.N., Berger R., McCollough C.H. Dynamic CT technique for assessment of wrist joint instabilities. Med Phys. 2010; 38, Suppl 1:S50
4. Amrami K, Felmlee J 3 Tesla imaging of the wrist and hand. Seminars in Musculoskeletal Radiology 2008;12:223–237
5. Gheno R., Buck F.M., Nico M.A, Trudell D.J., Resnick D. Differences between radial and ulnar deviation of the wrist in the study of the intrinsic intercarpal ligaments: magnetic resonance imaging and gross anatomic inspection in cadavers. Skeletal Radiol. 2010; 39,8:799–805
6. Moser T, Dosch J-C, Moussaoui A, Dietemann J-L. Wrist ligament tears: Evaluation of MRI and combined MDCT and MR arthrorarphy. American Journal of Roentgenology 2007;188:1278–1286
7. Rainbow M.J., Crisco J.J., Moore D.C., Kamal R.N., Laidlaw D.H., Akelman E., Wolfe S.W. Elongation of the dorsal carpal ligaments: a computational study of in vivo carpal kinematics. J Hand Surg Am. 2012; 37,7:1393–1399.
8. Shahabpour M, De Maeseneer M, Pouders C, Van Overstraeten L, Ceuterick P, Fierens Y, Goubau J, De Mey J MR imaging of normal extrinsic ligaments using thin slices with clinical and surgical correlation. European Journal of Radiology 2001;77:196–201
9. Theumann N, Pfirrmann C, Antonio G, Chung C, Gilula L, Trudell D, Resnick D. Extrinsic carpal ligaments: Normal MR arthrographic appearance in cadavers. Radiology 2003;226:171–179
10. Taljanovic M, Malan J, Sheppard J Normal anatomy of the extrinsic capsular wrist ligaments by 3_T MRI and high-resolution ultrasonography. Seminars in Musculoskeletal Radiology 2012;16:104–114
11. Tai T.W., Wu C.Y., Su F.C., Chern T.C., Jou I.M. Ultrasonography for diagnosing carpal tunnel syndrome: a meta-analysis of diagnostic test accuracy. Ultrasound Med Biol. 2012 Apr 27.
12. Deniz F.E., Oksüz E., Sarikaya B., Kurt S., Erkorkmaz U., Ulusoy H., Arslan S. Comparison of the diagnostic utility of electromyography, ultrasonography, computed tomography, and magnetic resonance imaging in idiopathic carpal tunnel syndrome determined by clinical findings. Neurosurgery. 2012; 70,3:610–616
13. Shen Z.L., Li Z.M. Ultrasound assessment of transverse carpal ligament thickness:a validity and reliability study. Ultrasound Med Biol. 2012; 38,6:982–988
14. von Schroeder H.P., Botte M.J. The extensor medii proprius and anomalous extensor tendons to the long finger. J Hand Surg Am. 1991; 16,6:1141–1145
15. von Schroeder H.P., Botte M.J. Anatomy of the extensor tendons of the fingers: variations and multiplicity. J Hand Surg Am. 1995; 20,1:27–34
16. von Schroeder H.P., Botte M.J., Gellman H. Anatomy of the juncturae tendinum ofthe hand. J Hand Surg Am. 1990; 15,4:595–602
17. von Schroeder H.P., Botte M.J. The functional significance of the long extensors and juncturae tendinum in finger extension. J Hand Surg Am. 1993; 18,4:641–647
18. Morley J, Bidwell J, Bransby-Zachary M. A comparison of the findings of wrist arthroscopy and magnetic resonance imaging in the investigation of wrist pain. Journal of Hand Surgery 2001;26B:544–546
19. Moser T, Khoury V, Harris P, Bureau N, Cardinal E, Dosch J-C. MDCT arthrography or MR arthrography for imaging of the wrist joint. Seminars in Musculoskeletal Radiology 2009;13:39–54
20. Smith T.O., Drew B., Toms A.P., Jerosch-Herold C., Chojnowski A.J. Diagnostic accuracy of magnetic resonance imaging and magnetic resonance arthrography for triangular fibrocartilaginous complex injury: a systematic review and meta-analysis. J Bone Joint Surg Am. 2012; 94, 9:824–832
21. Haims A, Schweitzer M, Morrison W, Deely D, Lange R, Osterman A, Bednar J, Taras J, Culp R. Limitations of MR imaging in the diagnosis of peripheral tears of the triangular fibrocartilage of the wrist. American Journal of Roentgenology 2002;178:419–422
22. Burns J, Tanaka T, Ueno T, Nakamura T, Yoshioka H. Pitfalls that may mimic injuries of the triangular fibrocartilage and proximal intrinsic wrist ligaments at MR imagning. Radiographics 2011; 31:63–78
23. Coggins C. Imaging of ulnar-sided wrist pain. Clinics in Sports Medicine 2006;25:505–526
24. Botte M.J., Cohen M.S., Lavernia C.J., von Schroeder H.P., Gellman H., Zinberg E.M. The dorsal branch of the ulnar nerve: an anatomic study. J Hand Surg Am. 1990; 15,4:603–607

Index

Note: Page numbers set in **bold** or *italic* indicate headings or figures, respectively.